Cognitive and Brain Plasticity: Advances in Neuroscience

Cognitive and Brain Plasticity: Advances in Neuroscience

Edited by Ronnie Turner

STATES
ACADEMIC PRESS
www.statesacademicpress.com

States Academic Press,
109 South 5th Street,
Brooklyn, NY 11249, USA

Visit us on the World Wide Web at:
www.statesacademicpress.com

ISBN: 978-1-63989-116-0

Cataloging-in-Publication Data

Cognitive and brain plasticity : advances in neuroscience / edited by Ronnie Turner.
p. cm.
Includes bibliographical references and index.
ISBN 978-1-63989-116-0
1. Neuroplasticity. 2. Cognitive neuroscience. 3. Developmental neurobiology. 4. Neurosciences. I. Turner, Ronnie.
QP363.3 .C64 2021
612.82--dc23

Table of Contents

Preface

In my initial years as a student, I used to run to the library at every possible instance to grab a book and learn something new. Books were my primary source of knowledge and I would not have come such a long way without all that I learnt from them. Thus, when I was approached to edit this book; I became understandably nostalgic. It was an absolute honor to be considered worthy of guiding the current generation as well as those to come. I put all my knowledge and hard work into making this book most beneficial for its readers.

A person's hidden cognitive potential or capacity within a particular set of situations is termed as cognitive plasticity. Brain plasticity, also known as neuroplasticity, refers to the capacity of the neural networks of the brain to develop and reorganize. The two major types of neuroplasticity are functional neuroplasticity and structural neuroplasticity. The capacity of the brain to adapt and alter the neurons' functional attributes is termed as functional neuroplasticity. Structural neuroplasticity is used to define the ability of the brain to alter its neuronal connections. On the basis of structural neuroplasticity, new neurons are continuously produced and integrated into the central nervous system. This book elucidates the concepts and innovative models around prospective developments with respect to cognitive and brain plasticity. It presents researches and studies performed by experts across the globe. The book is appropriate for students seeking detailed information in this area as well as for experts.

I wish to thank my publisher for supporting me at every step. I would also like to thank all the authors who have contributed their researches in this book. I hope this book will be a valuable contribution to the progress of the field.

Editor

1

Recruitment of Muscle Activity by the EEG-Neurofeedback Trainings of High Frequencies

Katarzyna Paluch[1†], Katarzyna Jurewicz[1*†], Jacek Rogala[1], Rafał Krauz[2], Marta Szczypińska[3], Mirosław Mikicin[3], Andrzej Wróbel[1] and Ewa Kublik[1]*

[1]Department of Neurophysiology, Nencki Institute of Experimental Biology of Polish Academy of Science, Warsaw, Poland, [2]Centre for Physical Education and Sport, Military University of Technology, Warsaw, Poland, [3]Department of Physical Education, University of Physical Education, Warsaw, Poland

Edited by:
Soledad Ballesteros,
National University of Distance Education, Spain

Reviewed by:
Felix Darvas,
University of Washington, USA
José Luis Ulloa,
Ghent University, Belgium

***Correspondence:**
Katarzyna Paluch
k.paluch@nencki.gov.pl
Katarzyna Jurewicz
k.jurewicz@nencki.gov.pl

†These authors have contributed equally to this work.

EEG-neurofeedback (NFB) became a very popular method aimed at improving cognitive and behavioral performance. However, the EMG frequency spectrum overlies the higher EEG oscillations and the NFB trainings focusing on these frequencies is hindered by the problem of EMG load in the information fed back to the subjects. In such a complex signal, it is highly probable that the most controllable component will form the basis for operant conditioning. This might cause different effects in the case of various training protocols and therefore needs to be carefully assessed before designing training protocols and algorithms. In the current experiment a group of healthy adults (n = 14) was trained by professional trainers to up-regulate their beta1 (15–22 Hz) band for eight sessions. The control group (n = 18) underwent the same training regime but without rewards for increasing beta. In half of the participants trained to up-regulate beta1 band (n = 7) a systematic increase in tonic EMG activity was identified offline, implying that muscle activity became a foundation for reinforcement in the trainings. The remaining participants did not present any specific increase of the trained beta1 band amplitude. The training was perceived effective by both trainers and the trainees in all groups. These results indicate the necessity of proper control of muscle activity as a requirement for the genuine EEG-NFB training, especially in protocols that do not aim at the participants' relaxation. The specificity of the information fed back to the participants should be of highest interest to all therapists and researchers, as it might irreversibly alter the results of the training.

Keywords: artifacts, attention, beta rhythm, biofeedback, muscle control, placebo

INTRODUCTION

In the last two decades, EEG-based neurofeedback (EEG-NFB) received vast popularity in clinical and paramedical practice, even though the therapeutic usage of this method was precariously ahead of the careful, systematic examination of its physiological mechanisms, confounding factors and possible side effects.

The method belongs to a broader category of biofeedback techniques aimed at altering various physiological parameters such as heart rate (ECG-feedback), muscle tension (EMG-feedback)

and others. The trainings are based on the assumption that one can learn to change her/his brain physiological activity in a chosen oscillatory frequency by virtue of continuous feedback about its amplitude. On the contrary to research on brain computer interfaces (BCI) which concentrates on finding easily detectable and modifiable signals that can be reliably used by machine control algorithms, the EEG-NFB training is directed toward lasting changes of brain activity and behavioral improvement. The trainings aim to induce systematic increases/decreases of predefined specific EEG frequencies reflecting particular cognitive or behavioral functions.

The EEG-NFB has been tested as a treatment in a vast domain of neurological and psychiatric disorders, e.g., epilepsy (Sterman and Friar, 1972; Kotchoubey et al., 2001), attention deficit hyperactivity disorder (ADHD; Kaiser and Othmer, 2000; Fuchs et al., 2003; Kropotov et al., 2007), schizophrenia (Gruzelier et al., 1999; Surmeli et al., 2012) and even in traumatic brain injury (TBI) and stroke rehabilitation (for the review of clinical applications, see Yucha and Montgomery, 2008). In healthy subjects the EEG-NFB has been applied expecting behavioral and/or cognitive improvements (Arns et al., 2008; Reiner et al., 2014) and as a supportive training of cognitive performance in the elderly (Becerra et al., 2012; Staufenbiel et al., 2014).

All traditionally discriminated EEG bands have been used as a feedback source, i.e., slow cortical potentials (<2 Hz; Birbaumer, 1999; Heinrich et al., 2004; Strehl et al., 2006; Leins et al., 2007), theta (4–7 Hz; Egner et al., 2002; Raymond et al., 2005; de Zambotti et al., 2012), alpha (8–12 Hz; Egner et al., 2002; Raymond et al., 2005; Zoefel et al., 2011; Gruzelier et al., 2014), lower and higher beta (12–30 Hz; Cannon et al., 2009; Egner and Gruzelier, 2001, 2004) and gamma (>30 Hz; Keizer et al., 2010a,b; Staufenbiel et al., 2014). This large diversity of protocols (i.e., sets of frequency bands used to up- or down-regulate their amplitudes or their ratios) resulted from a belief that each frequency range is related to some specific cognitive functions. Even though instances of such frequency-to-function mapping have been documented (Wróbel, 2000, 2014; Wang, 2010; Anguera et al., 2013), their complex interactions do not allow for simplifying generalizations and require further investigations. Among others, the beta band has been posited to be an attention carrier (Wróbel, 2000, 2014), with specific, local increases of amplitude during attentional tasks positively correlating with correct performance in animals and humans (Bekisz and Wróbel, 1993; Buschman and Miller, 2007; Wróbel et al., 2007; Kamiński et al., 2012; Gola et al., 2013). The up-regulation of this band has been applied in more complex EEG-NFB training protocols as a supplementary treatment in ADHD (e.g., Lévesque et al., 2006; Leins et al., 2007) and as skill enhancement for sportsmen and the elderly (e.g., Rostami et al., 2012; Staufenbiel et al., 2014).

Research focusing on beta and gamma bands confronts the problem of EEG contamination by muscle activity. Electromyographic activity recorded on the surface of the skin is composed of high frequencies with most of the power concentrating between 20 Hz and 150 Hz (Criswell, 2011). In consequence, muscles located on the head (e.g., temporal, occipitofrontal and auricular muscles) or even more distally can interfere with the EEG, sometimes constituting a majority of the power in the higher frequencies (Goncharova et al., 2003; Whitham et al., 2007) and influencing most of the electrodes on the scalp (Goncharova et al., 2003; Yilmaz et al., 2014). The relation between these signals is further complicated by the fact that facial EMG was shown to be sensitive to numerous cognitive and affective processes, including cognitive load (Waterink and van Boxtel, 1994; Whitham et al., 2008). Muscle interference has been widely discussed in the context of EEG and EMG data analysis (for review see McMenamin et al., 2011; Muthukumaraswamy, 2013) but is not sufficiently recognized and controlled in EEG-NFB trainings (see "Discussion" Section and Enriquez-Geppert et al., 2017). The EEG signal analyzed offline can be iteratively examined and cleaned of any obscuring components. However, in the EEG-NFB the signal is analyzed online and transformed into stimuli immediately fed back to a trained person. All undetected artifacts modify the feedback signal. This might cause different effects in the case of various training protocols and therefore needs to be carefully considered while designing training protocols and algorithms.

Here we report a particular instance of this problem concerning the NFB up-regulation of the beta band. Since there is vast research on clinical and normal population reporting no control or one with doubtful effectiveness (e.g., Leins et al., 2007; Gevensleben et al., 2009a,b; Keizer et al., 2010a,b; Logemann et al., 2010; Meisel et al., 2014; see "Discussion" Section), we conducted an experiment to assess the possible impact of muscle activity on EEG-NFB results. We applied the beta up-regulation set-up, commonly used as training aimed at improving attention (Egner and Gruzelier, 2001; Vernon et al., 2003; Egner et al., 2004; Logemann et al., 2010; Ghaziri et al., 2013). Healthy, young participants were trained to voluntarily increase the amplitude of beta1 band oscillations (15–22 Hz) recorded from the leads overlying the areas of the frontoparietal attention network. Examination of the raw signal revealed in a subgroup of participants a substantial muscle employment which increased systematically in the course of the session, mimicking the expected increase in the beta1 band. If the muscle related effects had gone unnoticed, the conclusion of our study would have been falsely positive stating a successful upregulation of the beta1 band. We discuss the need for proper muscle control for a reliable NFB training in the light of the current EEG-NFB literature.

MATERIALS AND METHODS

Participants

Thirty-two male healthy university students, age $m = 21.97 \pm 1.88$ years (mean $\pm$ standard deviation), were recruited for the experiment. The experiments were approved by the local ethics committee (Bioethical Committee at the Military Institute of Hygiene and Epidemiology). All subjects were informed about the study and gave their written informed consent for participation in the experiment in accordance with the Declaration of Helsinki.

The EEG-Neurofeedback Training

The subjects were randomly assigned to one of the three training groups: beta plus (B+), aimed at increasing the amplitude of beta1 (15–22 Hz) oscillations (n = 14), beta minus (B−) dedicated to down-regulation of the beta1 oscillatory activity (n = 6) and sham (SH) group, receiving pseudo-feedback (generated by a computer algorithm), unrelated to the brain's EEG signals (n = 12). The participants were unaware of their group affiliation and uninformed about the existence of the sham group to prevent loss of motivation.

The training sessions were performed using a customized version of the commercial EEG DigiTrack Biofeedback system (ELMIKO MEDICAL Sp. z o. o.). Each participant had a personal code, which was recognized by the program and started group-dependent feedback protocol. At the user (trainer) level, the program displayed set-ups only for two groups: beta plus and beta minus. Sham protocols were run under facade of these set-ups (half as B+ and the other half as B−). The trainings were conducted by hired professional NFB trainers. In order to reduce possible nonspecific effects trainers were instructed not to additionally motivate the trainees. Over a period of 1–2 months the subjects underwent eight training sessions (one to two trainings per week). During the session subjects were seated in a chair in front of a 17″ computer LCD screen (~70 cm from the screen). Each session consisted of 10 blocks of 3 min duration each. The session started after mounting the EEG electrodes with a short (*ca.* 2 min) resting period in order to accustom the participants with the training situations and screen the control sample of the EEG signal.

EEG was recorded from F3, F4, P3 and P4 sites in 10–20 standard, with linked ears as a reference and ground electrode placed at the Pz. Thus, the electrodes were positioned over the frontoparietal attention network nodes (Gross et al., 2004; Donner et al., 2007; Siegel et al., 2008). The signal was sampled at 250 Hz and band-pass filtered between 0.16 Hz and 70 Hz, with a notch filter at 50 Hz. A fast Fourier transform (FFT) spectrogram was computed for each electrode. The feedback parameter was obtained by averaging the FFT amplitudes over the beta1 range and across the electrodes. The FFT window of 2.07 s (512 point, giving 0.49 Hz resolution) was sliding with 92% or 77% overlap and, accordingly, the amplitude values presented to the trainer and used for feedback were updated with 200 or 500 ms delay. Windows overlap and the feedback delay varied between subjects (due to two software versions used in the study) but were constant for each person and randomly distributed among the experimental groups. There was no difference in results of participants trained with these two settings.

The training display consisted of a shooting target presented in the background and four green dots moving inwards and outwards along vertical and horizontal axes (**Figure 1**). The feedback information about the amplitude of beta1, was provided by the synchronized movement of the dots in B+ and B− groups. In the sham group a predefined algorithm controlled the movement of the dots. When the amplitude changed in the intended direction (towards the threshold value set manually by the trainers) all dots moved inwards. The subject's goal was to make the green dots meet in the center. To boost the participants' motivation and to make the training more involving additional reinforcements were provided. When the beta1 amplitude reached 43% of the threshold, the display was complemented with black rings within the high-scored area of the shooting target. When the beta1 amplitude reached 75% of the threshold value, a red ring in the center of the shooting target was presented, signaling achievement of the goal. The threshold defining the required value of the beta1 band amplitude was adjusted manually by the trainers during the session to provide a relatively constant rate of reward, thus encouraging the subjects to continuously improve their performance.

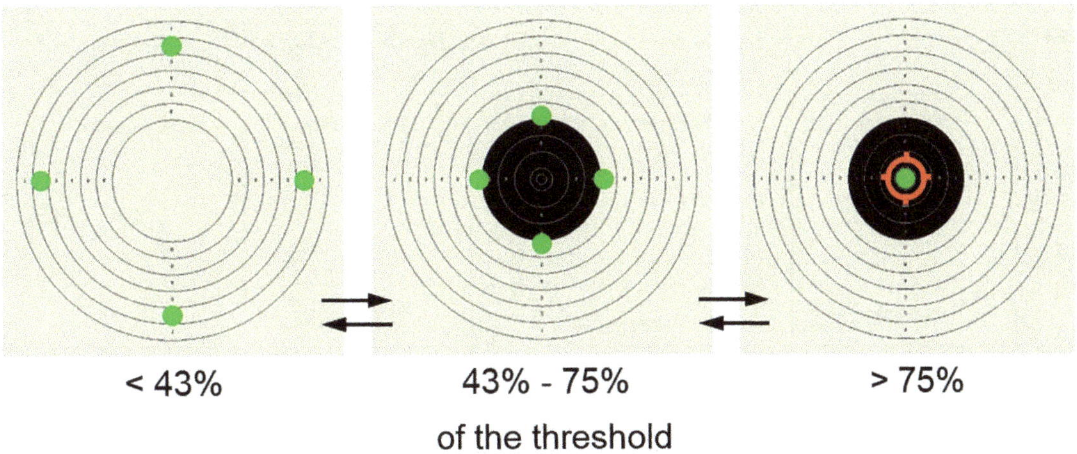

FIGURE 1 | Screen-stimulus used for the neurofeedback (NFB) training. Participants' goal was to move the four dots initially located on the outer edges of the shooting target to its center. The reward was provided in two steps—when the amplitude of trained band reached over 43% of the pre-set threshold the shooting target was filled in with black central rings, when it exceeded 75% the dots met in the center and the shooting aim appeared as a sign of successful performance.

Processing of the EEG Data

Raw EEG data were exported from the DigiTrack environment to the European Data Format (EDF) and further analyzed using the EEGLAB software (Delorme and Makeig, 2004) and self-written MATLAB scripts. The off-line analysis involved similar preprocessing of the data as the online feedback computation, to obtain the same frequency bands to those produced by the EEG-NFB apparatus. The continuous data recorded during training session were mean corrected and filtered to remove frequencies lower than 0.5 Hz and higher than 70 Hz. Notch filtering was applied at 50 Hz. The signal was split into 1 s epochs, which in turn were searched for artifacts with the EEGLAB function *pop_autorej*. An epoch was rejected from all the channels if any data point in this epoch exceeded 5 standard deviations from the amplitude of the signal on any of the channels. The algorithm proceeded iteratively—if the number of epochs classified for exclusion exceeded 5% of the data, the procedure was repeated with a more liberal exclusion criterion (increased by 0.5 standard deviation). Furthermore, to remove muscle artifacts, for every subject we removed whole training blocks, in which higher frequencies (22–45 Hz, referred to in DigiTrack software as beta2 band) diverged by more than 3 standard deviations from the individual mean of that participant. The procedure ran iteratively until no such cases were found. In effect, 3.05% of the data was removed, including three full sessions (belonging to two subjects). The FFT analysis was computed separately for each 3 min training block with a sliding Hanning window 512 points-long with a 92% overlap.

The visual inspection of the raw signal and the FFT spectra (performed after all cleaning steps described above) revealed, that the signals of some participants were dominated by frequencies above 15 Hz (**Figure 2**). Since such oscillations constituted the majority of some participants' signal, cleaning algorithms relaying on signal distribution parameters e.g., mean and standard deviation were unable to detect and reject them during offline automatic data processing. These signals were characterized by long sweeps of sharp high frequency oscillations characteristic for EMG (Criswell, 2011). In these cases, a typical logarithmic-like shape of the FFT curve was substantially distorted by an elevation spanning from higher to lower parts of the spectrum.

Therefore, we asked three independent judges to visually inspect the raw signals and the FFT spectra from all blocks and sessions of each participant and to classify the sessions as contaminated by muscle activity if FFT spectrum was distorted above 15 Hz in the majority of blocks (**Figure 2**; Criswell, 2011). The judges listed the participants who exhibited such a pattern in more than half of their sessions as muscle employing ones.

To confirm that it is possible to distinguish muscle-employing participants from the whole sample in an automated approach we applied two additional methods of classification: k-means clustering and logistic regression. For both these methods we used solely the amplitudes of beta2 as the bases of classification.

When applying the k-means method we asked for two clusters, to prove that our division into muscle employers and others is the most prevalent pattern in the data. The analysis was performed with the use of beta2 amplitudes from all

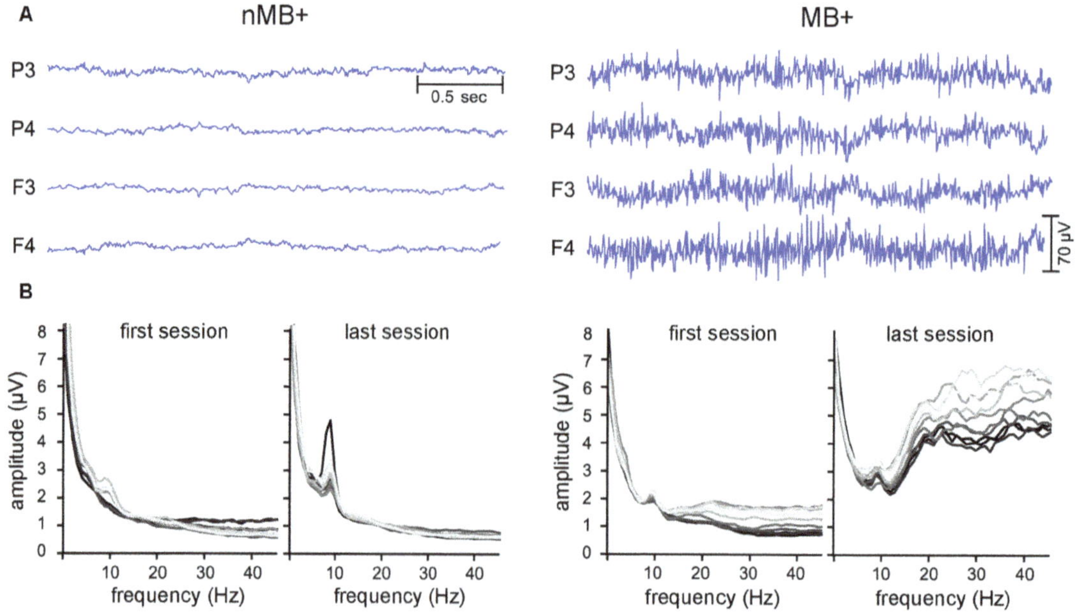

FIGURE 2 | Examples of the EEG data with and without the EMG contamination. (A) Raw EEG signal from four electrodes used for training. **(B)** Frequency spectra (fast Fourier transform (FFT)) averaged for all four NFB electrodes. Each line corresponds to a one 3-min block in the session, with each consecutive block marked with a brighter color (the darkest line—the first block, the lightest one—the tenth block). On the left: data from an exemplar subject with the EEG spectrum undistorted in the high frequency range (nMB+). On the right: data from a subject with increased amplitudes at high frequency part of the spectrum identified as originating from muscle activity (MB+).

available recordings (10 blocks × 8 sessions for each subject, 3.05% of blocks were missing, due to previous data cleaning and were substituted with the average of a given participant). The algorithm was set to minimize absolute deviations within clusters by calculating the median along predefined dimensions (Manhattan distance).

The logistic regression was applied as a supervised method of data classification. The binary classifier (muscle-employing/other) was guided by the classification made by independent judges. The mean beta2 amplitude from all available recordings for each participant constituted the predictor value. The regression line, fitted to the data, quantified the relationship between beta2 amplitude and the probability of belonging to one of the two categories. The decision criterion was established at a probability of 0.5.

In addition to the trained beta1 band (15–22 Hz), we reported on the alpha (8–12 Hz) and beta2 (22–45 Hz) flanking bands, as they are capable of showing potential specificity of the training effects.

Statistical Analyses

The amplitude values in each frequency band were averaged from the four electrodes (F3, F4, P3, P4) to reproduce the training setup averaging online the amplitudes from all channels. We confirmed with a three-way ANOVA of group, session and electrode that there were no significant differences between individual electrodes with respect to amplitudes of analyzed bands (no significant effects of electrode or interactions including this factor, all $p > 0.201$).

The main goal of the analysis was to compare the effects of the training in the participants employing and not employing muscles in their performance. The most prominent characteristic of the muscle-employing subjects was a pronounced elevation of high frequency amplitudes and their high variability among different blocks. In order to maintain the relations between individual subjects, as present in the raw data, we chose to perform a between-subject standardization (by subtracting the mean and dividing by standard deviation from all blocks/sessions across all participants). This procedure performed for each band separately enables a direct comparison of different frequency bands as it shifts the values to a common range (*z* space). Additionally, to ensure that the observed effects, even if different in absolute size, are common for the group and not driven by single cases we repeated our analysis with the within-subject *z*-scores (using individual mean and deviation for each subject).

We verified the effects of the EEG-NFB during the course of the session (the within session effects) and in consecutive sessions (the between session effects). For the within session effects, the values for each of the 10 blocks were obtained by averaging across all the sessions. For the between-session effects, the values were obtained by averaging all the blocks constituting each session. The missing session averages (only 3 per all 256 data points in all participants) were substituted with mean values interpolated from the directly preceding and following sessions.

Considering the small number of participants assigned to the B− protocol for the sake of further analyses we decided to combine it with the sham group to create a single control condition, further referred to as control group (CON). Before combining the groups we confirmed with three-way ANOVA of group, session and band that there were no significant differences between these groups (no significant effect of group or interactions including this factor, all $p > 0.208$). Since seven participants identified to have a steady EMG contamination belonged to the B+ protocol (50% of this group), we split this group into MB+ (muscle-employing participants from B+ group, $n = 7$) and nMB+ (participants not employing muscles from B+ group, $n = 7$). Their performance was compared to the results of the control group (CON, $n = 18$). The three-way ANOVAs were computed for within and between session effects with "time" (blocks 1–10 or sessions 1–8), "band" (alpha, beta1, beta2) as within subject factors and training "group" (MB+, nMB+, CON) as between subject factors. The Greenhouse-Geisser correction (G-G) was applied when the data did not meet the sphericity. We considered the results to be significant when the *p* value was below 0.05. For significant interactions *post hoc* pairwise comparisons were provided. For clarity of the presentation, from multiple pairwise comparisons between consecutive time points, we show the comparison of the first and the last blocks/sessions and prove the gradual character of the change by fitting a linear trend.

Self-Reports

After completing the training the participants were asked to assess: (1) the effectiveness of the NFB training; (2) the influence of the training on their functioning outside the sessions; (3) their ability to evoke the state from the trainings outside the sessions; (4) their progress in the ability to control visual stimulus during the trainings; and (5) their implemented strategies (if any).

RESULTS

Electroencephalographic Data

Fourteen healthy subjects took part in eight sessions of the EEG-NFB training that aimed to up-regulate the beta1 band amplitude. Another 18 participants who underwent the same training regime but were not rewarded for increasing beta1 amplitude formed the control group to account for the unspecific training factors.

To assess the possible impact of muscle activity on the EEG-NFB results we divided the participants into subgroups based on the presence of the extended muscle contamination in their EEG signal. To assure the validity and consistency of the ensuing division three different classification methods were used. Based on the screening of the raw signal and the shape of the FFT spectra competent judges marked nine subjects as muscle-employing. Their assessments agreed in 91% of cases (eight participants were identified by all three judges, and one by two judges).

K-means clustering with assumed two clusters divided the data into groups of eight and 24 participants. Eight out of nine subjects marked as muscle-employing during the visual inspection were classified as such by the k-means algorithm (see

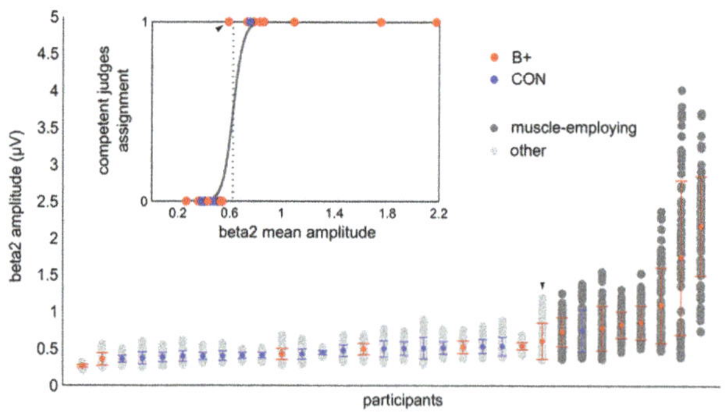

FIGURE 3 | Automatic classification of the participants based on beta2 amplitude: k-means (main graph) and logistic regression (insert). In the main graph the light and the dark gray dots correspond to the values of the beta2 amplitude from the single training blocks. The vertical bundles of dots display all of the training data of the individual participants, which constituted the basis for k-means clustering. The graph summarizes the results of the k-means classification: dark gray dots—muscle employing participants, light gray dots—others. The colored dots (in both graphs) correspond to the grand average beta2 of the person with red indicating the participants from the beta up-training group (B+) and blue those from the control group (CON). The participants are sorted by the increasing average of their beta2 amplitude. The error bars represent standard deviations. The embedded graph shows the result of a logistic regression analysis supervised by competent judges group assignments (code 1—muscle employing participants, code 0—others). The dotted vertical line marks the decision criterion. The participants whose grand mean exceeded this value were classified as muscle employing. Both automatic methods provided concurring results. Note the ambiguous case which was classified by competent judges as muscle employing but did not reach the decision criterion in both automatic classifications (marked on the graph with the arrow head).

Figure 3). All 23 participants judged not to employ muscles were in the second cluster. The same result was obtained with logistic regression (**Figure 3**). The increase in beta2 amplitude significantly raised the probability of a subject being classified as muscle employing ($\beta = 25.92$; $t = 3.87$; $p < 0.001$). It is worth noticing that while visual inspection was based on raw signals as well as on the shape of entire FFT spectrum, automatic classifications, relying exclusively on the amplitude of beta2 band lead to very similar results, proving that changes in the high frequencies are the critical feature distinguishing these two groups. All approaches resulted in the same outcome in 31/32 cases. In the single ambiguous case we leaned toward the automatic classification and included this subject in the control group.

We compared the effects of the training on the muscle employing participants trained to upregulate the beta band with other groups. The analysis of the within session effects (**Figure 4A**) revealed a significant three-way interaction of block, band and group factors ($F_{(36,522)} = 4.23$, $p = 0.001$, $\eta^2 = 0.226$). The statistics for the main and the interaction effects are shown in **Table 1**. We observed a general increase of amplitudes in MB+ during training session, with the magnitude varying between the bands. The most pronounced increase was in beta1 (first block: $m = 0.58$, last block: $m = 1.59$, $p < 0.001$, linear trend at $p = 0.029$) and beta2 (first block: $m = 0.77$, last block: $m = 1.81$, $p < 0.001$, linear trend at $p = 0.029$). In both of these bands the amplitudes during entire training session were significantly higher in this group than in nMB+ or CON (all $p < 0.001$). A smaller, yet significant increase was also present in the alpha band (first block: $m = -0.23$, last block: $m = 0.15$, $p = 0.001$, linear trend at $p = 0.018$). The mean alpha amplitude did not significantly differ between groups (all $p > 0.745$). MB+ was the only group that exhibited any amplitude changes during the training session. All comparisons between the first and the last blocks, for all bands in the remaining groups turned out insignificant (all $p > 0.361$).

In the analogous analysis performed for the between session effects (**Figure 4B**) the three-way interaction of session, band and group factors appeared insignificant ($F_{(28,406)} = 1.39$, $p = 0.215$, $\eta^2 = 0.087$), demonstrating a lack of systematic changes in the EEG amplitudes across sessions similar to those observed within sessions. However, beta1 and beta2 amplitudes were significantly higher across sessions (all $p < 0.001$) in MB+ (beta1 $m = 1.05 \pm 1.09$; beta2 $m = 1.23 \pm 1.152$) than in nMB+ (beta1 $m = -0.48 \pm 0.40$; beta2 $m = -0.35 \pm 0.25$) and CON (beta1 $m = -0.53 \pm 0.50$; beta2 $m = -0.40 \pm 0.21$), as shown in the significant interaction of band and group factor ($F_{(4,58)} = 6.06$, $p = 0.004$, $\eta^2 = 0.295$). There was no difference between groups in the alpha band amplitude (all $p > 0.764$).

The same analyses performed on the *z*-scores computed for each participant separately confirmed the effects previously observed in the beta1 and beta2 bands. The amplitude of these two bands increased within session in the MB+ group and did not change significantly in the other two groups as revealed by the interaction effect ($F_{(18,261)} = 2.38$, $p = 0.032$, $\eta^2 = 0.141$). The increase of the alpha amplitude visible in the previous approach appeared to be equal to the one observed in higher frequencies after its normalization to the subject-specific variability range. This is evidenced by the lack of significant differences between the bands in the MB+ group (interaction of band and group for the within session: $F_{(4,58)} = 0.27$, $p = 0.827$, $\eta^2 = 0.018$; between session: $F_{(4,58)} = 0.31$, $p = 0.744$, $\eta^2 = 0.021$).

The impact of muscle activity on the EEG spectrum increased with frequency. However, the training related increase in amplitude was proportional to the amount of muscle contamination in the particular frequency. The results showed that after separating muscle-employing participants from the group trained to increase beta1 band we were unable to observe any effects of the NFB training as indicated by no significant differences between the nMB+ and control group participants.

Self-Reports

The participants expressed their opinion about the EEG-NFB trainings on a Likert scale (1—not effective, 5—effective). The assessment of the effectiveness of the training varied between groups ($F_{(2,29)} = 5.65$, $p = 0.008$, $\eta^2 = 0.280$). Subjects assigned to the control group expressed a more positive opinion about the effectiveness of the training ($m = 4.17 \pm 0.71$) than those from the MB+ ($m = 3.29 \pm 0.76$) and nMB+ ($m = 3.00 \pm 1.29$). Consistently, the majority of subjects from the CON group (13 out of 18) declared that the trainings had positive influence on their functioning outside the sessions, the same was true only

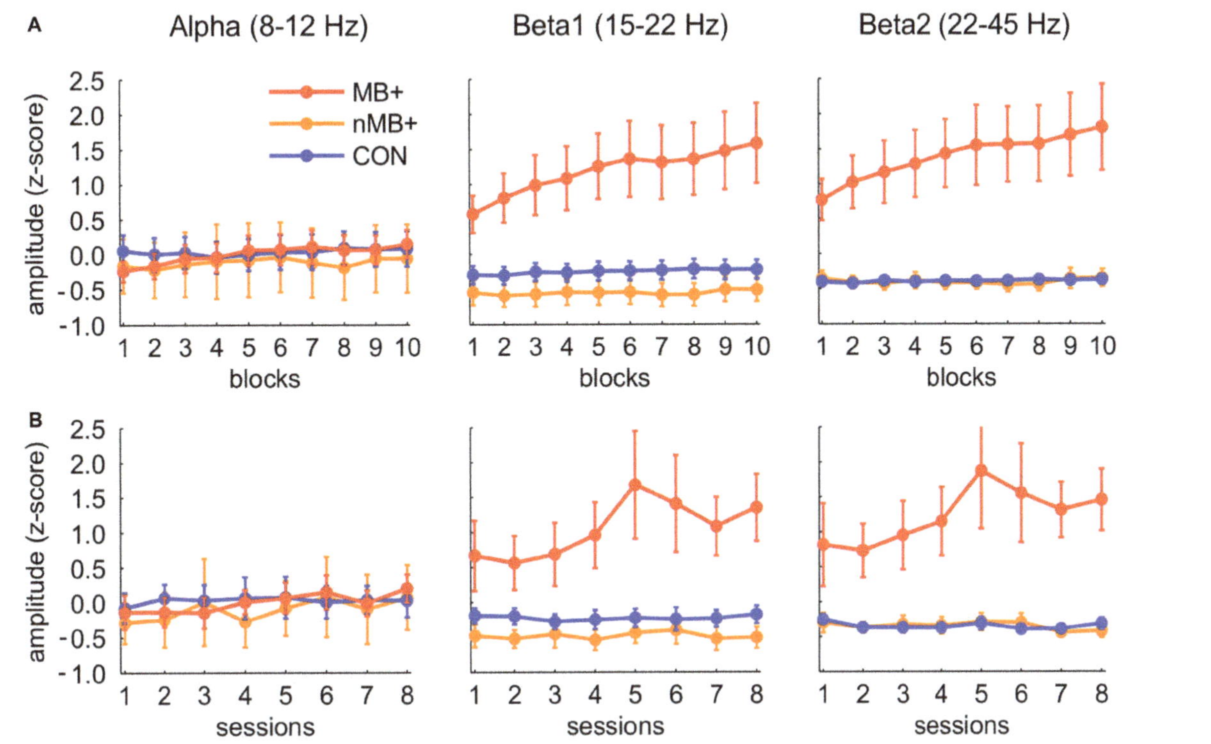

FIGURE 4 | Standardized (between subjects, see "Materials and Methods" Section) amplitudes of the three frequency bands in the three training groups (MB+, $n = 7$; nMB+, $n = 7$; CON, $n = 18$; for statistical significance see "Results" Section). (A) Consecutive 10 blocks averaged across sessions. **(B)** Means of eight consecutive sessions. Error bars represent standard error of the mean.

TABLE 1 | Results of a three-way ANOVA with time, band and group factors.

	Within sessions				Between sessions			
	F	*df1*	*df2*	*p*	*F*	*df1*	*df2*	*p*
Time	13.79	9	261	0.000	2.13	7	203	0.112
Band	0.90	2	58	0.368	0.82	2	58	0.391
Group	7.35	2	29	0.003	5.605	2	29	0.009
Time × Band	2.88	18	522	0.041	0.91	14	406	0.453
Time × Group	8.58	18	261	0.000	1.45	14	203	0.215
Band × Group	6.70	4	58	0.002	6.06	4	58	0.004
Time × Band × Group	4.23	36	522	0.001	1.39	28	406	0.215

for two out of seven subjects in the MB+ and only two subjects in the nMB+ group ($\chi^2_{(2,32)} = 6.03$, $p = 0.049$). About half of all the participants declared their ability to transfer the state maintained during the sessions onto other situations (half of the nMB+, two thirds of the CON and only one person form the MB+ group, $\chi^2_{(2,31)} = 5.55$, $p = 0.063$).

There were no differences between the groups in the reported ability to control the visual stimulus ($F_{(2,29)} = 2.26$, $p = 0.122$, $\eta^2 = 0.135$). All groups declared that their ability to control the visual stimulus increased during the trainings (CON: $m = 4.33 \pm 0.97$, MB+: $m = 4.14 \pm 0.69$, nMB+: $m = 3.43 \pm 1.13$). During the trainings the participants were left without any specific instruction. In post trainings self-reports, we asked them if they implemented any strategies to control the visual stimulus. In all groups the majority of subjects declared to apply some strategies during the NFB sessions ($\chi^2_{(2,32)} = 0.169$, $p = 0.919$). The participants indicated strategies such as: (1) looking at one point; (2) solving logical puzzles; (3) visualizing places; (4) relaxing; (5) focusing and calming down; and (6) singing songs in their minds. Four subjects from the MB+ group and one from nMB+ mentioned in their reports changing the muscle tension. Therefore, about half of the participants from MB+ were aware of the possibility to use muscle tension to control the feedback and half were not. However, these numbers are too small for direct statistical comparisons. The self-aware subjects had a slightly better opinion about the effectiveness of the training and perceived ability to control the visual stimulus than MB+ who were unaware of their muscle employment (effectiveness $m = 3.00 \pm 0.816$ vs. $m = 3.67 \pm 0.58$, perceived control $m = 3.75 \pm 0.50$ vs. $m = 4.67 \pm 0.58$).

DISCUSSION

In the present experiment performed on healthy adults, we failed to observe a change of the EEG activity in the trained beta1 (15–22 Hz) band despite the positive reception of the trainings effects reported by both the trainers and the trainees. However, we observed extensive muscle employment, which increased during the training sessions. We argue that in the reported experiment, in the subgroup of participants the EEG-NFB training was taken over by the EMG signal, which became the foundation for incentive-based learning. This conclusion is supported by reports showing that EMG is more susceptible to feedback modification than EEG (DeGood and Chisholm, 1977; Maurizio et al., 2013). Indeed, all but one participants who increased muscle activity belonged to the training group up-regulating the beta1 band. This group was rewarded for amplifying amplitude of beta1, which is at the lower edge of the EMG spectrum (Criswell, 2011). On the contrary, such excessive artifacts were not present in participants trained to down-regulate beta1 activity and present only in 1 out of 12 subjects trained in the sham protocol. In that participant the muscle activity did not change systematically in the course of the training.

We cannot eliminate the possibility that in the beta1 activity recorded from the participants identified as the muscle employing group (MB+) there was also a contribution of a neuronal origin overshadowed by muscular activity. However, in the analysis restricted to the subjects who did not employ muscles for trainings, no modifications in the beta1 range were detected, suggesting ineffectiveness of the performed EEG-NFB training. The susceptibility of the beta1 band for the NFB training has yet to be established with larger sample sizes.

Subjects generally declared that their ability to control the visual stimulus increased during the course of the trainings. Surprisingly, the participants from the control group (who did not show any changes in the EEG during the trainings) were most positive about the training effects. This counter-intuitive result may point out the presence of a placebo effect in the NFB trainings. It acted as if the effect was most pronounced when undisturbed by real control of the ongoing feedback (the case of MB+, which was less pleased with the effectiveness of the NFB). A majority of participants reported using various strategies during the trainings. The employment of muscle tension to control the visual feedback stimulus was reported post-training by four participants from MB+, the remaining subjects were unaware of using this strategy or failed to mention it in their reports. At the beginning of the experiment the participants were informed about the basic mechanisms of the EEG-NFB e.g., its relation to the ongoing brain activity. To assure a high quality of the recorded signals they were asked to sit still, and trainers intervened whenever they noticed excessive movement or other type of undesirable behavior. The fact that half of subjects trained to up-regulate the beta1 band managed to increase their muscle activity (in half of the cases unwittingly) shows that such behavior cannot be efficiently controlled and eliminated by trainers alone.

Our experiment strongly supports the need for effective automatic on-line control of muscle activity during the EEG-NFB trainings, in particular in the protocols aiming to up-regulate higher frequency bands. Proper muscle control is a requirement not solely to acquire a high quality EEG signal but primarily to accomplish a genuine EEG-NFB training. Muscle control must be recognized as standard part of the NFB procedure, to successfully prevent participants from unintentionally using muscle tension to change the signals registered by the EEG electrodes during the training. Various mathematical algorithms were proposed and validated as effective in removing the EMG components from the EEG signal (McMenamin et al., 2011; Fitzgibbon et al., 2016), however, most of them require high density multichannel recordings and as such are not applicable in the case of typical NFB setups. It was also proposed to model, fit and subtract individual EMG spikes from the EEG channels (Nottage et al., 2013)—such an approach does not require multiple recording channels but needs powerful computers and sophisticated software.

The strategy suggested in NFB guidebooks (Demos, 2005) is based on the intervention of the trainer, who is expected to instruct the trainee to relax, adopt a proper, comfortable position and to avoid muscles contraction. Trainers are expected to visually screen the recorded EEG and FFT spectra to detect sweeps of EMG activity and to instruct the trainees to correct their behavior. While this is the demanded minimum that can be done without adequate hardware and software support, present experiment shows that such a strategy may be inefficient at least in the trainings aiming to up-regulate high frequencies. Surprisingly, the reports provided by the authors in a clinical research concerning mostly the NFB applications for ADHD treatment in children do not refer to the issue of muscle control (Lévesque et al., 2006; Leins et al., 2007; for review see Lofthouse et al., 2012). It remains widely neglected also in the research conducted on healthy participants in which high frequency (beta and gamma) training is used in e.g., for cognitive improvement (Keizer et al., 2010a,b; Logemann et al., 2010). The articles presenting various control procedures are noticeable exceptions (e.g., Bird et al., 1978; Berner et al., 2006; Hoedlmoser et al., 2008; Kober et al., 2013; Witte et al., 2013). Based on this research three main approaches to control muscle activity can be distinguished.

Probably the most common, although only incidentally described as serving for artifact control, is the usage of multiband protocols aiming at simultaneous manipulation of two or more bands, or maximization of their proportion (e.g., up-regulating SMR while simultaneously decreasing theta and beta2). Rarely was such protocol claimed as serving for the eye blink (theta) and muscle (beta2) control (Kober et al., 2013; Witte et al., 2013). Even though such an approach can be effective in controlling muscle-related activity it is threatened by physiological invalidity when the contrasted bands are directly flanking (Ros et al., 2013). It is highly plausible that (at least) the edges of the neighboring bands are mutually interdependent and if left unconstrained, they tend to change their amplitude in the same direction. The interdependence of the flanking frequency bands (on the example of theta, alpha and beta) was demonstrated as moderate to strong (by means of correlation of the within-subject changes during training, $0.5 < r < 0.7$ (Ros et al., 2013). Thus, implementation of such protocols, although effective for the control of muscle artifacts, might lower the effectiveness of training.

Our study shows that the classification based solely on the beta2 amplitude proved that the changes in this frequency are a feature distinguishing the subjects who train based on the EMG activity from others. Thus, controlling this single parameter is sufficient to assure good quality of the feedback information. It can be implemented as an amplitude threshold on one of the high frequency bands, as the signal of the muscle origin have an amplitude far bigger than the neuronal one (procedure employed i.a. by Hoedlmoser et al., 2008). When the signal exceeds this threshold the participants are left without a reward and the training is interrupted. This method can be easily implemented in commercial software, but it does not completely exclude the risk of under threshold manipulation of muscle tension. Many of the articles that implement these solutions, report the use of an amplitude threshold in the range of 100–120 μV (e.g., Gevensleben et al., 2009a,b; Meisel et al., 2014). Our data clearly shows that it is perfectly feasible to gain control over the NFB apparatus with muscle activity in the range of 70 μV or lower (**Figure 2**). Since different apparatus and online signal processing settings influence the range of the recorded EEG values the amplitude threshold should not be generic but separately calibrated.

Finally, some authors used additional EMG recordings of facial muscles (Berner et al., 2006), neck-muscles (Bird et al., 1978) or the chest belt measuring the chest wall movements (Berner et al., 2006). In these experiments positive feedback was conditional upon ongoing EMG activity and provided only if the latter did not exceed established threshold. As this method unambiguously distinguishes between neuronal and muscular signals, it is the most precise one but also the most demanding in implementation (requiring additional hardware and software facilities and prolonging the preparation time).

Muscle activity can differently influence various training protocols, so it should be specifically approached with regard to the training band and behavioral goal. In the case of the protocols aiming to up-regulate high frequency bands, the EMG signal can result from a head or upper body muscle strain. It is especially plausible in trainings focusing on attention (which constitute many of high frequency protocols, e.g., Egner and Gruzelier, 2004; Cannon et al., 2006, 2009), as they do not instruct subjects to relax during the trainings. The situation is different for the NFB trainings aiming at subjects' relaxation, most often related to alpha protocols (e.g., Egner et al., 2002; van Boxtel et al., 2012). Interestingly, few articles directly comparing the EEG and EMG feedback employed the alpha band and have shown that down-regulating the amplitude of the muscle signal in the EMG-feedback can be equally or even more effective in increasing the alpha amplitude when compared to the direct alpha training (DeGood and Chisholm, 1977; Moore et al., 2000). Both these procedures resulted in subjects' relaxation as supported by physiological indices such as heart and respiratory rates (DeGood and Chisholm, 1977). In this comparison, the EMG training was explicitly described by participants as easier in the post training survey. Thus, the EMG-feedback can be considered as a valid replacement of the EEG-NFB protocols aiming at the alpha band up-regulation.

We conclude that the activity from the EEG electrodes might be overwhelmed by the stronger and easier to control EMG signals, which in turn becomes a foundation for the feedback reinforcement. This might cause different effects in various training protocols and therefore needs to be carefully considered while designing training protocols and algorithms. Online data analysis and quality of information fed back to the participants should be of the highest interest to all therapists and researchers, as any shortcomings at this stage irreversibly alter the training and cannot be fixed in further offline data processing. Extensive effort should be undertaken within the NFB community to develop, validate and implement in experimental and commercial setups efficient automatic artifact detection algorithms.

AUTHOR CONTRIBUTIONS

KP and KJ: data analyses, main conclusions, article drafting (equal contribution). JR: interpretation of the results, proofreading. RK and MS: data collection. MM: experimental setup, data collection. AW and EK: verification of main concept and conclusions, proofreading.

ACKNOWLEDGMENTS

We thank ELMIKO MEDICAL Sp. z o. o. for technical support. The study was supported by the Polish National Science Centre grant 2012/07/B/NZ7/04383 and by the National Centre for Research and Development grant POIR 01.01.01-00-178/15.

REFERENCES

Anguera, J. A., Boccanfuso, J., Rintoul, J. L., Al-Hashimi, O., Faraji, F., Janowich, J., et al. (2013). Video game training enhances cognitive control in older adults. *Nature* 501, 97–101. doi: 10.1038/nature12486

Arns, M., Kleinnijenhuis, M., Fallahpour, K., and Breteler, R. (2008). Golf performance enhancement and real-life neurofeedback training using personalized event-locked EEG profiles. *J. Neurother.* 11, 11–18. doi: 10.1080/10874200802149656

Becerra, J., Fernández, T., Roca-Stappung, M., Díaz-Comas, L., Galán, L., Bosch, J., et al. (2012). Neurofeedback in healthy elderly human subjects with electroencephalographic risk for cognitive disorder. *J. Alzheimers Dis.* 28, 357–367. doi: 10.3233/JAD-2011-111055

Bekisz, M., and Wróbel, A. (1993). 20 Hz rhythm of activity in visual system of perceiving cat. *Acta Neurobiol. Exp. (Wars)* 53, 175–182.

Berner, I., Schabus, M., Wienerroither, T., and Klimesch, W. (2006). The significance of sigma neurofeedback training on sleep spindles and aspects of declarative memory. *Appl. Psychophysiol. Biofeedback* 31, 97–114. doi: 10.1007/s10484-006-9013-7

Birbaumer, N. (1999). Slow cortical potentials: plasticity, operant control and behavioral effects. *Neuroscientist* 5, 74–78. doi: 10.1177/1073858499 00500211

Bird, B. L., Newton, F. A., Sheer, D. E., and Ford, M. (1978). Biofeedback training of 40-Hz EEG in humans. *Biofeedback Self Regul.* 3, 1–11. doi: 10.1007/bf00998559

Buschman, T. J., and Miller, E. K. (2007). Top-down versus bottom-up control of attention in the prefrontal and posterior parietal cortices. *Science* 315, 1860–1862. doi: 10.1126/science.1138071

Cannon, R., Congedo, M., Lubar, J., and Hutchens, T. (2009). Differentiating a network of executive attention: LORETA neurofeedback in anterior cingulate and dorsolateral prefrontal cortices. *Int. J. Neurosci.* 119, 404–441. doi: 10.1080/00207450802480325

Cannon, R., Lubar, J., Gerke, A., Thornton, K., Hutchens, T., and McCammon, V. (2006). EEG spectral-power and coherence: LORETA neurofeedback training in the anterior cingulate gyrus. *J. Neurother.* 10, 5–31. doi: 10.1300/j184v10n01_02

Criswell, E. (2011). *Cram's Introduction to Surface Electromyography.* 2nd Edn. Sudbury, MA: Jones and Bartlett Publishers.

DeGood, D. E., and Chisholm, R. C. (1977). Multiple response comparison of parietal EEG and frontalis EMG biofeedback. *Psychophysiology* 14, 258–265. doi: 10.1111/j.1469-8986.1977.tb01171.x

Delorme, A., and Makeig, S. (2004). EEGLAB: an open source toolbox for analysis of single-trial EEG dynamics including independent component analysis. *J. Neurosci. Methods* 134, 9–21. doi: 10.1016/j.jneumeth.2003.10.009

Demos, J. N. (2005). *Getting Started with Neurofeedback.* New York, NY: W.W. Norton & Company.

de Zambotti, M., Bianchin, M., Magazzini, L., Gnesato, G., and Angrilli, A. (2012). The efficacy of EEG neurofeedback aimed at enhancing sensory-motor rhythm theta ratio in healthy subjects. *Exp. Brain Res.* 221, 69–74. doi: 10.1007/s00221-012-3148-y

Donner, T. H., Siegel, M., Oostenveld, R., Fries, P., Bauer, M., and Engel, A. K. (2007). Population activity in the human dorsal pathway predicts the accuracy of visual motion detection. *J. Neurophysiol.* 98, 345–359. doi: 10.1152/jn.01141.2006

Egner, T., and Gruzelier, J. H. (2001). Learned self-regulation of EEG frequency components affects attention and event-related brain potentials in humans. *Neuroreport* 12, 4155–4159. doi: 10.1097/00001756-200112210-00058

Egner, T., and Gruzelier, J. H. (2004). EEG Biofeedback of low beta band components: frequency-specific effects on variables of attention and event-related brain potentials. *Clin. Neurophysiol.* 115, 131–139. doi: 10.1016/s1388-2457(03)00353-5

Egner, T., Strawson, E., and Gruzelier, J. H. (2002). EEG signature and phenomenology of alpha/theta neurofeedback training versus mock feedback. *Appl. Psychophysiol. Biofeedback* 27, 261–270. doi: 10.1023/A:102106 3416558

Egner, T., Zech, T. F., and Gruzelier, J. H. (2004). The effects of neurofeedback training on the spectral topography of the electroencephalogram. *Clin. Neurophysiol.* 115, 2452–2460. doi: 10.1016/j.clinph.2004.05.033

Enriquez-Geppert, S., Huster, R. J., and Herrmann, C. S. (2017). EEG-neurofeedback as a tool to modulate cognition and behavior: a review tutorial. *Front. Hum. Neurosci.* 11:51. doi: 10.3389/fnhum.2017.00051

Fitzgibbon, S. P., DeLosAngeles, D., Lewis, T. W., Powers, D. M. W., Grummett, T. S., Whitham, E. M., et al. (2016). Automatic determination of EMG-contaminated components and validation of independent component analysis using EEG during pharmacologic paralysis. *Clin. Neurophysiol.* 127, 1781–1793. doi: 10.1016/j.clinph.2015.12.009

Fuchs, T., Birbaumer, N., Lutzenberger, W., Gruzelier, J. H., and Kaiser, J. (2003). Neurofeedback treatment for attention-deficit/hyperactivity disorder in children: a comparison with methylphenidate. *Appl. Psychophysiol. Biofeedback* 28, 1–12. doi: 10.1023/A:1022353731579

Gevensleben, H., Holl, B., Albrecht, B., Schlamp, D., Kratz, O., Studer, P., et al. (2009a). Distinct EEG effects related to neurofeedback training in children with ADHD: a randomized controlled trial. *Int. J. Psychophysiol.* 74, 149–157. doi: 10.1016/j.ijpsycho.2009.08.005

Gevensleben, H., Holl, B., Albrecht, B., Vogel, C., Schlamp, D., Kratz, O., et al. (2009b). Is neurofeedback an efficacious treatment for ADHD? A randomised controlled clinical trial. *J. Child Psychol. Psychiatry* 50, 780–789. doi: 10.1111/j.1469-7610.2008.02033.x

Ghaziri, J., Tucholka, A., Larue, V., Blanchette-Sylvestre, M., Reyburn, G., Gilbert, G., et al. (2013). Neurofeedback training induces changes in white and gray matter. *Clin. EEG Neurosci.* 44, 265–272. doi: 10.1177/1550059413476031

Gola, M., Magnuski, M., Szumska, I., and Wróbel, A. (2013). EEG beta band activity is related to attention and attentional deficits in the visual performance of elderly subjects. *Int. J. Psychophysiol.* 89, 334–341. doi: 10.1016/j.ijpsycho.2013.05.007

Goncharova, I. I., McFarland, D. J., Vaughan, T. M., and Wolpaw, J. R. (2003). EMG contamination of EEG: spectral and topographical characteristics. *Clin. Neurophysiol.* 114, 1580–1593. doi: 10.1016/s1388-2457(03)00093-2

Gross, J., Schmitz, F., Schnitzler, I., Kessler, K., Shapiro, K., Hommel, B., et al. (2004). Modulation of long-range neural synchrony reflects temporal limitations of visual attention in humans. *Proc. Natl. Acad. Sci. U S A* 101, 13050–13055. doi: 10.1073/pnas.0404944101

Gruzelier, J., Hardman, E., Wild, J., and Zaman, R. (1999). Learned control of slow potential interhemispheric asymmetry in schizophrenia. *Int. J. Psychophysiol.* 34, 341–348. doi: 10.1016/s0167-8760(99)00091-4

Gruzelier, J. H., Thompson, T., Redding, E., Brandt, R., and Steffert, T. (2014). Application of alpha/theta neurofeedback and heart rate variability training to young contemporary dancers: state anxiety and creativity. *Int. J. Psychophysiol.* 93, 105–111. doi: 10.1016/j.ijpsycho.2013.05.004

Heinrich, H., Gevensleben, H., Freisleder, F. J., Moll, G. H., and Rothenberger, A. (2004). Training of slow cortical potentials in attention-deficit/hyperactivity disorder: evidence for positive behavioral and neurophysiological effects. *Biol. Psychiatry* 55, 772–775. doi: 10.1016/j.biopsych.2003.11.013

Hoedlmoser, K., Pecherstorfer, T., Gruber, G., Anderer, P., Doppelmayr, M., Klimesch, W., et al. (2008). Instrumental conditioning of human sensorimotor rhythm (12–15 Hz) and its impact on sleep as well as declarative learning. *Sleep* 31, 1401–1408.

Kaiser, D. A., and Othmer, S. (2000). Effect of neurofeedback on variables of attention in a large multi-center trial. *J. Neurother.* 4, 5–15. doi: 10.1300/j184v04n01_02

Kamiński, J., Brzezicka, A., Gola, M., and Wróbel, A. (2012). β band oscillations engagement in human alertness process. *Int. J. Psychophysiol.* 85, 125–128. doi: 10.1016/j.ijpsycho.2011.11.006

Keizer, A. W., Verment, R. S., and Hommel, B. (2010a). Enhancing cognitive control through neurofeedback: a role of gamma-band activity in managing episodic retrieval. *Neuroimage* 49, 3404–3413. doi: 10.1016/j.neuroimage.2009.11.023

Keizer, A. W., Verschoor, M., Verment, R. S., and Hommel, B. (2010b). The effect of gamma enhancing neurofeedback on the control of feature bindings and intelligence measures. *Int. J. Psychophysiol.* 75, 25–32. doi: 10.1016/j.ijpsycho.2009.10.011

Kober, S. E., Witte, M., Ninaus, M., Neuper, C., and Wood, G. (2013). Learning to modulate one's own brain activity: the effect of spontaneous mental strategies. *Front. Hum. Neurosci.* 7:695. doi: 10.3389/fnhum.2013.00695

Kotchoubey, B., Strehl, U., Uhlmann, C., Holzapfel, S., König, M., Fröscher, W., et al. (2001). Modification of slow cortical potentials in patients with refractory epilepsy: a controlled outcome study. *Epilepsia* 42, 406–416. doi: 10.1046/j.1528-1157.2001.22200.x

Kropotov, J. D., Grin-Yatsenko, V. A., Ponomarev, V. A., Chutko, L. S., Yakovenko, E. A., and Nikishena, I. S. (2007). Changes in EEG spectrograms, event-related potentials and event-related desynchronization induced by relative beta training in ADHD children. *J. Neurother.* 11, 3–11. doi: 10.1300/j184v11n02_02

Leins, U., Goth, G., Hinterberger, T., Klinger, C., Rumpf, N., and Strehl, U. (2007). Neurofeedback for children with ADHD: a comparison of SCP and Theta/Beta protocols. *Appl. Psychophysiol. Biofeedback* 32, 73–88. doi: 10.1007/s10484-007-9031-0

Lévesque, J., Beauregard, M., and Mensour, B. (2006). Effect of neurofeedback training on the neural substrates of selective attention in children with attention-deficit/hyperactivity disorder: a functional magnetic resonance imaging study. *Neurosci. Lett.* 394, 216–221. doi: 10.1016/j.neulet.2005.10.100

Lofthouse, N., Arnold, L. E., Hersch, S., Hurt, E., and DeBeus, R. (2012). A review of neurofeedback treatment for pediatric ADHD. *J. Atten. Disord.* 16, 351–372. doi: 10.1177/1087054711427530

Logemann, H. N. A., Lansbergen, M. M., Van Os, T. W. D. P., Böcker, K. B. E., and Kenemans, J. L. (2010). The effectiveness of EEG-feedback on attention, impulsivity and EEG: a sham feedback controlled study. *Neurosci. Lett.* 479, 49–53. doi: 10.1016/j.neulet.2010.05.026

Maurizio, S., Liechti, M. D., Brandeis, D., Jäncke, L., and Drechsler, R. (2013). Differential EMG biofeedback for children with ADHD: a control method for neurofeedback training with a case illustration. *Appl. Psychophysiol. Biofeedback* 38, 109–119. doi: 10.1007/s10484-013-9213-x

McMenamin, B. W., Shackman, A. J., Greischar, L. L., and Davidson, R. J. (2011). Electromyogenic artifacts and electroencephalographic inferences revisited. *Neuroimage* 54, 4–9. doi: 10.1016/j.neuroimage.2010.07.057

Meisel, V., Servera, M., Garcia-Banda, G., Cardo, E., and Moreno, I. (2014). Reprint of "Neurofeedback and standard pharmacological intervention in ADHD: a randomized controlled trial with six-month follow-up". *Biol. Psychol.* 95, 116–125. doi: 10.1016/j.biopsycho.2013.09.009

Moore, J. P., Trudeau, D. L., Thuras, P. D., Rubin, Y., Stockley, H., and Dimond, T. (2000). Comparison of alpha-theta, alpha and EMG neurofeedback in the production of alpha-theta crossover and the occurrence of visualizations. *J. Neurother.* 4, 29–42. doi: 10.1300/j184v04n01_04

Muthukumaraswamy, S. D. (2013). High-frequency brain activity and muscle artifacts in MEG/EEG: a review and recommendations. *Front. Hum. Neurosci.* 7:138. doi: 10.3389/fnhum.2013.00138

Nottage, J. F., Morrison, P. D., Williams, S. C. R., and Ffytche, D. H. (2013). A novel method for reducing the effect of tonic muscle activity on the gamma band of the scalp EEG. *Brain Topogr.* 26, 50–61. doi: 10.1007/s10548-012-0255-9

Raymond, J., Varney, C., Parkinson, L. A., and Gruzelier, J. H. (2005). The effects of alpha/theta neurofeedback on personality and mood. *Cogn. Brain Res.* 23, 287–292. doi: 10.1016/j.cogbrainres.2004.10.023

Reiner, M., Rozengurt, R., and Barnea, A. (2014). Better than sleep: theta neurofeedback training accelerates memory consolidation. *Biol. Psychol.* 95, 45–53. doi: 10.1016/j.biopsycho.2013.10.010

Ros, T., Théberge, J., Frewen, P. A., Kluetsch, R., Densmore, M., Calhoun, V. D., et al. (2013). Mind over chatter: plastic up-regulation of the fMRI salience network directly after EEG neurofeedback. *Neuroimage* 65, 324–335. doi: 10.1016/j.neuroimage.2012.09.046

Rostami, R., Sadeghi, H., Karami, K., Abadi, M., and Salamati, P. (2012). The effects of neurofeedback on the improvement of rifle shooters' performance. *J. Neurother.* 16, 264–269. doi: 10.1080/10874208.2012.730388

Siegel, M., Donner, T. H., Oostenveld, R., Fries, P., and Engel, A. K. (2008). Neuronal synchronization along the dorsal visual pathway reflects the focus of spatial attention. *Neuron* 60, 709–719. doi: 10.1016/j.neuron.2008.09.010

Staufenbiel, S. M., Brouwer, A. M., Keizer, A. W., and van Wouwe, N. C. (2014). Effect of beta and gamma neurofeedback on memory and intelligence in the elderly. *Biol. Psychol.* 95, 74–85. doi: 10.1016/j.biopsycho.2013.05.020

Sterman, M. B., and Friar, L. (1972). Suppression of seizures in an epileptic following sensori motor EEG feedback training. *Electroencephalogr. Clin. Neurophysiol.* 33, 89–95. doi: 10.1016/0013-4694(72)90028-4

Strehl, U., Leins, U., Goth, G., Klinger, C., Hinterberger, T., and Birbaumer, N. (2006). Self-regulation of slow cortical potentials: a new treatment for children with attention-deficit/hyperactivity disorder. *Pediatrics* 118, e1530–e1540. doi: 10.1542/peds.2005-2478

Surmeli, T., Ertem, A., Eralp, E., and Kos, I. H. (2012). Schizophrenia and the efficacy of qEEG-guided neurofeedback treatment: a clinical case series. *Clin. EEG Neurosci.* 43, 133–144. doi: 10.1177/1550059411429531

van Boxtel, G. J. M., Denissen, A. J. M., Jäger, M., Vernon, D., Dekker, M. K. J., Mihajlovic, V., et al. (2012). A novel self-guided approach to alpha activity training. *Int. J. Psychophysiol.* 83, 282–294. doi: 10.1016/j.ijpsycho.2011.11.004

Vernon, D., Egner, T., Cooper, N., Compton, T., Neilands, C., Sheri, A., et al. (2003). The effect of training distinct neurofeedback protocols on aspects of cognitive performance. *Int. J. Psychophysiol.* 47, 75–85. doi: 10.1016/s0167-8760(02)00091-0

Wang, X.-J. (2010). Neurophysiological and computational principles of cortical rhythms in cognition. *Physiol. Rev.* 90, 1195–1268. doi: 10.1152/physrev.000 35.2008

Waterink, W., and van Boxtel, A. (1994). Facial and jaw-elevator EMG activity in relation to changes in performance level during a sustained information processing task. *Biol. Psychol.* 37, 183–198. doi: 10.1016/0301-0511(94)90001-9

Whitham, E. M., Lewis, T., Pope, K. J., Fitzgibbon, S. P., Clark, C. R., Loveless, S., et al. (2008). Thinking activates EMG in scalp electrical recordings. *Clin. Neurophysiol.* 119, 1166–1175. doi: 10.1016/j.clinph.2008.01.024

Whitham, E. M., Pope, K. J., Fitzgibbon, S. P., Lewis, T., Clark, C. R., Loveless, S., et al. (2007). Scalp electrical recording during paralysis: quantitative evidence that EEG frequencies above 20 Hz are contaminated by EMG. *Clin. Neurophysiol.* 118, 1877–1888. doi: 10.1016/j.clinph.2007.04.027

Witte, M., Kober, S. E., Ninaus, M., Neuper, C., and Wood, G. (2013). Control beliefs can predict the ability to up-regulate sensorimotor rhythm during neurofeedback training. *Front. Hum. Neurosci.* 7:478. doi: 10.3389/fnhum. 2013.00478

Wróbel, A. (2000). Beta activity: a carrier for visual attention. *Acta Neurobiol. Exp.* 60, 247–260.

Wróbel, A. (2014). "Attentional activation in cortico-thalamic loops of the visual system," in *New Visual Neurosciences*, eds L. M. Chalupa and J. S. Werner (Cambridge, MA: MIT Press), 339–350.

Wróbel, A., Ghazaryan, A., Bekisz, M., Bogdan, W., and Kaminski, J. (2007). Two streams of attention-dependent δ activity in the striate recipient zone of cat's lateral posterior—pulvinar complex. *J. Neurosci.* 27, 2230–2240. doi: 10.1523/JNEUROSCI.4004-06.2007

Yilmaz, G., Ungan, P., Sebik, O., Uginčius, P., and Türker, K. S. (2014). Interference of tonic muscle activity on the EEG: a single motor unit study. *Front. Hum. Neurosci.* 8:504. doi: 10.3389/fnhum.2014.00504

Yucha, C. B., and Montgomery, D. (2008). *Evidence-Based Practice in Biofeedback and Neurofeedback.* Wheat Ridge, CO: Association for Applied Psychophysiology and Biofeedback.

Zoefel, B., Huster, R. J., and Herrmann, C. S. (2011). Neurofeedback training of the upper alpha frequency band in EEG improves cognitive performance. *Neuroimage* 54, 1427–1431. doi: 10.1016/j.neuroimage.2010.08.078

2

Dancing or Fitness Sport? The Effects of Two Training Programs on Hippocampal Plasticity and Balance Abilities in Healthy Seniors

Kathrin Rehfeld[1,2†], Patrick Müller[1,3†], Norman Aye[1,2], Marlen Schmicker[1], Milos Dordevic[1,2], Jörn Kaufmann[4], Anita Hökelmann[2] and Notger G. Müller[1,3,5]*

[1] German Center for Neurodegenerative Diseases, Magdeburg, Germany, [2] Institute for Sport Science, Otto von Guericke University Magdeburg, Magdeburg, Germany, [3] Medical Faculty, Otto von Guericke University Magdeburg, Magdeburg, Germany, [4] Department of Neurology, Otto von Guericke University Magdeburg, Magdeburg, Germany, [5] Center for Behavioral Brain Sciences, Magdeburg, Germany

Edited by:
Claudia Voelcker-Rehage, Technische Universität Chemnitz, Germany

Reviewed by:
Dieter J. Meyerhoff, University of California, San Francisco, United States
Marco Taubert, Otto von Guericke University Magdeburg, Germany

***Correspondence:**
Kathrin Rehfeld
kathrin.rehfeld@ovgu.de

† These authors have contributed equally to this work.

Age-related degenerations in brain structure are associated with balance disturbances and cognitive impairment. However, neuroplasticity is known to be preserved throughout lifespan and physical training studies with seniors could reveal volume increases in the hippocampus (HC), a region crucial for memory consolidation, learning and navigation in space, which were related to improvements in aerobic fitness. Moreover, a positive correlation between left HC volume and balance performance was observed. Dancing seems a promising intervention for both improving balance and brain structure in the elderly. It combines aerobic fitness, sensorimotor skills and cognitive demands while at the same time the risk of injuries is low. Hence, the present investigation compared the effects of an 18-month dancing intervention and traditional health fitness training on volumes of hippocampal subfields and balance abilities. Before and after intervention, balance was evaluated using the Sensory Organization Test and HC volumes were derived from magnetic resonance images (3T, MP-RAGE). Fourteen members of the dance (67.21 ± 3.78 years, seven females), and 12 members of the fitness group (68.67 ± 2.57 years, five females) completed the whole study. Both groups revealed hippocampal volume increases mainly in the left HC (CA1, CA2, subiculum). The dancers showed additional increases in the left dentate gyrus and the right subiculum. Moreover, only the dancers achieved a significant increase in the balance composite score. Hence, dancing constitutes a promising candidate in counteracting the age-related decline in physical and mental abilities.

Keywords: dancing, fitness training, balance, hippocampus, aging

INTRODUCTION

The human hippocampus (HC) is affected not only by pathological aging such as in Alzheimer's disease but also by the normal aging process resulting in deficits in memory, learning, and spatial navigation at old age (Driscoll et al., 2003; Barnes et al., 2009). Magnetic resonance-studies indicate an atrophy rate of the hippocampus and the nearby parahippocampal gyrus of 2–3% per decade (Raz et al., 2004, 2005), which is further accelerated in the very old age where there is an annual loss of 1% over the age of 70 (Jack et al., 1998). On the other hand more recent research has shown that the HC counts among the few brain regions with the ability to generate new neurons throughout the lifespan (Kempermann et al., 2010; Spalding et al., 2013). In animal models physical activity has been identified as a key mechanism that can drive this adult neuroplasticity (van Praag et al., 1999; Kronenberg, 2003). In humans, research has focused on the effects of aerobic fitness and training on volumes and perfusion of the HC. Results reveal that higher cardiorespiratory fitness levels (VO_2 max) are associated with larger hippocampal volumes in late adulthood, and that larger hippocampal volumes may, in turn, contribute to better memory function (Erickson et al., 2011; Szabo et al., 2011; Bugg et al., 2012; Maass et al., 2015). Furthermore, some investigations also assessed possible physiological mediators of the observed neuroplasticity, such as brain-derived neurotrophic factor (BDNF), insulin-like growth factor 1 (IGF-1), and vascular endothelial growth factor (VEGF) (Flöel et al., 2010; Erickson et al., 2011; Ruscheweyh et al., 2011; Maass et al., 2016). Whereas Erickson et al. (2011) reported a positive correlation between levels of serum BDNF, hippocampal volume and cardiorespiratory fitness during 1 year of aerobic training, neither Ruscheweyh et al. (2011) nor Maass et al. (2016) found fitness-related BDNF changes after 6 or 3 months of training, respectively. Moreover, other studies failed to find correlations between volumes of the medial temporal lobe area or the hippocampus and cardiovascular fitness in healthy elderly (Honea et al., 2009; Smith et al., 2011). Therefore, the role of cardio-respiratory fitness in modulating hippocampal gray matter volume is still under debate.

The hippocampus is also involved in spatial navigation (O'Keefe, 1990) and in motor sequence consolidation (Albouy et al., 2008) suggesting that motor skill learning and motor fitness can have impact on hippocampal volume without any cardio-respiratory change. In this respect, Niemann et al. (2014) tested whether 12 months of cardiovascular or coordination training induces larger increases in hippocampal volume in healthy older participants. After training, the cardio-vascular group revealed a significant volume increase in the left HC of 4.22% and a non-significant increase of 2.98% for the right HC. Effects of the coordinative training were more pronounced in the right HC with an increase of 3.91%, whereas the changes in the left HC (1.78%) were non-significant. Further correlation analyses between motor fitness and hippocampal volume failed to reach significant results. Still there is compelling evidence that the human brain undergoes morphological alterations in response to motor-skill learning (Draganski et al., 2004; Boyke et al., 2008; Taubert et al., 2010; Sehm et al., 2014). Along these lines, a recent study demonstrated structural brain changes already after two sessions of dynamic balance training that correlated with the individual motor skill learning success of the participants (Taubert et al., 2010). Sehm et al. (2014) could demonstrate that 6 weeks of balance training induced increases in the gray matter of the left HC in healthy seniors. These findings highlight the behavioral relevance of structural brain plasticity in the HC for the learning process. Hüfner et al. (2011) stated that long-term balance training with its extensive vestibular, visual and sensorimotor stimulation is associated with altered hippocampal formation volumes in professional ballet dancers and slackliners. Hence, the HC seems not only crucial for long-term memory consolidation, learning and spatial navigation, but also for balancing. Intact balance is essential for social mobility and quality of life in aging (Dordevic et al., 2017). Hence, physical intervention programs should take this function into account, too.

In this respect dancing seems to be a promising intervention since it requires the integration of sensory information from multiple channels (auditory, vestibular, visual, somatosensory) and the fine-grained motor control of the whole body. Behavioral studies have already provided evidence of better performance in balance and memory tasks in elderly dancers (Kattenstroth et al., 2010, 2013; Rehfeld et al., 2014), but the underlying neural mechanisms have not been addressed comprehensively so far. Knowing that aerobic, sensorimotor and cognitive training contribute to hippocampal volume, which also seems to be associated with balancing capabilities, we initialized a prospective, randomized longitudinal trial over a period of 18 months in healthy seniors. Two interventions were compared: a specially designed dance program, during which subjects constantly had to learn new choreographies, and a traditional fitness program with mainly repetitive exercises, such as cycling on an ergometer or Nordic walking. Whole-brain analyzes of the acquired data using voxel based morphometry had shown dance-associated volume increases mainly in the precentral and the parahippocampal gyrus (Müller et al., 2016). Knowing that dancing/slacklining (Hüfner et al., 2011) and endurance sport (e.g., Erickson et al., 2011) have different impact on anterior and posterior parts of the hippocampus in the present analysis we ran a region of interest analysis of this specific brain region. To do so we first computed a restricted VBM analysis with a hippocampal mask. In the next step we divided the hippocampus in five subfields in order to allow a detailed analysis of the interventions' effects on different parts of the HC. The hippocampus is not a homogeneous structure but consists of histologically specialized subfields, such as the subiculum, cornu ammonis (CA) 1–4 and dentate gyrus (DG). The subiculum has been implicated in working memory and spatial relations (Riegert et al., 2004; O'Mara, 2005). CA3 and DG have been suggested to be involved in memory and early retrieval, whereas CA1 in late retrieval, consolidation and recognition. Especially the DG is one of the few regions of the adult brain where neurogenesis takes places, which is important in the formation of new memories and spatial memory (Saab et al., 2009). Nevertheless all these subfields are tightly interconnected (Duvernoy, 2005). Since dancing seems to promote spatial orientation, working memory and might promote neurogenesis, we expected volume changes in more subfields of the HC after this intervention. Moreover, given the importance of intact balance for successful aging on the one hand and its dependence on the hippocampus on the other hand, we also assessed effects of the interventions on balancing capabilities and their relation to hippocampal subfield volumes.

MATERIALS AND METHODS

Study Design and Subjects

This investigation, comprising hippocampal volume alterations and changes in balance abilities, is part of a large prospective longitudinal study which compares the effects of dancing versus aerobic training on brain structure and function, mediating neuroplasticity factors, such as BDNF, as well as cognitive and motor performances in healthy elderly seniors. The cognitive development and BDNF changes are highlighted in our recent report (see Müller et al., 2017). The intervention was provided for 18 months and contained three time-points of measurement: baseline pre-test, first post-test after 6 months of training and second post-test after 18 months of training (see **Figure 1**). Again, the temporal dynamics of gray matter brain plasticity are already stated by Müller et al. (2017), showing a significant increase of gray matter volume in parahippocampal gyrus only for the dancers. Based on that finding, we assume only changes from baseline to the second post-test (18 months).

The approval for the study was obtained from the ethics committee of the Otto von Guericke University, Magdeburg. All subjects signed a written informed consent and received a reimbursement for their participation.

The timeline of the study can be depicted from **Figure 1**. Primarily, we invited 62 healthy elderly volunteers aged 63–80 years for cognitive and physical screening as well as for verification of magnetic resonance imaging suitability. Exclusion criteria were defined as follows: any history of severe neurological conditions, metal implants, claustrophobia, tinnitus, intensive physical engagement (more than 1 h/week), cognitive impairments as evidenced in the MMSE (Folstein et al., 1975) and depressive symptoms (BDI-II > 13) (Beck et al., 2006). Fifty two seniors met the inclusion criteria and were then randomly assigned to the experimental dance group and the control sport group. After 18 months of training we were left with 26 complete data sets, including 14 dancers and 12 sportsmen. Both groups (mean age = 67.9 ± 3.3 years) did not differ concerning age, sex, education, and BMI. For detailed information about demographic data see **Table 1**.

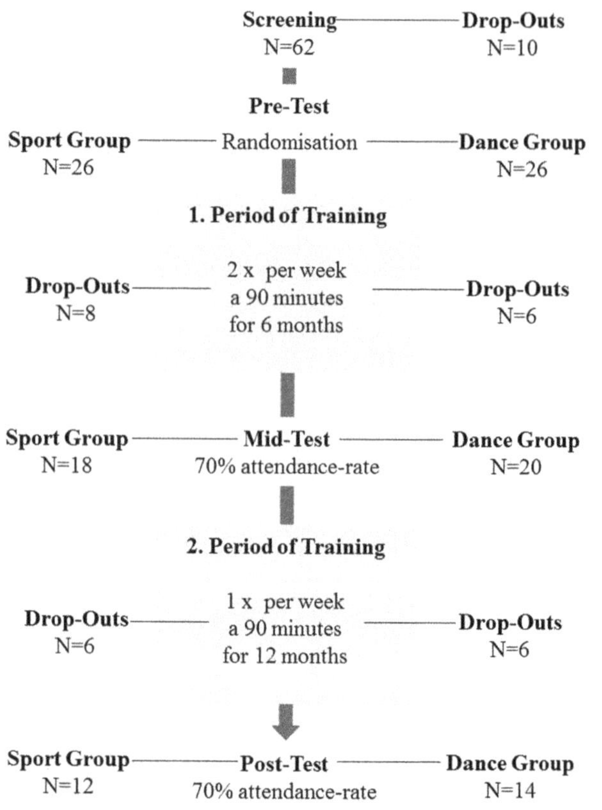

FIGURE 1 | Study design presenting: voluntary recruitment, drop-outs, time-points of measurement, duration of training periods.

Interventions

The precise description of the interventions is published elsewhere (Müller et al., 2016). In brief, the first period of training was provided for 6 months, twice a week for both groups. Each dancing or fitness class lasted 90 min. Because of organizational reasons we had to change the training frequency from twice a week to once a week after 6 months of training. The second training period was run for 12 months and the training sessions were reduced to once a week for 90 min in both groups. The content of the dance classes induced a permanent learning situation with constantly changing choreographies, which participants had to memorize accurately. The training focused on elementary longitudinal turns, head-spins, shifts of center of gravity (COG), single-leg stances, skips and hops, different steps like chassée, mambo, cha cha, grapevine, jazz square to challenge the balance system. Additional arm-patterns enforced imbalances (moving arms away from center of pressure).

The program for the sport group was adjusted according to the recommended guidelines for health sport (Brehm et al., 2006) and included endurance training, strength-endurance training, and flexibility training (stretching and mobility). Each part of the mentioned topics (endurance; strength-endurance; and flexibility) was exercised for 20 min, whereby a 10 min warm-up, a 10 min cool-down and short breaks between the different exercises adding to another 10 min completed each 90 min lasting session. So both groups exercised for 90 min in each training session. In the first 6 months, endurance training was performed on bicycle ergometers with the intensity adjusted to the individual training heart rate (HR) using the Karvonen Formula:

$$\text{Target training HR} =$$
$$\text{Resting HR} + (0.6[\text{maximum HR} - \text{resting HR}]).$$

The factor 0.6 is a representative for an extensive aerobic training (Davis and Convertino, 1975). In the second training period (12 months) the participants completed a Nordic Walking program. The strength-endurance training aimed to strengthen major muscles of the muscular skeleton. In this program we

TABLE 1 | Demographic information at baseline of analyzed participants ($N = 26$).

	Dance group [N = 14]		Sport group [N = 12]			
	M	*SD*	*M*	*SD*	*t*-value	*p*-value
Age [years]	67.21	3.78	68.67	2.57	−1.12	0.272
Sex [%]	50% male		58% male		0.154	0.695
MMSE [points]	28.07	0.92	29.17	0.58	−3.011	0.003
BDI-II [points]	4.5/5.54	3.37/2.97	3.75/3.39	3.79/3.77	0.53	0.598
Education [years]	15.40	2.05	16.10	1.45	−1.395	0.175
BMI [kg/m^2]	27.51	3.87	27.24	2.94	−0.275	0.786

BMI, Body-Mass-Index; BDI-II, Becks-Depressions-Inventar II; MMSE, Mini Mental State Examination; M, Mean; SD, Standard deviation; $p \leq 0.05$ = statistical significance.

avoided combined arm and leg movements in order to keep coordinative demands low.

Structural MRI Acquisition, Preprocessing, and Analysis

Magnetic resonance (MR) images were acquired on a 3 Tesla Siemens MAGNETOM Verio (Syngo MR B17) using a 32-channel head coil. T-1 weighted MPRAGE sequence (224 sagittal slices, voxel size: 0.8 mm × 0.8 mm × 0.8 mm, TR: 2500 ms, TE: 3.47 ms, TI: 1100 ms, flip angle: 7°) were analyzed using region of interest (ROI) defined voxel-based morphometry with SPM 12 (Welcome Department of Cognitive Neurology, London, United Kingdom) running under Matlab (The Math Works). The data preprocessing involved gray matter segmentation, DARTEL based template creation, spatial normalization to MNI-Space and an 5 mm smoothing with a Gaussian kernel as previously described.

Voxel-Based Morphometry with Hippocampal Mask

In order to incorporate our *a priori* hypotheses concerning hippocampal gray matter volume changes we first conducted a ROI-VBM with hippocampal masks. The longitudinal analysis for hippocampal gray matter volume changes was performed using repeated measurement ANOVAs in a full factorial design. We applied a threshold of $p < 0.05$ (FDR corrected).

Hippocampal Subfield Volume Measurements

In a second step we analyzed volume changes in five subfields of the HC. Up to now there is no real gold standard in analyzing HC subfield volumes and each of the current manifold analytic techniques has its strengths and weaknesses (Bandettini, 2009; Kuhnt et al., 2013). Here for the hippocampal subfield segmentation in order to obtain ROI volumes we chose the SPM ANATOMY Toolbox v.2.2.c (Eickhoff et al., 2007) with normalized images. This segmentation included the cornu ammonis (CA1–CA3), the dentate gyrus (DG, including CA4) and the subiculum (**Figure 2**). In SPM Anatomy toolbox, definition of anatomical regions is based on maximum probability cytoarchitectonic maps.

Postural Control

Postural control was assessed with the Sensory Organization Test (SOT) implemented in the Balance Master System (Neurocom International, Inc., United States). This test provides information about the contribution of the visual, somatosensory, and vestibular system to the maintenance of balance. The system consists of a dual force platform including force transducers measuring the angular displacement of the COG under certain conditions and visual surround. Both, visual surround and platform enable anterior/posterior sway and this sway can be assessed under different conditions. The six conditions are: normal vision and fixed support (condition 1), absent vision and fixed support (condition 2), sway-referenced vision and fixed support (condition 3), normal vision and sway-referenced support (condition 4), absent vision and sway referenced support (condition 5), and sway-referenced vision and sway-referenced support (condition 6). These conditions were performed in three trials for 20 s, resulting in equilibrium scores. Those equilibrium scores range from 0% (balance loss) to 100% (perfect stability). From the equilibrium scores a sensory analysis was performed by calculating average scores of specific pairs of SOT conditions: the participant's ability to use input from the somatosensory system to maintain balance is reflected by the average of condition 2 divided by the average of condition 1, the contribution of the visual system by the average of condition 4 divided by the average of condition 1 and that of the vestibular system by the average of condition 5 divided by the average of condition 1.

The composite score was calculated by averaging the score for conditions 1 and 2; adding these two scores to the equilibrium scores from each trial of sensory conditions 3, 4, 5, and 6; and dividing that sum by the total number of trials (NeuroCom Natus Medical Incorporated, 2008).

Statistical Analysis

Statistical analysis of hippocampal volumes and balance data were performed with SPSS (SPSS 22, inc./IBM). Intervention effects were tested using repeated-measurement ANOVAs with group (dance, sport) as between-subject factor and time (pre, post) as within-subject factor. Hereby, age, gender, and total hippocampal volume were included as covariates. Additionally, hypothesis driven *t*-tests (with Bonferroni

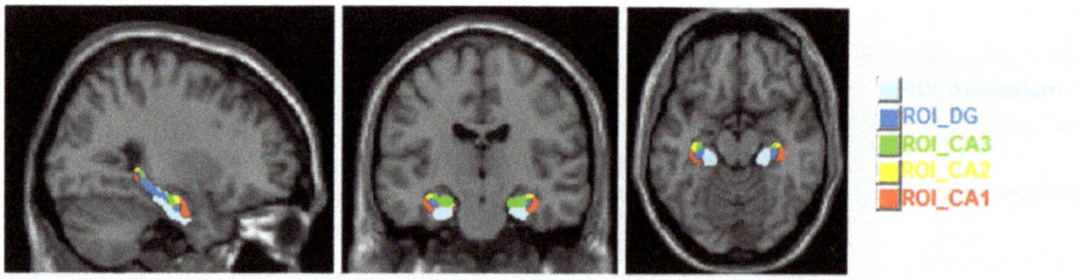

FIGURE 2 | Sagittal, coronal and axial views of the hippocampal subfields.

adjustment) were performed to determine longitudinal changes in the dance and the sports group separately. In case of missing normal distribution we used the Mann-Whitney-*U*-test or Wilcoxon instead of *t*-tests. Pearson-Correlation analysis was performed between percentage change of hippocampal subfield volumes and the balance composite score.

RESULTS

The presentation of the results is structured as follows. We first tested for hippocampal volume differences after intervention using both masked VBM and subfield volume measurements. In the next step we investigated balance data and finally we looked for correlations between improvements in balance and hippocampal volume.

Voxel-Based Morphometry with Hippocampal Mask

A two-sample *t*-test revealed no group differences at baseline. To explore hippocampal gray matter volume changes during intervention we used repeated measurement ANOVA for comparison between baseline and post-test. There was a significant interaction effect in the right hippocampus [MNI-coordinates: $x = 28$, $y = -16$, $z = -23$; $p(\text{FDR}) = 0.049$, $F = 17.03$]. *Post hoc* paired *t*-tests showed only in the dance group significant volume increases in the right hippocampus [MNI-coordinates: $x = 29$, $y = -16$, $z = -27$; $p(\text{FDR}) = 0.001$, $t = 6.10$] (**Figure 3**).

Hippocampal Subfield Volume Measurements

A two-sample *t*-test revealed no group differences of total hippocampal volumes at baseline [$t(25) = -1.078$, $p = 0.658$, $d = -0{,}424$]. The repeated measurement ANOVA of hippocampal subfield volumes showed a main effect of time regarding left CA1, left CA2, left and right subiculum and left CA4/dentate gyrus (**Table 2**). There were no significant interactions with group. Paired *t*-tests showed significant volume increases for the dancers in left CA1, left CA2, left CA4/dentate gyrus and left and right subiculum and for the sportsmen in the left CA1, left CA2, and left subiculum (**Figure 4**).

Postural Control

Repeated measurement ANOVAs of balance data showed an interaction effect with group for the composite equilibrium score (see **Table 3** and **Figure 5**).

There was a main effect of time regarding the somatosensory and vestibular contribution but no significant time × group interaction effects after 18 months of training (see **Table 3**). *Post hoc* tests revealed that the dancers improved in the use of all three sensory systems somatosensory system [$t(13) = -2.902$, $p = 0.004$], visual system [$t(12) = -2.525$, $p = 0.027$] vestibular system [$t(12) = -3.271$, $p = 0.007$] to maintain balance. Members of the sports group improved in the use of the somatosensory system [$t(9) = -3.579$, $p = 0.006$] and the vestibular system [$t(9) = -3.881$, $p = 0.004$] but not in the visual system. **Table 3** presents an overview of significant alterations related to employment of sensory information to maintain balance from baseline to post-intervention for both groups.

Correlation Analysis

Correlation analysis between all hippocampal subfields and balance did not yield any significant results irrespective of whether the groups were analyzed separately or jointly.

DISCUSSION

Animal research has shown that combining aerobic training with sensory enrichment has a superior effect on inducing neuroplasticity in the HC compared to physical exercise or sensory stimulation alone (Kempermann et al., 2010). This sparked our idea to investigate the impact on neuroplasticity in elderly humans of a specially designed, sensorimotor and cognitive challenging dance program in comparison to a classical cardiovascular fitness program. In addition to our previous work (Müller et al., 2017), in the present study we ran a dedicated ROI analysis, which was focused on subfield volumes of the HC. The HC is of special interest as this brain structure is (a) especially affected by normal and pathological aging and (b) plays a key role in major cognitive processes, e.g., memory and learning and (c) is also involved in keeping one's balance, a function which is crucial for well-being and quality of life.

We observed that both, dancing and fitness training led to increases in hippocampal subfield volumes. Although there was no significant group × time interaction in the ANOVA omnibus

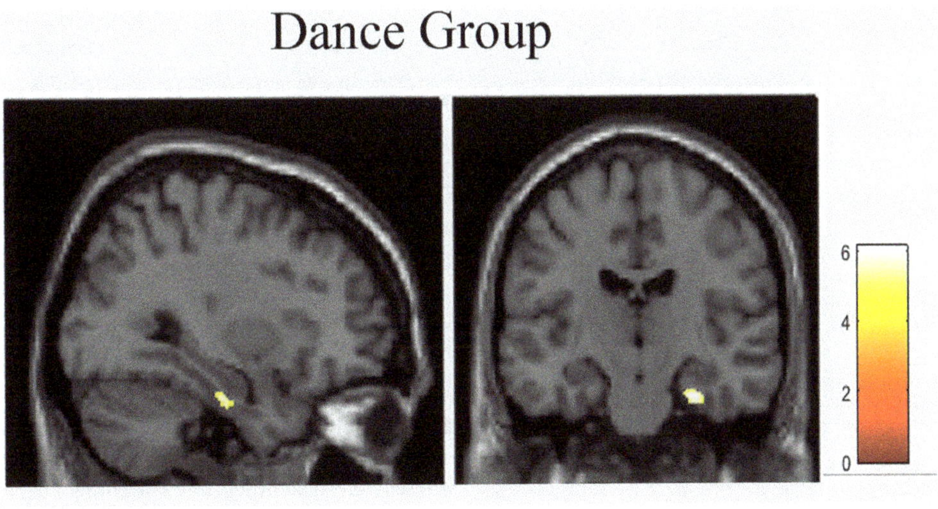

FIGURE 3 | Hippocampal volume increases after 18 month of intervention in dance group.

TABLE 2 | Statistical values of repeated-measures ANOVAs for hippocampal subfields.

Hippocampal subfield	Main effect of time				Main effect of group				Interaction (time × group)			
	F	df	*p*	η^2	*F*	df	*p*	η^2	*F*	df	*p*	η^2
Left CA1	16.920	1.25	**0.001*****	0.410	0.000	1.25	0.985	0.000	0.469	1.25	0.500	0.019
Right CA1	2.952	1.25	0.099	0.110	0.116	1.25	0.736	0.005	2.189	1.25	0.152	0.084
Left CA2	21.126	1.25	**0.001*****	0.468	0.427	1.25	0.520	0.017	0.941	1.25	0.342	0.038
Right CA2	2.020	1.25	0.162	0.078	0.212	1.25	0.650	0.009	1.431	1.25	0.243	0.056
Left CA3	4.237	1.25	0.51	0.150	0.347	1.25	0.561	0.014	0.986	1.25	0.331	0.039
Right CA3	2.680	1.25	0.115	0.100	0.011	1.25	0.918	0.000	1.370	1.25	0.252	0.054
Left subiculum	49.926	1.25	**0.001*****	0.675	0.959	1.25	0.337	0.038	0.094	1.25	0.762	0.004
Right subiculum	12.976	1.25	**0.001*****	0.351	2.025	1.25	0.168	0.079	0.001	1.25	0.976	0.000
Left CA4/DG	9.480	1.25	**0.005***	0.283	0.541	1.25	0.469	0.022	0.001	1.25	0.961	0.000
Right CA4/DG	0.002	1.25	0.963	0.000	0.595	1.25	0.448	0.024	2.32	1.25	0.141	0.088

*CA, cornu ammonis; DG, dentate gyrus; $p \leq 0.05$ = statistical significance. Level of significance: $0.01 \leq \alpha < 0.05$: * "significant"; $0.001 \leq \alpha < 0.01$: ** "high significant"; $\alpha < 0.001$: *** "highly significant".*

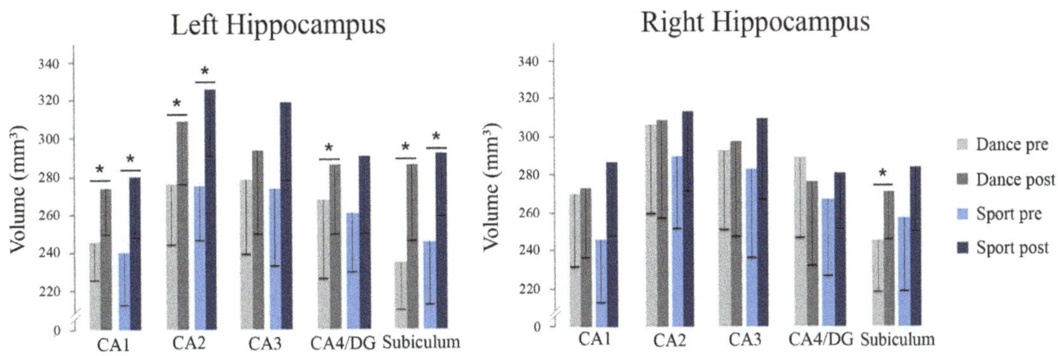

FIGURE 4 | Volumes of hippocampal subfields in dance and sport group at baseline and after 18 months of intervention including standard deviation (DG, dentate gyrus; CA, cornu ammonis; $^*p < 0.05$).

TABLE 3 | Statistical values of repeated-measures ANOVAs for sensory organization of balance.

Sensory organization of balance [%]	Time				Group				Interaction (time × group)			
	F	df	*p*	η^2	*F*	df	*p*	η^2	*F*	df	*p*	η^2
Somatosensory system	30.340	1,25	**0.001*** **	0.591	1.208	1,25	0.284	0.054	0.692	1,25	0.415	0.032
Visual system	6.094	1,25	0.022*	0.225	0.363	1,25	0.553	0.017	0.296	1,25	0.592	0.014
Vestibular system	17.722	1,25	**0.001*** **	0.458	0.229	1,25	0.637	0.011	1.326	1,25	0.262	0.059
Composite equilibrium score	0.514	1,25	0.481	0.024	0.092	1,25	0.764	0.004	4.851	1,25	0.039*	0.188

*Level of significance: 0.01 ≤ α < 0.05: * "significant"; 0.001 ≤ α < 0.01: ** "high significant"; α < 0.001: *** "highly significant".*

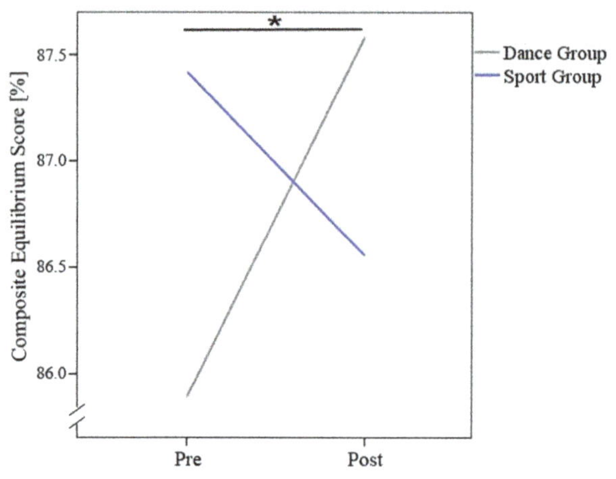

FIGURE 5 | Interaction-effect (time × group) for composite equilibrium score. *Means significant interaction-effect.

analysis, exploratory *post hoc t*-tests indicated that participants of the dance group showed volume increases in more subfields (four out of five, including the DG) of the left HC and that only dancing led to an increase in one subfield of the right HC, namely the subiculum. Regarding balance abilities dancing was superior to standard fitness as expressed by a larger increase in the composite score of our balance test and improved use of all three sensory systems. We, however, did not observe a correlation between changes in HC subfield volumes changes and those in balance; in other words whether the observed skill improvement can be attributed to the HC cannot be fully answered yet.

Regarding the HC volume increases observed in both groups, our results support the assumption that HC volume can be enhanced by physical fitness alone, as this was the overlapping feature of both trainings. Animal studies have shown that adult neurogenesis takes place mainly in the DG part of the HC (van Praag et al., 1999). Interestingly, only the dancers showed an increase in this brain region. Whether adult neurogenesis was indeed the basis of the here observed volume change, however, must remain an open question as there is no direct way in addressing this process in humans.

The dancers showed increases in some HC subfields where there was no change to be observed in the sports group. This indicates that apart from physical fitness, other factors inherent in dancing, contribute to HC volume changes, too. Animal research has suggested that sensory enrichment may be such a factor whereby physical fitness and enrichment have different effects on HC neurons: running in a wheel generates new neurons in the HC of mice but these only survive when sensory stimulation is also present (Kempermann et al., 2010). Again, with our own data we cannot differentiate between these different processes. We nevertheless can conclude that the additional challenges involved in our dance program, namely cognitive and sensorimotor stimulation, induced extra HC volume changes in addition to those attributable to physical fitness alone. It is noteworthy, that other studies in elderly humans, which did not boost physical fitness but which were sensorimotor demanding, such as learning to juggle (Boyke et al., 2008), have observed HC volume increases as well.

Only the dancers showed an increased balance composite score and they improved in all three involved sensory systems. This indicates that dancing drives all three senses and presumably also improves the integration of sensorimotor, visual and vestibular information. Balancing is an important everyday function, crucial for example for social mobility. Impaired balance often results in falls, which constitutes a major health risk factor with consequences both on morbidity (and even mortality) and health care costs (see also Dordevic et al., 2017). Although the ability to balance has been also linked to the HC and its connections, for example, to the vestibular system (Brandt et al., 2005), we did not observe a correlation between HC subfield volumes and improvements in balance. Given the small size of our sample, this needs to be interpreted with care but may suggest that other brain regions, probably those described in our earlier analysis (Müller et al., 2017) were involved in these improvements or that changes in the HC other than those expressed in measurable volumes, e.g., synaptic function, perfusion, etc. contributed to this effect.

There are other limitations in the present study which should not be left unmentioned. As already mentioned above (see Materials and Methods), we had to change the training intervention frequency from twice a week to once a week after 6 months of training. Hence, it must remain unclear whether more pronounced effects could have been observed if we had been able to stick to the initial training intensity. Next the ANOVAs failed to reach significant group interaction effects, only the exploratory *t*-tests became significant which may be a consequence of the large number of factors and levels in the ANOVAs on the one hand, and the small sample size on the other hand. A further limitation can be seen in the use of fully automated segmentation tools. Finally, the small sample size accompanied by a high drop-out rate as well as the highly selective inclusion, a missing inactive control group and exclusion criteria must be mentioned as they limit the generalizability of our results.

In sum, the present results indicate that both dance and fitness training can induce hippocampal plasticity in the elderly, but only dance training improved balance capabilities.

However, larger studies with more representative samples are required in the future. They should include additional analysis of mediating factors and they should try to find ways to optimally adjust the training protocol to an individual's needs and preferences. Most of all, it needs to be investigated in longitudinal randomized clinical trials whether the proposed interventions indeed have the potential to reduce or postpone the risk of neurodegenerative diseases such as Alzheimer's as suggested in large non-interventional studies (Verghese et al., 2003).

AUTHOR CONTRIBUTIONS

KR was responsible for the study organization and execution, as well as writing the text of the manuscript (Introduction, Discussion, and some parts of the Materials and Methods: Study Design and Subjects). PM contributes equally to this work. He has written some parts of the manuscript (Materials and Methods, Results, Discussion). NA assessed balance abilities and analyzed the data. He has written some parts of the Materials and Methods and Results (postural control). MS contributes to the Statistical Analysis and did some corrections of this manuscript. MD supported hippocampal subfield analysis and corrected this manuscript. JK contributes to the MRI measurements and for structural brain analysis. He corrected this manuscript. AH is the chief coordinator of this study and selected the motor skill tasks and organized the framework. NM is the second chief coordinator of this study and provided MRI measurements. He also worked on the Introduction and Discussion of this manuscript.

REFERENCES

Albouy, G., Sterpenich, V., Balteau, E., Vandewalle, G., Desseilles, M., Dang-Vu, T., et al. (2008). Both the hippocampus and striatum are involved in consolidation of motor sequence memory. *Neuron* 58, 261–272. doi: 10.1016/j.neuron.2008.02.008

Bandettini, P. A. (2009). What's new in neuroimaging methods? *Ann. N. Y. Acad. Sci.* 1156, 260–293. doi: 10.1111/j.1749-6632.2009.04420.x

Barnes, J., Bartlett, J. W., van de Pol, L. A., Loy, C. T., Scahill, R. I., Frost, C., et al. (2009). A meta-analysis of hippocampal atrophy rates in Alzheimer's disease. *Neurobiol. Aging* 30, 1711–1723. doi: 10.1016/j.neurobiolaging.2008.01.010

Beck, A. T., Brown, G. K., and Steer, R. A. (2006). *Beck Depressions-Inventar BDI-II, Manual.* 2. Auflage. Frankfurt: Harcourt Test Services.

Boyke, J., Driemeyer, J., Gaser, C., Büchel, C., and May, A. (2008). Training-induced brain structure changes in the elderly. *J. Neurosci.* 28, 7031–7035. doi: 10.1523/JNEUROSCI.0742-08.2008

Brandt, T., Schautzer, F., Hamilton, D. A., Brüning, R., Markowitsch, H. J., Kalla, R., et al. (2005). Vestibular loss causes hippocampal atrophy and impaired spatial memory in humans. *Brain* 128, 2732–2741. doi: 10.1093/brain/awh617

Brehm, W., Janke, A., Sygusch, R., and Wagner, P. (2006). *Gesund durch Gesundheitssport.* München: Juventa, 16–23.

Bugg, J. M., Shah, K., Villareal, D. T., and Head, D. (2012). Cognitive and neural correlates of aerobic fitness in obese older adults. *Exp. Aging Res.* 38, 131–145. doi: 10.1080/0361073X.2012.659995

Davis, J. A., and Convertino, V. A. (1975). A comparison of heart rate methods for predicting endurance training intensity. *Med. Sci. Sports* 7, 295–298. doi: 10.1249/00005768-197500740-00010

Dordevic, M., Hökelmann, A., Müller, P., Rehfeld, K., and Müller, N. G. (2017). Improvements in orientation and balancing abilities in response to one month of intensive slackline training. a randomized controlled feasibility study. *Front. Hum. Neurosci.* 11:55. doi: 10.3389/fnhum.2017.00055

Draganski, B., Gaser, C., Busch, V., Schuierer, G., Bogdahn, U., and May, A. (2004). Neuroplasticity: changes in grey matter induced by training. *Nature* 427, 311–312. doi: 10.1038/427311a

Driscoll, I., Hamilton, D. A., Petropoulos, H., Yeo, R. A., Brooks, W. M., Baumgartner, R. N., et al. (2003). The aging hippocampus: cognitive, biochemical and structural findings. *Cereb. Cortex* 13, 1344–1351. doi: 10.1093/cercor/bhg081

Duvernoy, H. M. (2005). *The Human Hippocampus: Functional Anatomy, Vascularization and Serial Sections with MRI.* Berlin: Springer Science and Business Media.

Eickhoff, S. B., Paus, T., Caspers, S., Grosbras, M. H., Evans, A. C., Zilles, K., et al. (2007). Assignment of functional activations to probabilistic cytoarchitectonic areas revisited. *Neuroimage* 36, 511–521. doi: 10.1016/j.neuroimage.2007.03.060

Erickson, K. I., Voss, M. W., Prakash, R. S., Basak, C., Szabo, A., Chaddock, L., et al. (2011). Exercise training increases size of hippocampus and improves memory. *Proc. Natl. Acad. Sci. U.S.A.* 108, 3017–3022. doi: 10.1073/pnas.1015950108

Flöel, A., Ruscheweyh, R., Krüger, K., Willemer, C., Winter, B., Völker, K., et al. (2010). Physical activity and memory functions: are neurotrophins and cerebral gray matter volume the missing link? *Neuroimage* 49, 2756–2763. doi: 10.1016/j.neuroimage.2009.10.043

Folstein, M. F., Folstein, S. E., and McHugh, P. R. (1975). "Mini-mental" state. A practical method for grading the state of patients for the clinician. *J. Psychiatr. Res.* 12, 189–198. doi: 10.1016/0022-3956(75)90026-6

Honea, R., Thomas, G. P., Harsha, A., Anderson, H. S., Donnelly, J. E., Brooks, W. M., et al. (2009). Cardiorespiratory fitness and preserved medial temporal lobe volume in Alzheimer's disease. *Alzheimer Dis. Assoc. Disord.* 23, 188–197. doi: 10.1097/WAD.0b013e31819cb8a2

Hüfner, K., Binetti, C., Hamilton, D. A., Stephan, T., Flanagin, V. L., Linn, J., et al. (2011). Structural and functional plasticity of the hippocampal formation in professional dancers and slackliners. *Hippocampus* 21, 855–865. doi: 10.1002/hipo.20801

Jack, C. R., Petersen, R. C., Xu, Y., O'Brien, P. C., Smith, G. E., Ivnik, R. J., et al. (1998). Rate of medial temporal lobe atrophy in typical aging and Alzheimer's disease. *Neurology* 51, 993–999. doi: 10.1212/WNL.51.4.993

Kattenstroth, J. C., Kalisch, T., Holt, S., Tegenthoff, M., and Dinse, H. R. (2013). Six months of dance intervention enhances postural, sensorimotor, and cognitive performance in elderly without affecting cardio-respiratory functions. *Front. Aging Neurosci.* 5:5. doi: 10.3389/fnagi.2013.00005

Kattenstroth, J. C., Kolankowska, I., Kalisch, T., and Dinse, H. R. (2010). Superior sensory, motor, and cognitive performance in elderly individuals with multi-year dancing activities. *Front. Aging Neurosci.* 2:31. doi: 10.3389/fnagi.2010.00031

Kempermann, G., Fabel, K., Ehninger, D., Babu, H., Leal-Galicia, P., Garthe, A., et al. (2010). Why and how physical activity promotes experience-induced brain plasticity. *Front. Neurosci.* 4:189. doi: 10.3389/fnins.2010.00189

Kronenberg, H. M. (2003). Developmental regulation of the growth plate. *Nature* 423, 332–336. doi: 10.1038/nature01657

Kuhnt, D., Bauer, M. H., Egger, J., Richter, M., Kapur, T., Sommer, J., et al. (2013). Fiber tractography based on diffusion tensor imaging compared with high-angular-resolution diffusion imaging with compressed sensing: initial experience. *Neurosurgery* 72 165–175. doi: 10.1227/NEU.0b013e318270d9fb

Maass, A., Düzel, S., Brigadski, T., Goerke, M., Becke, A., Sobieray, U., et al. (2016). Relationships of peripheral IGF-1, VEGF and BDNF levels to exercise-related changes in memory, hippocampal perfusion and volumes in older adults. *Neuroimage* 131, 142–154. doi: 10.1016/j.neuroimage.2015.10.084

Maass, A., Düzel, S., Goerke, M., Becke, A., Sobieray, U., Neumann, K., et al. (2015). Vascular hippocampal plasticity after aerobic exercise in older adults. *Mol. Psychiatry* 20, 585–593. doi: 10.1038/mp.2014.114

Müller, P., Rehfeld, K., Lüders, A., Schmicker, M., Hökelmann, A., Kaufman, J., et al. (2016). Effekte eines Tanz-und eines Gesundheitssporttrainings auf die graue Hirn-substanz gesunder Senioren. *Sportwissenschaft* 46, 213–222. doi: 10.1007/s12662-016-0411-6

Müller, P., Rehfeld, K., Schmicker, M., Hökelmann, A., Dordevic, M., Lessmann, V., et al. (2017). Evolution of neuroplasticity in response to physical activity in old age: the case for dancing. *Front. Aging Neurosci.* 9:56. doi: 10.3389/fnagi.2017.00056

NeuroCom Natus Medical Incorporated (2008). *Balance Manager Systems, Clinical Interpretation Guide.* Clackamas, OR: NeuroCom International, Inc.

Niemann, C., Godde, B., and Voelcker-Rehage, C. (2014). Not only cardiovascular, but also coordinative exercise increases hippocampal volume in older adults. *Front. Aging Neurosci.* 6:120. doi: 10.3389/fnagi.2014.00170

O'Keefe, J. (1990). A computational theory of the hippocampal cognitive map. *Prog. Brain Res.* 83, 301–312. doi: 10.1016/S0079-6123(08)61258-3

O'Mara, S. (2005). The subiculum: what it does, what it might do, and what neuroanatomy has yet to tell us. *J. Anat.* 207, 271–282. doi: 10.1111/j.1469-7580.2005.00446.x

Raz, N., Lindenberger, U., Rodrigue, K. M., Kennedy, K. M., Head, D., Williamson, A., et al. (2005). Regional brain changes in aging healthy adults: general trends, individual differences and modifiers. *Cereb. Cortex* 15, 1676–1689. doi: 10.1093/cercor/bhi044

Raz, N., Rodrigue, K. M., Head, D., Kennedy, K. M., and Acker, J. D. (2004). Differential aging of the medial temporal lobe a study of a five-year change. *Neurology* 62, 433–438. doi: 10.1212/01.WNL.0000106466.09835.46

Rehfeld, K., Hökelmann, A., Lehmann, W., and Blaser, P. (2014). Auswirkungen einer Tanz- und Kraft-Ausdauer-Intervention auf kognitive Fähigkeiten älterer Menschen. *Z. Neuropsychol.* 25, 99–108. doi: 10.1024/1016-264X/a000124

Riegert, C., Galani, R., Heilig, S., Lazarus, C., Cosquer, B., and Cassel, J. C. (2004). Electrolytic lesions of the ventral subiculum weakly alter spatial memory but potentiate amphetamine-induced locomotion. *Behav. Brain Res.* 152, 23–34.

Ruscheweyh, R., Willemer, C., Krüger, K., Duning, T., Warnecke, T., Sommer, J., et al. (2011). Physical activity and memory functions: an interventional study. *Neurobiol. Aging* 32, 1304–1319. doi: 10.1016/j.neurobiolaging.2009.08.001

Saab, B. J., Georgiou, J., Nath, A., Lee, F. J., Wang, M., Michalon, A., et al. (2009). NCS-1 in the dentate gyrus promotes exploration, synaptic plasticity, and rapid acquisition of spatial memory. *Neuron* 63, 643–656. doi: 10.1016/j.neuron.2009.08.014

Sehm, B., Taubert, M., Conde, V., Weise, D., Classen, J., Dukart, J., et al. (2014). Structural brain plasticity in Parkinson's disease induced by balance training. *Neurobiol. Aging* 35, 232–239. doi: 10.1016/j.neurobiolaging.2013.06.021

Smith, J. C., Nielson, K. A., Woodard, J. L., Seidenberg, M., Durgerian, S., Antuono, P., et al. (2011). Interactive effects of physical activity and APOE-ε4 on BOLD semantic memory activation in healthy elders. *Neuroimage* 54, 635–644. doi: 10.1016/j.neuroimage.2010.07.070

Spalding, K. L., Bergmann, O., Alkass, K., Bernard, S., Salehpour, M., Huttner, H. B., et al. (2013). Dynamics of hippocampal neurogenesis in adult humans. *Cell* 153, 1219–1227. doi: 10.1016/j.cell.2013.05.002

Szabo, A. N., McAuley, E., Erickson, K. I., Voss, M., Prakash, R. S., Mailey, E. L., et al. (2011). Cardiorespiratory fitness, hippocampal volume, and frequency of forgetting in older adults. *Neuropsychology* 25, 545–553. doi: 10.1037/a0022733

Taubert, M., Draganski, B., Anwander, A., Müller, K., Horstmann, A., Villringer, A., et al. (2010). Dynamic properties of human brain structure: learning-related changes in cortical areas and associated fiber connections. *J. Neurosci.* 30, 11670–11677. doi: 10.1523/JNEUROSCI.2567-10.2010

van Praag, H., Christie, B. R., Sejnowski, T. J., and Gage, F. H. (1999). Running enhances neurogenesis, learning, and long-term potentiation in mice. *Proc. Natl. Acad. Sci. U.S.A.* 96, 13427–13431. doi: 10.1073/pnas.96.23.13427

Verghese, J., Lipton, R. B., Katz, M. J., Hall, C. B., Dervy, C. A., Kuslansky, G., et al. (2003). Leisure activities and the risk of dementia in the elderly. *N. Engl. J. Med.* 348, 2508–2516. doi: 10.1056/NEJMoa022252

3

A Possible Role of Prolonged Whirling Episodes on Structural Plasticity of the Cortical Networks and Altered Vertigo Perception: The Cortex of Sufi Whirling Dervishes

Yusuf O. Cakmak[1]*, *Gazanfer Ekinci*[2], *Armin Heinecke*[3] *and Safiye Çavdar*[4]

[1]Department of Anatomy, School of Biomedical Sciences, University of Otago, Dunedin, New Zealand, [2]Radiology Department, School of Medicine, Marmara University, Istanbul, Turkey, [3]Brain Innovation BV, Biopartner Center, Maastricht, Netherlands, [4]Department of Anatomy, School of Medicine, Koc University, Istanbul, Turkey

Edited by:
Claudia Voelcker-Rehage,
Chemnitz University of Technology,
Germany

Reviewed by:
Hidenao Fukuyama,
Kyoto University, Japan
Xin Di,
New Jersey Institute of Technology,
USA

***Correspondence:**
Yusuf O. Cakmak
yusuf.cakmak@otago.ac.nz

Although minutes of a spinning episode may induce vertigo in the healthy human, as a result of a possible perceptional plasticity, Sufi Whirling Dervishes (SWDs) can spin continuously for an hour without a vertigo perception.This unique long term vestibular system stimulation presents a potential human model to clarify the cortical networks underlying the resistance against vertigo. This study, therefore, aimed to investigate the potential structural cortical plasticity in SWDs. Magnetic resonance imaging (MRI) of 10 SWDs and 10 controls were obtained, using a 3T scanner. Cortical thickness in the whole cortex was calculated. Results demonstrated significantly thinner cortical areas for SWD subjects compared with the control group in the hubs of the default mode network (DMN), as well as in the motion perception and discrimination areas including the right dorsolateral prefrontal cortex (DLPFC), the right lingual gyrus and the left visual area 5 (V5)/middle temporal (MT) and the left fusiform gyrus. In conclusion, this is the first report that warrants the potential relationship of the motion/body perception related cortical networks and the prolonged term of whirling ability without vertigo or dizziness.

Keywords: cortex, whirling, meditation, vertigo, vestibular, plasticity

INTRODUCTION

Most studies to date that have investigated brain networks for vertigo or vestibular system have used or focused on the sole stimulation of the vestibular system, such as caloric or galvanic stimulation. However, these methodological approaches lack an engagement of proprioception and vestibular organ stimulation that would mimic motion perception based vertigo. To date, there is not a study that has investigated the structural plasticity induced by a prolonged period of stimulation using both systems, together. The Mevleviye Semazens,

---

Abbreviations: DLPFC, Dorsolateral Prefrontal Cortex; DMN, Default Mode Network; fMRI, Functional Magnetic Resonance Imaging; LH, Left hemisphere; MT, Middle Temporal; PCC, posterior cingulate cortex; POI, Patch of Interest; RH, Right hemisphere; SWDs, Sufi Whirling Dervishes; TAL, Talairach; TMS, Transcranial Magnetic Stimulation; V5, Visual area 5.

alternatively known as Sufi Whirling Dervishes (SWDs), have a unique meditation style that is termed as the Sema Ceremony which may provide a unique model to investigate cortical networks of motion perception and balance together with vestibular and proprioception sensory systems.

The Mevleviye is an ascetic Sufi order founded in 1273 in Konya, Turkey (Smeets, 2006). In the Sema Ceremony, a SWD rotates anti-clockwise around the vertical axis of their body, while also rotating around the other SWDs. Whirling intends to be a travel of soul awareness and loosening of the material self. To become trained for the Sema Ceremony so that they can able to rotate up to 1 h without vertigo or dizziness perception, Sufis traditionally receive up to 1000 days of training within the Mevlevi houses. At the end of that time, the Sufis are now trained as SWD. They re-join their families and return to their jobs, but gather together for Sema ceremony for several days in a week (Smeets, 2006). This unique whirling based meditation style of SWDs achieves extraordinary physiological outcomes that overcome vertigo and balance impairment, which would be expected after prolonged times of whirling.

It has been argued that alternating self-localization is caused by abnormal integration of vestibular signals. Additionally, it has been shown that vestibular processing is involved in space perception and locomotion (somatosensory processing) as well as the cognitive aspects of own-body representations, the consciousness of the own-body and bistable visual perception (Lopez et al., 2010, 2012).

The default mode of functioning was initially defined on particular areas of the brain that decrease activity when subjects focus on goal-directed tasks in comparison to simply resting (Raichle and Snyder, 2007). In the following years, the default mode definition extends to default mode network (DMN; Raichle and Snyder, 2007). The DMN of the brain has been observed to be related to self-awareness, consciousness, embodiment and also unhappiness (Killingsworth and Gilbert, 2010; Brewer et al., 2011). Therefore, it may also be theorized that prolonged periods of whirling based meditation of the Sufi dervishes contribute to structural changes in the networks of the DMN and self-perception, as well as motion perception related networks. A recent analysis of research on DMN that included anatomical connectivity and task-evolved neuroimaging revealed hubs of the resting state activity, including posterior cingulate cortex (PCC) and Precuneus areas (Gramann et al., 2006; Andrews-Hanna, 2012). It is relevant to note that in Kang's study, the reported regions of decreased cortical thickness in meditators' brains were the precuneus and PCC of the DMN (Kang et al., 2013). Additionally, a study that looked at functional magnetic resonance imaging (fMRI) scans of all meditation types but not including SWDs (Brewer et al., 2011) demonstrated that experienced meditators compared with controls showed decreased activity in the DMN including the main hub precuneus (Laird et al., 2009).

Previous studies demonstrated that long-term meditation practice is associated with altered resting brain activity which suggests long lasting activity changes persist in the brain (Lutz et al., 2004). The following cross-sectional studies demonstrated that meditation and experience dependent differences are correlated with cortical thickness (Maguire et al., 2000; Mechelli et al., 2004; Lazar et al., 2005). Significant positive associations were also evidenced between the cognitive ability factor and cortical thickness in most multimodal association areas in a large sample of healthy children and adults (Karama et al., 2009). Moreover, a relationship between cortical thickness and functional activation in the early blind have also been demonstrated recently (Anurova et al., 2014). A recent research (Burge et al., 2016) demonstrated that cortical thickness in human V1 is associated with central vision loss in 10 macular degeneration patients in comparison to 10 controls in a cross-sectional study that underlines the functional relationship with the cortical thickness. Considering the motionless but embodiment-related meditation study results that demonstrated a functional depression on cortical hubs of body perception networks, cortical thickness changes in experienced based cross-sectional studies and loss of visual input reflections on thinner relevant cortical areas, we theorized that there might also be a decrease in cortical thickness of precuneus and PCC of the DMN in SWDs as a results of the depressed or altered perceptions of motion and embodiment inputs to induce the cortical neuronal changes, resulting in the thinning of responsible cortices. Any additional structural plasticity findings of the SWDs' cortical areas may also have the possibility to highlight the plasticity of the motion related networks that may be responsible for the alterations of the vertigo perception of SWDs. Improvement of navigation softwares for non-invasive brain stimulation techniques like Transcranial Magnetic Stimulation (TMS) have enabled structural and functional mapping of the brain and targetted stimulation of the specific cortical areas to be performed. This study aimed to map the structural cortical plasticity induced by Sufi whirling meditation as a unique human model of vestibular system stimulation and plasticity to clarify a network that may alter vertigo perception in SWDs and it may also provide a potential cortical map for non-invasive brain stimulation modalities to alleviate vertigo.

MATERIALS AND METHODS

Participants

It is noted that far fewer SWD ceremonies are performed in Mevlevi-houses, as a result of secularization policies enforced by government in the early 20th Century. Although, in the late 20th Century, the Turkish government did again allow performances, most of these have been confined to public tourist audiences and are simplified to meet commercial requirements (Smeets, 2006). Consequently, it is difficult to select SWDs who perform the whirling ceremony using the traditional physical and spiritual method.

Ten (8 male, 2 female adults) right-handed traditional SWDs with greater than 8 years and an average of 10.5 years of whirling meditation (regular two whirling sessions each week) and 10 (8 male, 2 female adults) meditation naive right-handed controls were included into our study. The controls were case-matched for the country of origin and location (Turkey, Istanbul), primary language (Turkish) and demographics such as sex, age, race, education and employment status (SWD mean age: 32 years (range: 26–44), 8 male, 2 female. Control group mean age: 33 years (range: 26–44), 8 male, 2 female). Exclusion criteria for all subjects were abnormalities in magnetic resonance imaging (MRI), MRI incompatible implants and implanted devices and general medical disorders or any clinically relevant abnormalities. All subjects were free of medical, neurological and psychiatric disorders.

All procedures of this study were carried according to the principles and procedures outlined in the Declaration of Helsinki for Medical Research involving human subjects. The study was approved by the Ethics Committee (Prof. Ihsan Solaroglu - Head of the ethical committee for non-invasive human research. Institutional Review Board) at the Koç University. Each Participant provided written informed consent before entering the study and understood that s/he could discontinue the study at any time.

Scanning Sequence

MRI scans of the participants were carried out on a 3T scanner with an 8-channel head coil (MAGNETOM Verio, Siemens Healthcare, Erlangen, Germany). The three-dimensional magnetization prepared rapid acquisition gradient echo sequence (3D T1-weighted MPRAGE). This was used to acquire the volume data of the whole brain of all the participants. 3D T1-weighted MP-RAGE protocol (42) was used with the following parameters: TR = 1670 ms, TE = 2.47 ms, TI = 900 ms, flip angle 9°, 176 slices scanned for sagittal plane with 1.0 mm slice thickness and the scanning matrix was 256 × 256 with a field of view of 250 mm, resulting in a voxel size of 1.0 mm × 1.0 mm × 1.0 mm. Total scan time for 3D T1-weighted imaging was 3.47 min.

Anatomical Data Processing

Data Import, Preprocessing and Normalization

Raw MRI data from each subject was provided in DICOM format. It was then imported and converted into BrainVoyager's internal "VMR" data format. Correction for inherent spatial intensity inhomogeneities was applied according to Vaughan et al. (2001). The data was then transformed into AC-PC position and Talairach (TAL) standard space.

Cortex Segmentation

Segmentation of the gray/white matter boundaries was achieved using the method of Kriegeskorte and Goebel, 2001. This included automatic segmentation routines, followed by a "bridge removal" algorithm, which ensured the creation of topologically correct mesh representations. For the two resulting segmented subvolumes, borders were tessellated to produce a surface reconstruction of the left hemisphere (LH) and right hemisphere (RH; Kriegeskorte and Goebel, 2001). All processing steps for segmentation as well as cortical thickness calculation have been thoroughly checked and evaluated by an expert. This is an important part of the preparation for the cortical thickness calculation in BrainVoyager, which is not directly comparable to automated analysis approaches in other analysis tools.

High-Resolution Intersubject Cortex Alignment

A high-resolution, multiscale cortex alignment procedure was performed following the method of van Atteveldt et al. (2004). This procedure substantially increased the statistical power and spatial specificity of group analyses. Before performing the group analysis on the basis of the subject-specific cortical thickness maps, all the single subject maps have been aligned using transformation matrices generated on the basis of cortical alignment (Fischl et al., 1999). The Cortex-based alignment approach (Fischl et al., 1999) has been specifically applied to the data to allow a proper comparability between cortical structures between subjects. Taken this into account, smoothing the cortical thickness data was not necessary. The addition of smoothing may even prove to be more harmful than helpful. In this context, multiple reference articles using BrainVoyager for analyzing cortical thickness data don't apply spatial smoothing (Davis et al., 2008; Geuze et al., 2008; Strenziok et al., 2011; Van Swam et al., 2012; Thorns et al., 2013).

Cortical Thickness Analysis

The normalized version of each VMR was prepared in the following way to prepare the calculation of cortical thickness. First, the VMR data was interpolated to a higher resolution (0.5 mm * 0.5 mm * 0.5 mm) version using a sinc interpolation. In this new dataset, the ventricles and subcortical areas were filled, using a standard intensity value. Using an automatic detection approach, the cerebellum was removed. By applying a sigma filtering step, the tissue contrast of the data was enhanced.

Next, the boundary between gray and white matter was detected using a gradient-based adaptive approach. On the basis of a dilation procedure, the border between gray matter and Cerebrospinal fluid was detected. The final result of the preparatory steps consists of a VMR representing only gray and white matter in two grayscale/intensity values. To improve the quality of the procedure, this dataset was compared to the original VMR file in 0.5 mm resolution and corrected for potential errors.

To calculate the cortical thickness in the whole cortex, Laplace equations (Jones et al., 2000) were applied. The volumetric cortical thickness values were sampled to standardized surface meshes of the separate hemispheres using trilinear interpolation.

To correct the final result map showing group differences in cortical thickness, the automated cluster-level thresholding approach (Forman et al., 1995) was applied. This means that every patch of interest (POI) exceeding a calculated size (square mm on the surface mesh) is considered significant. The final result map has on average a corrected false alarm level of 5%. A cluster defining the threshold (CDT) of $p < 0.05$ was utilized. After applying the cluster level thresholding method, each contiguous regions of interest on the surface reaching a size beyond the calculated region size threshold (58 square mm for the left and 65 square mm for the RH) was turned into a POI. Based on the idea that there was no specific assumption about the direction of a difference in cortical thickness between groups, a two-sided t-test was performed to analyze the group differences.

For the surface-based analysis, a standardized mesh size was applied to the cortical surface of every subject. The standardized mesh has exactly "40961" vertices per hemisphere (identical for every subject) and thus solves a potential mapping issue between regions and between subjects. For the group comparison of the subject-specific cortical thickness surface maps, a simple subtraction of the cortically aligned thickness values was performed between two cohorts (Sufi dervishes and a control cohort). The analysis was performed specifically for each of the hemispheres based on the standard approach of segmentation and cortex-based alignment in BrainVoyager QX. The separation of hemispheres also allows for a more specific evaluation and analysis of hemisphere-specific effects. The variability within and between groups was also checked besides just using a *t*-test to compare the groups. It is still important to check the details within globally "detected" regions of interest. We have done this to perform a "sanity check" of the data included within the analysis and to explore the variability within and between groups.

RESULTS

Figure 1 shows regional differences in cortical thickness between Sufi dervishes and control group displayed on the average surface mesh (after applying the cortex-based alignment procedure to obtain optimal fitting of cortical structures). An average difference in cortical thickness of 0.10 mm for the LH and 0.15 mm for the RH was found. We compared the average cortical thickness within each hemisphere between the groups and found no significant differences within either of the hemispheres (LH: $t = 1.56$, $p = 0.14$, RH: $t = 2.07$, $p = 0.055$).

Table 1 shows the cortical thickness differences between Sufis and Controls for the whole brain and **Table 2** shows the significant clusters with their *t, p* values, *X,Y,Z* coordinates and areas on both hemispheres.

On the basis of the detected POIs on the surface mesh, corresponding TAL coordinates were extracted. This is based on the referential connection between the underlying TAL VMR and the cortical surface meshes created afterwards.

Based on external analysis of the coordinates using the "Talairach daemon" database (Lancaster et al., 1997) was performed. The results are displayed in **Table 2**. **Figure 1** demonstrates surface maps for the statistically significant differences of cortical thickness between groups (Sufi–Controls) in both hemispheres : four POIs for the RH and five POIs for the LH.

TABLE 1 | The cortical thickness differences between Sufis and Controls for the whole brain.

	Sufis	Controls	Difference
LH			
Average thickness (mm)	2.92	3.02	−0.10
Maximum thickness (mm)	3.11	3.28	−0.17
Standard deviation	0.16	0.15	0.01
RH			
Average thickness (mm)	2.90	3.05	−0.15
Maximum thickness (mm)	3.20	3.22	−0.02
Standard deviation	0.19	0.13	0.06

LH, Left hemisphere; RH, Right hemisphere.

DISCUSSION

The present study demonstrates differences in cortical thickness analysis between the 10 SWDs brain and 10 control cases as a proof of structural plasticity potentially induced by whirling meditation of SWDs.

Cortical thickness analysis, as structural plasticity reflection, is considered one of the best tools to reveal prolonged effects of meditation on the cerebral cortex. It has been well documented in the literature that meditation exercises including Zen meditation induce cortical plasticity in specific cortical zones as thickened gray matter (Lazar et al., 2005; Pagnoni and Cekic, 2007; Hölzel et al., 2008, 2010; Luders et al., 2009; Vestergaard-Poulsen et al., 2009; Grant et al., 2010, 2013). While the study by Lazar et al. (2005) demonstrated increased cortical thickness in the insula and prefrontal regions, yet Kang et al. (2013) demonstrated increased cortical thickness in the frontal and temporal regions only, and decreased cortical thickness in the DMN including the main hubs precuneus and PCC with different type of meditations. These findings are supported by fMRI studies by Brewer et al. (2011). Brewer et al. (2011) demonstrated decreased activity in the hubs of the DMN after numerous types of meditation. Cortical thickness results of the SWDs in this study showed similar results to Brewer et al. (2011) and Kang et al. (2013) reports for the DMN plasticity. There were four thinner cortical areas in the RH, and five thinner in the LH including the hubs of DMN as precuneus and PCC. There were no thicker cortical areas compared with the control group. The thinner cortical zones of SWDs were the Precuneus, PCC and on both hemispheres and middle temporal (MT)/visual area 5 (V5) and fusiform gyrus on the left and Dorsolateral Prefrontal cortex (DLPFC) and lingual gyrus on the RH. With the SWDs having meditation practice combined with movement, the results obtained in the left MT/V5, fusiform gyrus and Right DLPFC and DMN hubs may all underline the altered vertigo perception in whirling motion of SWDs.

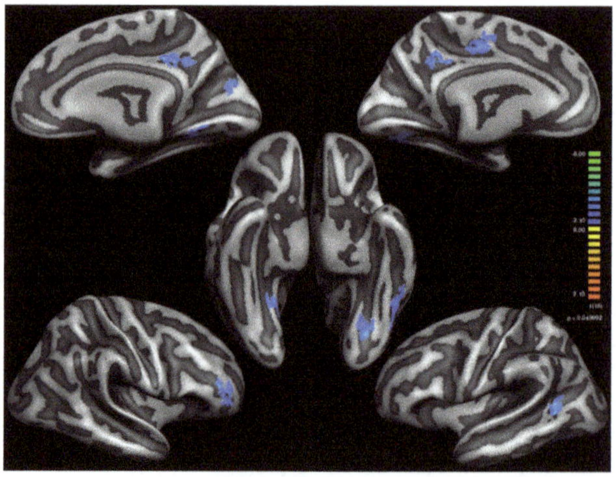

FIGURE 1 | Thinner Cortical areas in Sufi Dervishes (Sufi > Controls). All regions are based on cluster thresholding.

TABLE 2 | The significant clusters with their *t*, *p* values, X, *Y*, *Z* coordinates and areas on both hemispheres.

	Cortical area	TAL *X*	TAL *Y*	TAL *Z*	*t*	*p*	Square mm
Left hemisphere							
POI 1	Fusiform gyrus, temporal lobe	−42	−48	−10	−3.9369	0.0010	76.90
POI 2	Fusiform gyrus, occipital lobe	−27	−66	−5	−3.9400	0.0010	111.90
POI 3	MT/V5	−48	−50	5	−4.6672	0.0002	61.15
POI 4	PCC	−12	−19	43	−4.0061	0.0008	92.80
POI 5	Precuneus, PCC	−8	−35	33	−3.8878	0.0011	65.33
Right hemisphere							
POI 1	Lingual gyrus	14	−53	−2	−4.2423	0.0005	80.88
POI 2	precuneus, parieto-occipital sulcus	11	−66	19	−3.8815	0.0011	74.91
POI 3	PCC, precuneus	5	−33	36	−4.6599	0.0002	88.32
POI 4	DLPFC	39	35	20	−3.9253	0.0010	76.8

Altered Perception of Motion and Vertigo

Left MT/V5

Our results demonstrated a thinner Left MT/V5 in the LH of the SWDs. In previous studies that have explored V5/MT, the left MT/V5 was shown to have more robust involvement in motion detection (Beckers and Hömberg, 1992; Stewart et al., 1999; Antal et al., 2004; Schwarzkopf et al., 2011; Tadin et al., 2011; Murd et al., 2012).

The dominance of left V5/MT may explain the thinner V5/MT on the LH of the SWDs. With the depressed function of left V5/MT, the perception of the movement during whirling meditation may be depressed and as a consequence, the possible physiological and motor responses to whirling motion perception may be inhibited. In addition to robust function of left V5/MT on motion perception, discrimination function is also found to be related with the left V5/MT rather than the right V5/MT (Cornette et al., 1998).

Fusiform Gyrus, Right DLPFC and Change Detection

Fusiform gyrus is well known for its face detection function but it also discriminates between places; particularly in the medial and anterior portions of the fusiform gyrus. Conscious detection of visual changes including face and place changes mostly relies on regions of the ventral visual cortex including the fusiform gyrus, but also the right DLPFC (Beck et al., 2001). The left fusiform gyrus is also found to be related with the non-face related visual changes (Rangarajan et al., 2014). Further, left fusiform gyrus showed greater activity when participants attended to changes in face parts than to changes in whole face. The opposite pattern was demonstrated in the right FFA (Rossion et al., 2000).

The role of right DLPFC in visual change awareness has been demonstrated by fMRI and TMS studies (Beck et al., 2001; Turatto et al., 2004). The right DLPFC is activated with place changes and it has been shown to be non-active in the cases of change blindness by fMRI and TMS studies (Beck et al., 2001). Additionally, it is demonstrated that activation of ventral occipitotemporal cortex, including lingual gyrus, is also related to the processing of visual information for human faces (McCarthy et al., 1991).

Our analyses showed that in the SWDs cortex, the fusiform gyrus were thinner on the left and lingual gyrus and DLPFC were thinner only on the right side. By doing so, SWDs may also have an altered state of place change perception, especially important for keeping the body stability in the case of a whirling meditation which includes a continuous place change stimulation for the place change detection areas of fusiform gyrus, lingual gyrus and right DLPFC.

Precuneus, Egocentric Framework and Default Network Hubs

In three dimensional spaces, humans navigate themselves with the aid of spatial relationship references. Two different type of spatial reference coding frameworks (or frame of reference) are *allocentric* and *egocentric* abilities. While the *allocentric* ability depends on object to object positional references and is independent from self-position, the *egocentric* ability depends on self to object positional references (Vogeley and Fink, 2003; Gramann et al., 2006). Research on the cortical regions related to these two distinct frameworks has revealed that egocentric conditions have activations exclusively within the precuneus in comparison to allocentric conditions (Gramann et al., 2006). The precuneus as a location of the egocentric representation does the updating during self-motion and it is demonstrated that it is the only region for working memory of directional updating (Land, 2014). The precuneus is considered as a machinery of self-perception that builds a conscious self-perception by providing continous data of external space to maintain a synchronous relationship with the body in the move and the objects in the environment (Land, 2014). In this study, bilateral thinner precuneus in SWDs was shown. Thinner precuneus may underline the role of egocentric framework depression to aid the extraordinary whirling ability of SWDs in addition to the role of depressed activations of left MT/V5 and fusiform gyrus and right DLPC and lingual gyrus. The last but not the least, it has been shown that the electrical cortical stimulation of the precuneus produce vestibular sensations and implicating the role of precuneus for vestibular information processing (Wiest et al., 2004).

The Default Mode and Subsystems

A recent analysis of the DMN neuroimaging studies suggests the precuneus is the core node or the hub of the DMN (Andrews-Hanna, 2012). Activation of both the DMN core hub precuneus and prefrontal cortex has been found to be related to self-perception and mind wandering (Kjaer and Lou, 2000; Kjaer et al., 2002). Imaging studies have shown that these areas are deactivated in the case of altered states of consciousness including vegetative state, hypnosis and sleeping (Maquet et al., 1997, 1999; Laureys et al., 1999; Hobson et al., 2000; Maquet, 2000). It has also been observed that the precuneus is one of the first zones to be reactivated in the case of a reconsciousness (Laureys et al., 2004, 2006).

In addition to bilateral thinner precuneus in SWDs, the posterior cingulate gyrus was thinner. In the context of thinner precuneus and posterior cingulate gyrus in SWDs's brains, it has been shown that these becomes progressively deactivated in anesthetic sedation states (Alkire et al., 1999; Fiset et al., 1999). Additionally, independent researchers have observed that coactivation of precuneus and PCC occurs when processing intentions related to self (Vogeley and Fink, 2003; den Ouden et al., 2005).

The outcomes of the present study may open a new era in the field of vertigo therapy. This is because if whirling based movement achieves inhibition of the self-perception and motion related regions such as left V5/MT, fusiform gyrus, right DLPFC precuneus and PCC and the DMN hub, then this may underline the cortical plasticity for a network of resistance to vertigo perception. Targeting these areas to inhibit by interventional non-invasive brain stimulation tools may achieve maintenance of balance when conditions of extreme spatial and proprioception information occur in addition to pathological conditions that trigger vertigo.

Mood

A possible mood enhancing effect of the defined structurally plastinated cortical areas in the present study is worth to give an attention.

In the theory of mind, the DMN activity as a self-awareness state is correlated with the neuronal representation of mind-wandering (Kjaer and Lou, 2000; Kjaer et al., 2002). This DMN is active at all times except when suppressed by other networks, stimulated by other states, and its activity is correlated with lower levels of Happiness (Killingsworth and Gilbert, 2010; Brewer et al., 2011). Gusnard and Raichle (2001) demonstrated that the goal-directed cognitive process can decrease the activity of precuneus, the core hub of the DMN or mind-wandering network of the brain. Therefore, it is theorized that prolonged periods of goal-directed cognitive processes may decrease the mind-wandering activity in the SWD's brain because the precuneus activity has been decreased. fMRI data results from the Brewer et al. (2011) study on the DMN of the experienced meditators showed that the DMN main nodes, including medial prefrontal cortex and PCC areas extending to precuneus were relatively deactivated. Further, precuneus and PCC have been observed as thinner and concluded to be so as a response to meditation (Kang et al., 2013). In line with these results, the structural cortical thickness analysis of the two cohorts in this study showed that the experienced SWDs had bilateral thinner PCC and precuneus zones. It can be therefore be theorized that the prolonged period of decreased activity in the PCC and precuneus may result in the thinner zones in the SWDs. As the DMN activity presented thinner in the SWDs, this is likely related to suppressed mind wandering, and as a consequence, this plasticity may improve the happiness level in SWDs. These results justify further studies to clarify the potential effects of SWDs's unique meditation on their moods and depression levels.

Behavior

In addition to potential mood enhancing effects by Whirling Meditation as achieved with decreased mind wandering, or by DMN activity as achieved with other types of meditation, decreased activity in the DLPFC may contribute to the behavioral attribute of honesty. As the precuneus stands as a core hub for the DMN, the DLPFC stands as a core hub for the executive network (Beaty et al., 2015). It has been shown that to achieve creative idea production, there is a coupling of the PCC and precuneus of the DMN with the right DLPFC of the executive network (Beaty et al., 2015). It has also been shown that increased task complexity or increased rule complexity is accompanied by increased activation in the right DLPFC and precuneus (Jia et al., 2015). In the case of lying, we need a creative idea production process and to consider long-term benefits. It has been shown that disruption of the right DLPFC leads to a greater selection of both gains and losses that have better immediate but worse long-term alternatives (Essex et al., 2012). It has also been shown that when the right DLPFC activity was disrupted using TMS, subjects were statistically less inclined to lie about the subject matter tested (Karton and Bachmann, 2011). Regarding the decreased thickness in the right DLPFC in SWDs, it may be theorized that this contributes to improve their behavioral attitude of honesty. It may also be speculated that the decrease in the thickness of fusiform and right DLPFC contributes to decreased discrimination of places and faces, and that such an altered perception of the world and people is also a result of SWDs's meditations. Further studies are needed to investigate whether the suppression of cortical areas related with discriminational perception leads to less selfish, egocentric behavior and increased level of happiness.

Neuroprotection

The DMN activity is also found to be related to Alzheimer's disease (Bero et al., 2011). Bero et al. (2011) demonstrated that increased amyloid-β deposition overlaps with the DMN, including the core hub, precuneus and PCC regions. This overlapping is attributed to the higher metabolic activity of the DMN. The decreased thicknesses of these regions in SWDs cortex that are shown in the present study may underline a possible whirling meditation protective effect of over Alzheimer disease by its possible effect of decreasing the amyloid-β deposition in these regions because of their decreased activity in SWDs.

Limitations

The current study used a cross-sectional design and it is performed on a small group of SWDs. As a result of the cross-sectional character of the study, the results are correlational and an absolute relationship between the cortical thinning and whirling experience can not be suggested. In addition, it may also be argued that individuals who have such cortical properties are more likely becoming a Sufi whirling Dervish. On the other hand, it is worth to note that there are numerous factors to consider that relate the outcomes of the present study to whirling experience. This is a cross-sectional study in a very unique (and rare) group who had traditional training for whirling (approximately 1 year in most of the cases) and each of them reported that they were falling down when they try to whirl in the first months of the whirling training sessions. This indicates that they did not have a unique previous ability that was superior to the predisposition of the control group. After the long-term training, they gained an ability to whirl without vertigo. The present cross-sectional study focused on experienced Sufis that passed through the same traditional whirling training that enabled them to whirl for an hour without falling. In this context, the detected structural differences are more likely to be specific to motion perception and body perception networks. As the analyses were performed without visual input, the outcomes of these areas are free of bias. Analyses within the article were almost not separated but discussed in the context of relevant networks. The structural cortical plasticity that was demonstrated in SWDs were distributed over the body/motion perception areas, therefore the discussion was focused on the possible relationships of the structural plasticity of the body/motion perception areas and their potential role to alter vertigo perception. In sum, we only explained the results on the basis of the previous work which was the most fitting way for the data obtained in this cross-sectional article. Longitudinal studies are needed to clarify the role of these areas in vertigo perception.

The outcomes of this cross-sectional study in a rare and unique group (whirling Sufi dervishes) warrants cortical zones which may have significant roles to alter vertigo/dizziness and address those areas for future studies. In conclusion, this is the first report that demonstrates correlations of the structural cortical plasticity and the prolonged period of vestibular system stimulation in humans.

AUTHOR CONTRIBUTIONS

YOC designed, performed the study, analyzed the data and wrote the manuscript and made critical review of the manuscript. GE performed the study, collected data, contributed analytical tool, made critical review of the manuscript. AH analyzed and interpreted data, contributed analytical tool, performed statistics and made critical review of the manuscript. SÇ contributed analytical tool, collected data, wrote manuscript and made critical review of the manuscript.

REFERENCES

Alkire, M. T., Pomfrett, C. J., Haier, R. J., Gianzero, M. V., Chan, C. M., Jacobsen, B. P., et al. (1999). Functional brain imaging during anesthesia in humans: effects of halothane on global and regional cerebral glucose metabolism. *Anesthesiology* 90, 701–709. doi: 10.1097/00000542-199903000-00011

Andrews-Hanna, J. R. (2012). The brain's default network and its adaptive role in internal mentation. *Neuroscientist* 18, 251–270. doi: 10.1177/1073858411403316

Antal, A., Varga, E. T., Nitsche, M. A., Chadaide, Z., Paulus, W., Kovács, G., et al. (2004). Direct current stimulation over MT+/V5 modulates motion aftereffect in humans. *Neuroreport* 15, 2491–2494. doi: 10.1097/00001756-200411150-00012

Anurova, I., Renier, L. A., De Volder, A. G., Carlson, S., and Rauschecker, J. P. (2014). Relationship between cortical thickness and functional activation in the early blind. *Cereb. Cortex* 25, 2035–2048. doi: 10.1093/cercor/bhu009

van Atteveldt, N., Formisano, E., Goebel, R., and Blomert, L. (2004). Integration of letters and speech sounds in the human brain. *Neuron* 43, 271–282. doi: 10.1016/j.neuron.2004.06.025

Beaty, R. E., Benedek, M., Kaufman, S. B., and Silvia, P. J. (2015). Default and executive network coupling supports creative idea production. *Sci. Rep.* 5:10964. doi: 10.1038/srep10964

Beck, D. M., Rees, G., Frith, C. D., and Lavie, N. (2001). Neural correlates of change detection and change blindness. *Nat. Neurosci.* 4, 645–650. doi: 10.1038/88477

Beckers, G., and Hömberg, V. (1992). Cerebral visual motion blindness: transitory akinetopsia induced by transcranial magnetic stimulation of human area V5. *Proc. Biol. Sci.* 249, 173–178. doi: 10.1098/rspb.1992.0100

Bero, A. W., Yan, P., Roh, J. H., Cirrito, J. R., Stewart, F. R., Raichle, M. E., et al. (2011). Neuronal activity regulates the regional vulnerability to amyloid-β deposition. *Nat. Neurosci.* 14, 750–756. doi: 10.1038/nn.2801

Brewer, J. A., Worhunsky, P. D., Gray, J. R., Tang, Y.-Y., Weber, J., and Kober, H. (2011). Meditation experience is associated with differences in default mode network activity and connectivity. *Proc. Natl. Acad. Sci. U S A* 108, 20254–20259. doi: 10.1073/pnas.1112029108

Burge, W. K., Griffis, J. C., Nenert, R., Elkhetali, A., DeCarlo, D. K., ver Hoef, L. W., et al. (2016). Cortical thickness in human V1 associated with central vision loss. *Sci. Rep.* 6:23268. doi: 10.1038/srep23268

Cornette, L., Dupont, P., Rosier, A., Sunaert, S., Van Hecke, P., Michiels, J., et al. (1998). Human brain regions involved in direction discrimination. *J. Neurophysiol.* 79, 2749–2765.

Davis, K. D., Pope, G., Chen, J., Kwan, C. L., Crawley, A. P., and Diamant, N. E. (2008). Cortical thinning in IBS: implications for homeostatic, attention, and pain processing. *Neurology* 70, 153–154. doi: 10.1212/01.WNL.0000295509.30630.10

Essex, B. G., Clinton, S. A., Wonderley, L. R., and Zald, D. H. (2012). The impact of the posterior parietal and dorsolateral prefrontal cortices on the optimization of long-term versus immediate value. *J. Neurosci.* 32, 15403–15413. doi: 10.1523/JNEUROSCI.6106-11.2012

Fischl, B., Sereno, M. I., Tootel, R. B. H., and Dale, A. M. (1999). High-resolution intersubject averaging and a coordinate system for the cortical surface. *Hum. Brain Mapp.* 8, 272–284. doi: 10.1002/(SICI)1097-0193(1999)8:4<272::AID-HBM10 >3.0.CO;2-4

Fiset, P., Paus, T., Daloze, T., Plourde, G., Meuret, P., Bonhomme, V., et al. (1999). Brain mechanisms of propofol-induced loss of consciousness in humans: a positron emission tomographic study. *J. Neurosci.* 19, 5506–5513.

Forman, S. D., Cohen, J. D., Fitzgerald, M., Eddy, W. F., Mintun, M. A., and Noll, D. C. (1995). Improved assessment of significant activation in functional magnetic resonance imaging (fMRI): use of a cluster-size threshold. *Magn. Reson. Med.* 33, 636–647. doi: 10.1002/mrm.1910330508

Geuze, E., Westenberg, H. G., Heinecke, A., de Kloet, C. S., Goebel, R., and Vermetten, E. (2008). Thinner prefrontal cortex in veterans with posttraumatic stress disorder. *Neuroimage* 41, 675–681. doi: 10.1016/j.neuroimage.2008.03.007

Gramann, K., Müller, H. J., Schönebeck, B., and Debus, G. (2006). The neural basis of ego- and allocentric reference frames in spatial navigation: evidence from spatio-temporal coupled current density reconstruction. *Brain Res.* 1118, 116–129. doi: 10.1016/j.brainres.2006.08.005

Grant, J. A., Courtemanche, J., Duerden, E. G., Duncan, G. H., and Rainville, P. (2010). Cortical thickness and pain sensitivity in zen meditators. *Emotion* 10, 43–53. doi: 10.1037/a0018334

Grant, J. A., Duerden, E. G., Courtemanche, J., Cherkasova, M., Duncan, G. H., and Rainville, P. (2013). Cortical thickness, mental absorption and meditative practice: possible implications for disorders of attention. *Biol. Psychol.* 92, 275–281. doi: 10.1016/j.biopsycho.2012.09.007

Gusnard, D. A., and Raichle, M. E. (2001). Searching for a baseline: functional imaging and the resting human brain. *Nat. Rev. Neurosci.* 2, 685–694. doi: 10.1038/35094500

Hobson, J. A., Pace-Schott, E. F., and Stickgold, R. (2000). Dreaming and the brain: toward a cognitive neuroscience of conscious states. *Behav. Brain Sci.* 23, 793–842; discussion 904–1121. doi: 10.1017/s0140525x00003976

Hölzel, B. K., Carmody, J., Evans, K. C., Hoge, E. A., Dusek, J. A., Morgan, L., et al. (2010). Stress reduction correlates with structural changes in the amygdala. *Soc. Cogn. Affect. Neurosci.* 5, 11–17. doi: 10.1093/scan/nsp034

Hölzel, B. K., Ott, U., Gard, T., Hempel, H., Weygandt, M., Morgen, K., et al. (2008). Investigation of mindfulness meditation practitioners with voxel-based morphometry. *Soc. Cogn. Affect. Neurosci.* 3, 55–61. doi: 10.1093/scan/nsm038

Jia, X., Liang, P., Shi, L., Wang, D., and Li, K. (2015). Prefrontal and parietal activity is modulated by the rule complexity of inductive reasoning and can be predicted by a cognitive model. *Neuropsychologia* 66, 67–74. doi: 10.1016/j.neuropsychologia.2014.10.015

Jones, S. E., Buchbinder, B. R., and Aharon, I. (2000). Three-dimensional mapping of cortical thickness using Laplace's equation. *Hum. Brain Mapp.* 11, 12–32. doi: 10.1002/1097-0193(200009)11:1<12::AID-HBM20 >3.0.CO;2-K

Kang, D. H., Jo, H. J., Jung, W. H., Kim, S. H., Jung, Y. H., Choi, C. H., et al. (2013). The effect of meditation on brain structure: cortical thickness mapping and diffusion tensor imaging. *Soc. Cogn. Affect. Neurosci.* 8, 27–33. doi: 10.1093/scan/nss056

Karama, S., Ad-Dab'bagh, Y., Haier, R. J., Deary, I. J., Lyttelton, O. C., Lepage, C., et al. (2009). Positive association between cognitive ability and cortical thickness in a representative US sample of healthy 6 to 18 year-olds. *Intelligence* 37, 145–155. doi: 10.1016/s1053-8119(09)70678-0

Karton, I., and Bachmann, T. (2011). Effect of prefrontal transcranial magnetic stimulation on spontaneous truth-telling. *Behav. Brain Res.* 225, 209–214. doi: 10.1016/j.bbr.2011.07.028

Killingsworth, M. A., and Gilbert, D. T. (2010). A wandering mind is an unhappy mind. *Science* 330:932. doi: 10.1126/science.1192439

Kjaer, T. W., and Lou, H. C. (2000). Interaction between precuneus and dorsolateral prefrontal cortex may play a unitary role in consciousness-A principal component analysis of rCBF. *Conscious. Cogn.* 9, S59.

Kjaer, T. W., Nowak, M., and Lou, H. C. (2002). Reflective self-awareness and conscious states: PET evidence for a common midline parietofrontal core. *Neuroimage* 17, 1080–1086. doi: 10.1016/s1053-8119(02)91230-9

Kriegeskorte, N., and Goebel, R. (2001). An efficient algorithm for topologically correct segmentation of the cortical sheet in anatomical mr volumes. *Neuroimage* 14, 329–346. doi: 10.1006/nimg.2001.0831

Laird, A. R., Eickhoff, S. B., Li, K., Robin, D. A., Glahn, D. C., and Fox, P. T. (2009). Investigating the functional heterogeneity of the default mode network using coordinate-based meta-analytic modeling. *J. Neurosci.* 29, 14496–14505. doi: 10.1523/JNEUROSCI.4004-09.2009

Lancaster, J. L., Rainey, L. H., Summerlin, J. L., Freitas, C. S., Fox, P. T., Evans, A. C., et al. (1997). Automated labeling of the human brain: a preliminary report on the development and evaluation of a forward-transform method. *Hum. Brain Mapp.* 5, 238–242. doi: 10.1002/(SICI)1097-0193(1997)5:4<238::AID-HBM6>3.3.CO;2-3

Land, M. F. (2014). Do we have an internal model of the outside world? *Philos. Trans. R. Soc. Lond. B Biol. Sci.* 369:20130045. doi: 10.1098/rstb.2013.0045

Laureys, S., Boly, M., and Maquet, P. (2006). Tracking the recovery of consciousness from coma. *J. Clin. Invest.* 116, 1823–1825. doi: 10.1172/jci29172

Laureys, S., Goldman, S., Phillips, C., Van Bogaert, P., Aerts, J., Luxen, A., et al. (1999). Impaired effective cortical connectivity in vegetative state: preliminary investigation using PET. *Neuroimage* 9, 377–382. doi: 10.1006/nimg.1998.0414

Laureys, S., Owen, A. M., and Schiff, N. D. (2004). Brain function in coma, vegetative state and related disorders. *Lancet Neurol.* 3, 537–546. doi: 10.1016/s1474-4422(04)00852-x

Lazar, S. W., Kerr, C. E., Wasserman, R. H., Gray, J. R., Greve, D. N., Treadway, M. T., et al. (2005). Meditation experience is associated with increased cortical thickness. *Neuroreport* 16, 1893–1897. doi: 10.1097/01.WNR.0000186598.66243.19

Lopez, C., Lenggenhager, B., and Blanke, O. (2010). How vestibular stimulation interacts with illusory hand ownership. *Conscious. Cogn.* 19, 33–47. doi: 10.1016/j.concog.2009.12.003

Lopez, C., Schreyer, H. M., Preuss, N., and Mast, F. W. (2012). Vestibular stimulation modifies the body schema. *Neuropsychologia* 50, 1830–1837. doi: 10.1016/j.neuropsychologia.2012.04.008

Luders, E., Toga, A. W., Lepore, N., and Gaser, C. (2009). The underlying anatomical correlates of long-term meditation: larger hippocampal and frontal volumes of gray matter. *Neuroimage* 45, 672–678. doi: 10.1016/j.neuroimage.2008.12.061

Lutz, A., Greischar, L. L., Rawlings, N. B., Ricard, M., and Davidson, R. J. (2004). Long-term meditators self-induce high-amplitude gamma synchrony during mental practice. *Proc. Natl. Acad. Sci. U S A* 101, 16369–16373. doi: 10.1073/pnas.0407401101

Maguire, E. A., Gadian, D. G., Johnsrude, I. S., Good, C. D., Ashburner, J., Frackowiak, R. S. J., et al. (2000). Navigation-related structural change in the hippocampi of taxi drivers. *Proc. Natl. Acad. Sci. U S A* 97, 4398–4403. doi: 10.1073/pnas.070039597

Maquet, P. (2000). Functional neuroimaging of normal human sleep by positron emission tomography. *J. Sleep Res.* 9, 207–231. doi: 10.1046/j.1365-2869.2000.00214.x

Maquet, P., Degueldre, C., Delfiore, G., Aerts, J., Péters, J. M., Luxen, A., et al. (1997). Functional neuroanatomy of human slow wave sleep. *J. Neurosci.* 17, 2807–2812.

Maquet, P., Faymonville, M. E., Degueldre, C., Delfiore, G., Franck, G., Luxen, A., et al. (1999). Functional neuroanatomy of hypnotic state. *Biol. Psychiatry* 45, 327–333. doi: 10.1016/s0006-3223(97)00546-5

McCarthy, G., Puce, A., Belger, A., and Allison, T. (1991). Electrophysiological studies of human face perception. II: response properties of face-specific potentials generated in occipitotemporal cortex. *Cereb. Cortex* 9, 431–444. doi: 10.1093/cercor/9.5.431

Mechelli, A., Crinion, J. T., Noppeney, U., O'Doherty, J., Ashburner, J., Frackowiak, R. S., et al. (2004). Neurolinguistics: structural plasticity in the bilingual brain. Proficiency in a second language and age at acquisition affect grey-matter density. *Nature* 431:757. doi: 10.1038/431757a

Murd, C., Einberg, A., and Bachmann, T. (2012). Repetitive TMS over V5/MT shortens the duration of spatially localized motion aftereffect: the effects of pulse intensity and stimulation hemisphere. *Vision Res.* 68, 59–64. doi: 10.1016/j.visres.2012.07.009

den Ouden, H. E. M., Frith, U., Frith, C., and Blakemore, S. J. (2005). Thinking about intentions. *Neuroimage* 28, 787–796. doi: 10.1016/j.neuroimage.2005.05.001

Pagnoni, G., and Cekic, M. (2007). Age effects on gray matter volume and attentional performance in Zen meditation. *Neurobiol. Aging* 28, 1623–1627. doi: 10.1016/j.neurobiolaging.2007.06.008

Raichle, M. E., and Snyder, A. Z. (2007). A default mode of brain function: a brief history of an evolving idea. *Neuroimage* 37, 1083–1090; discussion 1097–1099. doi: 10.1016/j.neuroimage.2007.02.041

Rangarajan, V., Hermes, D., Foster, B. L., Weiner, K. S., Jacques, C., Grill-Spector, K., et al. (2014). Electrical stimulation of the left and right human fusiform gyrus causes different effects in conscious face perception. *J. Neurosci.* 34, 12828–12836. doi: 10.1523/JNEUROSCI.0527-14.2014

Rossion, B., Dricot, L., Devolder, A., Bodart, J. M., Crommelinck, M., De Gelder, B., et al. (2000). Hemispheric asymmetries for whole-based and part-based face processing in the human fusiform gyrus. *J. Cogn. Neurosci.* 12, 793–802. doi: 10.1162/089892900562606

Schwarzkopf, D. S., Silvanto, J., and Rees, G. (2011). Stochastic resonance effects reveal the neural mechanisms of transcranial magnetic stimulation. *J. Neurosci.* 31, 3143–3147. doi: 10.1523/JNEUROSCI.4863-10.2011

Smeets, R. (Ed.) (2006). "Mevlevi sema ceremony," in *Masterpieces of the Oral and Intangible Heritage of Humanity: Proclamations 2001, 2003 and 2005*, (Paris: UNESCO and Snoeck- Ducaju and Zoon), 90.

Stewart, L., Battelli, L., Walsh, V., and Cowey, A. (1999). Motion perception and perceptual learning studied by magnetic stimulation. *Electroencephalogr. Clin. Neurophysiol. Suppl.* 51, 334–350.

Van Swam, C., Federspiel, A., Hubl, D., Wiest, R., Boesch, C., Vermathen, P., et al. (2012). Possible dysregulation of cortical plasticity in auditory verbal hallucinations-A cortical thickness studyin schizophrenia. *J. Psychiatr. Res.* 8, 1015–1023. doi: 10.1016/j.jpsychires.2012.03.016

Strenziok, M., Krueger, F., Heinecke, A., Lenroot, R. K., Knutson, K. M., van der Meer, E., et al. (2011). Developmental effects of aggressive behavior in male adolescents assessed with structural and functional brain imaging. *Soc. Cogn. Affect. Neurosci.* 6, 2–11. doi: 10.1093/scan/nsp036

Tadin, D., Silvanto, J., Pascual-Leone, A., and Battelli, L. (2011). Improved motion perception and impaired spatial suppression following disruption of cortical area MT/V5. *J. Neurosci.* 31, 1279–1283. doi: 10.1523/JNEUROSCI.4121-10.2011

Thorns, J., Jansma, H., Peschel, T., Grosskreutz, J., Mohammadi, B., Dengler, R., et al. (2013). Extent of cortical involvement in amyotrophic lateral sclerosis an analysis based on cortical thickness. *BMC Neurol.* 13:148. doi: 10.1186/1471-2377-13-148

Turatto, M., Sandrini, M., and Miniussi, C. (2004). The role of the right dorsolateral prefrontal cortex in visual change awareness. *Neuroreport* 15, 2549–2552. doi: 10.1097/00001756-200411150-00024

Vaughan, J. T., Garwood, M., Collins, C. M., Liu, W., DelaBarre, L., Adriany, G., et al. (2001). 7T vs. 4T: RF power, homogeneity and signal-to-noise comparison in head images. *Magn. Reson. Med.* 46, 24–30. doi: 10.1002/mrm.1156

Vestergaard-Poulsen, P., van Beek, M., Skewes, J., Bjarkam, C. R., Stubberup, M., Bertelsen, J., et al. (2009). Long-term meditation is associated with increased gray matter density in the brain stem. *Neuroreport* 20, 170–174. doi: 10.1097/WNR.0b013e328320012a

Vogeley, K., and Fink, G. R. (2003). Neural correlates of the first-person-perspective. *Trends Cogn. Sci.* 7, 38–42. doi: 10.1016/s1364-6613(02)00003-7

Wiest, G., Zimprich, F., Prayer, D., Czech, T., Serles, W., and Baumgartner, C. (2004). Vestibular processing in human paramedian precuneus as shown by electrical cortical stimulation. *Neurology* 62, 473–475. doi: 10.1212/01.WNL.0000106948.17561.55

4

Cognitive Training for Post-Acute Traumatic Brain Injury

*Harry Hallock[1], Daniel Collins[1], Amit Lampit[1,2], Kiran Deol[3], Jennifer Fleming[4,5,6] and Michael Valenzuela[1]**

[1] Regenerative Neuroscience Group, Brain and Mind Centre, University of Sydney, Sydney, NSW, Australia, [2] School of Psychology, University of Sydney, Sydney, NSW, Australia, [3] Sydney Medical School, University of Sydney, Sydney, NSW, Australia, [4] School of Health and Rehabilitation Sciences, University of Queensland, Brisbane, QLD, Australia, [5] Occupational Therapy Department, Princess Alexandra Hospital, Brisbane, QLD, Australia, [6] Centre for Functioning and Health Research, Metro South Hospital and Health Service, Brisbane, QLD, Australia

Edited by:
Soledad Ballesteros, National University of Distance Education, Spain

Reviewed by:
Pierluigi Zoccolotti, Sapienza University of Rome, Italy
José Manuel Reales, National University of Distance Education, Spain

****Correspondence:***
Michael Valenzuela
michael.valenzuela@sydney.edu.au

Objective: To quantitatively aggregate effects of cognitive training (CT) on cognitive and functional outcome measures in patients with traumatic brain injury (TBI) more than 12-months post-injury.

Design: We systematically searched six databases for non-randomized and randomized controlled trials of CT in TBI patients at least 12-months post-injury reporting cognitive and/or functional outcomes.

Main Measures: Efficacy was measured as standardized mean difference (Hedges' g) of post-training change. We investigated heterogeneity across studies using subgroup analyses and meta-regressions.

Results: Fourteen studies encompassing 575 patients were included. The effect of CT on overall cognition was small and statistically significant ($g = 0.22$, 95%CI 0.05 to 0.38; $p = 0.01$), with low heterogeneity ($I^2 = 11.71\%$) and no evidence of publication bias. A moderate effect size was found for overall functional outcomes ($g = 0.32$, 95%CI 0.08 to 0.57, $p = 0.01$) with low heterogeneity ($I^2 = 14.27\%$) and possible publication bias. Statistically significant effects were also found only for executive function ($g = 0.20$, 95%CI 0.02 to 0.39, $p = 0.03$) and verbal memory ($g = 0.32$, 95%CI 0.14 to 0.50, $p < 0.01$).

Conclusion: Despite limited studies in this field, this meta-analysis indicates that CT is modestly effective in improving cognitive and functional outcomes in patients with post-acute TBI and should therefore play a more significant role in TBI rehabilitation.

Keywords: traumatic brain injury, TBI, closed head injury, cognitive training, cognitive outcome, neuropsychological outcome, rehabilitation

INTRODUCTION

Traumatic brain injury (TBI) causes ongoing disability for millions worldwide (Wilson et al., 2014), with cognitive impairment and psychosocial issues presenting major barriers to positive social outcomes such as community reintegration and employment (Rice-Oxley and Turner-Stokes, 1999). Cognitive impairment in TBI frequently affects the domains of attention, memory, executive functions, processing speed, language, and visuospatial skills (Dikmen et al., 2009). Reviews (Gordon et al., 2006; Cicerone et al., 2011; Lu et al., 2012) have suggested that cognitive rehabilitation for TBI, which encompasses several therapeutic strategies and interventions, can be beneficial for improving these cognitive domains and even community functioning. These interventions may include education, goal-setting, counseling, and internal and external compensation strategies targeting specific cognitive domains.

An on-going issue within the wider field of cognitive rehabilitation is a lack of a consensus for taxonomy of cognitive interventions, including of cognitive training (CT), but here we utilize a working definition consistent across key contributors to the literature (Clare et al., 2003; Buschert et al., 2010; Gates and Valenzuela, 2010). Here, we define and assess the impact of one specific form of cognitive rehabilitation which is seen to be cost-effective, scalable, adaptive (Gates and Valenzuela, 2010): CT. We and others have operationally defined CT to include four main characteristics: (1) repeated practice, (2) on problem-orientated tasks, (3) using standardized stimuli, and (4) targeting specified cognitive domains (Gates and Valenzuela, 2010; Bahar-Fuchs et al., 2013). CT aims to restore impaired skills or harness compensatory mechanisms (Buschert et al., 2010) and can include drill and practice exercises or applied mnemonic strategies. It can be administered either in paper-and-pen format, typically facilitated on a one-on-one basis by a therapist, or computer-assisted CT that can be supervised in a group setting or delivered at home at the individual level. It is therefore important to distinguish CT from the more holistic concept of cognitive rehabilitation that may include aspects of CT targeted to improve cognitive deficits, but also includes non-CT interventions aimed at improving psychological, emotional, motivational, and interpersonal functioning (Gordon et al., 2006).

Restorative treatments and compensatory strategies are generically recommended for the rehabilitation of TBI patients displaying cognitive deficits (INCOG guidelines; (Bayley et al., 2014)). Based on efficacy in other clinical populations (Wykes et al., 2011; Lampit et al., 2014; Leung et al., 2015), CT may have therapeutic potential for TBI. Yet prior reviews of cognitive interventions (Cicerone et al., 2005, 2011; Rees et al., 2007) have not specifically addressed the efficacy of CT for TBI patients. These reviews have attempted to synthesize across mixed samples with various kinds of acquired brain injury (ABI), as well as combine different types of cognitive therapies, and permitted a diversity of study designs. A recent meta-analysis (Rohling et al., 2009) highlights the potential therapeutic benefits of CT for specific brain injury deficits, but similar to the reviews, their study is of mixed etiology and also combines samples of varying time since injury, which although is inevitable, potentially introduces spontaneous recovery as a confounder. However, this could be attenuated by confining research to before or after 12 months post injury.

Accordingly, using a meta-analytic approach, this study aims to systematically evaluate whether operationally defined CT is effective in improving cognitive and functional outcomes at least one-year post-TBI, and to analyze potential moderators that may affect treatment outcomes. The study will analyze individual cognitive and functional domains, as well as overall cognition and overall functioning by pooling the individual domains together, respectively. Investigation of individual domains allows for identification of specific training effects, whilst pooling together individual domains allows for the identification of more general or overall effects that may not be apparent at the individual level for a multitude of reasons such as low sample size or poor study design. Additionally, to investigate potential moderators of training, a sub-group analysis will be conducted. Studies in this field are often small, underpowered and vary in design, thus a meta-analysis can add clarity, as it allows for amalgamation of these small studies to produce an overall analysis with greater statistical power and further reaching conclusions. Thus, as the field of cognitive rehabilitation in TBI is still in its infancy and much more research is required, a meta-analysis could prove crucial in identifying the future direction of CT, and potential design factors that may prove most effective.

MATERIALS AND METHODS

This systematic review and meta-analysis adheres to the Preferred Reporting Items for Systematic Reviews and Meta-Analyses (PRISMA) guidelines (Supplementary Table S1), (Liberati et al., 2009) was prospectively registered with PROSPERO (CRD42014013274) and largely follows methods established in our previous meta-analyses (Lampit et al., 2014; Leung et al., 2015).

Eligibility Criteria

We included both non randomized and randomized controlled trials (RCTs) provided they investigated the effects of a CT intervention on cognitive and/or functional outcomes in individuals (both intervention and controls groups) with post-acute TBI (time since injury $\geq$12 months, study mean). Thus we excluded studies that included healthy or acute TBI controls. Eligible outcomes were baseline and post-training performance on measures of cognition, Instrumental Activities of Daily Living (IADL) or dysexecutive functioning, defined as holistic disruptions to frontal lobe functions such as behavior, executive functions and cognition. CT was defined as any intervention incorporating computer-assisted CT, pencil-and-paper-administered CT, or cognitive strategy training, practiced systematically for a minimum of 4 hours. Studies that used combined interventions (e.g., CT with standard physical rehabilitation) were eligible if CT comprised at least 50% of the total intervention duration.

Search Methodology

We searched CINAHL, the Cochrane Database of Systematic Reviews, EMBASE, MEDLINE, PsycBITE, and PsycINFO databases from inception to July 27, 2015 using a comprehensive search strategy (Supplementary Datasheet 1).

Relevant articles were downloaded to an EndNote library, duplicates were removed and articles from other sources (e.g., references from systematic reviews) were manually added. HH and DC conducted initial screening for eligibility using title and abstract, and then independently examined full-text articles for inclusion.

Study Appraisal and Risk of Bias Within Studies

A modified form of the Physiotherapy Evidence Database (PEDro) scale (Maher et al., 2003), designed for rating the quality of RCTs, was used by HH and DC to assess the methodological rigor of included studies. As blinding of participants and therapists is impractical in CT trials, these two PEDro items were not assessed, and the maximum overall score (i.e., highest study quality) became 9 (Lampit et al., 2014). Risk of bias resulted from lack of assessor blinding or adherence to intention-to-treat analysis was assessed using the Cochrane's risk of bias tool (Higgins and Green, 2011). RCTs with high or unclear risk of bias for either of these categories were defined as having a high risk of bias.

Data Extraction

Cognitive and functional outcome data were extracted in the form of means and standard deviations for each group immediately pre- and post-intervention using a correlation of 0.6 between timepoints or mean group change, and entered into Comprehensive Meta-Analysis version 2 (CMA, Biostat, Englewood, NJ, USA). Coding of outcomes into cognitive domains and effect direction were performed using the *Compendium of Neuropsychological Tests* (Strauss et al., 2006) or by consensus.

Data Analysis

The dependent variable was standardized mean differences (SMD) (calculated as Hedges' g to correct for small sample sizes) of change from baseline to post-intervention between CT and control groups. Precision of SMD was estimated using 95% confidence intervals (CI). Analyses were conducted on individual cognitive (executive functions, verbal memory, working memory, attention, processing speed, non-verbal memory, visuospatial, language) and functional domains (IADL and dysexecutive functions). Analyses were also conducted on Overall Cognition and Overall Function, which were a result of combining or pooling the respective individual cognitive or functional domains together (Wykes et al., 2011; Lampit et al., 2014). An effect size of $g < 0.30$ was considered small, $g \geq 0.30$ moderate, and $g \geq 0.60$ large.

To avoid selective analyses of outcomes, study-level SMDs from the same cognitive domain were combined into a single effect estimate, corrected for inter-correlation across outcomes using a correlation of 0.7 (Gleser and Olkin, 2009). Pooling of outcomes across studies was conducted using random effects model. Heterogeneity across studies was quantified using the I^2 statistic, which quantifies the proportion of variance due to heterogeneity in true effects rather than random error (Higgins et al., 2003). I^2 values of 25, 50, and 75% imply low, moderate, and large heterogeneity, respectively.

To assess publication bias (small-study effect), funnel plots were visually inspected and formally tested using Egger's Test of the Intercepts if at least 10 studies were available for analysis (Egger et al., 1997; Sterne et al., 2011). If significant asymmetry was detected ($p < 0.1$), we estimated the magnitude of small-study effect using Duval and Tweedie's Trim and Fill method (Duval and Tweedie, 2000).

In order to detect design factors that may affect CT efficacy, we performed subgroup meta-analyses based on mixed-effects model. Between-subgroup heterogeneity was tested using Cochrane's Q statistic (significant at $p < 0.05$). Analyses were performed for overall cognitive and overall functional outcomes based on the following study characteristics: study design (randomized or non-randomized), intervention type (combined, strategy or training), control type (active or passive), total hours of training ($\leq$20 or >20 h), session length ($\leq$60 or >60 mins), and session frequency (<4 or $\geq$4 a week). Univariate meta-regressions were used to detect relationships between cognitive results and PEDro score, sample size and year of publication. All analyses were conducted in CMA.

RESULTS

Study Selection

After removal of duplicates, 3464 articles were screened for inclusion based on published title and abstract. 421 articles were suitable for full-text screening, including one manually added study (**Figure 1**). After full-text screening, 15 studies were eligible for review, however one focused solely on children and adolescence (Thomas-Stonell et al., 1994) and was therefore excluded, leaving 14 studies for analysis. Age was not a screening criterion, but given the fact that TBI can manifest quite differently during adolescent brain development, it was deemed appropriate to exclude this study.

Characteristics of Included Studies

Data from 575 participants and 169 outcomes were included. The mean number of participants per study was 41.07, with a mean participant age of 38.79 years. Brain injury severity ranged from mild to severe. Time since injury ranged from 1.01 to 14.4 years (*mean* = 5.3 years, *SD* = 3.78). Strategy-based interventions were used in four studies (O'Neil-Pirozzi et al., 2010; Vas et al., 2011; Dawson et al., 2013; Twamley et al., 2014), drill and practice training (including computer-assisted training) in six (Ryan and Ruff, 1988; Baribeau et al., 1989; Ruff et al., 1989; Rattok et al., 1992; Potvin et al., 2011; Nelson et al., 2013), and a combination of both in four studies (Goranson et al., 2003; Tiersky et al., 2005; Wai-Kwong Man et al., 2006; Cantor et al., 2014). An active control group was used in seven studies (**Table 1**). The average PEDro score was 5.64/9 (*SD* = 0.84). Seven studies were RCTs (Ryan and Ruff, 1988; Ruff et al., 1989; Tiersky et al., 2005; Vas et al., 2011; Nelson et al., 2013; Twamley et al., 2014) and seven were non-randomized controlled studies (Baribeau et al., 1989; Rattok et al., 1992; Goranson et al., 2003; Wai-Kwong Man et al., 2006; O'Neil-Pirozzi et al., 2010; Potvin et al., 2011; Dawson et al., 2013; Cantor et al., 2014). Four of the studies

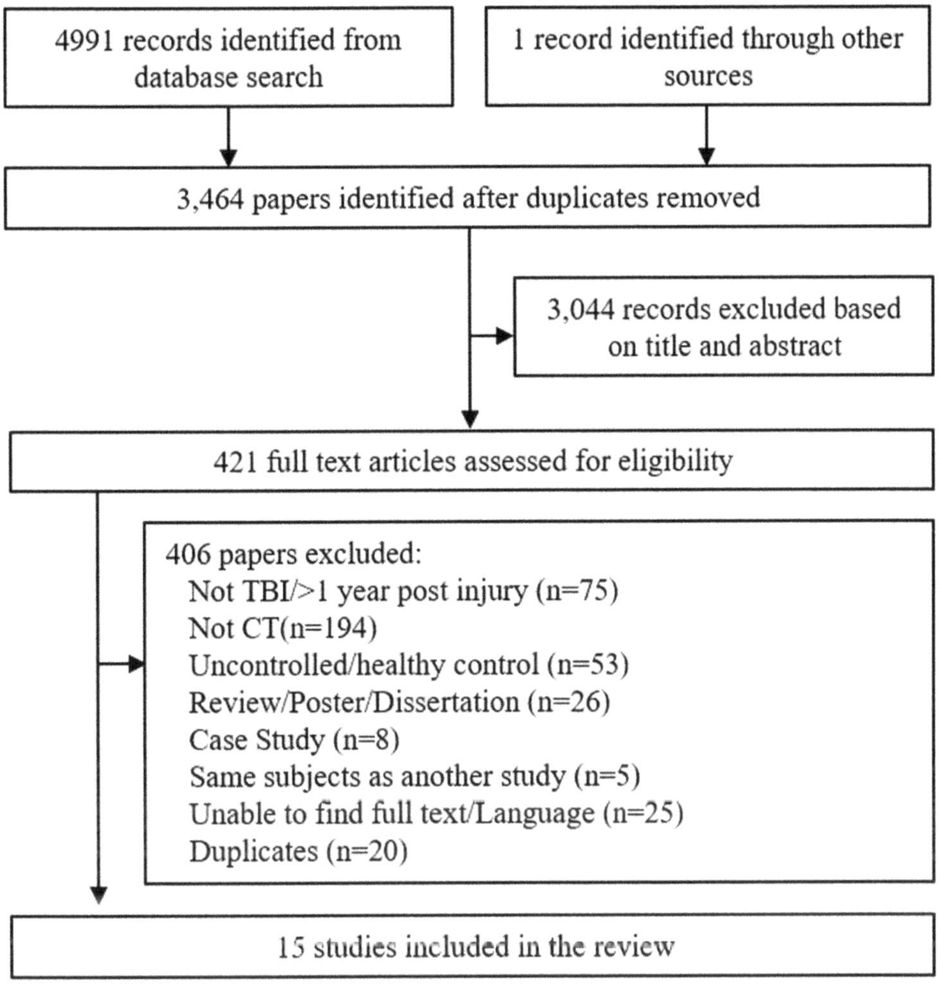

FIGURE 1 | Flowchart of trial identification and selection. Note that a single study could be excluded on more than one criterion, but appears only once in the chart.

confirmed assessor blinding, whilst three reported intention-to-treat.

Efficacy on Overall Cognitive Outcomes

There was a small, statistically significant positive effect of CT on overall cognitive outcomes ($k = 12$, $g = 0.22$, 95% CI 0.05 to 0.38, $p = 0.01$; **Figure 2A**). Heterogeneity across studies was low ($I^2 = 11.71\%$, 95% CI 0% to 51.39%). A funnel plot of results did not reveal asymmetry (Egger's intercept = −0.93, $p = 0.51$; **Figure 3**) suggesting no significant evidence of systematic bias toward including positive (or negative) outcomes.

Efficacy on Specific Cognitive Domains

Executive Function

The effect size was small and statistically significant ($k = 8$, $g = 0.20$, 95% CI 0.02 to 0.39, $p = 0.03$; **Figure 2B**). Statistical heterogeneity across studies was zero ($I^2 = 0$, 95% CI 0% to 0%), and the funnel plot did not show evidence of asymmetry (**Figure 3**).

Verbal Memory

The effect size was moderate and statistically significant ($k = 10$, $g = 0.32$, 95% CI 0.14 to 0.50, $p < 0.01$; **Figure 2C**). Statistical heterogeneity across studies was small ($I^2 = 3.40$, 95% CI 0% to 63.84%), and the funnel plot did not show evidence of asymmetry (Egger's intercept = −1.69, $p = 0.21$; **Figure 3**).

Working Memory

The effect size was small and statistically non-significant ($k = 7$, $g = 0.06$, 95% CI −0.21 to 0.34, $p = 0.94$; **Figure 4A**). Statistical heterogeneity across studies was moderate ($I^2 = 36.88$, 95% CI 0% to 73.44%), and the funnel plot did not show evidence of asymmetry (**Figure 3**).

Attention

The effect size was small and statistically non-significant ($k = 6$, $g = 0.14$, 95% CI −0.09 to 0.37, $p = 0.22$; **Figure 4B**). Statistical heterogeneity across studies was zero ($I^2 = 0$, 95% CI 0% to

TABLE 1 | Characteristics of included studies.

Author and year	Study design	Mean age (treatment, control)	Injury characteristics	Mean time since injury (treatment, control-years)	Intervention type; total duration (h)	Control type	Outcomes	PEDro score	Risk of bias
Baribeau et al., 1989 (*N* = 41)	Non-randomized controlled trial	27, 27	All severe Closed-head injury	6.58, 5.92	CCT	Active (standard rehab)	Attention	6	N/A
Cantor et al., 2014 (*N* = 91)	Non- RCT	46.7, 43.9	Mixed TBI severity (mild 50%, moderate 19%, severe 31%)	10.7, 14.4	Strategy/CT for executive dysfunction; 90	Passive (wait-list)	Cognitive functioning (multiple domains), IADL, dysexecutive functions	7	N/A
Dawson et al., 2013 (*N* = 13)	Non- RCT	42.6, 40.5	Mixed TBI severity (mild 15%, moderate to severe 85%)	9.8, 10.8	Strategy training for occupational performance; 20	Passive; matched control group	IADL, dysexecutive functions	6	N/A
Goranson et al., 2003 (*N* = 42)	Non-randomized case-control study	34.71, 36.57	Mild to moderate TBI; PTA < 24 h	1.01, 1.12	CT/Strategy training within multidisciplinary rehab; avg. 352	Passive (no rehab)	Community integration	5	N/A
Nelson et al., 2013 (*N* = 36)	RCT	34.8, 31.1	Blast-related mild to moderate TBI; avg. 2.9 blast injuries	2.92, 1.83	CT plus standard rehab; 15	Active (standard rehab)	Cognitive functioning (multiple domains)	6	High
O'Neil-Pirozzi et al., 2010 (*N* = 94)	Non-RCT	47.3, 47	Mixed TBI severity (mild 20%, moderate 22%, severe 47%)	11.8, 13.4	Strategy for memory; 18	Passive (no rehab)	Verbal memory	6	N/A
Potvin et al., 2011 (*N* = 30)	Non-RCT	35.0, 30.9	Mixed TBI severity (moderate 10%, severe 90%)	3.62, 2.83	CT/CCT for prospective memory rehab; 15	Active (education); matched control group	Cognitive functioning (multiple domains), IADL	6	N/A
Rattok et al., 1992[a] (*N* = 36)	Non-RCT	28.5, 27.1	Severe TBI; days in coma: 36.9 (treatment), 38.9 (control)	3.35, 2.82	CT/CCT within multidisciplinary rehab; 200	Active (multidimensional rehab)	Cognitive functioning (multiple domains)	5	N/A
Ruff et al., 1989 (*N* = 40)	RCT	29.9, 31.7	Moderate to severe TBI; days in coma: 32.1 (treatment), 48.8 (control)	3.18, 4.37	CCT/CT within structured cognitive rehab; 160	Active (non-structured rehab)	Cognitive functioning (multiple domains)	5	High
Ryan and Ruff, 1988 (*N* = 20)	RCT	34.3, 31.4	Head injury with mild to moderate neuropsychological impairment; GCS ≤8 at time of injury	4.54, 4.78	CT/CCT within structured memory rehab; 132	Active (psychosocial rehab)	Cognitive functioning (multiple domains)	4	High
Tiersky et al., 2005 (*N* = 20)	RCT	47.55, 46	Mixed TBI severity (mild 90%)	5.01, 5.47	CT/CBT	Passive (wait-list)	Cognitive functioning (multiple domains), IADL	7	High

(Continued)

TABLE 1 | Continued

Author and year	Study design	Mean age (treatment, control)	Injury characteristics	Mean time since injury (treatment, control-years)	Intervention type; total duration (h)	Control type	Outcomes	PEDro score	Risk of bias
Twamley et al., 2014 ($N = 34$)	RCT	29.4, 34.3	Mild to moderate TBI; loss of consciousness <24 hrs	3.6, 5.1	Strategy training within supported employment program; 12	Active (supported employment)	Cognitive functioning (multiple domains), daily functioning,	5	High
Vas et al., 2011 ($N = 28$)	RCT	39.0, 47.0	Mild to severe TBI; PTA: 2.1 & 2.46 weeks; moderate functional impairment.	1.39, 1.36	Strategy training for higher-order reasoning; 18	Active (psychoeducation)	Cognitive functioning (multiple domains), IADL	6	High
Wai-Kwong Man et al., 2006 ($N = 50$)	Non-RCT	44.87, 48.55	Not specified	3.48, 4.13	CCT/Strategy training for problem-solving; 20 sessions	Passive (no treatment); matched control group	Executive function, IADL	5	N/A

RCT, randomized controlled trial; TBI, traumatic brain injury; IADL, Instrumental Activities of Daily Living; CT, cognitive training; CCT, computerized cognitive training; GCS, Glasgow coma scale; PTA, Post-traumatic amnesia. [a] *Three treatment groups - 1 group excluded, 95% TBI and 5% cerebral anoxia.*

61.04%), and the funnel plot did not show evidence of asymmetry (**Figure 3**).

Processing Speed

The effect size was small and statistically non-significant ($k = 5$, $g = 0.22$, 95% CI −0.01 to 0.46, $p = 0.06$; **Figure 4C**). Statistical heterogeneity across studies was zero ($I^2 = 0$, 95% CI 0% to 62.91%), and the funnel plot did not show evidence of asymmetry (**Figure 3**).

Non-verbal Memory

The effect size was negative, small and statistically non-significant ($k = 4$, $g = -0.08$, 95% CI −0.40 to 0.24, $p = 0.63$; **Figure 5A**). Statistical heterogeneity across studies was zero ($I^2 = 0$, 95% CI 0% to 0%), and the funnel plot did not show evidence of asymmetry.

Visuospatial

The effect size was small and statistically non-significant ($k = 4$, $g = 0.01$, 95% CI −0.29 to 0.31, $p = 0.94$; **Figure 5B**). Statistical heterogeneity across studies was zero ($I^2 = 0$, 95% CI 0% to 62.81%), and the funnel plot did not show evidence of asymmetry.

Language

The effect size was small and statistically non-significant ($k = 3$, $g = 0.08$, 95% CI −0.27 to 0.43, $p = 0.66$; **Figure 5C**). Statistical heterogeneity across studies was small ($I^2 = 24.57$, 95% CI 0% to 97.47%), and the funnel plot did not show evidence of asymmetry.

Efficacy on Overall Functional Outcomes

A pooled analysis of the seven studies reporting functional outcomes revealed a moderate and statistically significant effect size ($g = 0.32$, 95% CI 0.08 to 0.57, $p = 0.01$; **Figure 6A**). Heterogeneity across studies was low ($I^2 = 14.27\%$, 95% CI 0% to 75.39%). The funnel plot revealed asymmetry, indicating more positive results in smaller studies. A trim and fill analysis revealed a smaller and statistically non-significant effect size ($g = 0.23$, 95% CI −0.05 to 0.51, $p = 0.11$ **Figure 3**).

Efficacy on Specific Functional Domains

Instrumental Activities of Daily Living (IADL)

The effect size was moderate and statistically non-significant ($k = 7$, $g = 0.36$, 95% CI −0.04 to 0.75, $p = 0.08$; **Figure 6B**). Statistical heterogeneity across studies was moderate ($I^2 = 62.07\%$, 95% CI 13.59% to 83.35%). The funnel plot showed evidence of asymmetry, but trim and fill analysis did not alter the effect size (**Figure 3**).

Dysexecutive Functions

The effect size was small and statistically non-significant ($k = 2$, $g = 0.23$, 95% CI −0.11 to 0.57, $p = 0.19$; **Figure 6C**). Statistical heterogeneity across studies was zero ($I^2 = 0$).

Moderators of CT Efficacy

Possible moderators of training effects on overall cognitive (**Figure 7A**) and functional (**Figure 7B**) outcomes were investigated using sub-group analyses. For overall cognition,

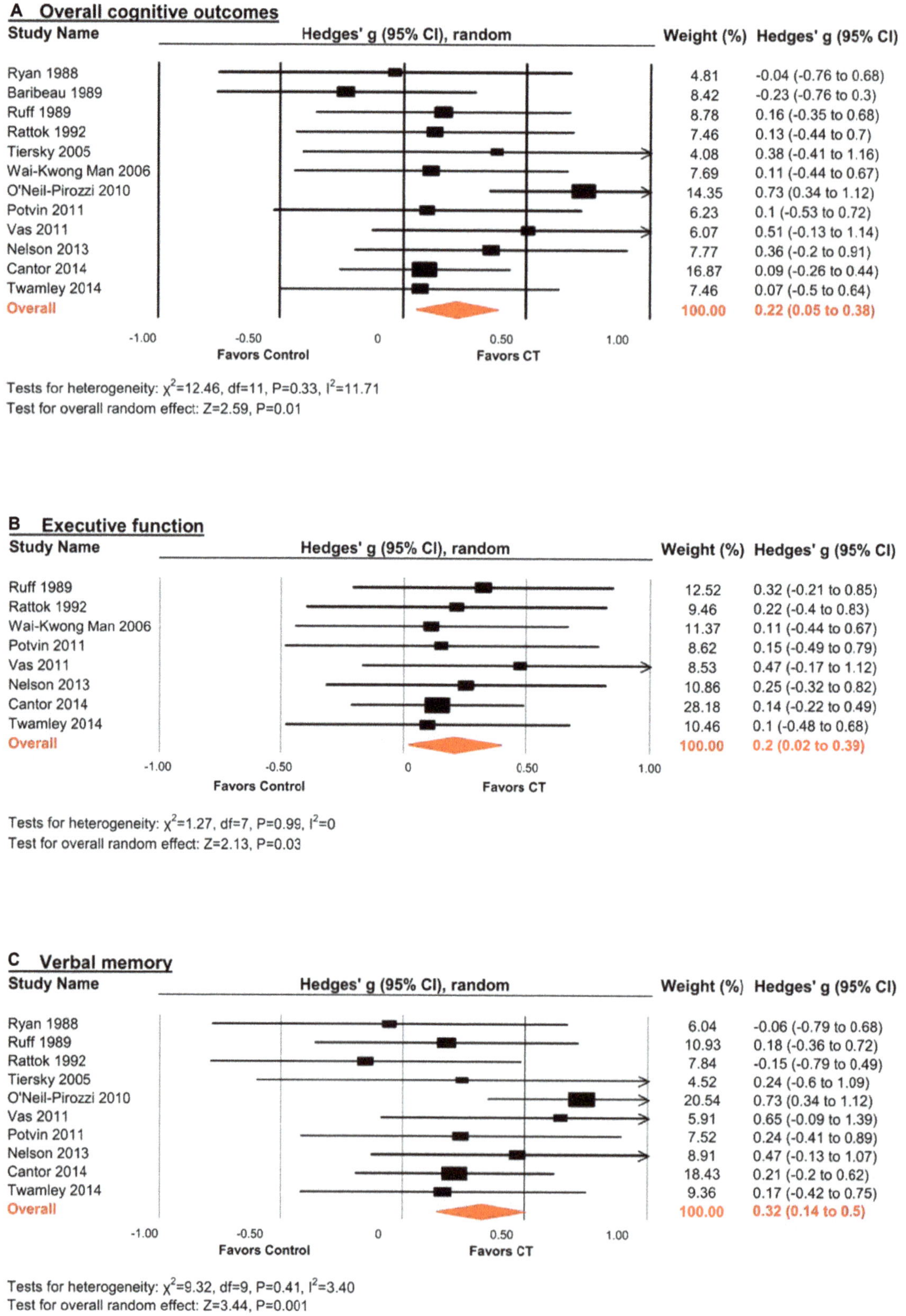

FIGURE 2 | Efficacy of cognitive training (CT) on (A) overall cognitive outcomes; (B) executive function; and (C) verbal memory. Effect estimates are based on a random-effects model.

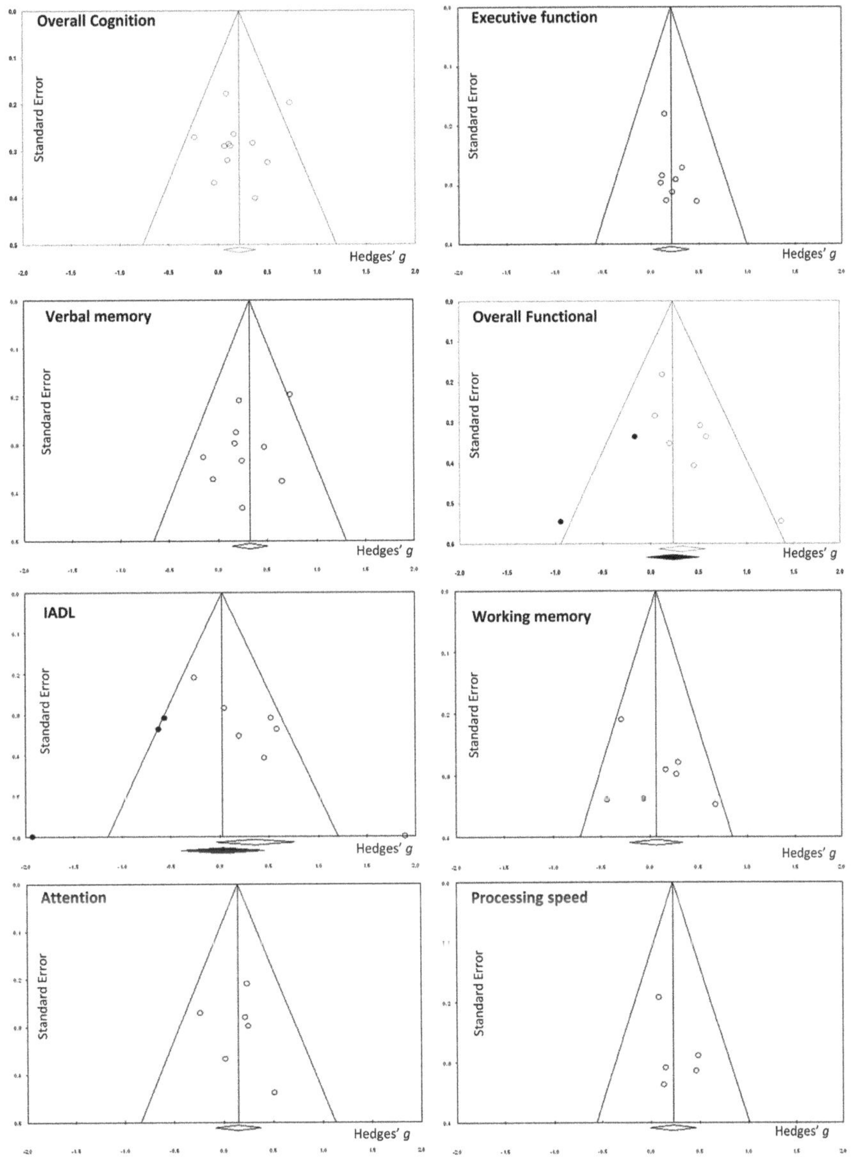

FIGURE 3 | Funnel plots.

we did not find significant between group differences for study design, intervention type, control type, total hours of training, session length or session frequency. However there was a strong trend toward less training being more effective on overall cognition, with studies providing 20 h or less of training ($g = 0.41$, 95% CI 0.14 to 0.68, $p < 0.01$, $I^2 = 21.40\%$) being more effective than those that provided more than 20 hours ($g = 0.06$, 95% CI −0.15 to 0.28, $p = 0.55$; $Q = 3.80$, df = 1, $p = 0.05$). To further investigate this trend, we conducted an analysis on a *post hoc* basis. This correlation comparing length of training and severity of injury was found to be non-significant ($r = 0.26$, $p = 0.44$, $n = 11$). There were no significant between-subgroup differences with overall functional outcomes for any of these moderators. As both IADL and working memory outcomes had moderate heterogeneity, subgroup analyses were conducted, but no significant differences were found for either. For other domains, heterogeneity was close to zero, thus subgroup analyses were not warranted.

Meta-regression showed no statistically significant relationships between overall cognitive effects and PEDro score ($\beta = 0.06$, $p = 0.57$), sample size ($\beta = 0.004$, $p = 0.23$), or year of publication ($\beta = 0.01$, $p = 0.18$).

A matrix was constructed to investigate whether the content of training (the domain/s that were trained) moderated outcomes on specific cognitive domains outcomes, i.e., if there was transfer. A summary of these cognitive outcomes is presented in **Figure 8**, and categorized by study and cognitive domain trained. No

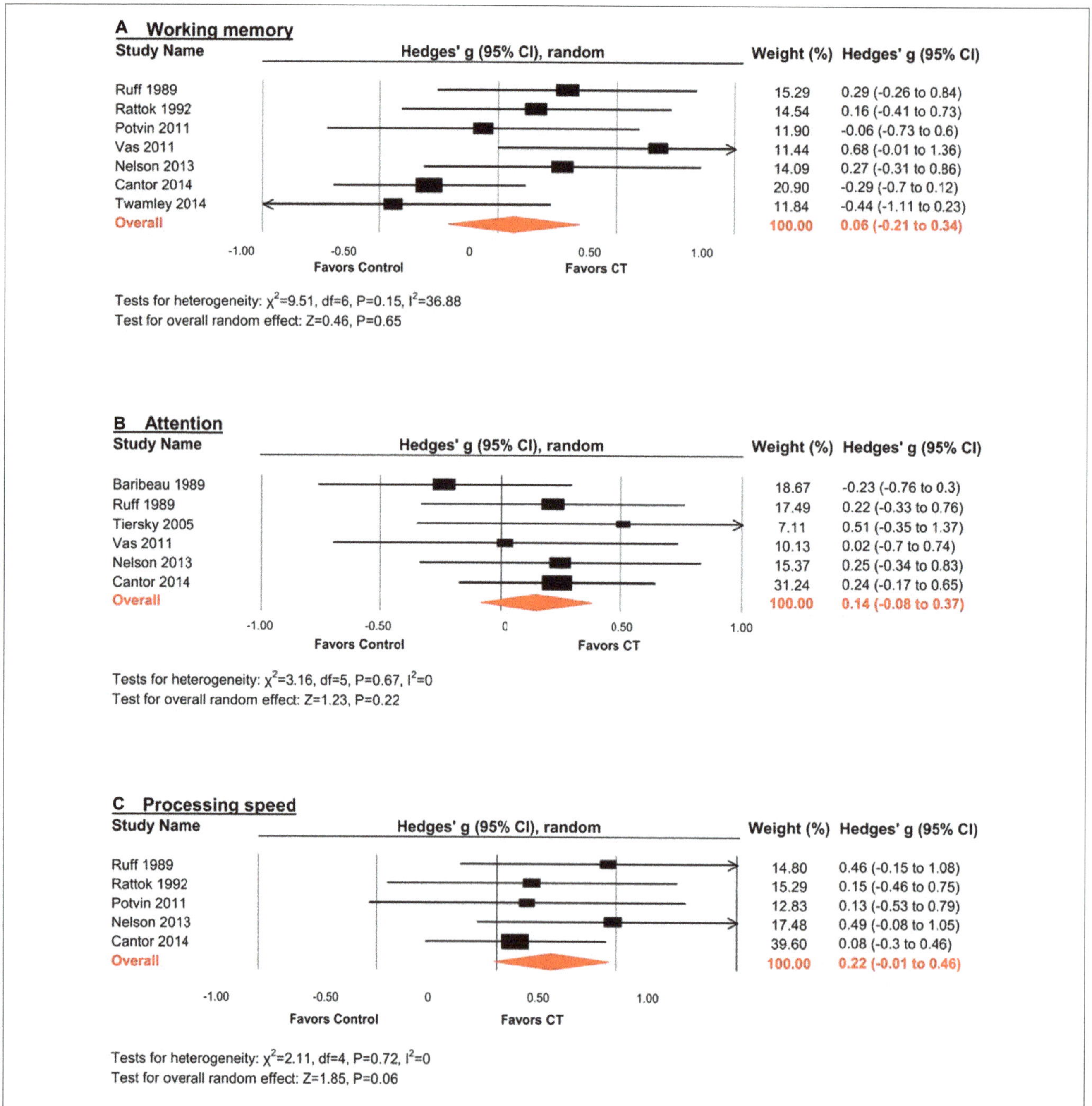

FIGURE 4 | Efficacy of CT on (A) working memory; (B) attention; and (C) processing speed. Effect estimates are based on a random-effects model.

statistical analysis was run on this data, but the matrix illustrates which cognitive domains were trained (gray color cells), and the effect sizes at a study level or pooled together at a domain level.

DISCUSSION

Cognitive-based interventions are effective in several clinical populations (Wykes et al., 2011; Lampit et al., 2014; Leung et al., 2015), and here we expand the evidence base to include post-acute TBI. CT was particularly effective on overall cognition, as well as the cognitive domains of verbal memory and executive function, and jointly improved individuals' IADLs whilst reducing severity of dysexecutive signs and symptoms.

TBI is extremely heterogeneous in its etiology and origins. Accordingly, patients present with a variety of cognitive deficits (Dikmen et al., 2009), with information processing speed and verbal memory most commonly affected (Skandsen et al., 2010). It is therefore promising that this study found not only general

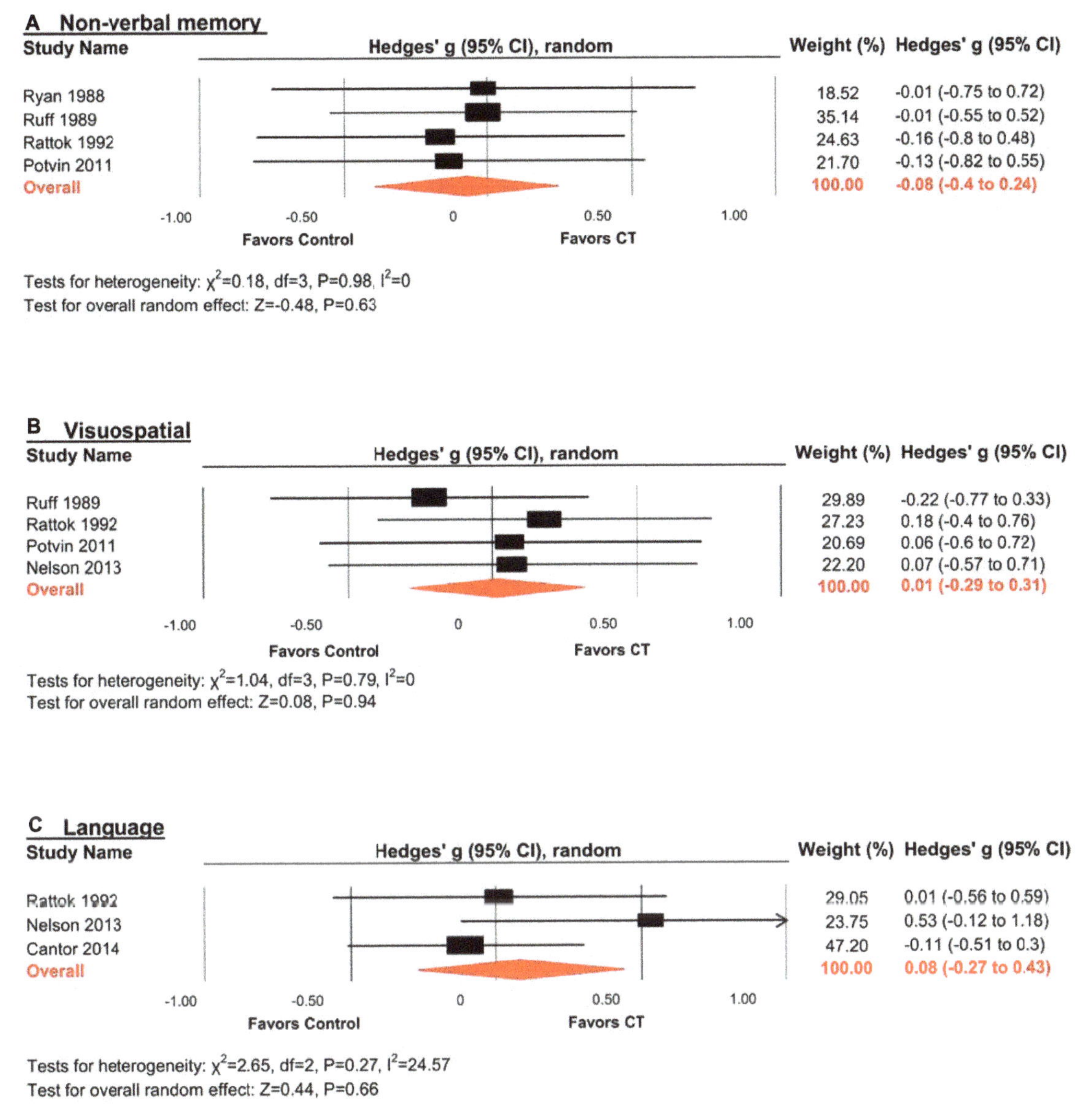

FIGURE 5 | Efficacy of CT on (A) non-verbal memory; (B) visuospatial; and (C) language. Effect estimates are based on a random-effects model.

cognitive efficacy, but specific efficacy for executive function and verbal memory. Contrary to this, a previous meta-analysis (Rohling et al., 2009) found that cognitive rehabilitation was not effective in TBI patients. However, that study combined several different types of cognitive interventions and patients varied greatly in the time since injury. As mentioned, cognitive rehabilitation encompasses a variety of therapeutic approaches, and here we aim to focus on CT as operationally defined in the introduction. Moreover, timing of intervention may well be critical. TBI often progresses through stages of unconsciousness and emerging consciousness; confusion with dense anterograde amnesia that can vary from days to several weeks; and a long-term period of restoration of cognitive, neuropsychological and social functioning that can last for several years (Povlishock and Katz, 2005). Here we have clarified the literature to some extent and shown that one approach to cognitive rehabilitation, CT, is effective for certain cognitive domains in the post-acute phase.

Cognitive rehabilitation, which can include CT, is known to improve community functioning even several years after TBI (Gordon et al., 2006). Our analyses suggest that CT may itself be sufficient to retrain functional skills or facilitate compensatory mechanisms that can translate into everyday outcomes. In the TBI literature, functionality is often measured by IADL scales and assessment of dysexecutive syndrome. Given the importance of both IADLs and dysexecutive syndrome to everyday life, it is noteworthy that CT produced a moderate effect size on these outcomes when combined. Furthermore, the low heterogeneity surrounding this estimate indicates that the result is subject to little explainable variation and is thus an accurate estimate of effect size. Whilst the combination of these two outcomes

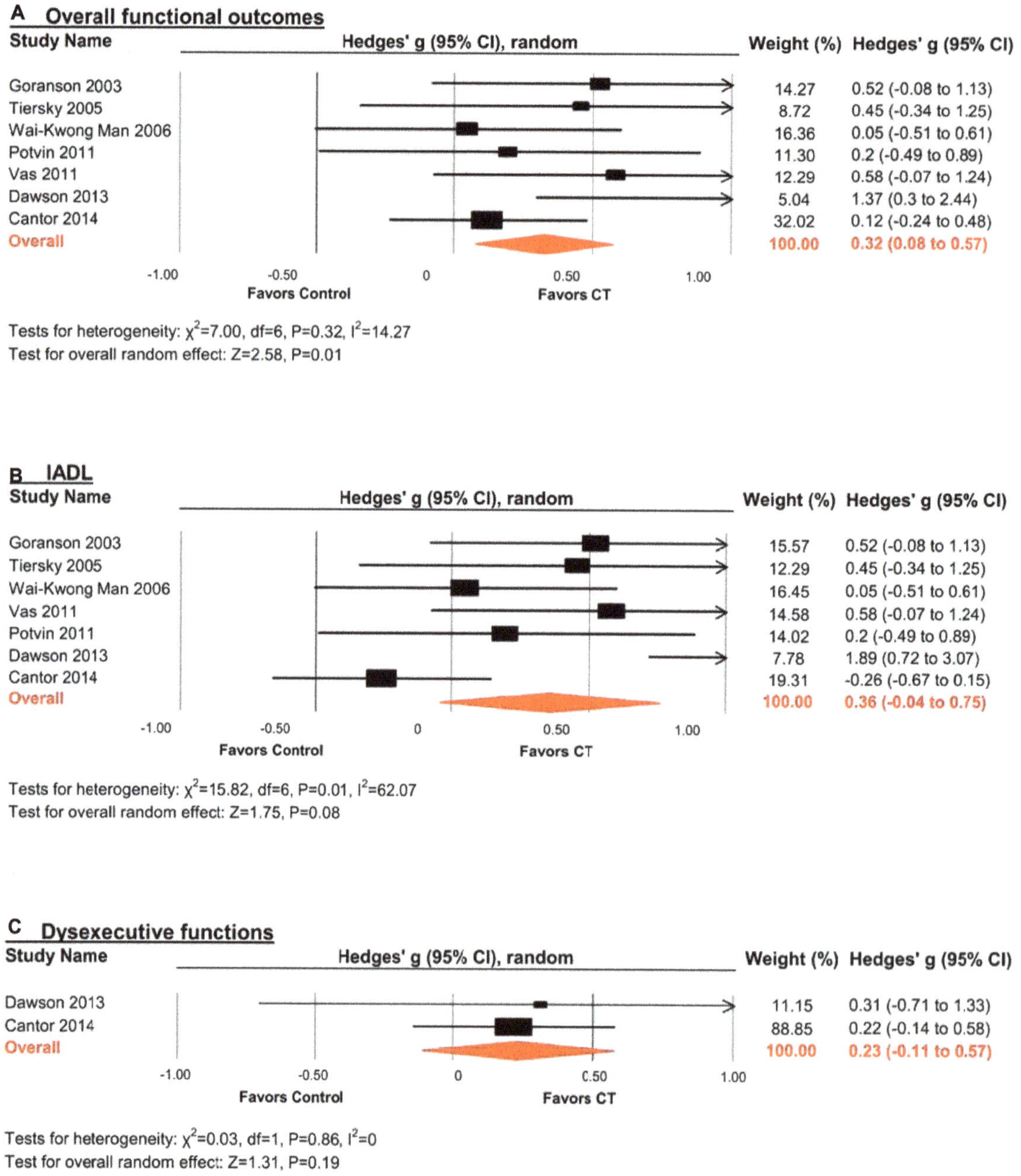

FIGURE 6 | Efficacy of CT on (A) overall functional outcomes; (B) instrumental activities of daily living (IADL); and (C) dysexecutive functions. Effect estimates are based on a random-effects model.

may appear to be novel, previous studies have shown loose connections between the two (Pa et al., 2009; Marshall et al., 2011). Importantly, this result suggests that CT has the potential to achieve so-called "far-transfer" (Barnett and Ceci, 2002) to positively influence real world issues faced by TBI patients.

Despite these combined results, IADL or dysexecutive functioning did not produce significant improvements when considered separately. This may be due to insufficient power, as not only were there limited studies examining these outcomes, and small sample sizes, but a separate analysis of the two domains displayed larger CI. Positive effects on daily function were restricted to a pooled analysis of combined dysexecutive and IADL outcomes. Whilst this approach has some precedence (Pa et al., 2009; Marshall et al., 2011) and was planned a priori, when each type of outcome was considered individually no significant effects were observed. This therefore brings up the issue as to what can be reasonably combined in terms of outcomes measures within a meta-analysis – a topic treated in detail by

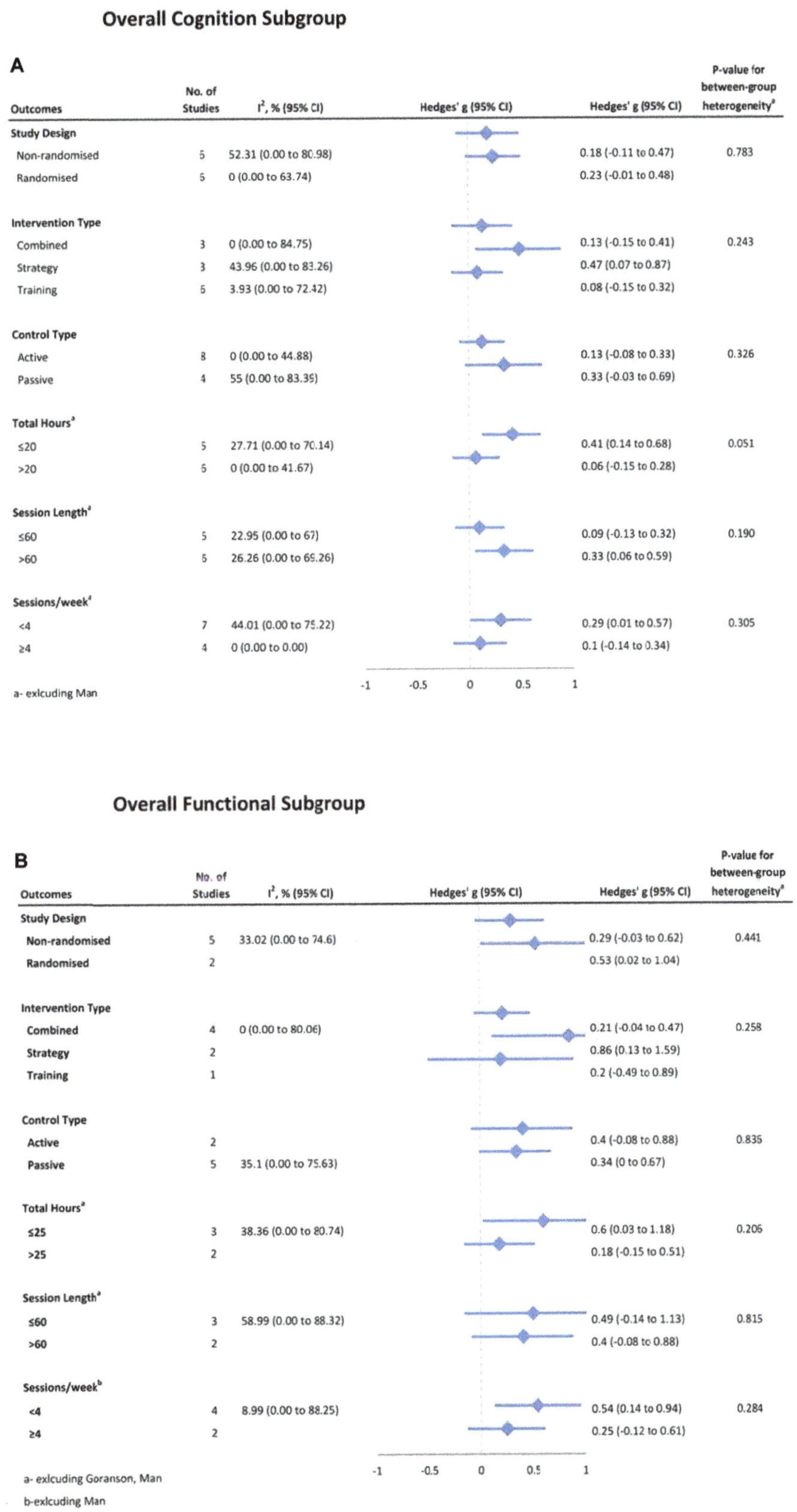

FIGURE 7 | Subgroup analysis of moderators for (A) overall cognitive outcomes, and (B) overall functional outcomes.

Study	Attention CT	Verbal Memory CT	Non-verbal Memory CT	Speed CT	Visuospatial CT	Language CT	EF CT	WM CT
Baribeau 1989	-0.23							
Cantor 2014	0.24	0.21		0.08		-0.11	0.14	-0.29
Dawson 2013								
Goranson 2003								
Nelson 2013	0.25	0.47		0.49	0.07	0.53	0.25	0.27
O'Neil-Pirozzi 2010		0.73**						
Potvin 2011		0.24	-0.13	0.13	0.06		0.15	-0.06
Rattok 1992		-0.15	-0.16	0.15	0.18	0.01	0.22	0.16
Ruff 1989	0.22	0.18	-0.01	0.46	-0.22		0.32	0.29
Ryan 1988		-0.06	-0.01					
Tiersky 2005	0.51	0.24						
Twamley 2014		0.17					0.10	-0.44
Vas 2011	0.02	0.65					0.47	0.68
Wai-Kwong Man 2006							0.11	
Domains	0.14	0.32**	-0.08	0.22	0.01	0.08	0.20**	0.06

FIGURE 8 | Matrix of training content against effect size of each cognitive outcome from the individual studies. Gray cells indicate the study trained in the domain. EF = executive functions; WM = working memory. $^{**}p < 0.05$

Borenstein et al. (2009). In their example, combining tests of Maths and English is justified, "If our goal is to assess the impact on performance in general, then the answer is Yes." (Borenstein et al., 2009, p. 357). Our goal was to assess the impact of CT on those areas that most impact day to day function in TBI rehabilitation, inclusive of both dysexecutive syndrome (Rao and Lyketsos, 2000) and impaired IADLs (Colantonio et al., 2004). Hence, there are promising indications that CT can help support daily function in chronic TBI patients, but clearly more research is required to parse these effects out.

Interestingly, CT had a significant effect on executive function but not dysexecutive outcomes. This may appear paradoxical given the two outcomes are intrinsically (and inversely) related (Ardila, 2013). However, this pattern of results can be explained by the nature of the data. Executive outcomes originate from neuropsychological tests that are generally objective, quantitative and continuous, and thus sensitive to change, whilst dysexecutive instruments are generally subjective, qualitative and ordinal. By nature these instruments are therefore of lower resolution and require much larger behavioral change before detection. Further research is therefore required to determine whether CT can improve not just psychometric executive function but also minimize the presentation or severity of dysexecutive symptoms in post-acute TBI.

Of the potential moderators analyzed, a strong trend was found only for training hours. Studies where subjects trained for ≤ 20 h showed improvements in overall cognition compared to studies where patients trained more. This is consistent with evidence of weaker effect sizes in studies that provided intense training schedules (Lampit et al., 2014) or long training durations (Toril et al., 2014) in healthy older adults. A possible explanation for this trend could be the heterogeneity in injury severity amongst the population, whereby those with more severe injuries required more training, with the assumption that increased severity means lower improvement. We conducted a *post hoc* analysis to test this theory, but we did not find a relationship between length of training and injury severity across studies. However given that this *post hoc* analysis was conducted on such a small sample size, and thus lacks power, we cannot completely rule out that the trend in training time is linked with injury severity. Nonetheless, it is intriguing that across different clinical cohorts there may be converging evidence for the importance of avoiding over-dosing, or over-training participants. This concept is even more salient in the field of TBI, where rehabilitation is often guided by the principle that greater intensity or number of repetitions is better. Here, we conclude that CT at a circumscribed dose, at the right time in the post-acute stage, is preferable.

Other possible moderators analyzed were found to be non-significant, consistent with the small number of studies and minimal explainable between-study variance – a concept we have previously discussed (Leung et al., 2015). More specifically, our data suggests that an important study design factor, whether randomization occurred or not, did not impact CT efficacy in post-acute TBI. However, we cannot rule out that this could be due to a lack of power, a notion counter-weighed by similar effect sizes from the two design methods. This finding supports our decision to combine both non randomized and RCTs into a single analysis.

To further explore moderating or driving factors of cognitive outcomes, we investigated whether there was a link between training content and cognitive outcomes (**Figure 8**). For this population, cross-transfer, the idea that training in one domain can result in improvements in another untrained domain, appears to be unlikely. This is evident when looking at the columns for working memory, speed, language and executive functions. We can see here, as indicated by the gray cells, or lack thereof, that there was minimal training on these domains, however there was training in many other domains. The fact that there are no significant results, in addition to the obvious lack of power, suggests a lack of cross transfer, a sentiment mirrored in previous research (Edwards et al., 2002). Importantly, we cannot conclude that certain domains, such as working memory, speed, language, and executive functions are ineffective or non-responsive in this population. Instead, this figure suggests that there is need for more trials that are training or targeting multiple different cognitive domains.

Limitations include potential selection bias that may have influenced results. Our narrow eligibility criteria and decision to include only studies published in English, resulted in well-controlled CT studies being excluded from this analysis, such as trials implemented before 12 months post-injury. We chose this temporal window for clinical reasons, namely to minimize the confounding effects of spontaneous recovery of function that can occur during the acute and sub-acute stages (Sohlberg and Mateer, 2001). A caveat to this criterion was a reliance on study-level characteristic. Some studies included participants from 3 months post-injury and onward, resulting in large variations in time since injury, despite the reported study average being >12 months post injury. To further clarify the specificity of our findings to this temporal window, a patient-level meta-analysis is required. In addition, our decision to only include functional outcomes that could be categorized as IADL or dysexecutive functioning was a potential source of selection bias, but a decision we consider clinically principled since functional outcomes from three studies e.g., 'Life-3' (Dawson et al., 2013; Cantor et al., 2014; Twamley et al., 2014) were idiosyncratic and deemed incomparable.

A notable limitation of our analysis is the heterogeneity in injury severity, but this is reflective of the state of the field. Indeed, many of the included studies themselves comprised patients of varying TBI severity (from mild to severe). However, low statistical heterogeneity indicates that there was no other important source of bias between study variance besides total hours of training. Average PEDro quality scores were relatively low, but this was mainly attributable to two points being allocated for randomization procedures. We specifically tested this factor and found it was not influencing effect size estimates. Perhaps the largest limitation of our study is the relative infancy of the field. With only six of the studies included being RCTs, the field is somewhat nascent, thus our results must be viewed with some skepticism. Nonetheless there is enough power to show effectiveness of CT on overall cognitive and functional outcomes, however, clearly future research with more rigorous trial design and reporting is required.

TBI is fundamentally heterogeneous and manifests in complex and unpredictable patterns, resulting in diverse physical, behavioral, cognitive and functional outcomes. Discerning therapeutic efficacy in this population is therefore challenging. Despite this potential for background 'noise' and the limited studies in a still developing field, we found encouraging results with implications for clinical practice. Namely, significant cognitive gains were seen as a result of CT more than one-year post-injury when spontaneous neurological recovery is assumed to have stabilized. It is encouraging to see that there may be a possible link between training intensity and overall efficacy, but further studies with larger sample sizes and more heterogeneous populations are required to explore this relationship. Small samples and lack of power have meant that the effectiveness of CT in TBI has been inconclusive in individual studies - this is precisely the condition when a meta-analysis can add value and clarity to a field (Borenstein et al., 2009). This meta-analysis thereby provides evidence that CT may be modestly effective in promoting cognitive and functional gains in everyday life. Accordingly, further investigation of different approaches to CT is required along with health economic analyses of the costs and benefits of CT for post-acute TBI.

AUTHOR CONTRIBUTIONS

HH, DC, KD and MV: Design and/or conceptualization of the study. HH, DC, JF, AL and MV: Analysis and/or interpretation of the data. HH, DC, KD, JF, AL and MV: Drafting and/or revising the manuscript.

REFERENCES

Ardila, A. (2013). There are two different dysexecutive syndromes. *J. Neurol. Disord.* 1, 1–4. doi: 10.4172/2329-6895.1000114

Bahar-Fuchs, A., Clare, L., and Woods, B. (2013). Cognitive training and cognitive rehabilitation for mild to moderate Alzheimer's disease and vascular dementia. *Cochrane Database Syst. Rev.* 6, CD003260. doi: 10.1002/14651858.CD003260.pub2

Baribeau, J., Ethier, M., and Braun, C. (1989). A neurophysiological assessment of selective attention before and after cognitive remediation in patients with severe closed head injury. *J. Neurol. Rehabil.* 3, 71–92.

Barnett, S. M., and Ceci, S. J. (2002). When and where do we apply what we learn? A taxonomy for far transfer. *Psychol. Bull.* 128, 612–637. doi: 10.1037/0033-2909.128.4.612

Bayley, M. T., Tate, R., Douglas, J. M., Turkstra, L. S., Ponsford, J., Stergiou-Kita, M., et al. (2014). Incog guidelines for cognitive rehabilitation following traumatic brain injury: methods and overview. *J. Head Trauma Rehabil.* 29, 290–306. doi: 10.1097/HTR.0000000000000070

Borenstein, M., Hedges, L., Higgins, J. P., and Rothstein, H. R. (2009). *Introduction to Meta-Analysis*. Chichester: Wiley.

Buschert, V., Bokde, A. L., and Hampel, H. (2010). Cognitive intervention in Alzheimer disease. *Nat. Rev. Neurol.* 6, 508–517. doi: 10.1038/nrneurol.2010.113

Cantor, J., Ashman, T., Dams-O'connor, K., Dijkers, M. P., Gordon, W., Spielman, L., et al. (2014). Evaluation of the short-term executive plus intervention for executive dysfunction after traumatic brain injury: a randomized controlled trial with minimization. *Arch. Phys. Med. Rehabil.* 95, 1.e–9.e. doi: 10.1016/j.apmr.2013.08.005

Cicerone, K. D., Dahlberg, C., Malec, J. F., Langenbahn, D. M., Felicetti, T., Kneipp, S., et al. (2005). Evidence-based cognitive rehabilitation: updated review of the literature from 1998 through 2002. *Arch. Phys. Med. Rehabil.* 86, 1681–1692. doi: 10.1016/j.apmr.2005.03.024

Cicerone, K. D., Langenbahn, D. M., Braden, C., Malec, J. F., Kalmar, K., Fraas, M., et al. (2011). Evidence-based cognitive rehabilitation: updated review of the literature from 2003 through 2008. *Arch. Phys. Med. Rehabil.* 92, 519–530. doi: 10.1016/j.apmr.2010.11.015

Clare, L., Woods, R. T., Moniz Cook, E. D., Orrell, M., and Spector, A. (2003). Cognitive rehabilitation and cognitive training for early-stage Alzheimer's disease and vascular dementia. *Cochrane Database Syst. Rev.* 4:CD003260.

Colantonio, A., Ratcliff, G., Chase, S., Kelsey, S., Escobar, M., and Vernich, L. (2004). Long-term outcomes after moderate to severe traumatic brain injury. *Disabil. Rehabil.* 26, 253–261. doi: 10.1080/09638280310001639722

Dawson, D. R., Binns, M. A., Hunt, A., Lemsky, C., and Polatajko, H. J. (2013). Occupation-based strategy training for adults with traumatic brain injury: a pilot study. *Arch. Phys. Med. Rehabil.* 94, 1959–1963. doi: 10.1016/j.apmr.2013.05.021

Dikmen, S. S., Corrigan, J. D., Levin, H. S., Machamer, J., Stiers, W., and Weisskopf, M. G. (2009). Cognitive outcome following traumatic brain injury. *J. Head Trauma Rehabil.* 24, 430–438. doi: 10.1097/HTR.0b013e3181c133e9

Duval, S., and Tweedie, R. (2000). Trim and fill: a simple funnel-plot-based method of testing and adjusting for publication bias in meta-analysis. *Biometrics* 56, 455–463. doi: 10.1111/j.0006-341X.2000.00455.x

Edwards, J., Wadley, V., Myers, R., Roenker, D. L., Cissell, G., and Ball, K. (2002). Transfer of a speed of processing intervention to near and far cognitive functions. *Gerontology* 48, 329–340. doi: 10.1159/000065259

Egger, M., Davey Smith, G., Schneider, M., and Minder, C. (1997). Bias in meta-analysis detected by a simple, graphical test. *BMJ* 315:629. doi: 10.1136/bmj.315.7109.629

Gates, N., and Valenzuela, M. J. (2010). Cognitive exercise and its role in cogitive function in older adults. *Curr. Psychiatry Rep.* 12, 20–27. doi: 10.1007/s11920-009-0085-y

Gleser, L. J., and Olkin, I. (2009). "Stochastically dependent effect sizes," in *The Handbook of Research Synthesis and Meta-Analysis*, 2nd Edn, eds H. Cooper, L. Hedges, and J. Valentine (New York, NY: Russell Sage Foundation).

Goranson, T. E., Graves, R. E., Allison, D., and La Freniere, R. (2003). Community integration following multidisciplinary rehabilitation for traumatic brain injury. *Brain Injury* 17, 759–774. doi: 10.1080/0269905031000088513

Gordon, W. A., Zafonte, R., Cicerone, K., Cantor, J., Brown, M., Lombard, L., et al. (2006). Traumatic brain injury rehabilitation: state of the science. *Am. J. Phys. Med. Rehabil.* 85, 343–382. doi: 10.1097/01.phm.0000202106.01654.61

Higgins, J., and Green, S. (eds) (2011). *Cochrane Handbook for Systematic Reviews of Interventions Version 5.1.0: The Cochrane Collaboration.* Available at: http://www.cochrane-handbook.org [accessed Nov 14, 2011]

Higgins, J. P., Thompson, S. G., Deeks, J. J., and Altman, D. G. (2003). Measuring inconsistency in meta-analyses. *BMJ* 327:557. doi: 10.1136/bmj.327.7414.557

Lampit, A., Hallock, H., and Valenzuela, M. (2014). Computerized cognitive training in cognitively healthy older adults: a systematic review and meta-analysis of effect modifiers. *PLoS Med.* 11:e1001756. doi: 10.1371/journal.pmed.1001756

Leung, I. H. K., Walton, C. C., Hallock, H., Lewis, S. J. G., Valenzuela, M., and Lampit, A. (2015). Cognitive training in Parkinson disease: a systematic review and meta-analysis. *Neurology* 85, 1843–1851. doi: 10.1212/WNL.0000000000002145

Liberati, A., Altman, D. G., Tetzlaff, J., Mulrow, C., Gotzsche, P. C., Ioannidis, J. P., et al. (2009). The Prisma statement for reporting systematic reviews and meta-analyses of studies that evaluate healthcare interventions: explanation and elaboration. *BMJ* 339:b2700. doi: 10.1136/bmj.b2700

Lu, J., Gary, K. W., Neimeier, J. P., Ward, J., and Lapane, K. L. (2012). Randomized controlled trials in adult traumatic brain injury. *Brain Inj.* 26, 1523–1548. doi: 10.3109/02699052.2012.722257

Maher, C. G., Sherrington, C., Herbert, R. D., Moseley, A. M., and Elkins, M. (2003). Reliability of the Pedro scale for rating quality of randomized controlled trials. *Phys. Ther.* 83, 713–721.

Marshall, G. A., Rentz, D. M., Frey, M. T., Locascio, J. J., Johnson, K. A., and Sperling, R. A. (2011). Executive function and instrumental activities of daily living in MCI and AD. *Alzheimers Dement.* 7, 300–308. doi: 10.1016/j.jalz.2010.04.005

Nelson, L. A., Macdonald, M., Stall, C., and Pazdan, R. (2013). Effects of interactive metronome therapy on cognitive functioning after blast-related brain injury: a randomized controlled pilot trial. *Neuropsychology* 27, 666–679. doi: 10.1037/a0034117

O'Neil-Pirozzi, T. M., Strangman, G. E., Goldstein, R., Katz, D. I., Savage, C. R., Kelkar, K., et al. (2010). A controlled treatment study of internal memory strategies (I-Mems) following traumatic brain injury. *J. Head Trauma Rehabil.* 25, 43–51. doi: 10.1097/HTR.0b013e3181bf24b1

Pa, J., Boxer, A., Chao, L. L., Gazzaley, A., Freeman, K., Kramer, J., et al. (2009). Clinical-neuroimaging characteristics of dysexecutive mild cognitive impairment. *Ann. Neurol.* 65, 414–423. doi: 10.1002/ana.21591

Potvin, M. J., Rouleau, I., Senechal, G., and Giguere, J. F. (2011). Prospective memory rehabilitation based on visual imagery techniques. *Neuropsychol. Rehabil.* 21, 899–924. doi: 10.1080/09602011.2011.630882

Povlishock, J. T., and Katz, D. I. (2005). Update of neuropathology and neurological recovery after traumatic brain injury. *J. Head Trauma Rehabil.* 20, 76–94. doi: 10.1097/00001199-200501000-00008

Rao, V., and Lyketsos, C. (2000). Neuropsychiatric sequelae of traumatic brain injury. *Psychosomatics* 41, 95–103. doi: 10.1176/appi.psy.41.2.95

Rattok, J., Ross, B., Ben-Yishay, Y., Ezrachi, O., Silver, S., Lakin, P., et al. (1992). Outcome of different treatment mixes in a multidimensional neuropsychological rehabilitation program. *Neuropsychology* 6, 395–415. doi: 10.1037/0894-4105.6.4.395

Rees, L., Marshall, S., Hartridge, C., Mackie, D., and Weiser, M. (2007). Cognitive interventions post acquired brain injury. *Brain Inj.* 21, 161–200. doi: 10.1080/02699050701201813

Rice-Oxley, M., and Turner-Stokes, L. (1999). Effectiveness of brain injury rehabilitation. *Clin. Rehabil.* 13(Suppl. 1), 7–24. doi: 10.1191/026921599668051623

Rohling, M. L., Faust, M. E., Beverly, B., and Demakis, G. (2009). Effectiveness of cognitive rehabilitation following acquired brain injury: a meta-analytic re-examination of Cicerone et al.'s (2000, 2005) systematic reviews. *Neuropsychology* 23, 20–39. doi: 10.1037/a0013659

Ruff, R. M., Baser, C. A., Johnston, J. W., Marshall, L. F., Klauber, S. K., Klauber, M. R., et al. (1989). Neuropsychological rehabilitation: an experimental study with head-injured patients. *J. Head Trauma Rehabil.* 4, 20–36. doi: 10.1097/00001199-198909000-00006

Ryan, T. V., and Ruff, R. M. (1988). The efficacy of structured memory retraining in a group comparison of head trauma patients. *Arch. Clin. Neuropsychol.* 3, 165–179. doi: 10.1016/0887-6177(88)90061-3

Skandsen, T., Finnanger, T. G., Andersson, S., Lydersen, S., Brunner, J. F., and Vik, A. (2010). Cognitive impairment 3 months after moderate, and severe traumatic brain injury: a prospective follow-up study. *Arch. Phys. Med. Rehabil.* 91, 1904–1913. doi: 10.1016/j.apmr.2010.08.021

Sohlberg, M. M., and Mateer, C. A. (2001). *Cognitive Rehabilitation: An Integrative Neuropsychological Approach.* New York, NY: The Guilford Press.

Sterne, J. A., Sutton, A. J., Ioannidis, J. P., Terrin, N., Jones, D. R., Lau, J., et al. (2011). Recommendations for examining and interpreting funnel plot asymmetry in meta-analyses of randomised controlled trials. *BMJ* 343:d4002. doi: 10.1136/bmj.d4002

Strauss, S., Sherman, E., and Spreen, O. (2006). *A compendium of Neuropsychological Tests: Administration, Norms and Commentary.* Oxford: Oxford University Press.

Thomas-Stonell, N., Johnson, P., Schuller, R., and Jutai, J. (1994). Evaluation of a computer-based program for remediation of cognitive-communication skills. *J. Head Trauma Rehabil.* 9, 25–37. doi: 10.1097/00001199-199412000-00005

Tiersky, L. A., Anselmi, V., Johnston, M. V., Kurtyka, J., Roosen, E., Schwartz, T., et al. (2005). A trial of neuropsychologic rehabilitation in mild-spectrum traumatic brain injury. *Arch. Phys. Med. Rehabil.* 86, 1565–1574. doi: 10.1016/j.apmr.2005.03.013

Toril, P., Reales, J. M., and Ballesteros, S. (2014). Video game training enhances cognition of older adults: a meta-analytic study. *Psychol. Aging* 29, 706–716. doi: 10.1037/a0037507

Twamley, E. W., Jak, A. J., Delis, D. C., Bondi, M. W., and Lohr, J. B. (2014). Cognitive symptom management and rehabilitation therapy (cogSMART) for veterans with traumatic brain injury: pilot randomized controlled trial. *J. Rehabil. Res. Dev.* 51, 59–70. doi: 10.1682/JRRD.2013.01.0020

Vas, A. K., Chapman, S. B., Cook, L. G., Elliott, A. C., and Keebler, M. (2011). Higher-order reasoning training years after traumatic brain injury in adults. *J. Head Trauma Rehabil.* 26, 224–239. doi: 10.1097/HTR.0b013e318218dd3d

Wai-Kwong Man, D., Soong, W. Y. L., Tam, S. F., and Hui-Chan, C. W. Y. (2006). Development and evaluation of a pictorial-based analogical problem-solving programme for people with traumatic brain injury. *Brain Inj.* 20, 981–990. doi: 10.1080/13561820600909852

Wilson, M., Zolfaghari, P., Griffin, C., Lockey, D., Tolias, C., and Verma, V. (2014). The future of traumatic brain injury research. *Scand. J. Trauma Resusc. Emerg. Med.* 22(Suppl. 1):A7. doi: 10.1186/1757-7241-22-S1-A7

Wykes, T., Huddy, V., Cellard, C., Mcgurk, S. R., and Czobor, P. (2011). A meta-analysis of cognitive remediation for schizophrenia: methodology and effect sizes. *Am. J. Psychiatry* 168, 472–485. doi: 10.1176/appi.ajp.2010.10060855

5

Aerobic Exercise as a Tool to Improve Hippocampal Plasticity and Function in Humans: Practical Implications for Mental Health Treatment

Aaron Kandola[1,2], Joshua Hendrikse[1], Paul J. Lucassen[3] and Murat Yücel[1]**

[1] Brain and Mental Health Lab, School of Psychological Sciences and Monash Institute of Cognitive and Clinical Neurosciences, Monash University, Melbourne, VIC, Australia, [2] Amsterdam Brain and Cognition, University of Amsterdam, Amsterdam, Netherlands, [3] Centre for Neuroscience, Swammerdam Institute of Life Sciences, University of Amsterdam, Amsterdam, Netherlands

Edited by:
Claudia Voelcker-Rehage,
Chemnitz University of Technology,
Germany

Reviewed by:
Yvonne Nolan,
University College Cork, Ireland
Dieter J. Meyerhoff,
University of California,
San Francisco, USA

***Correspondence:**
Aaron Kandola
aaron.kandola@gmail.com
Murat Yücel
murat.yucel@monash.edu

Aerobic exercise (AE) has been widely praised for its potential benefits to cognition and overall brain and mental health. In particular, AE has a potent impact on promoting the function of the hippocampus and stimulating neuroplasticity. As the evidence-base rapidly builds, and given most of the supporting work can be readily translated from animal models to humans, the potential for AE to be applied as a therapeutic or adjunctive intervention for a range of human conditions appears ever more promising. Notably, many psychiatric and neurological disorders have been associated with hippocampal dysfunction, which may underlie the expression of certain symptoms common to these disorders, including (aspects of) cognitive dysfunction. Augmenting existing treatment approaches using AE based interventions may promote hippocampal function and alleviate cognitive deficits in various psychiatric disorders that currently remain untreated. Incorporating non-pharmacological interventions into clinical treatment may also have a number of other benefits to patient well being, such as limiting the risk of adverse side effects. This review incorporates both animal and human literature to comprehensively detail how AE is associated with cognitive enhancements and stimulates a cascade of neuroplastic mechanisms that support improvements in hippocampal functioning. Using the examples of schizophrenia and major depressive disorder, the utility and implementation of an AE intervention to the clinical domain will be proposed, aimed to reduce cognitive deficits in these, and related disorders.

Keywords: aerobic fitness, hippocampus, plasticity, schizophrenia, depression, dementia, memory, neurogenesis

INTRODUCTION

The brain is continuously balancing two conflicting demands: it must retain enough structural integrity to maintain proper neurotransmission, and function efficiently, whilst remaining malleable enough to restructure itself and adapt to changing environmental demands. The dynamic nature of the brain is underpinned by the concept of neuroplasticity, which refers to the brains capacity to change and reorganize itself in response to internal and/or external influences. The impact and eventual consequences of brain plasticity can be twofold; i.e., these influences can be adaptive, such as during skill learning, when they help the individual to survive, or can be maladaptive, when plasticity is insufficient to meet a specific demand, which may then contribute toward disease conditions.

To some extent, brain disorders can be considered maladies of neuroplasticity (Krystal et al., 2009). As such, stimulating neuroplasticity is becoming a popular approach aimed to counteract pathological harm (Kays et al., 2012). Interestingly, a stimulus as peripheral as aerobic exercise (AE) has been demonstrated to have a strong influence on inducing neuroplasticity (Voss et al., 2013a) and promoting cognitive performance (Smith et al., 2010). Given its general benefits to ones physical health, low risk profile and relative ease of implementation, AE represents a promising therapeutic target for a range of brain pathologies.

One brain region with a high degree of endogenous neuroplasticity is the hippocampus (Bavelier and Neville, 2002). The hippocampus is heavily involved in learning and memory processes and is particularly vulnerable to damage in various pathological conditions like major depressive disorder (MDD), Alzheimer's disease and schizophrenia (Adriano et al., 2012; Bartsch and Wulff, 2015; Schmaal et al., 2016). Conversely, the positive influence of AE on neuroplasticity is more pronounced within the hippocampus than in any other brain region (Gomez-Pinilla and Hillman, 2013). AE has been suggested as a promising approach in remediating hippocampal harm and cognitive deficits caused by neurodegenerative disorders like AD (Intlekofer and Cotman, 2013), but AE may also be a promising approach for various psychiatric disorders like schizophrenia or MDD (Oertel-Knöchel et al., 2014).

This paper will review the cognitive benefits associated with AE and focus on aspects of cognition that are particularly dependent hippocampal functioning such as episodic memory formation. We further discuss the capacity of AE to stimulate macro- and micro-scale neuroplastic mechanisms relating to hippocampal functioning. Finally, we address the suitability of AE to be used as a novel therapeutic intervention for psychiatric disorders. Both schizophrenia and MDD are associated with hippocampal deterioration and cognitive dysfunctions, so we take these two conditions as examples to discuss the potential utility of AE-based interventions.

EXERCISE AND COGNITION

The interest in how AE influences cognitive performance has exploded in the past decade. AE generally refers to exercise that improve the efficiency of aerobic energy producing systems by increasing maximal oxygen uptake and cardiorespiratory endurance (Voss et al., 2013a). Large-scale epidemiological studies have consistently correlated high levels of aerobic fitness with greater academic achievement and IQ scores (Sibley and Etnier, 2003; Tomporowski et al., 2008, 2014; Howie and Pate, 2012) as well as with a greater preservation of cognitive function in old age (Yaffe et al., 2001; Barnes et al., 2003; Middleton et al., 2008; Wendell et al., 2014) and fewer incidences of dementia (Hamer and Chida, 2009). The capacity to promote cognitive performance in this way implies that AE may have an important clinical relevance in counteracting the cognitive decline associated with aging or dementia (Kramer et al., 2006) and has catalyzed its systematic investigation. Many randomized controlled trials (RCTs) have now been conducted using AE interventions of a moderate intensity (such as 30 min of Nordic walking) that generally span for 3–12 months and are mostly conducted in older adults. Meta-analyses have found AE interventions to improve cognitive performance across a variety of domains, including attention, executive functioning, processing speed, motor functioning, and memory in healthy young and middle aged adults (Etnier et al., 1997; Smith et al., 2010; Chang et al., 2012; Roig et al., 2013; Verburgh et al., 2013) but mostly in older age groups (Etnier et al., 1997; Colcombe and Kramer, 2003; Angevaren et al., 2008; van Uffelen et al., 2008; Smith et al., 2010; Snowden et al., 2011; Chang et al., 2012), as well as in older individuals with mild cognitive impairments or dementia (Heyn et al., 2004; van Uffelen et al., 2008; Gates et al., 2013).

The available evidence strongly suggests that AE has a positive influence on cognition in individuals of all age groups, particularly in older adults. However, the exact nature of how AE impacts upon cognition is not yet clear. Some RCTs have stipulated that AE influences divergent cognitive domains, whereas others have suggested AE had no significant impact on cognition at all (Etnier et al., 2006; van Uffelen et al., 2008; Snowden et al., 2011; Gates et al., 2013; Kelly et al., 2014; Young et al., 2015). Such inconsistencies may partially be explained by the methodological variation between RCTs, making it difficult to systematically compare their findings in meta-analyses (Angevaren et al., 2008; Young et al., 2015).

On a neural level, findings have been consistent in demonstrating that AE has a strong, positive influence on the structure of the hippocampus, which is not seen to the same extent in any other brain regions (Gomez-Pinilla and Hillman, 2013). As will be discussed below, it has been extensively demonstrated in animal models that AE stimulates a cascade of neuroplastic mechanisms within the hippocampus that are often paralleled by functional improvements (Voss et al., 2013a; Opendak and Gould, 2015). A large cohort of animal studies have assessed the functional impact of AE using tasks designed to specifically assess hippocampus dependent processing such as spatial (Vaynman et al., 2004) or contextual memory (Radak et al., 2006). Using hippocampus dependent paradigms, AE has been reliably demonstrated to improve task performance in animal models (van Praag, 2009; Voss et al., 2013a), although this does also depend on others aspects of AE such as the duration and intensity of AE (Naylor et al., 2005; Ploughman et al., 2007; O'Callaghan et al., 2009).

Until recently, human studies had primarily focussed on examining the impact of AE on performance in frontal-executive or attentional tasks rather than on specific hippocampus dependent forms of cognition (Ruscheweyh et al., 2011). It is possible that this may have contributed toward the inconsistent findings when investigating the effect of AE on human cognition. Based on the profound impact of AE on the hippocampus, this bottom-up focus on hippocampus dependent processing may also be a useful approach in specifying the impact of AE on human cognition and will be adopted here.

A Hippocampus-Centric Approach

The hippocampus plays an important role in both learning and memory (Jarrard, 1993) and affective processing (Phillips et al., 2003). The dichotomous functioning of the hippocampus is thought to be reflected in its structure, with affective processing being largely attributed to the ventral hippocampus and learning and memory processes mostly occurring through the dorsal hippocampus (Moser and Moser, 1998). Given that cognition is a central theme of this paper, the following sections will predominantly focus on the role of the hippocampus in learning and memory processing.

Several meta-analyses have denoted the tendency for RCTs to report improvements in memory-based task performance following an AE intervention (Colcombe and Kramer, 2003; van Uffelen et al., 2008; Smith et al., 2010; Chang et al., 2012; Roig et al., 2013). However, some domains of memory are more reliant on hippocampal functioning than others (see **Box 1**) and therefore, it is possible that the most consistent cognitive improvements may be found in these specific domains of memory.

Some human studies have focussed on assessing the influence of AE on hippocampus dependent cognition and shown in older adults that AE was associated with improved performances in both episodic (Richards et al., 2003; Stewart et al., 2003; Sabia et al., 2009; Flöel et al., 2010; Ruscheweyh et al., 2011) and spatial (Erickson and Kramer, 2009; Erickson et al., 2010, 2011) memory tasks as well as in pattern separation tasks in young adults (Déry et al., 2013). Moreover, some studies have demonstrated in preadolescent children and young adults that AE is selectively associated with improved performances on contextual (Chaddock et al., 2010, 2011; Monti et al., 2012) and spatial (Stroth et al., 2009; Herting and Nagel, 2012) memory tasks and not with less hippocampus dependent tasks such as attention, verbal memory, or item recognition tasks.

Despite a limited selection of studies, these findings indicate that AE may have a positive influence on hippocampus dependent forms of cognition in healthy human participants, similar to what has been consistently shown in animal models. Pertaining to its highly neuroplastic nature (Bavelier and Neville, 2002), the hippocampus is particularly vulnerable to structural and functional deterioration in a wide range of neurological and psychiatric disorders (Bartsch and Wulff, 2015). The aforementioned studies demonstrate that AE could have a positive influence on hippocampal functioning, but a significantly greater cohort of systematic investigations using human participants will be necessary to outline this relationship on a broader cognitive level. A growing body of evidence is also accumulating to suggest that AE may have a prominent impact on hippocampal structure in humans as well as in animal models. The following sections will first discuss the relationship between AE and gross structural changes related to the hippocampus in humans. We will then discuss both animal and human work, which indicates that these structural changes may be driven by a cascade of micro-scale neuroplastic mechanisms within the hippocampus that are stimulated by AE.

BOX 1 | Hippocampus dependent memory. The human hippocampus plays a vital role in the formation of declarative memories, most prominently of which, in the formation of episodic and spatiotemporal memories (Burgess et al., 2002). Episodic memory refers to the recollection of autobiographical events and is related to spatial memory, which refers to one's environment and spatial orientation. Spatial and episodic memory processes are inherently related given their specific reliance on the hippocampus (Bird and Burgess, 2008) and the fact that episodic memories are encoded in a spatio-temporal context (Tulving, 1993), making spatial information important in episodic memory formation. Also, the hippocampus, and particularly the DG, is crucial in selecting and separating similar events in space and time, and hence pattern separation is a main function attributed to the hippocampus (Yassa and Stark, 2011; Oomen et al., 2013, 2014). It is important to note that given the requirement of a conscious experience to form an episodic memory, at present episodic memory cannot be directly studied in animals given the lack of behavioral markers for their conscious experience (Clayton et al., 2001). Contextual memory is a process strongly related to episodic memory that is also highly dependent on the hippocampus and refers to the capacity for an animal to make associations with salient landmark objects and their environmental context (Eichenbaum et al., 2005). As there is currently no objective proxy for studying episodic-like memory processing in animals (Templer and Hampton, 2013), hippocampal functioning shall be considered here as a function of contextual and spatial memory task performance when referring to animal literature and episodic and spatial memory task performance in human literature.

MACRO-SCALE CHANGES

Directly studying structural changes in the human brain *in vivo* is currently limited to the use of neuroimaging techniques, like magnetic resonance imaging (MRI), to detect macro-scale changes such as in grey-matter volume or white-matter integrity.

Gray-Matter

A number of cross-sectional studies have used both voxel-based morphometric (VBM) and region of interest (ROI) techniques on structural MRI data to estimate volume changes associated with AE. Higher levels of aerobic fitness have been consistently associated with larger hippocampal or temporal lobe volumes in healthy adolescent (Chaddock et al., 2010) and older adults (Colcombe et al., 2003; Bugg and Head, 2011; Head et al., 2012; Niemann et al., 2014). Several studies have also shown that hippocampal growth induced by AE correlates with a greater performance on spatial memory tasks such as a virtual Morris Water Maze task (Erickson and Kramer, 2009; Szabo et al., 2011; Herting and Nagel, 2012) and on contextual memory tasks (Chaddock et al., 2010) with correlations ranging from $r = 0.12$ to $r = 0.36$. Cross-sectional data has also indicated that AE may also be beneficial to non-healthy individuals as higher levels of aerobic fitness have also been correlated with larger hippocampal volumes in patients with obesity (Bugg et al., 2012), anorexia (Beadle et al., 2015), mild cognitive impairments (Gates et al., 2013; Makizako et al., 2014), MDD (Travis et al., 2015),

Alzheimer's disease (Honea et al., 2009), and multiple sclerosis (Prakash et al., 2010; Motl et al., 2015).

Several RCTs have extended upon these findings in healthy and non-healthy samples, which have mostly implemented AE interventions of a moderate intensity for 3–12 months. RCTs in healthy samples have demonstrated that AE interventions were associated with increases in hippocampal volume in young and middle aged (Thomas et al., 2016) and older adults (Colcombe et al., 2006; Erickson et al., 2011; Niemann et al., 2014; Kleemeyer et al., 2015; Maass et al., 2015; Sexton et al., 2015a). In some cases the AE induced growth in hippocampal volume was correlated with improved performances on a computerized spatial memory task ($r = 0.28$; Erickson et al., 2011) or on a complex figure test of spatial object recognition ($r = 0.37$; Maass et al., 2015). AE interventions have also been shown to increase hippocampal volume in patients with mild cognitive impairments (ten Brinke et al., 2015), schizophrenia (Pajonk et al., 2010), and multiple sclerosis (Leavitt et al., 2014). While some RCTs have found that AE did not have an impact on hippocampal volume (Ruscheweyh et al., 2011; Scheewe et al., 2013; Krogh et al., 2014; Rosenbaum et al., 2015; Malchow et al., 2016), it is possible that such discrepancies are caused by a lack of consistency in AE protocols used (Prakash et al., 2015) or in the methods of calculating hippocampal volume (Niemann et al., 2014).

White-Matter

The majority of the current literature has focussed on assessing gray-matter changes, but some studies have investigated the impact of AE on white-matter integrity. A recent systematic review concluded that AE was associated with global and localized improvements in white-matter volume and microstructural integrity in older adults (Sexton et al., 2015b). It would be reasonable to expect AE to have a specific impact on hippocampal connectivity, but such findings were not supported in this review (Sexton et al., 2015b). However, some studies have found AE to be associated with greater white-matter volume in the temporal lobes that surround the hippocampus in older adults (Colcombe et al., 2003, 2006; Tseng et al., 2013; Burzynska et al., 2014). In addition, one RCT that assessed a 12-month AE intervention did demonstrate that greater changes in aerobic fitness were associated with greater improvements in temporal lobe white-matter integrity in healthy, older adults (Voss et al., 2013b). White-matter alterations may also occur in non-healthy individuals as one recent RCT demonstrated a 6-month AE intervention to improve global white-matter integrity in patients with schizophrenia (Svatkova et al., 2015).

Structural Benefits of AE

There is a growing cohort of evidence to suggest that AE is associated with increases in hippocampal gray-matter volume in both healthy and non-healthy individuals (Hötting and Röder, 2013; Hamilton and Rhodes, 2015), and with increases in hippocampal microstructural integrity (Kleemeyer et al., 2015). In some cases, these AE-induced gray-matter changes have been directly correlated with improvements in hippocampal functioning (Prakash et al., 2015). AE appears to have a beneficial impact on global white-matter integrity (Sexton et al., 2015b) and potentially on hippocampal connectivity.

These studies support the idea that AE may be beneficial to hippocampal integrity but it is important to note that these human imaging techniques may only directly assess macro-scale changes and not the functional changes or biological mechanisms that may underlie these changes. Without information relating to the specific substrates underlying changes in tissue composition, it is difficult to determine the exact functional significance of a change in volume (Czéh and Lucassen, 2007; Thomas et al., 2012; Biedermann et al., 2016). For example, volume growth could be driven by a regional increase in dendritic length or density, but it could also be driven by changes that are likely to be less functionally relevant, such as expanding interstitial space between cells or changes in relative water distributions. Alternatively, increases in the proliferation of stem cells, glia, or the birth of new neurons that are added to existing hippocampal circuitry could also influence hippocampal volume over time. Furthermore, the additional energy demands from new neurons or synaptic changes may also require greater metabolic support. This could induce gliogenesis or changes in vasculature, i.e., angiogenesis, that may further contribute to fluctuations in volume (Anderson, 2011). In many respects, such structural adaptations resemble some of the opposite changes seen after exposure to (chronic) stress, that are generally associated with hippocampal volume reductions and represents a risk factor for depression (Czéh and Lucassen, 2007). Whether the same substrates underlie both the atrophy and the growth of a brain region is not clear and in principle, different mechanisms may be responsible for such opposing effects.

Micro-scale changes on a molecular or cellular level can be directly studied using histological approaches in animal models *in vivo*. Therefore, the following section will focus predominantly on animal literature to outline the micro-scale impact of AE on hippocampal neuroplasticity that may drive these macro-scale structural and functional improvements seen in human studies.

MICRO-SCALE CHANGES

Aerobic exercise has been linked to changes in a range of independent and interdependent mechanisms of neuroplasticity within the hippocampus (for comprehensive reviews, see: van Praag, 2009; Gomez-Pinilla and Hillman, 2013; Voss et al., 2013a; Bolijn and Lucassen, 2015; Opendak and Gould, 2015). Key mechanisms at both the cellular and molecular level will be discussed below in terms of their contribution to AE-induced enhancements in hippocampal functioning.

Neurogenesis

Adult neurogenesis is a form of structural hippocampal plasticity that refers to the process of stem cells forming new neurons within a few, distinct sub-regions of the adult brain. These stem cells undergo subsequent stages of proliferation, migration and neuronal differentiation, eventually producing adult-generated, fully functional, neurons that are well integrated into existing neural circuits (Kempermann et al., 2015). The subgranular zone of the hippocampal dentate gyrus (DG) is one of the just two primary locations where neurogenesis is known to occur in the adult rodent and human brain (Spalding et al., 2013; Kempermann et al., 2015). AE increases the rate of hippocampal neurogenesis, i.e., both the rate of cell proliferation as well as the survival of newborn granule cells (Cotman et al., 2007; Kempermann et al., 2010; Lucassen et al., 2010; Vivar et al., 2013) and despite being difficult to study in humans (Manganas et al., 2007; Ho et al., 2013; Jessberger and Gage, 2014), AE may also stimulate cell proliferation and DG volume growth in the human brain (Pereira et al., 2007; Erickson et al., 2011; Demirakca et al., 2014).

The proliferation of adult-born granule cells is thought to play an important role in hippocampal functioning (Deng et al., 2010; Oomen et al., 2014). It has been extensively demonstrated that the process of neurogenesis modifies the excitation of hippocampal neurons (Ikrar et al., 2013). Animal models have demonstrated that the inhibition or ablation of neurogenesis impairs performance on spatial and contextual memory tasks while improved performances on these tasks are seen when neurogenesis is stimulated (Deng et al., 2010; Snyder and Cameron, 2012; Aimone et al., 2014; Vadodaria and Jessberger, 2014; Kent et al., 2015). Furthermore, manipulating the rate of proliferation in rodents has been shown to selectively effect hippocampus dependent task performance, such as in spatial and contextual memory or pattern separation tasks, but not in tasks that are less hippocampus dependent, such as delay conditioning (Gould et al., 1999; Shors et al., 2002; Snyder et al., 2005, 2011; Deng et al., 2009; Sahay et al., 2011; Lucassen et al., 2013).

While there is still debate as to the exact role that adult-born granule cells play in hippocampal functioning, the process of neurogenesis forms a substrate for experience-dependent change (Opendak and Gould, 2015; Lucassen and Oomen, 2016), which has been implicated in fear and anxiety and depression like-behavior (Sahay and Hen, 2007; Besnard and Sahay, 2015; Lucassen et al., 2015; Hu et al., 2016). This primarily occurs through the role that neurogenesis plays in facilitating memory formation by dictating a computational mechanism known as *pattern separation* (Aimone et al., 2011; Sahay et al., 2011). Pattern separation is an essential mechanism for the DG to efficiently process and store sensory inputs to enable the formation of episodic, contextual or spatial memories (Lazarov and Hollands, 2016), and its importance in AE induced cognitive enhancement is epitomized by correlative studies that manipulate neurogenesis (Kent et al., 2015; Lucassen and Oomen, 2016). For example, inhibiting the rate of cell proliferation in mice was sufficient to impair pattern separation (Deng et al., 2010) and block AE-induced improvements in spatial (Clark et al., 2009) and contextual (Wojtowicz et al., 2008) memory performance, but only in conditions in which the task required fine spatial discriminations (i.e., where pattern separation was necessary; Creer et al., 2010). Therefore, AE may augment hippocampal memory formation by minimizing the interference between highly similar inputs through increasing the rate of cell proliferation (Déry et al., 2013).

While pattern separation is a popular example of DG function, adult-born granule cells have also been associated with a number of other theoretical DG frameworks important to memory formation that are not discussed here, such as memory resolution or encoding temporal context (see Aimone et al., 2014 for a comprehensive review). While neurogenesis is a crucial process to the spatiotemporal aspect of hippocampal functioning and is likely to be a key mediator of the hippocampal enhancement stimulated by AE (Cotman et al., 2007), more research is needed to elucidate the exact role that adult-born granule cells play in DG and general hippocampal functioning.

Stimulating neurogenesis and promoting DG function is one mechanism through which AE may promote hippocampal function and some recent findings suggest this mechanisms may be driving the macro-scale increases in hippocampal volume found in human imaging studies (Erickson et al., 2011; Fuss et al., 2014). However, AE also induces a variety of other neuroplastic mechanisms that work both independently and in tandem with neurogenesis to improve hippocampal functioning.

Synaptic Plasticity

Learning and memory is reliant upon the efficient communication between neural cells through their synapses and AE is thought to enhance this efficiency through promoting synaptic plasticity in a number of ways (Vivar et al., 2013), such as through facilitating long-term potentiation (LTP). LTP is one model of synaptic plasticity that refers to the strengthening of synaptic connections between neurons (Bliss and Collingridge, 1993). Forming an episodic memory involves the association of an event or feature with a particular location in space and occurs through this LTP mechanism in the hippocampus (Bannerman et al., 2014). AE has been demonstrated to stimulate LTP in young rodents and reverse the age-related decline of LTP within the DG of aged rodents compared to sedentary controls (van Praag, 2009; Voss et al., 2013a). Interestingly, these changes appear to be specific to the DG region and may be directly related to the stimulation of neurogenesis by AE (van Praag, 2008). Indeed, immature granule cells are particularly suited to participate in the learning process as they have a lower threshold for LTP induction (Schmidt-Hieber et al., 2004) and demonstrate enhanced LTP compared to surrounding mature granule cells (Lee S.W. et al., 2012). Being hypersensitive to influence on their synaptic plasticity has led to the idea that these adult-born granule cells mediate the enhancement of LTP in the DG from AE (Voss et al., 2013a).

Aerobic exercise has also been associated with certain morphological changes to the structure of neural cells, which may be important in facilitating hippocampal learning and memory (Lang et al., 2004). The dendrites of granule cells within the DG have been shown to increase in length, complexity, and spine density in response to AE (Eadie et al., 2005; Redila and Christie, 2006) as well as spine density in surrounding pyramidal cells of the entorhinal cortex and CA1 regions (Stranahan et al., 2007). AE also interacts with the glutamatergic system through increasing the expression of *N*-methyl-D-aspartic acid (NMDA) receptors in the hippocampus (specifically, both NR2A and NR2B subtypes), which contributes toward the synaptic plasticity of the region (Molteni et al., 2002; Farmer et al., 2004). These morphological changes are associated with higher rates of LTP induction and facilitate changes in dendritic strength (van Praag, 2008).

While certain morphological changes enhance synaptic plasticity within the CA1 and entorhinal cortex, AE seems to have a particularly potent impact on the granule cells of the DG. Through generating a greater influx of adult-born granule cells that have an enhanced propensity for LTP and fine-grained morphological changes, AE stimulates an environment within the hippocampus that promotes LTP and facilitates improvements in hippocampus-dependent cognition (Boecker et al., 2012).

Vasculature

Cerebral blood flow is important in providing oxygen and essential nutrients that facilitate brain functioning. Improving cerebral blood flow may be an important mediator of AE induced changes in hippocampal functioning (Christie et al., 2008). It has been demonstrated in animal models that AE stimulates the sprouting of new capillaries (angiogenesis) and improves vasculature within the hippocampus (Trejo et al., 2001; van Praag et al., 2005). This coincides with studies that have demonstrated a greater cerebral blood flow in the human hippocampus (Pereira et al., 2007; Burdette et al., 2010; Maass et al., 2015), some of which have correlated this increase with improved performance on episodic memory tasks (Pereira et al., 2007; Maass et al., 2015). The positive influence of improving vascularization may extend beyond a greater supply of oxygen and glucose through prompting the release of neurotrophic factors (the influence of which will be discussed below; Maass et al., 2015) or through facilitating other neuroplastic mechanisms like synaptic plasticity (Christie et al., 2008) or neurogenesis (Palmer et al., 2000; Pereira et al., 2007; Boecker et al., 2012; Bolijn and Lucassen, 2015; Biedermann et al., 2016). In fact, one recent human RCT found that the improvements in hippocampus dependent task performance and growth in hippocampal volume, which occurred following a 3-month AE intervention were predominantly attributable to a greater cerebral blood flow in the hippocampus (Maass et al., 2015). The authors suggested that these changes were either a direct consequence of vascularization or an indirect consequence of changes in synaptic plasticity or neurogenesis that were stimulated by the improvements in cerebral blood flow.

Quantifying the impact that changes in vasculature induced by AE have on hippocampal functioning is increasingly attracting attention, but the relative contribution of changes in vasculature is still in contention. For example, some animal models have suggested that angiogenesis may underlie improvements in spatial memory tasks independent of other neuroplastic mechanisms (van Praag et al., 2007; Kerr et al., 2010), whereas others have found improvements in spatial learning to be driven by neurogenesis with no influence at all from angiogenesis (van Praag et al., 2005). Changes in vasculature may indeed stimulate other neuroplastic mechanisms like synaptogenesis or neurogenesis and promote hippocampal tissue growth (Kleemeyer et al., 2015), but a greater investigation is required to outline the direct relationship between vascularization and enhancements in hippocampal functioning stimulated by AE (Davenport et al., 2012). Interestingly, AE is specifically associated with an increase the density of small, rather than large-diameter blood vessels in both humans (Bullitt et al., 2009) and animals (Bloor, 2005; Van der Borght et al., 2009). Increasing microvasculature density may be protective against white-matter hyperintensities, which itself may reduce gray-matter atrophy and cognitive dysfunction (Voss et al., 2013a). Therefore, in additional to promoting hippocampal function, the influence of AE on vasculature may also preserve structural integrity in the hippocampus and other regions of the brain.

On a cellular level, both animal and human literature has suggested that neurogenesis, synaptic plasticity and vascularization within the hippocampus represent the three primary neuroplastic mechanisms that are stimulated by AE to promote hippocampal functioning. These cellular changes are in turn influenced by a number of changes that occur on a molecular level in response to AE and the relevance of these molecular factors to hippocampal functioning will be considered below.

Neurotrophic Factors

Neurotrophins are important to the development and maintenance of functioning neural cells in the brain (Barbacid, 1995) and are likely to play a crucial role in mediating the impact of AE on hippocampal neuroplasticity and functioning (Cotman et al., 2007; Voss et al., 2013a; Bolijn and Lucassen, 2015). Brain-derived neurotrophic factor (BDNF) is a centrally produced neurotrophin of particular interest due to its high concentration within the hippocampus and its integral role in supporting neuronal survival and growth, and synaptic plasticity (Cotman et al., 2007; Cowansage et al., 2010). Animal models have shown AE to be associated with a region-specific up-regulation of BDNF in the hippocampus (Neeper et al., 1995; Marlatt et al., 2012; Uysal et al., 2015). Similarly, in human models AE has been associated with an increase in BDNF serum (Coelho et al., 2013) with some indication of this up-regulation occurring specifically within the hippocampus (Erickson et al., 2011; Voss et al., 2013a).

Brain-derived neurotrophic factor may be the most important factor that is upregulated by AE given its extensive involvement in both synaptic plasticity and neurogenesis (Cotman et al., 2007). The protein is thought to interact with energy metabolism to facilitate both pre- and post-synaptic mechanisms and the induction of LTP (Gomez-Pinilla and Hillman, 2013; Edelmann et al., 2014), as well as promoting the proliferation and survival of adult-born granule cells (Korol et al., 2013; Park and Poo, 2013). The importance of BDNF to hippocampal neuroplasticity is epitomized by animal studies, which have found that the manipulation of BDNF expression directly impacts upon performance in spatial and contextual memory tasks (Linnarsson et al., 1997; Alonso et al., 2002; Heldt et al., 2007; Peters et al., 2010), and also that the downregulation of BDNF inhibits AE induced improvements in spatial memory performance (Vaynman et al., 2004).

Recently, a number of human studies have also demonstrated that the increased BDNF serum levels associated with AE are directly correlated with improved performances in various domains of memory including on spatial memory tasks (Piepmeier and Etnier, 2015). In line with the molecules' interaction with neurogenesis and particularly high concentration within the DG subfield of the hippocampus (Farmer et al., 2004), BDNF may play an important role in pattern separation. Recent studies have shown that BDNF is required for the pattern separation to occur in memory encoding and consolidation, and specifically that BDNF acts on adult-born granule cells within the DG to facilitate pattern separation (Bekinschtein et al., 2013, 2014).

Vascular endothelial derived growth factor (VEGF) and insulin growth factor 1 (IGF-1) are growth factors that are produced peripherally and are implicated in both angiogenesis and neurogenesis (Gomez-Pinilla and Hillman, 2013). Human studies have shown that AE is associated with peripheral increases in VEGF and IGF-1 serum concentrations (Schobersberger et al., 2000; Llorens-Martín et al., 2010), and both molecules are known to cross the blood brain barrier and interact with hippocampal cells (Ding et al., 2006; Tang et al., 2010). VEGF is a hypoxia-inducible protein that stimulates angiogenesis (Krum et al., 2002). By facilitating vascularization in this way, particularly within the DG (Clark et al., 2009), the molecule also supports the AE induced stimulation of neurogenesis (Gomez-Pinilla and Hillman, 2013). Similarly, IGF-1 is known to support alterations in vascularization that are induced by AE (Lopez-Lopez et al., 2004) and promotes the proliferation and survival of newborn neural cells (Gomez-Pinilla and Hillman, 2013). Indeed, the inhibition of VEGF or IGF-1 has been demonstrated to impair the promotional impact of AE on the rate of neurogenesis (Trejo et al., 2001; Fabel et al., 2003; Ding et al., 2006) and spatial memory performance (Ding et al., 2006). Conversely, up-regulating either VEGF or IGF-1 can stimulate neurogenesis independently of AE (Aberg et al., 2000; Carro et al., 2000; Trejo et al., 2001; Cao et al., 2004).

While a number of other biochemical changes occur in response to AE (see Bolijn and Lucassen, 2015), BDNF, VEGF, and IGF-1 are considered to be key proteins upregulated by AE that induce hippocampal neuroplasticity. The important contribution that these neurotrophins make to the neuroplasticity induced by AE is underscored by animal models, which demonstrate their direct and significant impact on hippocampal functioning (Cotman et al., 2007; Llorens-Martín et al., 2010; Voss et al., 2013a; Piepmeier and Etnier, 2015). Subsequently, human studies are starting to take a step further than only assessing the impact of AE in terms of macro-scale structural changes by attempting to indirectly study underlying biological processes.

Inferring Micro-Scale Changes Using Human Imaging

An important approach has been to supplement volumetric changes with recordings of peripheral biomarkers as a proxy for measuring changes in neurotrophin regulation within the brain. Results using this approach have thus far have been mixed, with some AE studies findings a positive correlation between hippocampal volume or connectivity changes and serum concentrations of BDNF, VEGF, and IGF-1 (Erickson et al., 2011; Coelho et al., 2013; Voss et al., 2013b), while others have failed to replicate such findings (Maass et al., 2016).

Another promising approach has been to combine multimodal imaging techniques to estimate the micro-scale processes that underlie volumetric changes associated with AE. For example, one study demonstrated that AE stimulated hippocampal volume growth and then utilized a range of multi-modal MRI techniques to indirectly suggest that this growth may be supported by changes in myelination, rather than in vasculature (Thomas et al., 2016). Some studies have used diffusion tensor imaging (DTI) to demonstrate that the growth in hippocampal volume induced by AE is correlated with improvements in the microstructural integrity of hippocampal gray-matter, based on the assumption that a low mean diffusivity is indicative of an increased gray-matter tissue density (Kleemeyer et al., 2015). Another multimodal approach that is growing in popularity is the use of MR spectroscopy (MRS) to measure microscale changes in local metabolite composition. *N*-acetylaspartate (NAA) is a metabolite indicative of neuronal integrity and a number of AE studies have demonstrated that the growth in hippocampal volume (Pajonk et al., 2010; Erickson et al., 2012; Gonzales et al., 2013; Wagner et al., 2015) and in some cases, improvements in working memory performance (Erickson et al., 2011) are both correlated with higher concentrations of NAA. One of these studies found that an AE intervention led to a 2% decrease in hippocampal volume but the MRS data indicated there was no change in NAA (Wagner et al., 2015). Therefore, given the approximation that 50% of gray-matter is composed of neuropil (Thomas et al., 2012), the authors suggested that the volumetric decline is unlikely to have resulted from a loss of neurons (which would have been indicated by a lower NAA value) and may be due to other factors such as changes in glial cells (Wagner et al., 2015). This analysis and others (Dennis et al., 2015) illustrate the utility of using multimodal imaging such as MRI with MRS to assess the functional relevance of volumetric alterations that is not possible using one modality alone. Future research would benefit from adopting methods similar to those outlined above to aid in the translation between animal and human models and help provide a more comprehensive account detailing the impact of AE on the human brain.

Animal studies have demonstrated that AE stimulates a cascade of interdependent cellular and molecular mechanisms of neuroplasticity that mediate the associated enhancements in hippocampal functioning. In humans, AE is associated with increases in hippocampal volume and some indirect indicators of neuroplasticity (e.g., increased cerebral blood flow or BDNF serum concentration), which correlate with improved performances on hippocampus dependent tasks, indicative of an enhanced hippocampal functioning. These findings suggest that AE can stimulate hippocampal neuroplasticity and promote the regions functioning in humans in a similar way to that which has been demonstrated using animal models. Considerably more research will be necessary to substantiate this relationship and methods such as multimodal imaging and assessing peripheral biomarkers represent promising ways that future RCTs can help to bridge the gap between animal and human models. Based on the available evidence outlined above, AE does appear to have a highly beneficial impact on hippocampal integrity and the following sections will discuss whether AE thus represents a viable clinical intervention.

CLINICAL APPLICATION

The capacity for AE to induce neuroplastic changes that improve both hippocampal integrity and promote hippocampus dependent cognition may be of particularly clinical importance for two reasons. Firstly, a number of psychiatric and neurological disorders seem to have a particularly potent influence on hippocampal structure (Bartsch and Wulff, 2015) and its deterioration may underlie certain aspects of their symptomatology. Secondly, psychiatric symptoms can be dichotomously described as being either affective or cognitive in nature, yet a disproportionate amount of the current literature has exclusively focussed on ameliorating affective symptoms (Millan et al., 2012). Currently, no effective treatments have been developed to alleviate cognitive deficits associated with psychiatric or neurological disorders (Wallace et al., 2011; Keefe et al., 2013, 2014; Solé et al., 2015). Promoting neuroplastic changes that enhance hippocampal functioning may be useful in remediating certain domains of cognitive dysfunction (e.g., in learning and memory), which occur in disorders that have a particularly detrimental impact on hippocampal integrity. The efficacy of AE is already being investigated as a therapeutic intervention to counteract cognitive decline and deteriorating hippocampal integrity associated with aging or neurological disorders like dementia (Ahlskog et al., 2011). Comparatively little attention has been afforded to the potential application of AE in treating psychiatric disorders that have a similarly deleterious impact on the hippocampus and are associated with severe cognitive deficits. The following sections will outline the need to develop effective interventions that remediate cognitive symptoms, which can have a debilitating impact on psychiatric patients, using the examples of schizophrenia and MDD. The capacity for AE to aid in the alleviation of cognitive symptoms and improve the efficacy of current treatment will then be discussed in the context of both MDD and schizophrenia.

Cognitive Dysfunction in Psychiatric Disorders

Behaviors observed in animal models of anxiety/MDD have indicated that MDD can cause deficits in several areas of cognition, many of which are strongly related to hippocampal function (Darcet et al., 2016). A number of animal studies have shown models of anxiety/MDD to be associated with poorer performances on tasks of working memory (Mizoguchi et al., 2000; Henningsen et al., 2009) and attention (Baudin et al., 2012; Wilson et al., 2012; Wallace et al., 2014), as well as on tasks reliant on hippocampal functioning such as episodic-like memory (Orsetti et al., 2007; Baudin et al., 2012; Naninck et al., 2015) and spatial memory (Markham et al., 2010; Darcet et al., 2014). Similarly, human patients with MDD have consistently demonstrated clinically relevant deficits in domains of executive functioning, psychomotor speed, attention, and memory (McDermott and Ebmeier, 2009; Lee R.S. et al., 2012; McIntyre et al., 2013; Rock et al., 2013). Even after remission following successful antidepressant treatment, most patients continue to experience cognitive deficits, particularly within domains of executive function, memory, and attention (Hammar and Ardal, 2009; Bora et al., 2013; Rock et al., 2013; Popovic et al., 2015; Solé et al., 2015). Individuals with MDD who continue to experience these cognitive symptoms are more likely to relapse and display worse psychosocial functioning outcomes (Papakostas et al., 2008; Bortolato et al., 2016), which can impact their capacity to socialize or to function well at work (Jaeger et al., 2006; McIntyre et al., 2013). Consequentially, the importance of alleviating cognitive dysfunction to enhance the success of MDD treatment is increasingly being recognized (Solé et al., 2015; Bortolato et al., 2016).

The heterogeneity of schizophrenia makes the disorder extremely difficult to model in animals and most approaches have focussed on replicating certain groups of schizophrenia-like behaviors in animals (Nestler and Hyman, 2010). For example, disrupting NMDA receptors with phencyclidine (PCP) is known to produce a range of symptoms associated with schizophrenia (Nestler and Hyman, 2010) and has subsequently been shown to cause a number of cognitive deficits including in cognitive flexibility (Abdul-Monim et al., 2007), attention (Amitai et al., 2007) and episodic-like memory (Grayson et al., 2007; Nagai et al., 2009). Cognitive dysfunction in human patients with schizophrenia is rapidly being considered amongst the most debilitating aspects of schizophrenia (Nuechterlein et al., 2011) and the severity of cognitive dysfunction is a key determinant of the functional outcome following treatment (Goldberg and Green, 2002). Schizophrenia is associated with deficits in cognitive domains of executive functioning, processing speed, memory and attention (Mesholam-Gately et al., 2009; Keefe and Harvey, 2012). The persistence of these deficits has a significant impact on an individual's quality of life and ability to attain and maintain employment (Archer and Kostrzewa, 2015) making the amelioration of cognitive deficits a highly prioritized therapeutic goal in schizophrenia treatment (Malchow et al., 2013).

The Underlying Neuroplasticity of Cognitive Dysfunction

Both MDD and schizophrenia have a detrimental impact on neuroplasticity, particularly within the hippocampus. A reduced hippocampal volume is one of the most consistently reported structural abnormalities in patients of MDD (Schmaal et al., 2016) and of schizophrenia (Ellison-Wright and Bullmore, 2010; Adriano et al., 2012). In patients with schizophrenia, these hippocampal abnormalities have been correlated with deficits in memory (Gur et al., 2000) and aspects of executive functioning involving inhibitory control (Bilder et al., 1995; Szeszko et al., 2002), demonstrating the importance of hippocampal abnormalities to cognitive dysfunction. Both disorders seem to have a particularly deleterious impact on DG volume (Tamminga et al., 2010; Huang et al., 2013; Travis et al., 2015), which is reminiscent of the reduced level of neurogenesis found in animal models of both disorders (Eisch and Petrik, 2012; Lucassen et al., 2015; Allen et al., 2016). Schizophrenia and MDD also inhibit other important neuroplastic mechanisms such as synaptic plasticity (Law and Deakin, 2001; Kolomeets et al., 2007; Kobayashi, 2009; McEwen et al., 2012; Sanderson et al., 2012) and BDNF expression (Krishnan and Nestler, 2008; Green et al., 2011; Favalli et al., 2012) within the hippocampus. The inhibition of such key neuroplastic mechanisms in the hippocampus is likely to be an important factor contributing toward the cognitive deficits associated with MDD (Perera et al., 2008; Kaymak et al., 2010; Nagahara and Tuszynski, 2011; Turner et al., 2012) and schizophrenia (Ranganath et al., 2008; Schobel et al., 2009; Heckers and Konradi, 2010; Zhang et al., 2012).

Targeting neuroplasticity has recently become an important approach in treating psychiatric symptoms (Kays et al., 2012) and may be useful in counteracting this hippocampal harm to remediate cognitive deficits. For example, deficits in episodic memory have been consistently found in patients with MDD (McDermott and Ebmeier, 2009) and schizophrenia (Barch and Ceaser, 2012), and given the role of the hippocampus in episodic memory formation this may be somewhat attributable to its dysfunction. Indeed, aspects of hippocampal dysfunction such as a lower basal rate of neurogenesis are thought to inhibit one's capacity for pattern separation in patients with MDD (Déry et al., 2013; Shelton and Kirwan, 2013) or schizophrenia (Das et al., 2014) and the negative impact that this has on episodic memory formation may have broad implications for the symptomology of both disorders (Dere et al., 2010; Tamminga et al., 2010).

To illustrate this point, deficits in pattern separation could negatively influence one's capacity to correctly discriminate between stimuli and lead to a tendency for overgeneralization (Kheirbek et al., 2012; Shelton and Kirwan, 2013). The predisposition for individuals with MDD to make negative self-inferences coupled with the tendency to overgeneralize could result in negative overgeneralizations in the formation of episodic memories, which may contribute toward affective symptoms such as anhedonia (Eisch and Petrik, 2012; Shelton and Kirwan, 2013). In the case of schizophrenia, the added complication of a reduced synaptic connectivity between the DG and CA3 subfields (Kolomeets et al., 2007) to a lower basal rate of neurogenesis may contribute toward psychosis to some extent. Patients with schizophrenia show a disproportionately low level of pattern separation relative to pattern completion (Tamminga et al., 2010). Pattern completion is a complimentary process to pattern separation whereby through the activation of associative networks in the CA3 region, partial information can act as a recall cue to return the full representation of a previously stored memory (Nakashiba et al., 2012). It is possible that this overactivation of the pattern completion mechanism could lead to the inappropriate associations and representations causing the encoding or retrieval of false episodic memories with psychotic content (Tamminga et al., 2010; Das et al., 2014).

These two theoretical examples illustrate how hippocampal dysfunction in either disorder may disrupt the correct formation of episodic memories and potentially exasperate other psychiatric symptoms. Within this framework, the stimulation of neuroplastic mechanisms like neurogenesis might help to alleviate deficits in episodic memory, subsequently help to reduce the expression of other psychiatric symptoms. Furthermore, given the regions importance to learning and memory processing, it is possible that improving hippocampal functioning would also contribute toward the alleviation of other cognitive deficits than episodic memory. For example, deficits in working memory represent an aspect of executive functioning impaired in MDD (Lee R.S. et al., 2012; Rock et al., 2013) and schizophrenia (Forbes et al., 2009). As hippocampal functioning may be an important factor supporting working memory (Fell and Axmacher, 2011; Chaieb et al., 2015) promoting hippocampal integrity may indirectly contribute toward alleviating working memory deficits and improving executive functioning.

While it has not been the focus of this paper, it is also worth noting that altered hippocampal functioning can directly influence other, non-cognitive processes that are important in the pathology of certain psychiatric disorders like MDD. Through its dense connectivity with the prefrontal cortex and the amygdala, the hippocampus is also implicated in emotional regulation (O'Donnell and Grace, 1995; Seidenbecher et al., 2003; Lisman and Grace, 2005; Maren and Hobin, 2007) as well as playing an important role in regulating feedback inhibition from the hypothalamic-pituitary-adrenal axis (Jacobson and Sapolsky, 1991). Hippocampal dysfunctioning may therefore contribute toward deficits in the regulation of emotional processing and stress responses that are often seen in patients with MDD (Sapolsky, 2000; Davidson et al., 2002).

The role of these deficits in neuroplasticity within the hippocampus may be a crucial factor underlying hippocampal dysfunction in psychiatric disorders like MDD and schizophrenia. Directly targeting these deficits to enhance hippocampal functioning may help to improve deficient cognitive processes whose underlying etiology are particularly localized to the hippocampus. Furthermore, it is possible that promoting hippocampal functioning may have a beneficial impact on alleviating other cognitive or affective symptoms, which are more broadly related to dysfunctional networks that involve the hippocampus.

Current Treatment Approaches

Psychiatric disorders like schizophrenia and MDD have been primarily treated using pharmacotherapy such as with antipsychotic or antidepressant medications, both of which have been shown to reduce psychiatric symptoms (Leucht et al., 2012; Undurraga and Baldessarini, 2012). However, several large-scale meta-analyses have recently suggested that the effectiveness of antipsychotic and antidepressant medications is only marginally different from that of a placebo (Leucht et al., 2009; Rief et al., 2009), and neither have been able to successfully remediate cognitive dysfunction (Keefe et al., 2013, 2014; Solé et al., 2015). These approaches are generally not designed to target neuroplasticity, but rather to remediate other aspects of a psychiatric disorder such as dysfunctional neurotransmitter systems. Neither antipsychotics nor antidepressants have been consistently shown to induce any lasting neuroplastic changes in the brain (Rief et al., 2015). With the growing importance that is being placed on deficits in neuroplasticity to the underlying etiology of psychiatric disorders, it may be necessary to stimulate underlying neuroplastic changes in order to induce lasting structural alterations and effectively alleviate cognitive dysfunctions.

For example, there have been equivocal findings regarding the impact of antipsychotic medications like haloperidol (typical) and olanzapine (atypical) on macro-scale hippocampal structure, with studies finding chronic use to cause volumetric increases (Schmitt et al., 2004), decreases (Barr et al., 2013), and no impact at all (Navari and Dazzan, 2009; Smieskova et al., 2009; Vernon et al., 2011). Micro-scale changes associated with the chronic use of antipsychotics have also been mixed, for example it remains unclear whether any antipsychotic has a consistent impact on hippocampal neurogenesis (Schoenfeld and Cameron, 2015). Even in cases where antipsychotics like olanzapine were found to increase the number of adult-born cells in the DG, these cells were likely to be endothelial cells and oligodendrocytes rather than granule cells (Kodama et al., 2004), which may not promote DG function and mechanisms like pattern separation in the same way. The impact of both types of antipsychotics on synaptic plasticity is also ambiguous, with some studies showing drugs like olanzapine to promote dendritic growth (Park et al., 2013), while others have found that various typical and atypical antipsychotics are associated with a general reduction in dendritic complexity and impaired LTP (Frost et al., 2010; Price et al., 2014). Finally, BDNF is considered to be an important factor underlying the pathophysiology of schizophrenia. However, typical antipsychotics have been largely associated with reductions in BDNF expression and the impact of atypical antipsychotics remains unclear, with many studies finding it to have no impact on BDNF expression in the hippocampus and across other regions (Favalli et al., 2012).

Furthermore, no antipsychotic medication (Goldberg et al., 2007; Tybura et al., 2013) or other pharmacological intervention (Keefe et al., 2013) has been consistently demonstrated to alleviate the cognitive deficits associated with schizophrenia and in cases where the medication is anticholinergic, cognitive deficits have been shown to worsen (Tandon, 2011). The most promising approach in restoring cognitive deficits in schizophrenia may in fact, be through cognitive remediation which has produced some significant improvements in a number of cognitive domains and functional outcomes (McGurk et al., 2007; Reddy et al., 2014), however, effect sizes remain only small to moderate (Wykes et al., 2011). Currently, cognitive deficits are one of the most debilitating aspects of schizophrenia that remain the least effectively treated (Gibbons and Dean, 2016).

In the case of treating MDD, widely prescribed antidepressant medications such as selective serotonin reuptake inhibitors (SSRIs) have been more convincingly demonstrated to induce neuroplastic changes. SSRI medications have been shown to stimulate the rate of hippocampal neurogenesis (Malberg et al., 2000; Boldrini et al., 2009), but again this may not be representative of increased granule cells. It has been suggested that this effect is likely due to a 'dematuration' of mature granule cells in the DG rather than increased cell proliferation and it is unclear what impact this would have on hippocampal functioning (Kobayashi et al., 2010). For example, mature granule cells are intrinsic to pattern completion (Nakashiba et al., 2012) so this dematuration of granule cells caused by SSRIs could lead to an underactivation of pattern separation and inhibit proper episodic memory formation. However, various antidepressant treatments have reliably been shown to up-regulate hippocampal BDNF (Duman and Monteggia, 2006; Musazzi et al., 2009), which appears to be promoting synaptic plasticity within the region (Bath et al., 2012). Despite this, antidepressant medications are encumbered with slow response rates, a modest therapeutic efficacy and little or no impact on the cognitive deficits associated with MDD (Duman and Aghajanian, 2012; McIntyre et al., 2013; Rosenblat et al., 2015; Solé et al., 2015; Bortolato et al., 2016). Despite the increasing importance placed on alleviating cognitive dysfunction in MDD, research has continued to focus on treating affective symptoms (Baune and Renger, 2014). Subsequently, there are currently no prescribed treatments available that effectively alleviate cognitive deficits in MDD (Keefe et al., 2014; Solé et al., 2015; Bortolato et al., 2016).

Through directly targeting neuroplasticity in crucial areas like the hippocampus, it may be possible to induce lasting structural changes that promote the region's functioning and contribute toward the alleviation of cognitive dysfunction in psychiatric disorders. With the global pharmaceutical industry being estimated to reach a value of US$1.3 trillion by 2018 (CMR International, 2015), bridging the gap between neuroplasticity and functional outcomes in treating psychiatric disorders will likely be dominated by a pharmacological approach. Indeed, a great amount of research is being conducted into developing an effective pharmacological intervention to treat cognitive deficits in psychiatric disorders (Wallace et al., 2011). However, none of the most promising pharmacological agents have been able to achieve more than a moderate effect size in treating most cognitive deficits, at least within MDD (Keefe et al., 2014; Solé et al., 2015) and schizophrenia (Keefe et al., 2013). Therefore, it may be worth considering the inclusion of non-pharmacological approaches such as AE, as an adjunction to pharmacotherapy that may improve treatment of cognitive dysfunction.

The Prospect of an AE Intervention

While its therapeutic potential has only been explored very recently, AE has been demonstrated to counteract pathologically induced hippocampal harm and improve the region's functioning in a range of animal disease models including fetal alcohol spectrum disorders, traumatic brain injury, stroke, and Parkinson's, Alzheimer's and Huntington's diseases (Patten et al., 2015). In humans, AE has been shown to stimulate hippocampal neuroplasticity and successfully counteract deteriorating hippocampal function caused by aging or Alzheimer's disease (Intlekofer and Cotman, 2013). However, whether these findings can be extended to individuals with psychiatric disorders is still unclear. Most of the existing human literature investigating the use of AE in the treatment of MDD or schizophrenia has only measured its impact on individual psychopathologies, such as depressive symptoms or positive and negative symptoms (Knöchel et al., 2012). In both cases, AE has been demonstrated to be effective in reducing both positive and negative symptoms of schizophrenia (Vancampfort et al., 2012; Firth et al., 2015; Rimes et al., 2015) and affective symptoms in MDD (Cooney et al., 2012), in some cases just as effectively as antidepressants (Blumenthal et al., 1999, 2007; Brosse et al., 2002), or in terms of neurogenesis, exceeding it (Marlatt et al., 2010). The efficacy of AE in reducing a range of psychiatric symptoms suggests that AE interventions could have a number of benefits to the treatment of disorders like MDD or schizophrenia. Importantly, AE appears to be able to stimulate neuroplasticity and promote hippocampal functioning in brains with both healthy and pathologically deteriorated hippocampi. It is plausible that AE interventions could be used to counteract hippocampal harm caused by disorders that profoundly impact upon hippocampal functioning, and through this approach, aid in the alleviation of certain aspects of cognitive dysfunction.

In recent years, AE has started to attract attention as a therapeutic target for schizophrenia treatment, but only a handful of studies have systematically investigated the capacity for an AE intervention to remediate cognitive deficits associated with the disorder (Knöchel et al., 2012; Sommer and Kahn, 2015). Both cross-sectional (Kimhy et al., 2014) and interventional studies (Pajonk et al., 2010; Oertel-Knöchel et al., 2014; Kimhy et al., 2015; McEwen et al., 2015) have demonstrated that AE can promote cognitive functioning in patients with schizophrenia across a range of cognitive domains including speed of processing, short-term and working memory and visual learning. Although one review was unable to find an association between AE and a reduction of cognitive symptoms in patients with schizophrenia (Dauwan et al., 2016) these early results are largely promising.

On a cellular level, some studies have used animal models of schizophrenia to demonstrate that AE can promote neurogenesis (Wolf et al., 2011), hippocampal BDNF concentration and the expression of NDMA receptors in the hippocampus (Kim T.W. et al., 2014; Park et al., 2014). One study using an animal model of schizophrenia also demonstrated AE to improve performance on a spatial working memory task (Kim T.W. et al., 2014). These initial results suggest that AE could be beneficial for improving hippocampal structure and functioning in schizophrenia but such findings must be interpreted with caution given the aforementioned difficulty of modeling complex disorders like schizophrenia in animals (Nestler and Hyman, 2010). Some recent studies in human patients with schizophrenia have shown AE interventions to be associated with increased BDNF serum concentrations (Kuo et al., 2013; Kim H. et al., 2014; Kimhy et al., 2015) and one study found that the increased BDNF concentration accounted for a significant proportion of the improvements they had observed in cognitive performance observed in following AE (Kimhy et al., 2015). Another study in patients with schizophrenia also demonstrated AE to counteract the deterioration of white-matter tract integrity that is associated with the disorder (Svatkova et al., 2015).

These findings are encouraging and some human imaging studies have suggested the positive impact of AE may be region-specific to the hippocampus. For example, in patients with schizophrenia a 12-week AE intervention has led to increased hippocampal volume, hippocampal NAA concentration and improved performances on short-term memory and working memory tasks (Pajonk et al., 2010; Lin et al., 2015; McEwen et al., 2015). However, other studies have found AE interventions to of had no impact on hippocampal volume or function in patients with schizophrenia (Scheewe et al., 2013; Rosenbaum et al., 2015). It is possible that these discrepancies are caused by systemic differences between the studies. Although data was not available for all studies (Rosenbaum et al., 2015) attendance rates for AE sessions were generally higher in those studies that did find improvements in hippocampal volume and function (Pajonk et al., 2010; Lin et al., 2015) than those which did not (Scheewe et al., 2013). Additionally, both studies that found no volume change used an automated algorithm to segment the hippocampus (Scheewe et al., 2013; Rosenbaum et al., 2015), which is known to be less accurate than the manual method (Morey et al., 2009) employed in the former study (Pajonk et al., 2010) – although this was not always the case (Lin et al., 2015).

In patients with MDD, several interventional studies have demonstrated that AE can promote cognitive performance in executive functioning, attention, inhibitory control, speed of processing, working and spatial memory and visual learning (Kubesch et al., 2003; Vasques et al., 2011; Oertel-Knöchel et al., 2014; Greer et al., 2015). Although one study did not find AE to have any positive impact on cognition (Hoffman et al., 2008), the results so far are promising and AE may represent a viable option in remediating cognitive dysfunction in MDD (Solé et al., 2015).

In animal models of stress/MDD, certain micro-scale changes have been recorded which demonstrate that AE can promote hippocampal neurogenesis, vascularization, BDNF expression (both brain-wide and within the hippocampus), IGF-1 expression, VEGF expression, and hippocampal synaptic plasticity (Adlard and Cotman, 2004; Zheng et al., 2006; Bjørnebekk et al., 2010; Nakajima et al., 2010; Sartori et al., 2011; Kiuchi et al., 2012; Yau et al., 2012; Lu et al., 2014). Animal models of stress/MDD have also shown that AE can reduce depressive-like behavioral and deficits in spatial memory (Zheng et al., 2006; Nakajima et al., 2010; Yau et al., 2012). In studies of human patients with MDD, AE has been associated with increased BDNF serum concentration (Gustafsson et al., 2009; Laske et al., 2010). Just one human study has sought to assess macro-scale structural changes and found no association between an AE intervention and hippocampal volume or neurotrophin circulation (Krogh et al., 2014). However, participant attendance rate to AE sessions was very low in this study, at less than half (one session per week) the attendance rate recorded by studies in other psychiatric populations who did demonstrate growth in hippocampal volume (2.6 sessions per week; Pajonk et al., 2010). Furthermore, participants in this study also showed no reduction in depressive symptoms. This indicates that there may not have been a sufficient level of engagement in AE for changes in hippocampal structure and neurobiology to be recorded.

In addition to promoting neuroplastic changes that could lead to cognitive enhancement, AE is also thought to interact with several neurotransmitter systems, including the monoamine system (Chaouloff, 1989). The action of the monoamine neurotransmitter serotonin (5-hydroxytryptamine, 5-HT) in the hippocampus is known to facilitate the process of hippocampal learning and memory (Riedel et al., 1999; Buhot et al., 2000). 5-HT transmission in the hippocampus is disrupted in schizophrenia and MDD (Naughton et al., 2000; Middlemiss et al., 2002) and this 5-HT dysfunction is likely to contribute deficits in learning and memory in these disorders (Meeter et al., 2006; Gray and Roth, 2007). The exact nature of this dysfunction is unclear given the diverging impact that agonists and antagonists have on each 5-HT receptor subtype within the hippocampus and the complex interactions between 5-HT and other neurotransmitter systems (Meneses, 1999). Targeting specific hippocampal 5-HT receptors, particularly the 5-HT_{1a} receptor subtype, is growing in popularity as a pharmacological approach designed to promote learning and memory in psychiatric disorders (Wallace et al., 2011) like schizophrenia (Meltzer and Sumiyoshi, 2008) or MDD (Meeter et al., 2006). Some animal studies have indicated that AE may also be associated with elevated levels of 5-HT in the hippocampus (Gomez-Merino et al., 2001) as well as an increase in tryptophan hydroxylase, a rate-limiting precursor of 5-HT produced in the raphe nucleus, which projects directly to the hippocampus (Chaouloff, 1989). It is unclear whether this interaction with hippocampal 5-HT would be beneficial or not, but some recent animal work has indicated that AE can specifically ameliorate dysfunction in the 5-HT_{1a} receptor subtype (Maniam and Morris, 2010; Kim M.H. et al., 2014). The impact of AE on the monoamine system has largely been discussed in terms of its antidepressant properties (Christie et al., 2008; van Praag, 2009), but it is possible that this interaction may also contribute toward cognitive enhancement. However, more work is needed to elucidate the exact role of 5-HT and 5-HT receptor subtypes in hippocampal learning and memory and whether this coincides with the actions of AE.

The inclusion of AE interventions into current treatment approaches could be useful to counteract hippocampal harm and alleviate cognitive dysfunctions caused by psychiatric disorders. The important role that AE could play in the treatment of cognitive dysfunction is starting to gain traction in relation to schizophrenia (Malchow et al., 2013; Sommer and Kahn, 2015; Vakhrusheva et al., 2016) and MDD (Malchow et al., 2013; Oertel-Knöchel et al., 2014). Despite this, there is a distinct lack of systematic investigations (both animal and human) into the relationship between AE and neuroplasticity, hippocampal functioning, and its impact on cognitive dysfunctions in psychiatric disorders such as MDD (Malchow et al., 2013) or schizophrenia (Sommer and Kahn, 2015). Based on the available evidence, the merits of AE are best capitulated as an adjunctive intervention to pharmacotherapy that could improve treatment efficacy through targeting cognitive dysfunctions that remain largely untreated. It is possible that pharmacotherapy may eventually develop a comprehensive treatment for cognitive dysfunction, but non-pharmacological approaches like AE have a number of distinct benefits to the patient (discussed below), which make these interventions worthy of further investigation by future research.

WHY ARE NON-PHARMACOLOGICAL INTERVENTIONS USEFUL?

The efficacy of both antidepressant and antipsychotic medications could be improved should more attention be afforded to relevant lifestyle factors such as AE engagement (Rief et al., 2015). There appears to be a degree of overlap in the underlying mechanisms that are stimulated by AE and certain pharmacological medications, such as with the antidepressant fluoxetine (Huang et al., 2012). It is possible that such a degree of overlap in their underlying mechanisms could mean that combining a traditional pharmacological intervention with an AE intervention would have a synergising impact on inducing neuroplasticity. For example, animal models have demonstrated that the combination of AE and antidepressant treatment had a stronger impact on up-regulating BDNF than either intervention had individually (Russo-Neustadt et al., 2001; Baj et al., 2012) – this is particularly important as BDNF regulation is thought to be crucial to the antidepressant mechanism (Duman and Aghajanian, 2012). Additionally, the inclusion of AE to a traditional antidepressant intervention has been shown to have greater impact on reducing depressive symptoms in patients with MDD, than antidepressant treatment alone (Knubben et al., 2007; Schuch et al., 2011; Legrand and Neff, 2016). Interestingly, MDD patients with higher basal levels of BDNF due to prior treatment with SSRI's experienced a more rapid reduction in symptoms following an AE intervention than those with lower basal BDNF levels (Toups et al., 2011). This suggests that antidepressant medications may be useful for 'priming' patients with MDD to respond better to a subsequent AE intervention (Toups et al., 2011). Additionally, in animals, AE was significantly more potent at increasing the survival of adult-born granule cells in comparison to SSRIs like fluoxetine and duloxetine (Marlatt et al., 2010). Therefore, the inclusion of AE to a traditional antidepressant intervention could also have an additive impact on promoting neurogenesis.

The use of AE as an adjunctive treatment to traditional antidepressant medication may have a synergising impact on neuroplasticity potentially resulting in a more effective approach toward remediating psychiatric symptoms. The possibility of an enhanced efficacy rate would be particularly useful in treating patients with MDD who do not respond to antidepressant treatment alone (Mura et al., 2014), which could be as many as 10-30% of patients with MDD (Joffe et al., 1996). An interesting direction for future research would be to investigate whether including AE as an adjunctive treatment to a traditional pharmacological approach would have a synergistic impact on neuroplasticity, resulting in a greater treatment efficacy than attainable by either intervention alone.

In addition to the potential benefits that a combined approach may have on symptom alleviation, the inclusion of AE interventions may have further benefits to the well being of patients. For example, the development of a psychiatric disorder significantly increases the risk of psychiatric comorbidity (Fusar-Poli et al., 2014; Avenevoli et al., 2015). AE is conversely associated with lowering the risk of various other conditions developing that range from age- and dementia-related cognitive decline to mood and anxiety disorders (Martinsen, 2008; Ahlskog et al., 2011; Mammen and Faulkner, 2013). For example, a recent systematic review concluded that AE was effective at reducing the risk of patients with schizophrenia developing a comorbid disorder (Firth et al., 2015). The inclusion of AE interventions could be useful in reducing the risk of patients developing other comorbidities, but AE may be of an even greater utility in helping to reduce the risk of pharmacologically induced side effects.

Side Effects in Pharmacology

Pharmacological treatments are generally associated with a higher risk of inducing adverse side effects than non-pharmacological interventions in patients of MDD or schizophrenia (Gartlehner et al., 2015, 2016). Both antipsychotic (De Hert et al., 2012) and antidepressant (Anderson et al., 2012) medications are associated with numerous adverse side effects that range from more common and less severe symptoms like headaches or nausea, to less common but more severe symptoms like cardiovascular or metabolic dysfunction. Independent of influences from medication, psychiatric populations are already at an elevated risk of cardiovascular, metabolic or respiratory dysfunction than the general population (Galletly et al., 2012; Vancampfort et al., 2013) and this risk may be heightened further by certain pharmacological treatments. Contrastingly, AE is known to elicit comparatively few adverse side effects and is associated with improvements in the social, physical and affective well being of individuals with psychiatric disorders (Fiuza-Luces et al., 2013). Moreover, AE is known to be preventative of cardiovascular, metabolic and respiratory dysfunction, which suggests that the inclusion of an AE intervention may be useful in stemming the risk of psychiatric patients developing these severe conditions (Caemmerer et al., 2012; Vancampfort et al., 2014). Some evidence of this can be drawn from recent animal studies that have demonstrated that AE ameliorates the metabolic, lipid peroxidation and extrapyramidal side effects of antipsychotic medication (Czéh et al., 2007; Teixeira et al., 2011; Baptista et al., 2013; Boyda et al., 2014).

Concerns are also mounting over the growing length of time in which a patient is subjected to pharmacotherapy, as the long-term impact of these medications is unclear. There is currently a distinct lack of longitudinal studies that systematically evaluate the impact of long-term treatment with widely used antidepressants like SSRI's on brain and behavior (Popovic et al., 2015). Some studies have suggested that long-term antidepressant treatment (generally lasting more than 6 months) can have a detrimental impact on executive function, memory, attention, and motivation in patients with MDD (Fava et al., 2006; Popovic et al., 2015; Bortolato et al., 2016). Worryingly, one recent animal study demonstrated that the long-term administration of fluoxetine at clinically relevant doses was associated with impaired dendritic spine morphology leading to deficits in hippocampal synaptic plasticity (Rubio et al., 2013). This is particularly concerning given the increasing importance that is being placed on the role of hippocampal synaptic plasticity in the effective treatment of MDD (Duman and Aghajanian, 2012). Evidence is also accumulating to suggest that long-term antipsychotic treatment in humans may be linked to a reduction in both global gray- and white-matter volumes (Navari and Dazzan, 2009; Ho et al., 2011; Vernon et al., 2011; Fusar-Poli et al., 2013) as well as region-specific reductions in hippocampal volume (Panenka et al., 2007).

There is an insufficient amount of data to make any definitive statements about the long-term impact these pharmacological interventions could be having on the brain. However, evidence may continue to emerge that shows the long-term application of widely used antidepressants and antipsychotics as having a detrimental impact on neuroplasticity and cognitive performance. The inclusion of AE interventions could be useful in counterbalancing some of these harms, at least with regard to the hippocampus, through the direct impact that AE has on promoting neuroplasticity and cognition. For example, recent animal studies have demonstrated that AE was able to reverse most of damage caused to hippocampal volume and hippocampal synaptic connectivity caused by antipsychotic medication (Barr et al., 2013; Ramos-Miguel et al., 2015). In addition, the aforementioned potential for a combined pharmacotherapy/AE approach to have an additive impact on symptom alleviating may mean that patients reach remission at a faster rate. Thereby, the inclusion of AE interventions may also reduce the total time a patient is exposed to pharmacotherapy, lowering their risk of any adversities associated with long-term use.

Developing further pharmacological interventions that effectively alleviate cognitive symptoms in medicated psychiatric populations will undoubtedly provide a more comprehensive treatment approach, but it could also elevate the risk of adverse side effects for the patient. AE has the potential to directly combat these adverse side effects as well as contributing toward the remediation of cognitive deficits, as well as various other psychiatric symptoms that may be related to hippocampal dysfunction. AE interventions are unlikely to represent a viable standalone treatment for cognitive dysfunction, but may make an important, low-risk adjunctive treatment to pharmacotherapy that promotes the effectiveness and reduces the harms associated with pharmacological interventions. However, this approach must be considered in light of some limitations associated with AE intervention.

Limitations of AE Interventions

Psychiatric patients often view pharmacological interventions more negatively than by the doctors who prescribe them (Nosè et al., 2012) and it is possible that patients may perceive a non-pharmacological adjunctive approach more favorably. Psychiatric patients have previously reported having a favorable perspective of AE treatment (Stanton and Reaburn, 2014), however, this is not necessarily reflected in actual AE engagement (Vancampfort et al., 2016). Motivating psychiatric patients to engage in regular AE is likely to be the greatest obstacle in both researching and implementing AE interventions in treatment, as epitomized by the high dropout rates in AE interventional studies in psychiatric samples (Stubbs et al., 2016; Vancampfort et al., 2016). Amongst those who are physically able to exercise, the lack of motivation is a significant factor preventing individuals with schizophrenia (Soundy et al., 2014) or MDD (Krämer et al., 2014) from adhering to AE interventions. It is possible that certain pharmacological treatments may contribute to this issue as psychiatric patients have previously reported medication side effects as a primary factor that inhibits their capacity to engage in regular exercise (Glover et al., 2013). While many studies investigating AE interventions in psychiatric patients do now incorporate motivational strategies (e.g., motivational interviews or goal setting) to encourage AE engagement, motivational factors are rarely included as a primary outcome measure (Farholm and Sørensen, 2016). Increasingly, efforts are being concentrated on promoting adherence to AE interventions in psychiatric patients (Knapen et al., 2015). For example, the integration of action video games with AE interventions has been shown as a promising method of enhancing the adherence of patients with schizophrenia to improving their aerobic fitness (Kimhy et al., 2016b). However, more research must be dedicated to directly studying the relationship between motivation and AE in psychiatric populations in order to measure and improve the effectiveness of motivational strategies.

Another issue in the conceptualization of AE treatments is the lack of consensus as to what type, intensity or length of exercise sessions has the strongest impact on the brain (Prakash et al., 2015). For example, some studies argue that a high-intensity exercise is optimal for reducing symptoms in MDD (Singh et al., 2005), while others have suggested that that a mild (Dunn et al., 2005) or a moderate intensity exercise intervention would be optimal (Stanton and Reaburn, 2014). It is possible that exercise intensities may vary depending on the purpose of the intervention, for example it has been suggested that improving cognitive performance may require high-intensity, interval training but preserving cognitive function in an aging brain may require a lower intensity, more continuous protocol (Duzel et al., 2016). Exercise type may also be an important factor. Although most of the current literature has focussed on AE, other forms of exercise such as yoga (Lin et al., 2015) or weight training (Suo et al., 2016) may also be beneficial in promoting brain health and cognition. Given the growing interest in exercise as a therapeutic intervention, it is surprising that only a handful of studies have attempted to systematically establish the most effective way in which it should be applied in psychiatric populations (Perraton et al., 2010; Stanton and Happell, 2014; Stanton and Reaburn, 2014; Kimhy et al., 2016a). It is important that future research concentrates on establishing the merits of different forms of exercise and fully outlining the dose-response relationship between the intensity and length of AE intervention and therapeutic outcome in each psychiatric population.

CONCLUSION

Research demonstrating the potential for AE to promote hippocampal structure and function is growing at an impressive rate as more and more work is translated from animal to human models. Importantly, the beneficial impact that AE has on the brain may have a useful clinical application in treating disorders in which hippocampal damage is a significant factor that underlies its symptomatology. There is currently a particular need to develop effective strategies that alleviate cognitive dysfunction and targeting deficits in the neuroplasticity of crucial areas to cognition like the hippocampus, is a promising approach to remediating cognitive dysfunction. AE interventions represent an effective method of promoting hippocampal neuroplasticity and function that encompasses few risks and several additional benefits to the patient, such as combating pharmacologically induced side effects. This paper has highlighted two promising examples of how AE interventions could improve the treatment of schizophrenia and MDD, but AE interventions could well have a broader application in mental health such as in treating substance abuse (Zschucke et al., 2012).

However, several issues must be addressed for AE to be successfully implemented as an adjunct to pharmacotherapy. Firstly, more RCTs are needed to systematically establish a causal relationship between AE with neural and cognitive outcomes. Future RCTs could benefit from a more hippocampus-focussed approach with particular regard to the choice of cognitive tasks used in the study. The use of techniques like multimodal imaging and peripheral biomarker assays should also be incorporated to build a comprehensive account of the impact that AE has on the brain. A greater focus should be placed on investigating the impact of AE in psychiatric populations both in terms of neuroplastic changes and therapeutic efficacy. An interesting avenue of research is to assess to what extent AE could interact with current pharmacological treatments to reduce side effects and have a synergistic impact on neuroplasticity and symptom reduction. Finally, future research should strive to establish standardized methodologies for investigating AE and the most effective method in which an AE intervention would be implemented to maximize therapeutic outcome. Improving our understanding of the role that lifestyle factors such as exercise play in maintaining and promoting brain functioning could have major implications for the way in which we treat, or even prevent, psychiatric and neurological disorders.

AUTHOR CONTRIBUTIONS

AK was responsible for the conception and writing of the review and received substantial, direct and intellectual contributions from JH, PL, and MY. All authors approved the paper for publication.

ACKNOWLEDGMENT

Thank you to Dr. Chao Suo for contributing toward the final revisions of the paper.

REFERENCES

Abdul-Monim, Z., Neill, J. C., and Reynolds, G. P. (2007). Sub-chronic psychotomimetic phencyclidine induces deficits in reversal learning and alterations in parvalbumin-immunoreactive expression in the rat. *J. Psychopharmacol.* 21, 198–205. doi: 10.1177/0269881107067097

Aberg, M. A., Aberg, N. D., Hedbäcker, H., Oscarsson, J., and Eriksson, P. S. (2000). Peripheral infusion of IGF-I selectively induces neurogenesis in the adult rat hippocampus. *J. Neurosci.* 20, 2896–2903.

Adlard, P. A., and Cotman, C. W. (2004). Voluntary exercise protects against stress-induced decreases in brain-derived neurotrophic factor protein expression. *Neuroscience* 124, 985–992. doi: 10.1016/j.neuroscience.2003.12.039

Adriano, F., Caltagirone, C., and Spalletta, G. (2012). Hippocampal volume reduction in first-episode and chronic schizophrenia: a review and meta-analysis. *Neuroscientist* 18, 180–200. doi: 10.1177/1073858410395147

Ahlskog, J. E., Geda, Y. E., Graff-Radford, N. R., and Petersen, R. C. (2011). Physical exercise as a preventive or disease-modifying treatment of dementia and brain aging. *Mayo Clinic Proc.* 86, 876–884. doi: 10.4065/mcp.2011.0252

Aimone, J. B., Deng, W., and Gage, F. H. (2011). Resolving new memories: a critical look at the dentate gyrus, adult neurogenesis, and pattern separation. *Neuron* 70, 589–596. doi: 10.1016/j.neuron.2011.05.010

Aimone, J. B., Li, Y., Lee, S. W., Clemenson, G. D., Deng, W., and Gage, F. H. (2014). Regulation and function of adult neurogenesis: from genes to cognition. *Physiol. Rev.* 94, 991–1026. doi: 10.1152/physrev.00004.2014

Allen, K. M., Fung, S. J., and Shannon Weickert, C. (2016). Cell proliferation is reduced in the hippocampus in schizophrenia. *Aust. N. Z. J. Psychiatry* 50, 473–480. doi: 10.1177/0004867415589793

Alonso, M., Vianna, M. R. M., Depino, A. M., Mello e Souza, T., Pereira, P., Szapiro, G., et al. (2002). BDNF-triggered events in the rat hippocampus are required for both short- and long-term memory formation. *Hippocampus* 12, 551–560. doi: 10.1002/hipo.10035

Amitai, N., Semenova, S., and Markou, A. (2007). Cognitive-disruptive effects of the psychotomimetic phencyclidine and attenuation by atypical antipsychotic medications in rats. *Psychopharmacology* 193, 521–537. doi: 10.1007/s00213-007-0808-x

Anderson, B. J. (2011). Plasticity of gray matter volume: the cellular and synaptic plasticity that underlies volumetric change. *Dev. Psychobiol.* 53, 456–465. doi: 10.1002/dev.20563

Anderson, H. D., Pace, W. D., Libby, A. M., West, D. R., and Valuck, R. J. (2012). Rates of 5 common antidepressant side effects among new adult and adolescent cases of depression: a retrospective US claims study. *Clin. Ther.* 34, 113–123. doi: 10.1016/j.clinthera.2011.11.024

Angevaren, M., Aufdemkampe, G., Verhaar, H. J., Aleman, A., and Vanhees, L. (2008). Physical activity and enhanced fitness to improve cognitive function in older people without known cognitive impairment. *Cochrane Database Syst. Rev.* 16:CD005381.

Archer, T., and Kostrzewa, R. M. (2015). Physical exercise alleviates health defects, symptoms, and biomarkers in schizophrenia spectrum disorder. *Neurotox. Res.* 28, 268–280. doi: 10.1007/s12640-015-9543-y

Avenevoli, S., Swendsen, J., He, J.-P., Burstein, M., and Merikangas, K. R. (2015). Major depression in the national comorbidity survey-adolescent supplement: prevalence, correlates, and treatment. *J. Am. Acad. Child Adolesc. Psychiatry* 54, 37.e2–44.e44. doi: 10.1016/j.jaac.2014.10.010

Baj, G., D'Alessandro, V., Musazzi, L., Mallei, A., Sartori, C. R., Sciancalepore, M., et al. (2012). Physical exercise and antidepressants enhance BDNF targeting in hippocampal CA3 dendrites: further evidence of a spatial code for BDNF splice variants. *Neuropsychopharmacology* 37, 1600–1611. doi: 10.1038/npp.2012.5

Bannerman, D. M., Sprengel, R., Sanderson, D. J., McHugh, S. B., Rawlins, J. N. P., Monyer, H., et al. (2014). Hippocampal synaptic plasticity, spatial memory and anxiety. *Nat. Rev. Neurosci.* 15, 181–192. doi: 10.1038/nrn3677

Baptista, P. P. A., de Senna, P. N., Paim, M. F., Saur, L., Blank, M., do Nascimento, P., et al. (2013). Physical exercise down-regulated locomotor side effects induced by haloperidol treatment in Wistar rats. *Pharmacol. Biochem. Behav.* 104, 113–118. doi: 10.1016/j.pbb.2012.12.020

Barbacid, M. (1995). Neurotrophic factors and their receptors. *Curr. Opin. Cell Biol.* 7, 148–155. doi: 10.1016/0955-0674(95)80022-0

Barch, D. M., and Ceaser, A. (2012). Cognition in schizophrenia: core psychological and neural mechanisms. *Trends Cogn. Sci.* 16, 27–34. doi: 10.1016/j.tics.2011.11.015

Barnes, D. E., Yaffe, K., Satariano, W. A., and Tager, I. B. (2003). A longitudinal study of cardiorespiratory fitness and cognitive function in healthy older adults. *J. Am. Geriatr. Soc.* 51, 459–465. doi: 10.1046/j.1532-5415.2003.51153.x

Barr, A. M., Wu, C. H., Wong, C., Hercher, C., Töpfer, E., Boyda, H. N., et al. (2013). Effects of chronic exercise and treatment with the antipsychotic drug olanzapine on hippocampal volume in adult female rats. *Neuroscience* 255, 147–157. doi: 10.1016/j.neuroscience.2013.10.010

Bartsch, T., and Wulff, P. (2015). The hippocampus in aging and disease: from plasticity to vulnerability. *Neuroscience* 309, 1–16. doi: 10.1016/j.neuroscience.2015.07.084

Bath, K. G., Jing, D. Q., Dincheva, I., Neeb, C. C., Pattwell, S. S., Chao, M. V., et al. (2012). BDNF Val66Met impairs fluoxetine-induced enhancement of adult hippocampus plasticity. *Neuropsychopharmacology* 37, 1297–1304. doi: 10.1038/npp.2011.318

Baudin, A., Blot, K., Verney, C., Estevez, L., Santamaria, J., Gressens, P., et al. (2012). Maternal deprivation induces deficits in temporal memory and cognitive flexibility and exaggerates synaptic plasticity in the rat medial prefrontal cortex. *Neurobiol. Learn. Mem.* 98, 207–214. doi: 10.1016/j.nlm.2012.08.004

Baune, B. T., and Renger, L. (2014). Pharmacological and non-pharmacological interventions to improve cognitive dysfunction and functional ability in clinical depression–a systematic review. *Psychiatry Res.* 219, 25–50. doi: 10.1016/j.psychres.2014.05.013

Bavelier, D., and Neville, H. J. (2002). Cross-modal plasticity: where and how? *Nat. Rev. Neurosci.* 3, 443–452. doi: 10.1038/nrn848

Beadle, J. N., Paradiso, S., Brumm, M., Voss, M., Halmi, K., and McCormick, L. M. (2015). Larger hippocampus size in women with anorexia nervosa who exercise excessively than healthy women. *Psychiatry Res. Neuroimag.* 232, 193–199. doi: 10.1016/j.pscychresns.2014.10.013

Bekinschtein, P., Kent, B. A., Oomen, C. A., Clemenson, G. D., Gage, F. H., Saksida, L. M., et al. (2013). BDNF in the dentate gyrus is required for consolidation of "pattern-separated" memories. *Cell Rep.* 5, 759–768. doi: 10.1016/j.celrep.2013.09.027

Bekinschtein, P., Kent, B. A., Oomen, C. A., Clemenson, G. D., Gage, F. H., Saksida, L. M., et al. (2014). Brain-derived neurotrophic factor interacts with adult-born immature cells in the dentate gyrus during consolidation of overlapping memories. *Hippocampus* 24, 905–911. doi: 10.1002/hipo.22304

Besnard, A., and Sahay, A. (2015). Adult hippocampal neurogenesis, Fear Generalization, and Stress. *Neuropsychopharmacology* 41, 24–44. doi: 10.1038/npp.2015.167

Biedermann, S. V., Fuss, J., Steinle, J., Auer, M. K., Dormann, C., Falfán-Melgoza, C., et al. (2016). The hippocampus and exercise: histological correlates of MR-detected volume changes. *Brain Struct. Funct.* 221, 1353–1363. doi: 10.1007/s00429-014-0976-5

Bilder, R. M., Bogerts, B., Ashtari, M., Wu, H., Alvir, J. M., Jody, D., et al. (1995). Anterior hippocampal volume reductions predict frontal lobe dysfunction in first episode schizophrenia. *Schizophr. Res.* 17, 47–58. doi: 10.1016/0920-9964(95)00028-K

Bird, C. M., and Burgess, N. (2008). The hippocampus and memory: insights from spatial processing. *Nat. Rev. Neurosci.* 9, 182–194. doi: 10.1038/nrn2335

Bjørnebekk, A., Mathé, A. A., and Brené, S. (2010). The antidepressant effects of running and escitalopram are associated with levels of hippocampal NPY and Y1 receptor but not cell proliferation in a rat model of depression. *Hippocampus* 20, 820–828. doi: 10.1002/hipo.20683

Bliss, T. V., and Collingridge, G. L. (1993). A synaptic model of memory: long-term potentiation in the hippocampus. *Nature* 361, 31–39. doi: 10.1038/361031a0

Bloor, C. M. (2005). Angiogenesis during exercise and training. *Angiogenesis* 8, 263–271. doi: 10.1007/s10456-005-9013-x

Blumenthal, J. A., Babyak, M. A., Doraiswamy, P. M., Watkins, L., Hoffman, B. M., Barbour, K. A., et al. (2007). Exercise and pharmacotherapy in the treatment of major depressive disorder. *Psychosom. Med.* 69, 587–596. doi: 10.1097/PSY.0b013e318148c19a

Blumenthal, J. A., Babyak, M. A., Moore, K. A., Craighead, W. E., Herman, S., Khatri, P., et al. (1999). Effects of exercise training on older patients with major depression. *Arch. Intern. Med.* 159, 2349–2356. doi: 10.1001/archinte.159.19.2349

Boecker, H., Hillman, C. H., Scheef, L., and Strüder, H. K. (2012). *Functional Neuroimaging in Exercise and Sport Sciences.* Berlin: Springer Science & Business Media.

Boldrini, M., Underwood, M. D., Hen, R., Rosoklija, G. B., Dwork, A. J., John Mann, J., et al. (2009). Antidepressants increase neural progenitor cells in the human hippocampus. *Neuropsychopharmacology* 34, 2376–2389. doi: 10.1038/npp.2009.75

Bolijn, S., and Lucassen, P. J. (2015). How the body talks to the brain; peripheral mediators of physical activity-induced proliferation in the adult hippocampus. *Brain Plast.* 1, 5–27. doi: 10.3233/BPL-150020

Bora, E., Harrison, B. J., Yücel, M., and Pantelis, C. (2013). Cognitive impairment in euthymic major depressive disorder: a meta-analysis. *Psychol. Med.* 43, 2017–2026. doi: 10.1017/S0033291712002085

Bortolato, B., Miskowiak, K. W., Köhler, C. A., Maes, M., Fernandes, B. S., Berk, M., et al. (2016). Cognitive remission: a novel objective for the treatment of major depression? *BMC Med.* 14:9. doi: 10.1186/s12916-016-0560-3

Boyda, H. N., Ramos-Miguel, A., Procyshyn, R. M., Töpfer, E., Lant, N., Choy, H. H. T., et al. (2014). Routine exercise ameliorates the metabolic side-effects of treatment with the atypical antipsychotic drug olanzapine in rats. *Int. J. Neuropsychopharmacol.* 17, 77–90. doi: 10.1017/S1461145713000795

Brosse, A. L., Sheets, E. S., Lett, H. S., and Blumenthal, J. A. (2002). Exercise and the treatment of clinical depression in adults. *Sports Med.* 32, 741–760. doi: 10.2165/00007256-200232120-00001

Bugg, J. M., and Head, D. (2011). Exercise moderates age-related atrophy of the medial temporal lobe. *Neurobiol. Aging* 32, 506–514. doi: 10.1016/j.neurobiolaging.2009.03.008

Bugg, J. M., Shah, K., Villareal, D. T., and Head, D. (2012). Cognitive and neural correlates of aerobic fitness in obese older adults. *Exp. Aging Res.* 38, 131–145. doi: 10.1080/0361073X.2012.659995

Buhot, M. C., Martin, S., and Segu, L. (2000). Role of serotonin in memory impairment. *Ann. Med.* 32, 210–221. doi: 10.3109/07853890008998828

Bullitt, E., Rahman, F. N., Smith, J. K., Kim, E., Zeng, D., Katz, L. M., et al. (2009). The effect of exercise on the cerebral vasculature of healthy aged subjects as visualized by MR angiography. *Am. J. Neuroradiol.* 30, 1857–1863. doi: 10.3174/ajnr.A1695

Burdette, J. H., Laurienti, P. J., Espeland, M. A., Morgan, A., Telesford, Q., Vechlekar, C. D., et al. (2010). Using network science to evaluate exercise-associated brain changes in older adults. *Front. Aging Neurosci.* 2:23. doi: 10.3389/fnagi.2010.00023

Burgess, N., Maguire, E. A., and O'Keefe, J. (2002). The human hippocampus and spatial and episodic memory. *Neuron* 35, 625–641. doi: 10.1016/S0896-6273(02)00830-9

Burzynska, A. Z., Chaddock-Heyman, L., Voss, M. W., Wong, C. N., Gothe, N. P., Olson, E. A., et al. (2014). Physical activity and cardiorespiratory fitness are beneficial for white matter in low-fit older adults. *PLoS ONE* 9:e107413. doi: 10.1371/journal.pone.0107413

Caemmerer, J., Correll, C. U., and Maayan, L. (2012). Acute and maintenance effects of non-pharmacologic interventions for antipsychotic associated weight gain and metabolic abnormalities: a meta-analytic comparison of randomized controlled trials. *Schizophr. Res.* 140, 159–168. doi: 10.1016/j.schres.2012.03.017

Cao, L., Jiao, X., Zuzga, D. S., Liu, Y., Fong, D. M., Young, D., et al. (2004). VEGF links hippocampal activity with neurogenesis, learning and memory. *Nat. Genet.* 36, 827–835. doi: 10.1038/ng1395

Carro, E., Nuñez, A., Busiguina, S., and Torres-Aleman, I. (2000). Circulating insulin-like growth factor I mediates effects of exercise on the brain. *J. Neurosci.* 20, 2926–2933.

Chaddock, L., Erickson, K. I., Prakash, R. S., Kim, J. S., Voss, M. W., Vanpatter, M., et al. (2010). A neuroimaging investigation of the association between aerobic fitness, hippocampal volume, and memory performance in preadolescent children. *Brain Res.* 1358, 172–183. doi: 10.1016/j.brainres.2010.08.049

Chaddock, L., Pontifex, M. B., Hillman, C. H., and Kramer, A. F. (2011). A review of the relation of aerobic fitness and physical activity to brain structure and function in children. *J. Int. Neuropsychol. Soc.* 17, 975–985. doi: 10.1017/S1355617711000567

Chaieb, L., Leszczynski, M., Axmacher, N., Höhne, M., Elger, C. E., and Fell, J. (2015). Theta-gamma phase-phase coupling during working memory maintenance in the human hippocampus. *Cogn. Neurosci.* 6, 149–157.

Chang, Y. K., Labban, J. D., Gapin, J. I., and Etnier, J. L. (2012). The effects of acute exercise on cognitive performance: a meta-analysis. *Brain Res.* 1453, 87–101. doi: 10.1016/j.brainres.2012.02.068

Chaouloff, F. (1989). Physical exercise and brain monoamines: a review. *Acta Physiol. Scand.* 137, 1–13. doi: 10.1111/j.1748-1716.1989.tb08715.x

Christie, B. R., Eadie, B. D., Kannangara, T. S., Robillard, J. M., Shin, J., and Titterness, A. K. (2008). Exercising our brains: how physical activity impacts synaptic plasticity in the dentate gyrus. *Neuromol. Med.* 10, 47–58. doi: 10.1007/s12017-008-8033-2

Clark, P. J., Brzezinska, W. J., Puchalski, E. K., Krone, D. A., and Rhodes, J. S. (2009). Functional analysis of neurovascular adaptations to exercise in the dentate gyrus of young adult mice associated with cognitive gain. *Hippocampus* 19, 937–950. doi: 10.1002/hipo.20543

Clayton, N. S., Griffiths, P. D., Emery, N. J., and Dickinson, A. (2001). Elements of episodic-like memory in animals. *Philos. Trans. R. Soc. Lond B Biol. Sci.* 356, 1483–1491. doi: 10.1098/rstb.2001.0947

CMR International (2015). *CMR International 2015 Pharmaceutical R&D Factbook.* Available at: http://www.techstreet.com/standards/cmr-international-2015-pharmaceutical-r-d-factbook?product_id=1899104#product

Coelho, F. G., de, M., Gobbi, S., Andreatto, C. A. A., Corazza, D. I., Pedroso, R. V., et al. (2013). Physical exercise modulates peripheral levels of brain-derived neurotrophic factor (BDNF): a systematic review of experimental studies in the elderly. *Arch. Gerontol. Geriatr.* 56, 10–15. doi: 10.1016/j.archger.2012.06.003

Colcombe, S., and Kramer, A. F. (2003). Fitness effects on the cognitive function of older adults: a meta-analytic study. *Psychol. Sci.* 14, 125–130. doi: 10.1111/1467-9280.t01-1-01430

Colcombe, S. J., Erickson, K. I., Raz, N., Webb, A. G., Cohen, N. J., McAuley, E., et al. (2003). Aerobic fitness reduces brain tissue loss in aging humans. *J. Gerontol. Ser. A Biol. Sci. Med. Sci.* 58, M176–M180. doi: 10.1093/gerona/58.2.M176

Colcombe, S. J., Erickson, K. I., Scalf, P. E., Kim, J. S., Prakash, R., McAuley, E., et al. (2006). Aerobic exercise training increases brain volume in aging humans. *J. Gerontol. Ser. A Biol. Sci. Med. Sci.* 61, 1166–1170. doi: 10.1093/gerona/61.11.1166

Cooney, G. M., Dwan, K., Greig, C. A., Lawlor, D. A., Rimer, J., Waugh, F. R., et al. (2012). Exercise for depression. *Cochrane Database Syst. Rev.* 11:CD004366. doi: 10.1002/14651858.CD004366.pub6

Cotman, C. W., Berchtold, N. C., and Christie, L.-A. (2007). Exercise builds brain health: key roles of growth factor cascades and inflammation. *Trends Neurosci.* 30, 464–472. doi: 10.1016/j.tins.2007.06.011

Cowansage, K. K., LeDoux, J. E., and Monfils, M.-H. (2010). Brain-derived neurotrophic factor: a dynamic gatekeeper of neural plasticity. *Curr. Mol. Pharmacol.* 3, 12–29. doi: 10.2174/1874467211003010012

Creer, D. J., Romberg, C., Saksida, L. M., van Praag, H., and Bussey, T. J. (2010). Running enhances spatial pattern separation in mice. *Proc. Natl. Acad. Sci. U.S.A.* 107, 2367–2372. doi: 10.1073/pnas.0911725107

Czéh, B., and Lucassen, P. J. (2007). What causes the hippocampal volume decrease in depression? Are neurogenesis, glial changes and apoptosis implicated? *Eur. Arch. Psychiatry Clin. Neurosci.* 257, 250–260. doi: 10.1007/s00406-007-0728-0

Czéh, B., Müller-Keuker, J. I. H., Rygula, R., Abumaria, N., Hiemke, C., Domenici, E., et al. (2007). Chronic social stress inhibits cell proliferation in the adult medial prefrontal cortex: hemispheric asymmetry and reversal by fluoxetine treatment. *Neuropsychopharmacology* 32, 1490–1503. doi: 10.1038/sj.npp.1301275

Darcet, F., Gardier, A., Gaillard, R., David, D., and Guilloux, J.-P. (2016). Cognitive dysfunction in major depressive disorder. A translational review in animal models of the disease. *Pharmaceuticals* 9:9. doi: 10.3390/ph9010009

Darcet, F., Mendez-David, I., Tritschler, L., Gardier, A. M., Guilloux, J.-P., and David, D. J. (2014). Learning and memory impairments in a neuroendocrine mouse model of anxiety/depression. *Front. Behav. Neurosci.* 8:136. doi: 10.3389/fnbeh.2014.00136

Das, T., Ivleva, E. I., Wagner, A. D., Stark, C. E. L., and Tamminga, C. A. (2014). Loss of pattern separation performance in schizophrenia suggests dentate gyrus dysfunction. *Schizophr. Res.* 159, 193–197. doi: 10.1016/j.schres.2014.05.006

Dauwan, M., Begemann, M. J. H., Heringa, S. M., and Sommer, I. E. (2016). Exercise improves clinical symptoms, quality of life, global functioning, and depression in schizophrenia: a systematic review and meta-analysis. *Schizophr. Bull.* 42, 588–599. doi: 10.1093/schbul/sbv164

Davenport, M. H., Hogan, D. B., Eskes, G. A., Longman, R. S., and Poulin, M. J. (2012). Cerebrovascular reserve: the link between fitness and cognitive function? *Exerc. Sport Sci. Rev.* 40, 153–158. doi: 10.1097/JES.0b013e3182553430

Davidson, R. J., Pizzagalli, D., Nitschke, J. B., and Putnam, K. (2002). Depression: perspectives from affective neuroscience. *Annu. Rev. Psychol.* 53, 545–574. doi: 10.1146/annurev.psych.53.100901.135148

De Hert, M., Detraux, J., van Winkel, R., Yu, W., and Correll, C. U. (2012). Metabolic and cardiovascular adverse effects associated with antipsychotic drugs. *Nat. Rev. Endocrinol.* 8, 114–126. doi: 10.1038/nrendo.2011.156

Demirakca, T., Brusniak, W., Tunc-Skarka, N., Wolf, I., Meier, S., Matthaus, F., et al. (2014). Does body shaping influence brain shape? Habitual physical activity is linked to brain morphology independent of age. *World J. Biol. Psychiatry* 15, 387–396. doi: 10.3109/15622975.2013.803600

Deng, W., Aimone, J. B., and Gage, F. H. (2010). New neurons and new memories: how does adult hippocampal neurogenesis affect learning and memory? *Nat. Rev. Neurosci.* 11, 339–350. doi: 10.1038/nrn2822

Deng, W., Saxe, M. D., Gallina, I. S., and Gage, F. H. (2009). Adult-born hippocampal dentate granule cells undergoing maturation modulate learning and memory in the brain. *J. Neurosci.* 29, 13532–13542. doi: 10.1523/JNEUROSCI.3362-09.2009

Dennis, A., Thomas, A. G., Rawlings, N. B., Near, J., Nichols, T. E., Clare, S., et al. (2015). An ultra-high field magnetic resonance spectroscopy study of post exercise lactate, glutamate and glutamine change in the human brain. *Front. Physiol.* 6:351. doi: 10.3389/fphys.2015.00351

Dere, E., Pause, B. M., and Pietrowsky, R. (2010). Emotion and episodic memory in neuropsychiatric disorders. *Behav. Brain Res.* 215, 162–171. doi: 10.1016/j.bbr.2010.03.017

Déry, N., Pilgrim, M., Gibala, M., Gillen, J., Wojtowicz, J. M., Macqueen, G., et al. (2013). Adult hippocampal neurogenesis reduces memory interference in humans: opposing effects of aerobic exercise and depression. *Front. Neurosci.* 7:66. doi: 10.3389/fnins.2013.00066

Ding, Q., Vaynman, S., Akhavan, M., Ying, Z., and Gomez-Pinilla, F. (2006). Insulin-like growth factor I interfaces with brain-derived neurotrophic factor-mediated synaptic plasticity to modulate aspects of exercise-induced cognitive function. *Neuroscience* 140, 823–833. doi: 10.1016/j.neuroscience.2006.02.084

Duman, R. S., and Aghajanian, G. K. (2012). Synaptic dysfunction in depression: potential therapeutic targets. *Science* 338, 68–72. doi: 10.1126/science.1222939

Duman, R. S., and Monteggia, L. M. (2006). A neurotrophic model for stress-related mood disorders. *Biol. Psychiatry* 59, 1116–1127. doi: 10.1016/j.biopsych.2006.02.013

Dunn, A. L., Trivedi, M. H., Kampert, J. B., Clark, C. G., and Chambliss, H. O. (2005). Exercise treatment for depression: efficacy and dose response. *Am. J. Prev. Med.* 28, 1–8. doi: 10.1016/j.amepre.2004.09.003

Duzel, E., van Praag, H., and Sendtner, M. (2016). Can physical exercise in old age improve memory and hippocampal function? *Brain* 139, 662–673. doi: 10.1093/brain/awv407

Eadie, B. D., Redila, V. A., and Christie, B. R. (2005). Voluntary exercise alters the cytoarchitecture of the adult dentate gyrus by increasing cellular proliferation, dendritic complexity, and spine density. *J. Comp. Neurol.* 486, 39–47. doi: 10.1002/cne.20493

Edelmann, E., Lessmann, V., and Brigadski, T. (2014). Pre- and postsynaptic twists in BDNF secretion and action in synaptic plasticity. *Neuropharmacology* 76(Pt C), 610–627. doi: 10.1016/j.neuropharm.2013.05.043

Eichenbaum, H., Fortin, N. J., Ergorul, C., Wright, S. P., and Agster, K. L. (2005). Episodic recollection in animals: "if it walks like a duck and quacks like a duck . . .." *Learn. Motiv.* 36, 190–207. doi: 10.1016/j.lmot.2005.02.006

Eisch, A. J., and Petrik, D. (2012). Depression and hippocampal neurogenesis: a road to remission? *Science (New York, N.Y.)* 338, 72–75. doi: 10.1126/science.1222941

Ellison-Wright, I., and Bullmore, E. (2010). Anatomy of bipolar disorder and schizophrenia: a meta-analysis. *Schizophr. Res.* 117, 1–12. doi: 10.1016/j.schres.2009.12.022

Erickson, K. I., and Kramer, A. F. (2009). Aerobic exercise effects on cognitive and neural plasticity in older adults. *Br. J. Sports Med.* 43, 22–24. doi: 10.1136/bjsm.2008.052498

Erickson, K. I., Raji, C. A., Lopez, O. L., Becker, J. T., Rosano, C., Newman, A. B., et al. (2010). Physical activity predicts gray matter volume in late adulthood: the cardiovascular health study. *Neurology* 75, 1415–1422. doi: 10.1212/WNL.0b013e3181f88359

Erickson, K. I., Voss, M. W., Prakash, R. S., Basak, C., Szabo, A., Chaddock, L., et al. (2011). Exercise training increases size of hippocampus and improves memory. *Proc. Natl. Acad. Sci. U.S.A.* 108, 3017–3022. doi: 10.1073/pnas.1015950108

Erickson, K. I., Weinstein, A. M., Sutton, B. P., Prakash, R. S., Voss, M. W., Chaddock, L., et al. (2012). Beyond vascularization: aerobic fitness is associated with N-acetylaspartate and working memory. *Brain Behav.* 2, 32–41. doi: 10.1002/brb3.30

Etnier, J. L., Nowell, P. M., Landers, D. M., and Sibley, B. A. (2006). A meta-regression to examine the relationship between aerobic fitness and cognitive performance. *Brain Res. Rev.* 52, 119–130. doi: 10.1016/j.brainresrev.2006.01.002

Etnier, J. L., Salazar, W., Landers, D. M., Petruzzello, S. J., Han, M., and Nowell, P. (1997). The influence of physical fitness and exercise upon cognitive functioning: a meta-analysis. *J. Sport Exerc. Psychol.* 19, 249–277. doi: 10.1523/JNEUROSCI.4975-05.2006

Fabel, K., Fabel, K., Tam, B., Kaufer, D., Baiker, A., Simmons, N., et al. (2003). VEGF is necessary for exercise-induced adult hippocampal neurogenesis. *Eur. J. Neurosci.* 18, 2803–2812. doi: 10.1111/j.1460-9568.2003.03041.x

Farholm, A., and Sørensen, M. (2016). Motivation for physical activity and exercise in severe mental illness: a systematic review of intervention studies. *Int. J. Mental Health Nursing* 25, 194–205. doi: 10.1111/inm.12214

Farmer, J., Zhao, X., van Praag, H., Wodtke, K., Gage, F. H., and Christie, B. R. (2004). Effects of voluntary exercise on synaptic plasticity and gene expression in the dentate gyrus of adult male Sprague-Dawley rats in vivo. *Neuroscience* 124, 71–79. doi: 10.1016/j.neuroscience.2003.09.029

Fava, M., Graves, L. M., Benazzi, F., Scalia, M. J., Iosifescu, D. V., Alpert, J. E., et al. (2006). A cross-sectional study of the prevalence of cognitive and physical symptoms during long-term antidepressant treatment. *J. Clin. Psychiatry* 67, 1754–1759. doi: 10.4088/JCP.v67n1113

Favalli, G., Li, J., Belmonte-de-Abreu, P., Wong, A. H. C., and Daskalakis, Z. J. (2012). The role of BDNF in the pathophysiology and treatment of schizophrenia. *J. Psychiatr. Res.* 46, 1–11. doi: 10.1016/j.jpsychires.2011.09.022

Fell, J., and Axmacher, N. (2011). The role of phase synchronization in memory processes. *Nat. Rev. Neurosci.* 12, 105–118. doi: 10.1038/nrn2979

Firth, J., Cotter, J., Elliott, R., French, P., and Yung, A. R. (2015). A systematic review and meta-analysis of exercise interventions in schizophrenia patients. *Psychol. Med.* 45, 1343–1361. doi: 10.1017/S0033291714003110

Fiuza-Luces, C., Garatachea, N., Berger, N. A., and Lucia, A. (2013). Exercise is the real polypill. *Physiology (Bethesda)* 28, 330–358. doi: 10.1152/physiol.00019.2013

Flöel, A., Ruscheweyh, R., Krüger, K., Willemer, C., Winter, B., Völker, K., et al. (2010). Physical activity and memory functions: are neurotrophins and cerebral gray matter volume the missing link? *Neuroimage* 49, 2756–2763. doi: 10.1016/j.neuroimage.2009.10.043

Forbes, N. F., Carrick, L. A., McIntosh, A. M., and Lawrie, S. M. (2009). Working memory in schizophrenia: a meta-analysis. *Psychol. Med.* 39, 889–905. doi: 10.1017/S0033291708004558

Frost, D. O., Page, S. C., Carroll, C., and Kolb, B. (2010). Early exposure to haloperidol or olanzapine induces long-term alterations of dendritic form. *Synapse (New York, N.Y.)* 64, 191–199. doi: 10.1002/syn.20715

Fusar-Poli, P., Nelson, B., Valmaggia, L., Yung, A. R., and McGuire, P. K. (2014). Comorbid depressive and anxiety disorders in 509 individuals with an at-risk mental state: impact on psychopathology and transition to psychosis. *Schizophr. Bull.* 40, 120–131. doi: 10.1093/schbul/sbs136

Fusar-Poli, P., Smieskova, R., Kempton, M. J., Ho, B. C., Andreasen, N. C., and Borgwardt, S. (2013). Progressive brain changes in schizophrenia related to antipsychotic treatment? A meta-analysis of longitudinal MRI studies. *Neurosci. Biobehav. Rev.* 37, 1680–1691. doi: 10.1016/j.neubiorev.2013.06.001

Fuss, J., Biedermann, S. V., Falfán-Melgoza, C., Auer, M. K., Zheng, L., Steinle, J., et al. (2014). Exercise boosts hippocampal volume by preventing early age-related gray matter loss. *Hippocampus* 24, 131–134. doi: 10.1002/hipo.22227

Galletly, C. A., Foley, D. L., Waterreus, A., Watts, G. F., Castle, D. J., McGrath, J. J., et al. (2012). Cardiometabolic risk factors in people with psychotic disorders: the second Australian national survey of psychosis. *Aust. N. Z. J. Psychiatry* 46, 753–761. doi: 10.1177/0004867412453089

Gartlehner, G., Gaynes, B. N., Amick, H. R., Asher, G., Morgan, L. C., Coker-Schwimmer, E., et al. (2015). *Nonpharmacological Versus Pharmacological Treatments for Adult Patients with Major Depressive Disorder. Comparative Effectiveness Review No. 161*. Rockville, MD: Agency for Healthcare Research and Quality (US).

Gartlehner, G., Gaynes, B. N., Amick, H. R., Asher, G. N., Morgan, L. C., Coker-Schwimmer, E., et al. (2016). Comparative benefits and harms of antidepressants, psychological, complementary, and exercise treatments for major depression: an evidence report for a clinical practice guideline from the american college of physicians. *Anna. Int. Med.* 164, 331–341. doi: 10.7326/M15-1813

Gates, N., Fiatarone Singh, M. A., Sachdev, P. S., and Valenzuela, M. (2013). The effect of exercise training on cognitive function in older adults with mild cognitive impairment: a meta-analysis of randomized controlled trials. *Am. J. Geriatr. Psychiatry* 21, 1086–1097. doi: 10.1016/j.jagp.2013.02.018

Gibbons, A., and Dean, B. (2016). The cholinergic system: an emerging drug target for schizophrenia. *Curr. Pharm. Des.* 22, 2124–2133.

Glover, C. M., Ferron, J. C., and Whitley, R. (2013). Barriers to exercise among people with severe mental illnesses. *Psychiatr. Rehabil. J.* 36, 45–47. doi: 10.1037/h0094747

Goldberg, T. E., Goldman, R. S., Burdick, K. E., Malhotra, A. K., Lencz, T., Patel, R. C., et al. (2007). Cognitive improvement after treatment with second-generation antipsychotic medications in first-episode schizophrenia: is it a practice effect? *Archives Gen. Psychiatry* 64, 1115–1122. doi: 10.1001/archpsyc.64.10.1115

Goldberg, T. E., and Green, M. F. (2002). "Neurocognitive functioning in patients with schizophrenia: an overview," in *Neuropsychopharmacology: The Fifth Generation of Progress*, eds K. L. Davis, D. Charney, J. T. Coyle, and C. Nemeroff (Philadelphia: Lippincott, Williams & Wilkins).

Gomez-Merino, D., Béquet, F., Berthelot, M., Riverain, S., Chennaoui, M., and Guezennec, C. Y. (2001). Evidence that the branched-chain amino acid L-valine prevents exercise-induced release of 5-HT in rat hippocampus. *Int. J. Sports Med.* 22, 317–322. doi: 10.1055/s-2001-15645

Gomez-Pinilla, F., and Hillman, C. H. (2013). The influence of exercise on cognitive abilities. *Compr. Physiol.* 3, 403–428. doi: 10.1002/cphy.c110063.The

Gonzales, M. M., Tarumi, T., Kaur, S., Nualnim, N., Fallow, B. A., Pyron, M., et al. (2013). Aerobic fitness and the brain: increased N-acetyl-aspartate and choline concentrations in endurance-trained middle-aged adults. *Brain Topogr.* 26, 126–134. doi: 10.1007/s10548-012-0248-8

Gould, E., Beylin, A., Tanapat, P., Reeves, A., and Shors, T. J. (1999). Learning enhances adult neurogenesis in the hippocampal formation. *Nat. Neurosci.* 2, 260–265. doi: 10.1038/6365

Gray, J. A., and Roth, B. L. (2007). Molecular targets for treating cognitive dysfunction in schizophrenia. *Schizophr. Bull.* 33, 1100–1119. doi: 10.1093/schbul/sbm074

Grayson, B., Idris, N. F., and Neill, J. C. (2007). Atypical antipsychotics attenuate a sub-chronic PCP-induced cognitive deficit in the novel object recognition task in the rat. *Behav. Brain Res.* 184, 31–38. doi: 10.1016/j.bbr.2007.06.012

Green, M. J., Matheson, S. L., Shepherd, A., Weickert, C. S., and Carr, V. J. (2011). Brain-derived neurotrophic factor levels in schizophrenia: a systematic review with meta-analysis. *Mol. Psychiatry* 16, 960–972. doi: 10.1038/mp.2010.88

Greer, T. L., Grannemann, B. D., Chansard, M., Karim, A. I., and Trivedi, M. H. (2015). Dose-dependent changes in cognitive function with exercise augmentation for major depression: results from the TREAD study. *Eur. Neuropsychopharmacol.* 25, 248–256. doi: 10.1016/j.euroneuro.2014.10.001

Gur, R. E., Turetsky, B. I., Cowell, P. E., Finkelman, C., Maany, V., Grossman, R. I., et al. (2000). Temporolimbic volume reductions in schizophrenia. *Arch. Gen. Psychiatry* 57, 769–775. doi: 10.1001/archpsyc.57.8.769

Gustafsson, G., Lira, C. M., Johansson, J., Wisén, A., Wohlfart, B., Ekman, R., et al. (2009). The acute response of plasma brain-derived neurotrophic factor as a result of exercise in major depressive disorder. *Psychiatry Res.* 169, 244–248. doi: 10.1016/j.psychres.2008.06.030

Hamer, M., and Chida, Y. (2009). Physical activity and risk of neurodegenerative disease: a systematic review of prospective evidence. *Psychol. Med.* 39, 3–11. doi: 10.1017/S0033291708003681

Hamilton, G. F., and Rhodes, J. S. (2015). Exercise regulation of cognitive function and neuroplasticity in the healthy and diseased brain. *Prog. Mol. Biol. Transl. Sci.* 135, 381–406. doi: 10.1016/bs.pmbts.2015.07.004

Hammar, A., and Ardal, G. (2009). Cognitive functioning in major depression–a summary. *Front. Hum. Neurosci.* 3:26. doi: 10.3389/neuro.09.026.2009

Head, D., Singh, T., and Bugg, J. M. (2012). The moderating role of exercise on stress-related effects on the hippocampus and memory in later adulthood. *Neuropsychol.* 26, 133–143. doi: 10.1037/a0027108

Heckers, S., and Konradi, C. (2010). Hippocampal pathology in schizophrenia. *Curr. Topics Behav. Neurosci.* 4, 529–553.

Heldt, S. A., Stanek, L., Chhatwal, J. P., and Ressler, K. J. (2007). Hippocampus-specific deletion of BDNF in adult mice impairs spatial memory and extinction of aversive memories. *Mol. Psychiatry* 12, 656–670. doi: 10.1038/sj.mp.4001957

Henningsen, K., Andreasen, J. T., Bouzinova, E. V., Jayatissa, M. N., Jensen, M. S., Redrobe, J. P., et al. (2009). Cognitive deficits in the rat chronic mild stress model for depression: relation to anhedonic-like responses. *Behav. Brain Res.* 198, 136–141. doi: 10.1016/j.bbr.2008.10.039

Herting, M. M., and Nagel, B. J. (2012). Aerobic fitness relates to learning on a virtual Morris Water Task and hippocampal volume in adolescents. *Behav. Brain Res.* 233, 517–525. doi: 10.1016/j.bbr.2012.05.012

Heyn, P., Abreu, B. C., and Ottenbacher, K. J. (2004). The effects of exercise training on elderly persons with cognitive impairment and dementia: a meta-analysis. *Arch. Phys. Med. Rehabil.* 85, 1694–1704. doi: 10.1016/j.apmr.2004.03.019

Ho, B.-C., Andreasen, N. C., Ziebell, S., Pierson, R., and Magnotta, V. (2011). Long-term antipsychotic treatment and brain volumes: a longitudinal study of first-episode schizophrenia. *Arch. Gen. Psychiatry* 68, 128–137. doi: 10.1001/archgenpsychiatry.2010.199

Ho, N. F., Hooker, J. M., Sahay, A., Holt, D. J., and Roffman, J. L. (2013). In vivo imaging of adult human hippocampal neurogenesis: progress, pitfalls and promise. *Mol. Psychiatry* 18, 404–416. doi: 10.1038/mp.2013.8

Hoffman, B. M., Blumenthal, J. A., Babyak, M. A., Smith, P. J., Rogers, S. D., Doraiswamy, P. M., et al. (2008). Exercise fails to improve neurocognition in depressed middle-aged and older adults. *Med. Sci. Sports Exerc.* 40, 1344–1352. doi: 10.1249/MSS.0b013e31816b877c

Honea, R. A., Thomas, G. P., Harsha, A., Anderson, H. S., Donnelly, J. E., Brooks, W. M., and Burns, J. M. (2009). Cardiorespiratory fitness and preserved medial temporal lobe volume in Alzheimer disease. *Alzheimer Dis. Assoc. Disord.* 23, 188–197. doi: 10.1097/WAD.0b013e31819cb8a2

Hötting, K., and Röder, B. (2013). Beneficial effects of physical exercise on neuroplasticity and cognition. *Neurosci. Biobehav. Rev.* 37, 2243–2257. doi: 10.1016/j.neubiorev.2013.04.005

Howie, E. K., and Pate, R. R. (2012). Physical activity and academic achievement in children: a historical perspective. *J. Sport Health Sci.* 1, 160–169. doi: 10.1016/j.jshs.2012.09.003

Hu, P., Wang, Y., Liu, J., Meng, F. -T., Qi, X. -R., Chen, L., et al. (2016). Chronic retinoic acid treatment suppresses adult hippocampal neurogenesis, in close correlation with depressive-like behavior. *Hippocampus* 26, 911–923. doi: 10.1002/hipo.22574

Huang, G.-J., Ben-David, E., Tort Piella, A., Edwards, A., Flint, J., and Shifman, S. (2012). Neurogenomic evidence for a shared mechanism of the antidepressant effects of exercise and chronic fluoxetine in mice. *PLoS ONE* 7:e35901. doi: 10.1371/journal.pone.0035901

Huang, Y., Coupland, N. J., Lebel, R. M., Carter, R., Seres, P., Wilman, A. H., et al. (2013). Structural changes in hippocampal subfields in major depressive disorder: a high-field magnetic resonance imaging study. *Biol. Psychiatry* 74, 62–68. doi: 10.1016/j.biopsych.2013.01.005

Ikrar, T., Guo, N., He, K., Besnard, A., Levinson, S., Hill, A., et al. (2013). Adult neurogenesis modifies excitability of the dentate gyrus. *Front. Neural Circ.* 7:204. doi: 10.3389/fncir.2013.00204

Intlekofer, K. A., and Cotman, C. W. (2013). Exercise counteracts declining hippocampal function in aging and Alzheimer's disease. *Neurobiol. Dis.* 57, 47–55. doi: 10.1016/j.nbd.2012.06.011

Jacobson, L., and Sapolsky, R. (1991). The role of the hippocampus in feedback regulation of the hypothalamic-pituitary-adrenocortical axis. *Endocr. Rev.* 12, 118–134. doi: 10.1210/edrv-12-2-118

Jaeger, J., Berns, S., Uzelac, S., and Davis-Conway, S. (2006). Neurocognitive deficits and disability in major depressive disorder. *Psychiatry Res.* 145, 39–48. doi: 10.1016/j.psychres.2005.11.011

Jarrard, L. E. (1993). On the role of the hippocampus in learning and memory in the rat. *Behav. Neural Biol.* 60, 9–26. doi: 10.1016/0163-1047(93)90664-4

Jessberger, S., and Gage, F. H. (2014). Adult neurogenesis: bridging the gap between mice and humans. *Trends Cell Biol.* 24, 558–563. doi: 10.1016/j.tcb.2014.07.003

Joffe, R. T., Levitt, A. J., and Sokolov, S. T. (1996). Augmentation strategies: focus on anxiolytics. *J. Clin. Psychiatry* 57(Suppl. 7), 25–31; discussion 32–3.

Kaymak, S. U., Demir, B., Sentürk, S., Tatar, I., Aldur, M. M., and Uluğ, B. (2010). Hippocampus, glucocorticoids and neurocognitive functions in patients with first-episode major depressive disorders. *Eur. Arch. Psychiatry Clin. Neurosci.* 260, 217–223. doi: 10.1007/s00406-009-0045-x

Kays, J. L., Hurley, R. A., and Taber, K. H. (2012). The dynamic brain: neuroplasticity and mental health. *J. Neuropsychiatry Clin. Neurosci.* 24, 118–124. doi: 10.1176/appi.neuropsych.12050109

Keefe, R. S. E., Buchanan, R. W., Marder, S. R., Schooler, N. R., Dugar, A., Zivkov, M., et al. (2013). Clinical trials of potential cognitive-enhancing drugs in schizophrenia: what have we learned so far? *Schizophr. Bull.* 39, 417–435. doi: 10.1093/schbul/sbr153

Keefe, R. S. E., and Harvey, P. D. (2012). Cognitive impairment in schizophrenia. *Handb. Exp. Pharmacol.* 213, 11–37. doi: 10.1007/978-3-642-25758-2_2

Keefe, R. S. E., McClintock, S. M., Roth, R. M., Doraiswamy, P. M., Tiger, S., and Madhoo, M. (2014). Cognitive effects of pharmacotherapy for major depressive disorder: a systematic review. *J. Clin. Psychiatry* 75, 864–876. doi: 10.4088/JCP.13r08609

Kelly, M. E., Loughrey, D., Lawlor, B. A., Robertson, I. H., Walsh, C., and Brennan, S. (2014). The impact of exercise on the cognitive functioning of healthy older adults: a systematic review and meta-analysis. *Ageing Res. Rev.* 16, 12–31. doi: 10.1016/j.arr.2014.05.002

Kempermann, G., Fabel, K., Ehninger, D., Babu, H., Leal-Galicia, P., Garthe, A., et al. (2010). Why and how physical activity promotes experience-induced brain plasticity. *Front. Neurosci.* 4:189. doi: 10.3389/fnins.2010.00189

Kempermann, G., Song, H., and Gage, F. H. (2015). Neurogenesis in the adult hippocampus. *Cold Spring Harb. Perspect. Med.* 5:a018812.

Kent, B. A., Oomen, C. A., Bekinschtein, P., Bussey, T. J., and Saksida, L. M. (2015). Cognitive enhancing effects of voluntary exercise, caloric restriction and environmental enrichment: a role for adult hippocampal neurogenesis and pattern separation? *Curr. Opin. Behav. Sci.* 4, 179–185. doi: 10.1016/j.cobeha.2015.06.009

Kerr, A. L., Steuer, E. L., Pochtarev, V., and Swain, R. A. (2010). Angiogenesis but not neurogenesis is critical for normal learning and memory acquisition. *Neuroscience* 171, 214–226. doi: 10.1016/j.neuroscience.2010.08.008

Kheirbek, M. A., Klemenhagen, K. C., Sahay, A., and Hen, R. (2012). Neurogenesis and generalization: a new approach to stratify and treat anxiety disorders. *Nat. Neurosci.* 15, 1613–1620. doi: 10.1038/nn.3262

Kim, H., Song, B., So, B., Lee, O., Song, W., and Kim, Y. (2014). Increase of circulating BDNF levels and its relation to improvement of physical fitness following 12 weeks of combined exercise in chronic patients with schizophrenia: a pilot study. *Psychiatry Res.* 220, 792–796. doi: 10.1016/j.psychres.2014.09.020

Kim, M. H., Leem, Y. H., Ader, R., Cohen, N., Praag, H., van Berton, O., et al. (2014). Chronic exercise improves repeated restraint stress-induced anxiety and depression through 5HT1A receptor and cAMP signaling in hippocampus. *J. Exer. Nutr. Biochem.* 18, 97–104. doi: 10.5717/jenb.2014.18.1.97

Kim, T.-W., Kang, H.-S., Park, J.-K., Lee, S.-J., Baek, S.-B., and Kim, C.-J. (2014). Voluntary wheel running ameliorates symptoms of MK-801-induced schizophrenia in mice. *Mol. Med. Rep.* 10, 2924–2930. doi: 10.3892/mmr.2014.2644

Kimhy, D., Lauriola, V., Bartels, M. N., Armstrong, H. F., Vakhrusheva, J., Ballon, J. S., et al. (2016a). Aerobic exercise for cognitive deficits in schizophrenia - the impact of frequency, duration, and fidelity with target training intensity. *Schizophr. Res.* 172, 213–215. doi: 10.1016/j.schres.2016.01.055

Kimhy, D., Khan, S., Ayanrouh, L., Chang, R. W., Hansen, M. C., Lister, A., et al. (2016b). Use of active-play video games to enhance aerobic fitness in schizophrenia: feasibility, Safety, and Adherence. *Psychiatr. Ser.* 67, 240–243. doi: 10.1176/appi.ps.201400523

Kimhy, D., Vakhrusheva, J., Bartels, M. N., Armstrong, H. F., Ballon, J. S., Khan, S., et al. (2015). The impact of aerobic exercise on brain-derived neurotrophic factor and neurocognition in individuals with schizophrenia: a single-blind, Randomized Clinical Trial. *Schizophr. Bull.* 41, 859–868. doi: 10.1093/schbul/sbv022

Kimhy, D., Vakhrusheva, J., Khan, S., Chang, R. W., Hansen, M. C., Ballon, J. S., et al. (2014). Emotional granularity and social functioning in individuals with schizophrenia: an experience sampling study. *J. Psychiatr. Res.* 53, 141–148. doi: 10.1016/j.jpsychires.2014.01.020

Kiuchi, T., Lee, H., and Mikami, T. (2012). Regular exercise cures depression-like behavior via VEGF-Flk-1 signaling in chronically stressed mice. *Neuroscience* 207, 208–217. doi: 10.1016/j.neuroscience.2012.01.023

Kleemeyer, M. M., Kühn, S., Prindle, J., Bodammer, N. C., Brechtel, L., Garthe, A., et al. (2015). Changes in fitness are associated with changes in hippocampal microstructure and hippocampal volume among older adults. *Neuroimage* 131, 155–161. doi: 10.1016/j.neuroimage.2015.11.026

Knapen, J., Vancampfort, D., Moriën, Y., and Marchal, Y. (2015). Exercise therapy improves both mental and physical health in patients with major depression. *Disabil. Rehabil.* 37, 1490–1495. doi: 10.3109/09638288.2014.972579

Knöchel, C., Oertel-Knöchel, V., O'Dwyer, L., Prvulovic, D., Alves, G., Kollmann, B., et al. (2012). Cognitive and behavioural effects of physical exercise in psychiatric patients. *Prog. Neurobiol.* 96, 46–68. doi: 10.1016/j.pneurobio.2011.11.007

Knubben, K., Reischies, F. M., Adli, M., Schlattmann, P., Bauer, M., and Dimeo, F. (2007). A randomised, controlled study on the effects of a short-term endurance training programme in patients with major depression. *Br. J. Sports Med.* 41, 29–33. doi: 10.1136/bjsm.2006.030130

Kobayashi, K. (2009). Targeting the hippocampal mossy fiber synapse for the treatment of psychiatric disorders. *Mol. Neurobiol.* 39, 24–36. doi: 10.1007/s12035-008-8049-5

Kobayashi, K., Ikeda, Y., Sakai, A., Yamasaki, N., Haneda, E., Miyakawa, T., et al. (2010). Reversal of hippocampal neuronal maturation by serotonergic antidepressants. *Proc. Natl. Acad. Sci. U.S.A.* 107, 8434–8439. doi: 10.1073/pnas.0912690107

Kodama, M., Fujioka, T., and Duman, R. S. (2004). Chronic olanzapine or fluoxetine administration increases cell proliferation in hippocampus and prefrontal cortex of adult rat. *Biol. Psychiatry* 56, 570–580. doi: 10.1016/j.biopsych.2004.07.008

Kolomeets, N. S., Orlovskaya, D. D., and Uranova, N. A. (2007). Decreased numerical density of CA3 hippocampal mossy fiber synapses in schizophrenia. *Synapse* 61, 615–621. doi: 10.1002/syn.20405

Korol, D. L., Gold, P. E., and Scavuzzo, C. J. (2013). Use it and boost it with physical and mental activity. *Hippocampus* 23, 1125–1135. doi: 10.1002/hipo.22197

Kramer, A. F., Erickson, K. I., and Colcombe, S. J. (2006). Exercise, cognition, and the aging brain. *J. Appl. Physiol.* 101, 1237–1242. doi: 10.1152/japplphysiol.00500.2006

Krämer, L. V., Helmes, A. W., Seelig, H., Fuchs, R., and Bengel, J. (2014). Correlates of reduced exercise behaviour in depression: the role of motivational and volitional deficits. *Psychol. Health* 29, 1206–1225. doi: 10.1080/08870446.2014.918978

Krishnan, V., and Nestler, E. J. (2008). The molecular neurobiology of depression. *Nature* 455, 894–902. doi: 10.1038/nature07455

Krogh, J., Rostrup, E., Thomsen, C., Elfving, B., Videbech, P., and Nordentoft, M. (2014). The effect of exercise on hippocampal volume and neurotrophines in patients with major depression–a randomized clinical trial. *J. Affect. Disord.* 165, 24–30. doi: 10.1016/j.jad.2014.04.041

Krum, J. M., Mani, N., and Rosenstein, J. M. (2002). Angiogenic and astroglial responses to vascular endothelial growth factor administration in adult rat brain. *Neuroscience* 110, 589–604. doi: 10.1016/S0306-4522(01)00615-7

Krystal, J. H., Tolin, D. F., Sanacora, G., Castner, S. A., Williams, G. V., Aikins, D. E., et al. (2009). Neuroplasticity as a target for the pharmacotherapy of anxiety disorders, mood disorders, and schizophrenia. *Drug Discov. Today* 14, 690–697. doi: 10.1016/j.drudis.2009.05.002

Kubesch, S., Bretschneider, V., Freudenmann, R., Weidenhammer, N., Lehmann, M., Spitzer, M., et al. (2003). Aerobic endurance exercise improves executive functions in depressed patients. *J. Clin. Psychiatry* 64, 1005–1012. doi: 10.4088/JCP.v64n0905

Kuo, F.-C., Lee, C.-H., Hsieh, C.-H., Kuo, P., Chen, Y.-C., and Hung, Y.-J. (2013). Lifestyle modification and behavior therapy effectively reduce body weight and increase serum level of brain-derived neurotrophic factor in obese non-diabetic patients with schizophrenia. *Psychiatry Res.* 209, 150–154. doi: 10.1016/j.psychres.2012.11.020

Lang, C., Barco, A., Zablow, L., Kandel, E. R., Siegelbaum, S. A., and Zakharenko, S. S. (2004). Transient expansion of synaptically connected dendritic spines upon induction of hippocampal long-term potentiation. *Proc. Natl. Acad. Sci. U.S.A.* 101, 16665–16670. doi: 10.1073/pnas.0407581101

Laske, C., Banschbach, S., Stransky, E., Bosch, S., Straten, G., Machann, J., et al. (2010). Exercise-induced normalization of decreased BDNF serum concentration in elderly women with remitted major depression. *Int. J. Neuropsychopharmacol.* 13, 595–602. doi: 10.1017/S1461145709991234

Law, A. J., and Deakin, J. F. (2001). Asymmetrical reductions of hippocampal NMDAR1 glutamate receptor mRNA in the psychoses. *Neuroreport* 12, 2971–2974. doi: 10.1097/00001756-200109170-00043

Lazarov, O., and Hollands, C. (2016). Hippocampal neurogenesis: learning to remember. *Prog. Neurobiol.* 138–140, 1–18. doi: 10.1016/j.pneurobio.2015.12.006

Leavitt, V. M., Cirnigliaro, C., Cohen, A., Farag, A., Brooks, M., Wecht, J. M., et al. (2014). Aerobic exercise increases hippocampal volume and improves memory in multiple sclerosis: preliminary findings. *Neurocase* 20, 695–697. doi: 10.1080/13554794.2013.841951

Lee, R. S. C., Hermens, D. F., Porter, M. A., and Redoblado-Hodge, M. A. (2012). A meta-analysis of cognitive deficits in first-episode major depressive disorder. *J. Affect. Disord.* 140, 113–124. doi: 10.1016/j.jad.2011.10.023

Lee, S. W., Clemenson, G. D., and Gage, F. H. (2012). New neurons in an aged brain. *Behav. Brain Res.* 227, 497–507. doi: 10.1016/j.bbr.2011.10.009

Legrand, F. D., and Neff, E. M. (2016). Efficacy of exercise as an adjunct treatment for clinically depressed inpatients during the initial stages of antidepressant pharmacotherapy: an open randomized controlled trial. *J. Affect. Disord.* 191, 139–144. doi: 10.1016/j.jad.2015.11.047

Leucht, S., Arbter, D., Engel, R. R., Kissling, W., and Davis, J. M. (2009). How effective are second-generation antipsychotic drugs? A meta-analysis of placebo-controlled trials. *Mol. Psychiatry* 14, 429–447. doi: 10.1038/sj.mp.4002136

Leucht, S., Tardy, M., Komossa, K., Heres, S., Kissling, W., Salanti, G., et al. (2012). Antipsychotic drugs versus placebo for relapse prevention in schizophrenia: a systematic review and meta-analysis. *Lancet* 379, 2063–2071. doi: 10.1016/S0140-6736(12)60239-6

Lin, J., Chan, S. K., Lee, E. H., Chang, W. C., Tse, M., Su, W. W., et al. (2015). Aerobic exercise and yoga improve neurocognitive function in women with early psychosis. *Npj Schizophr.* 1, 15047. doi: 10.1038/npjschz.2015.47

Linnarsson, S., Björklund, A., and Ernfors, P. (1997). Learning deficit in BDNF mutant mice. *Eur. J. Neurosci.* 9, 2581–2587. doi: 10.1111/j.1460-9568.1997.tb01687.x

Lisman, J. E., and Grace, A. A. (2005). The hippocampal-VTA loop: controlling the entry of information into long-term memory. *Neuron* 46, 703–713. doi: 10.1016/j.neuron.2005.05.002

Llorens-Martín, M., Torres-Alemán, I., and Trejo, J. L. (2010). Exercise modulates insulin-like growth factor 1-dependent and -independent effects on adult hippocampal neurogenesis and behaviour. *Mol. Cell. Neurosci.* 44, 109–117. doi: 10.1016/j.mcn.2010.02.006

Lopez-Lopez, C., LeRoith, D., and Torres-Aleman, I. (2004). Insulin-like growth factor I is required for vessel remodeling in the adult brain. *Proc. Natl. Acad. Sci. U.S.A.* 101, 9833–9838. doi: 10.1073/pnas.0400337101

Lu, J., Xu, Y., Hu, W., Gao, Y., Ni, X., Sheng, H., et al. (2014). Exercise ameliorates depression-like behavior and increases hippocampal BDNF level in ovariectomized rats. *Neurosci. Lett.* 573, 13–18. doi: 10.1016/j.neulet.2014.04.053

Lucassen, P. J., Fitzsimons, C. P., Korosi, A., Joels, M., Belzung, C., and Abrous, D. N. (2013). Stressing new neurons into depression? *Mol. Psychiatry* 18, 396–397. doi: 10.1038/mp.2012.39

Lucassen, P. J., Meerlo, P., Naylor, A. S., van Dam, A. M., Dayer, A. G., Fuchs, E., et al. (2010). Regulation of adult neurogenesis by stress, sleep disruption, exercise and inflammation: implications for depression and antidepressant action. *Eur. Neuropsychopharmacol.* 20, 1–17. doi: 10.1016/j.euroneuro.2009.08.003

Lucassen, P. J., and Oomen, C. A. (2016). Stress, hippocampal neurogenesis and cognition; functional correlations. *Front. Biol.* 11:182–192.

Lucassen, P. J., Oomen, C. A., Naninck, E. F. G., Fitzsimons, C. P., van Dam, A.-M., Czéh, B., et al. (2015). Regulation of adult neurogenesis and plasticity by (early) stress, glucocorticoids, and inflammation. *Cold Spring Harb. Perspect. Biol.* 7:a021303. doi: 10.1101/cshperspect.a021303

Maass, A., Düzel, S., Brigadski, T., Goerke, M., Becke, A., Sobieray, U., et al. (2016). Relationships of peripheral IGF-1, VEGF and BDNF levels to exercise-related changes in memory, hippocampal perfusion and volumes in older adults. *Neuroimage* 131, 142–154. doi: 10.1016/j.neuroimage.2015.10.084

Maass, A., Düzel, S., Goerke, M., Becke, A., Sobieray, U., Neumann, K., et al. (2015). Vascular hippocampal plasticity after aerobic exercise in older adults. *Mol. Psychiatry* 20, 585–593. doi: 10.1038/mp.2014.114

Makizako, H., Liu-Ambrose, T., Shimada, H., Doi, T., Park, H., Tsutsumimoto, K., et al. (2014). Moderate-intensity physical activity, hippocampal volume, and memory in older adults with mild cognitive impairment. *J. Gerontol. A Biol. Sci. Med. Sci.* 70, 1–7. doi: 10.1093/gerona/glu136

Malberg, J. E., Eisch, A. J., Nestler, E. J., and Duman, R. S. (2000). Chronic antidepressant treatment increases neurogenesis in adult rat hippocampus. *J. Neurosci.* 20, 9104–9110.

Malchow, B., Keeser, D., Keller, K., Hasan, A., Rauchmann, B.-S., Kimura, H., et al. (2016). Effects of endurance training on brain structures in chronic schizophrenia patients and healthy controls. *Schizophr. Res.* 173, 182–191. doi: 10.1016/j.schres.2015.01.005

Malchow, B., Reich-Erkelenz, D., Oertel-Knöchel, V., Keller, K., Hasan, A., Schmitt, A., et al. (2013). The effects of physical exercise in schizophrenia and affective disorders. *Eur. Arch. Psychiatry Clin. Neurosci.* 263, 451–467. doi: 10.1007/s00406-013-0423-2

Mammen, G., and Faulkner, G. (2013). Physical activity and the prevention of depression: a systematic review of prospective studies. *Am. J. Prev. Med.* 45, 649–657. doi: 10.1016/j.amepre.2013.08.001

Manganas, L. N., Zhang, X., Li, Y., Hazel, R. D., Smith, S. D., Wagshul, M. E., et al. (2007). Magnetic resonance spectroscopy identifies neural progenitor cells in the live human brain. *Science* 318, 980–985. doi: 10.1126/science.1147851

Maniam, J., and Morris, M. J. (2010). Voluntary exercise and palatable high-fat diet both improve behavioural profile and stress responses in male rats exposed to early life stress: role of hippocampus. *Psychoneuroendocrinology* 35, 1553–1564. doi: 10.1016/j.psyneuen.2010.05.012

Maren, S., and Hobin, J. A. (2007). Hippocampal regulation of context-dependent neuronal activity in the lateral amygdala. *Learn. Mem.* 14, 318–324. doi: 10.1101/lm.477007

Markham, J. A., Taylor, A. R., Taylor, S. B., Bell, D. B., and Koenig, J. I. (2010). Characterization of the cognitive impairments induced by prenatal exposure to stress in the rat. *Front. Behav. Neurosci.* 4:173. doi: 10.3389/fnbeh.2010.00173

Marlatt, M. W., Lucassen, P. J., and van Praag, H. (2010). Comparison of neurogenic effects of fluoxetine, duloxetine and running in mice. *Brain Res.* 1341, 93–99. doi: 10.1016/j.brainres.2010.03.086

Marlatt, M. W., Potter, M. C., Lucassen, P. J., and van Praag, H. (2012). Running throughout middle-age improves memory function, hippocampal neurogenesis, and BDNF levels in female C57BL/6J mice. *Dev. Neurobiol* 72, 943–952. doi: 10.1002/dneu.22009

Martinsen, E. W. (2008). Physical activity in the prevention and treatment of anxiety and depression. *Nord. J. Psychiatry* 62(Suppl. 4), 25–29. doi: 10.1080/08039480802315640

McDermott, L. M., and Ebmeier, K. P. (2009). A meta-analysis of depression severity and cognitive function. *J. Affect. Disord.* 119, 1–8. doi: 10.1016/j.jad.2009.04.022

McEwen, B. S., Eiland, L., Hunter, R. G., and Miller, M. M. (2012). Stress and anxiety: structural plasticity and epigenetic regulation as a consequence of stress. *Neuropharmacology* 62, 3–12. doi: 10.1016/j.neuropharm.2011.07.014

McEwen, S. C., Hardy, A., Ellingson, B. M., Jarrahi, B., Sandhu, N., Subotnik, K. L., et al. (2015). Prefrontal and hippocampal brain volume deficits: role of low physical activity on brain plasticity in first-episode schizophrenia patients. *J. Int. Neuropsychol. Soc.* 21, 868–879. doi: 10.1017/S1355617715000983

McGurk, S. R., Twamley, E. W., Sitzer, D. I., McHugo, G. J., and Mueser, K. T. (2007). A meta-analysis of cognitive remediation in schizophrenia. *Am. J. Psychiatry* 164, 1791–1802. doi: 10.1176/appi.ajp.2007.07060906

McIntyre, R. S., Cha, D. S., Soczynska, J. K., Woldeyohannes, H. O., Gallaugher, L. A., Kudlow, P., et al. (2013). Cognitive deficits and functional outcomes in major depressive disorder: determinants, substrates, and treatment interventions. *Depress. Anxiety* 30, 515–527. doi: 10.1002/da.22063

Meeter, M., Talamini, L., Schmitt, J. A. J., and Riedel, W. J. (2006). Effects of 5-HT on memory and the hippocampus: model and data. *Neuropsychopharmacology* 31, 712–720. doi: 10.1038/sj.npp.1300869

Meltzer, H. Y., and Sumiyoshi, T. (2008). Does stimulation of 5-HT1A receptors improve cognition in schizophrenia? *Behav. Brain Res.* 195, 98–102. doi: 10.1016/j.bbr.2008.05.016

Meneses, A. (1999). 5-HT system and cognition. *Neurosci. Biobehav. Rev.* 23, 1111–1125.

Mesholam-Gately, R. I., Giuliano, A. J., Goff, K. P., Faraone, S. V., and Seidman, L. J. (2009). Neurocognition in first-episode schizophrenia: a meta-analytic review. *Neuropsychol.* 23, 315–336. doi: 10.1037/a0014708

Middlemiss, D. N., Price, G. W., and Watson, J. M. (2002). Serotonergic targets in depression. *Curr. Opin. Pharmacol.* 2, 18–22. doi: 10.1016/S1471-4892(01)00116-3

Middleton, L. E., Mitnitski, A., Fallah, N., Kirkland, S. A., and Rockwood, K. (2008). Changes in cognition and mortality in relation to exercise in late life: a population based study. *PLoS ONE* 3:e3124. doi: 10.1371/journal.pone.0003124

Millan, M. J., Agid, Y., Brüne, M., Bullmore, E. T., Carter, C. S., Clayton, N. S., et al. (2012). Cognitive dysfunction in psychiatric disorders: characteristics, causes and the quest for improved therapy. *Nat. Rev. Drug Discov.* 11, 141–168. doi: 10.1038/nrd3628

Mizoguchi, K., Yuzurihara, M., Ishige, A., Sasaki, H., Chui, D. H., and Tabira, T. (2000). Chronic stress induces impairment of spatial working memory because of prefrontal dopaminergic dysfunction. *J. Neurosci.* 20, 1568–1574.

Molteni, R., Ying, Z., and Gómez-Pinilla, F. (2002). Differential effects of acute and chronic exercise on plasticity-related genes in the rat hippocampus revealed by microarray. *Eur. J. Neurosci.* 16, 1107–1116. doi: 10.1046/j.1460-9568.2002.02158.x

Monti, J. M., Hillman, C. H., and Cohen, N. J. (2012). Aerobic fitness enhances relational memory in preadolescent children: the FITKids randomized control trial. *Hippocampus* 22, 1876–1882. doi: 10.1002/hipo.22023

Morey, R. A., Petty, C. M., Xu, Y., Hayes, J. P., Wagner, H. R. II, Lewis, D. V., et al. (2009). A comparison of automated segmentation and manual tracing for quantifying hippocampal and amygdala volumes. *Neuroimage* 45, 855–866. doi: 10.1016/j.neuroimage.2008.12.033

Moser, M.-B., and Moser, E. I. (1998). Functional differentiation in the hippocampus. *Hippocampus* 8, 608–619. doi: 10.1002/(SICI)1098-1063(1998)8:6<608::AID-HIPO3>3.0.CO;2-7

Motl, R. W., Pilutti, L. A., Hubbard, E. A., Wetter, N. C., Sosnoff, J. J., and Sutton, B. P. (2015). Cardiorespiratory fitness and its association with thalamic, hippocampal, and basal ganglia volumes in multiple sclerosis. *Neuroimage* 7, 661–666. doi: 10.1016/j.nicl.2015.02.017

Mura, G., Moro, M. F., Patten, S. B., and Carta, M. G. (2014). Exercise as an add-on strategy for the treatment of major depressive disorder: a systematic review. *CNS Spectr.* 19, 496–508. doi: 10.1017/S1092852913000953

Musazzi, L., Cattaneo, A., Tardito, D., Barbon, A., Gennarelli, M., Barlati, S., et al. (2009). Early raise of BDNF in hippocampus suggests induction of posttranscriptional mechanisms by antidepressants. *BMC Neurosci.* 10:48. doi: 10.1186/1471-2202-10-48

Nagahara, A. H., and Tuszynski, M. H. (2011). Potential therapeutic uses of BDNF in neurological and psychiatric disorders. *Nat. Rev. Drug Discov.* 10, 209–219. doi: 10.1038/nrd3366

Nagai, T., Murai, R., Matsui, K., Kamei, H., Noda, Y., Furukawa, H., et al. (2009). Aripiprazole ameliorates phencyclidine-induced impairment of recognition memory through dopamine D1 and serotonin 5-HT1A receptors. *Psychopharmacology* 202, 315–328. doi: 10.1007/s00213-008-1240-6

Nakajima, S., Ohsawa, I., Ohta, S., Ohno, M., and Mikami, T. (2010). Regular voluntary exercise cures stress-induced impairment of cognitive function and cell proliferation accompanied by increases in cerebral IGF-1 and GST activity in mice. *Behav. Brain Res.* 211, 178–184. doi: 10.1016/j.bbr.2010.03.028

Nakashiba, T., Cushman, J. D., Pelkey, K. A., Renaudineau, S., Buhl, D. L., McHugh, T. J., et al. (2012). Young dentate granule cells mediate pattern separation, whereas old granule cells facilitate pattern completion. *Cell* 149, 188–201. doi: 10.1016/j.cell.2012.01.046

Naninck, E. F. G., Hoeijmakers, L., Kakava-Georgiadou, N., Meesters, A., Lazic, S. E., Lucassen, P. J., et al. (2015). Chronic early life stress alters developmental and adult neurogenesis and impairs cognitive function in mice. *Hippocampus* 25, 309–328. doi: 10.1002/hipo.22374

Naughton, M., Mulrooney, J. B., and Leonard, B. E. (2000). A review of the role of serotonin receptors in psychiatric disorders. *Hum. Psychopharmacol. Clin. Exp.* 15, 397–415. doi: 10.1002/1099-1077(200008)15:6<397::AID-HUP212>3.0.CO;2-L

Navari, S., and Dazzan, P. (2009). Do antipsychotic drugs affect brain structure? A systematic and critical review of MRI findings. *Psychol. Med.* 39, 1763–1777. doi: 10.1017/S0033291709005315

Naylor, A. S., Persson, A. I., Eriksson, P. S., Jonsdottir, I. H., and Thorlin, T. (2005). Extended voluntary running inhibits exercise-induced adult hippocampal progenitor proliferation in the spontaneously hypertensive rat. *J. Neurophysiol.* 93, 2406–2414. doi: 10.1152/jn.01085.2004

Neeper, S. A., Gómez-Pinilla, F., Choi, J., and Cotman, C. (1995). Exercise and brain neurotrophins. *Nature* 373, 109. doi: 10.1038/373109a0

Nestler, E. J., and Hyman, S. E. (2010). Animal models of neuropsychiatric disorders. *Nat. Neurosci.* 13, 1161–1169. doi: 10.1038/nn.2647

Niemann, C., Godde, B., and Voelcker-Rehage, C. (2014). Not only cardiovascular, but also coordinative exercise increases hippocampal volume in older adults. *Front. Aging Neurosci.* 6:170. doi: 10.3389/fnagi.2014.00170

Nosè, M., Mazzi, M. A., Esposito, E., Bianchini, M., Petrosemolo, P., Ostuzzi, G., et al. (2012). Adverse effects of antipsychotic drugs: survey of doctors' versus patients' perspective. *Soc. Psychiatry Psychiatr. Epidemiol.* 47, 157–164. doi: 10.1007/s00127-010-0320-1

Nuechterlein, K. H., Subotnik, K. L., Green, M. F., Ventura, J., Asarnow, R. F., Gitlin, M. J., et al. (2011). Neurocognitive predictors of work outcome in recent-onset schizophrenia. *Schizophr. Bull.* 37(Suppl. 2), S33–S40. doi: 10.1093/schbul/sbr084

O'Callaghan, R. M., Griffin, E. W., and Kelly, A. M. (2009). Long-term treadmill exposure protects against age-related neurodegenerative change in the rat hippocampus. *Hippocampus* 19, 1019–1029. doi: 10.1002/hipo.20591

O'Donnell, P., and Grace, A. A. (1995). Synaptic interactions among excitatory afferents to nucleus accumbens neurons: hippocampal gating of prefrontal cortical input. *J. Neurosci.* 15, 3622–3639.

Oertel-Knöchel, V., Mehler, P., Thiel, C., Steinbrecher, K., Malchow, B., Tesky, V., et al. (2014). Effects of aerobic exercise on cognitive performance and individual psychopathology in depressive and schizophrenia patients. *Eur. Arch. Psychiatry Clin. Neurosci.* 264, 589–604. doi: 10.1007/s00406-014-0485-9

Oomen, C. A., Bekinschtein, P., Kent, B. A., Saksida, L. M., and Bussey, T. J. (2014). Adult hippocampal neurogenesis and its role in cognition. *Wiley Interdiscipl. Rev. Cogn. Sci.* 5, 573–587. doi: 10.1002/wcs.1304

Oomen, C. A., Hvoslef-Eide, M., Heath, C. J., Mar, A. C., Horner, A. E., Bussey, T. J., et al. (2013). The touchscreen operant platform for testing working memory and pattern separation in rats and mice. *Nat. Protoc.* 8, 2006–2021. doi: 10.1038/nprot.2013.124

Opendak, M., and Gould, E. (2015). Adult neurogenesis: a substrate for experience-dependent change. *Trends Cogn. Sci.* 19, 151–161. doi: 10.1016/j.tics.2015.01.001

Orsetti, M., Colella, L., Dellarole, A., Canonico, P. L., and Ghi, P. (2007). Modification of spatial recognition memory and object discrimination after chronic administration of haloperidol, amitriptyline, sodium valproate or olanzapine in normal and anhedonic rats. *Int. J. Neuropsychopharmacol.* 10, 345–357. doi: 10.1017/S1461145706006705

Pajonk, F.-G., Wobrock, T., Gruber, O., Scherk, H., Berner, D., Kaizl, I., et al. (2010). Hippocampal plasticity in response to exercise in schizophrenia. *Arch. Gen. Psychiatry* 67, 133–143. doi: 10.1001/archgenpsychiatry.2009.193

Palmer, T. D., Willhoite, A. R., and Gage, F. H. (2000). Vascular niche for adult hippocampal neurogenesis. *J. Comp. Neurol.* 425, 479–494. doi: 10.1002/1096-9861(20001002)425:4<479::AID-CNE2>3.0.CO;2-3

Panenka, W. J., Khorram, B., Barr, A. M., Smith, G. N., Lang, D. J., Kopala, L. C., et al. (2007). A longitudinal study on the effects of typical versus atypical antipsychotic drugs on hippocampal volume in schizophrenia. *Schizophr. Res.* 94, 288–292. doi: 10.1016/j.schres.2007.05.002

Papakostas, G. I., Nelson, J. C., Kasper, S., and Möller, H.-J. (2008). A meta-analysis of clinical trials comparing reboxetine, a norepinephrine reuptake inhibitor, with selective serotonin reuptake inhibitors for the treatment of major depressive disorder. *Eur. Neuropsychopharmacol.* 18, 122–127. doi: 10.1016/j.euroneuro.2007.07.005

Park, H., and Poo, M. (2013). Neurotrophin regulation of neural circuit development and function. *Nat. Rev. Neurosci.* 14, 7–23. doi: 10.1038/nrn3379

Park, J. K., Lee, S. J., and Kim, T. W. (2014). Treadmill exercise enhances NMDA receptor expression in schizophrenia mice. *J. Exerc. Rehabil.* 10, 15–21. doi: 10.12965/jer.140088

Park, S. W., Lee, C. H., Cho, H. Y., Seo, M. K., Lee, J. G., Lee, B. J., et al. (2013). Effects of antipsychotic drugs on the expression of synaptic proteins and dendritic outgrowth in hippocampal neuronal cultures. *Synapse* 67, 224–234. doi: 10.1002/syn.21634

Patten, A. R., Yu, S., Fontaine, C. J., Meconi, A., and Wortman, R. C. (2015). The benefits of exercise on structural and functional plasticity in the rodent hippocampus of different disease models. *Track. Effects Exerc. Neuronal Plasticity* 1, 97–127. doi: 10.3233/BPL-150016

Pereira, A. C., Huddleston, D. E., Brickman, A. M., Sosunov, A. A., Hen, R., McKhann, G. M., et al. (2007). An in vivo correlate of exercise-induced neurogenesis in the adult dentate gyrus. *Proc. Natl. Acad. Sci. U.S.A.* 104, 5638–5643. doi: 10.1073/pnas.0611721104

Perera, T. D., Park, S., and Nemirovskaya, Y. (2008). Cognitive role of neurogenesis in depression and antidepressant treatment. *Neurosci. Rev. J. Bring. Neurobiol. Neurol. Psychiatry* 14, 326–338. doi: 10.1177/1073858408317242

Perraton, L. G., Kumar, S., and Machotka, Z. (2010). Exercise parameters in the treatment of clinical depression: a systematic review of randomized controlled trials. *J. Eval. Clin. Pract.* 16, 597–604. doi: 10.1111/j.1365-2753.2009.01188.x

Peters, J., Dieppa-Perea, L. M., Melendez, L. M., and Quirk, G. J. (2010). Induction of fear extinction with hippocampal-infralimbic BDNF. *Science* 328, 1288–1290. doi: 10.1126/science.1186909

Phillips, M. L., Drevets, W. C., Rauch, S. L., Lane, R., Adolphs, R., Tranel, D., et al. (2003). Neurobiology of emotion perception I: the neural basis of normal emotion perception. *Biol. Psychiatry* 54, 504–514. doi: 10.1016/S0006-3223(03)00168-9

Piepmeier, A. T., and Etnier, J. L. (2015). Brain-derived neurotrophic factor (BDNF) as a potential mechanism of the effects of acute exercise on cognitive performance. *J. Sport Health Sci.* 4, 14–23. doi: 10.1016/j.jshs.2014.11.001

Ploughman, M., Granter-Button, S., Chernenko, G., Attwood, Z., Tucker, B. A., Mearow, K. M., et al. (2007). Exercise intensity influences the temporal profile of growth factors involved in neuronal plasticity following focal ischemia. *Brain Res.* 1150, 207–216. doi: 10.1016/j.brainres.2007.02.065

Popovic, D., Vieta, E., Fornaro, M., and Perugi, G. (2015). Cognitive tolerability following successful long term treatment of major depression and anxiety disorders with SSRi antidepressants. *J. Affect. Disord.* 173, 211–215. doi: 10.1016/j.jad.2014.11.008

Prakash, R. S., Snook, E. M., Motl, R. W., and Kramer, A. F. (2010). Aerobic fitness is associated with gray matter volume and white matter integrity in multiple sclerosis. *Brain Res.* 1341, 41–51. doi: 10.1016/j.brainres.2009.06.063

Prakash, R. S., Voss, M. W., Erickson, K. I., and Kramer, A. F. (2015). Physical activity and cognitive vitality. *Annu. Rev. Psychol.* 66, 769–797. doi: 10.1146/annurev-psych-010814-015249

Price, R., Salavati, B., Graff-Guerrero, A., Blumberger, D. M., Mulsant, B. H., Daskalakis, Z. J., et al. (2014). Effects of antipsychotic D2 antagonists on long-term potentiation in animals and implications for human studies. *Prog. Neuro-Psychopharmacol. Biol. Psychiatry* 54, 83–91. doi: 10.1016/j.pnpbp.2014.05.001

Radak, Z., Toldy, A., Szabo, Z., Siamilis, S., Nyakas, C., Silye, G., et al. (2006). The effects of training and detraining on memory, neurotrophins and oxidative stress markers in rat brain. *Neurochem. Int.* 49, 387–392. doi: 10.1016/j.neuint.2006.02.004

Ramos-Miguel, A., Honer, W. G., Boyda, H. N., Sawada, K., Beasley, C. L., Procyshyn, R. M., et al. (2015). Exercise prevents downregulation of hippocampal presynaptic proteins following olanzapine-elicited metabolic dysregulation in rats: distinct roles of inhibitory and excitatory terminals. *Neuroscience* 301, 298–311. doi: 10.1016/j.neuroscience.2015.06.022

Ranganath, C., Minzenberg, M. J., and Ragland, J. D. (2008). The cognitive neuroscience of memory function and dysfunction in schizophrenia. *Biol. Psychiatry* 64, 18–25. doi: 10.1016/j.biopsych.2008.04.011

Reddy, L. F., Horan, W. P., Jahshan, C., and Green, M. F. (2014). Cognitive remediation for schizophrenia: a review of recent findings. *Curr. Treat. Options Psychiatry* 1, 121–133. doi: 10.1007/s40501-014-0011-8

Redila, V. A., and Christie, B. R. (2006). Exercise-induced changes in dendritic structure and complexity in the adult hippocampal dentate gyrus. *Neuroscience* 137, 1299–1307. doi: 10.1016/j.neuroscience.2005.10.050

Richards, M., Hardy, R., and Wadsworth, M. E. J. (2003). Does active leisure protect cognition? Evidence from a national birth cohort. *Soc. Sci. Med.* 56, 785–792. doi: 10.1016/S0277-9536(02)00075-8

Riedel, W. J., Klaassen, T., Deutz, N. E. P., van Someren, A., and van Praag, H. M. (1999). Tryptophan depletion in normal volunteers produces selective impairment in memory consolidation. *Psychopharmacology* 141, 362–369. doi: 10.1007/s002130050845

Rief, W., Barsky, A. J., Bingel, U., Doering, B., Schwarting, R., Wöhr, M., et al. (2015). Rethinking psychopharmacotherapy: the role of treatment context and brain plasticity in antidepressant and antipsychotic interventions. *Neurosci. Biobehav. Rev.* 60, 51–64. doi: 10.1016/j.neubiorev.2015.11.008

Rief, W., Nestoriuc, Y., Weiss, S., Welzel, E., Barsky, A. J., and Hofmann, S. G. (2009). Meta-analysis of the placebo response in antidepressant trials. *J. Affect. Disord.* 118, 1–8. doi: 10.1016/j.jad.2009.01.029

Rimes, R. R., de Souza Moura, A. M., Lamego, M. K., de Sá Filho, A. S., Manochio, J., Paes, F., et al. (2015). Effects of exercise on physical and mental health, and cognitive and brain functions in schizophrenia: clinical and experimental evidence. *CNS and Neurol. Disord. Drug Targets* 14, 1244–1254. doi: 10.2174/1871527315666151111130659

Rock, P. L., Roiser, J. P., Riedel, W. J., and Blackwell, A. D. (2013). Cognitive impairment in depression: a systematic review and meta-analysis. *Psychol. Med.* 44, 2029–2040. doi: 10.1017/S0033291713002535

Roig, M., Nordbrandt, S., Geertsen, S. S., and Nielsen, J. B. (2013). The effects of cardiovascular exercise on human memory: a review with meta-analysis. *Neurosci. Biobehav. Rev.* 37, 1645–1666. doi: 10.1016/j.neubiorev.2013.06.012

Rosenbaum, S., Lagopoulos, J., Curtis, J., Taylor, L., Watkins, A., Barry, B. K., et al. (2015). Aerobic exercise intervention in young people with schizophrenia spectrum disorders; improved fitness with no change in hippocampal volume. *Psychiatry Res. Neuroimag.* 232, 200–201. doi: 10.1016/j.pscychresns.2015.02.004

Rosenblat, J. D., Kakar, R., and McIntyre, R. S. (2015). The cognitive effects of antidepressants in major depressive disorder: a systematic review and meta-analysis of randomized clinical trials. *Int. J. Neuropsychopharmacol.* 19:pyv082. doi: 10.1093/ijnp/pyv082

Rubio, F. J., Ampuero, E., Sandoval, R., Toledo, J., Pancetti, F., and Wyneken, U. (2013). Long-term fluoxetine treatment induces input-specific LTP and LTD impairment and structural plasticity in the CA1 hippocampal subfield. *Front. Cell. Neurosci.* 7:66. doi: 10.3389/fncel.2013.00066

Ruscheweyh, R., Willemer, C., Krüger, K., Duning, T., Warnecke, T., Sommer, J., et al. (2011). Physical activity and memory functions: an interventional study. *Neurobiol. Aging* 32, 1304–1319. doi: 10.1016/j.neurobiolaging.2009.08.001

Russo-Neustadt, A., Ha, T., Ramirez, R., and Kesslak, J. P. (2001). Physical activity–antidepressant treatment combination: impact on brain-derived neurotrophic factor and behavior in an animal model. *Behav. Brain Res.* 120, 87–95. doi: 10.1016/S0166-4328(00)00364-8

Sabia, S., Nabi, H., Kivimaki, M., Shipley, M. J., Marmot, M. G., and Singh-Manoux, A. (2009). Health behaviors from early to late midlife as predictors of cognitive function: the Whitehall II study. *Am. J. Epidemiol.* 170, 428–437. doi: 10.1093/aje/kwp161

Sahay, A., and Hen, R. (2007). Adult hippocampal neurogenesis in depression. *Nat. Neurosci.* 10, 1110–1115. doi: 10.1038/nn1969

Sahay, A., Scobie, K. N., Hill, A. S., O'Carroll, C. M., Kheirbek, M. A., Burghardt, N. S., et al. (2011). Increasing adult hippocampal neurogenesis is sufficient to improve pattern separation. *Nature* 472, 466–470. doi: 10.1038/nature09817

Sanderson, T. M., Cotel, M.-C., O'Neill, M. J., Tricklebank, M. D., Collingridge, G. L., and Sher, E. (2012). Alterations in hippocampal excitability, synaptic transmission and synaptic plasticity in a neurodevelopmental model of schizophrenia. *Neuropharmacology* 62, 1349–1358. doi: 10.1016/j.neuropharm.2011.08.005

Sapolsky, R. M. (2000). Glucocorticoids and hippocampal atrophy in neuropsychiatric disorders. *Arch. Gen. Psychiatry* 57, 925–935. doi: 10.1001/archpsyc.57.10.925

Sartori, C. R., Vieira, A. S., Ferrari, E. M., Langone, F., Tongiorgi, E., and Parada, C. A. (2011). The antidepressive effect of the physical exercise correlates with increased levels of mature BDNF, and proBDNF proteolytic cleavage-related genes, p11 and tPA. *Neuroscience* 180, 9–18. doi: 10.1016/j.neuroscience.2011.02.055

Scheewe, T. W., van Haren, N. E. M., Sarkisyan, G., Schnack, H. G., Brouwer, R. M., de Glint, M., et al. (2013). Exercise therapy, cardiorespiratory fitness and their effect on brain volumes: a randomised controlled trial in patients with schizophrenia and healthy controls. *Eur. Neuropsychopharmacol.* 23, 675–685. doi: 10.1016/j.euroneuro.2012.08.008

Schmaal, L., Veltman, D. J., van Erp, T. G. M., Sämann, P. G., Frodl, T., Jahanshad, N., et al. (2016). Subcortical brain alterations in major depressive disorder: findings from the ENIGMA major depressive disorder working group. *Mol. Psychiatry* 21, 806–812. doi: 10.1038/mp.2015.69

Schmidt-Hieber, C., Jonas, P., and Bischofberger, J. (2004). Enhanced synaptic plasticity in newly generated granule cells of the adult hippocampus. *Nature* 429, 184–187. doi: 10.1038/nature02553

Schmitt, A., Weber, S., Jatzko, A., Braus, D. F., and Henn, F. A. (2004). Hippocampal volume and cell proliferation after acute and chronic clozapine or haloperidol treatment. *J. Neural Trans.* 111, 91–100. doi: 10.1007/s00702-003-0070-2

Schobel, S. A., Kelly, M. A., Corcoran, C. M., Van Heertum, K., Seckinger, R., Goetz, R., et al. (2009). Anterior hippocampal and orbitofrontal cortical structural brain abnormalities in association with cognitive deficits in schizophrenia. *Schizophr. Res.* 114, 110–118. doi: 10.1016/j.schres.2009.07.016

Schobersberger, W., Hobisch-Hagen, P., Fries, D., Wiedermann, F., Rieder-Scharinger, J., Villiger, B., et al. (2000). Increase in immune activation, vascular endothelial growth factor and erythropoietin after an ultramarathon run at moderate altitude. *Immunobiology* 201, 611–620. doi: 10.1016/S0171-2985(00)80078-9

Schoenfeld, T. J., and Cameron, H. A. (2015). Adult neurogenesis and mental illness. *Neuropsychopharmacology* 40, 113–128. doi: 10.1038/npp.2014.230

Schuch, F. B., Vasconcelos-Moreno, M. P., Borowsky, C., and Fleck, M. P. (2011). Exercise and severe depression: preliminary results of an add-on study. *J. Affect. Disord.* 133, 615–618. doi: 10.1016/j.jad.2011.04.030

Seidenbecher, T., Laxmi, T. R., Stork, O., and Pape, H.-C. (2003). Amygdalar and hippocampal theta rhythm synchronization during fear memory retrieval. *Science* 301, 846–850. doi: 10.1126/science.1085818

Sexton, C., Filippini, N., Betts, J., Zsoldos, E., Thomas, A., Dennis, A., Johansen-Berg, H. (2015a). Physical activity and anterior hippocampal volume in older adults. *Proc. Physiol. Soc.* 33:PC10

Sexton, C. E., Betts, J. F., Demnitz, N., Dawes, H., Ebmeier, K. P., and Johansen-Berg, H. (2015b). A systematic review of MRI studies examining the relationship between physical fitness and activity and the white matter of the ageing brain. *Neuroimage* 31, 81–90. doi: 10.1016/j.neuroimage.2015.09.071

Shelton, D. J., and Kirwan, C. B. (2013). A possible negative influence of depression on the ability to overcome memory interference. *Behav. Brain Res.* 256, 20–26. doi: 10.1016/j.bbr.2013.08.016

Shors, T. J., Townsend, D. A., Zhao, M., Kozorovitskiy, Y., and Gould, E. (2002). Neurogenesis may relate to some but not all types of hippocampal-dependent learning. *Hippocampus* 12, 578–584. doi: 10.1002/hipo.10103

Sibley, B. A., and Etnier, J. L. (2003). The relationship between physical activity and cognition in children: a meta-analysis. *Pediatr. Exerc. Sci.* 15, 243–256. doi: 10.1515/ijsl.2000.143.183

Singh, N. A., Stavrinos, T. M., Scarbek, Y., Galambos, G., Liber, C., and Fiatarone Singh, M. A. (2005). A randomized controlled trial of high versus low intensity weight training versus general practitioner care for clinical depression in older adults. *J. Gerontol. Ser. A Biol. Sci. Med. Sci.* 60, 768–776. doi: 10.1093/gerona/60.6.768

Smieskova, R., Fusar-Poli, P., Allen, P., Bendfeldt, K., Stieglitz, R. D., Drewe, J., et al. (2009). The effects of antipsychotics on the brain: what have we learnt from structural imaging of schizophrenia?–a systematic review. *Curr. Pharmac. Des.* 15, 2535–2549. doi: 10.2174/138161209788957456

Smith, P. J., Blumenthal, J. A., Hoffman, B. M., Cooper, H., Strauman, T. A., Welsh-Bohmer, K., et al. (2010). Aerobic exercise and neurocognitive performance: a meta-analytic review of randomized controlled trials. *Psychosom. Med.* 72, 239–252. doi: 10.1097/PSY.0b013e3181d14633

Snowden, M., Steinman, L., Mochan, K., Grodstein, F., Prohaska, T. R., Thurman, D. J., et al. (2011). Effect of exercise on cognitive performance in community-dwelling older adults: review of intervention trials and recommendations for public health practice and research. *J. Am. Geriatr. Soc.* 59, 704–716. doi: 10.1111/j.1532-5415.2011.03323.x

Snyder, J. S., and Cameron, H. A. (2012). Could adult hippocampal neurogenesis be relevant for human behavior? *Behav. Brain Res.* 227, 384–390. doi: 10.1016/j.bbr.2011.06.024

Snyder, J. S., Hong, N. S., McDonald, R. J., and Wojtowicz, J. M. (2005). A role for adult neurogenesis in spatial long-term memory. *Neuroscience* 130, 843–852. doi: 10.1016/j.neuroscience.2004.10.009

Snyder, J. S., Soumier, A., Brewer, M., Pickel, J., and Cameron, H. A. (2011). Adult hippocampal neurogenesis buffers stress responses and depressive behaviour. *Nature* 476, 458–461. doi: 10.1038/nature10287

Solé, B., Jiménez, E., Martinez-Aran, A., and Vieta, E. (2015). Cognition as a target in major depression: new developments. *Eur. Neuropsychopharmacol.* 25, 231–247. doi: 10.1016/j.euroneuro.2014.12.004

Sommer, I. E., and Kahn, R. S. (2015). The magic of movement; the potential of exercise to improve cognition. *Schizophr. Bull.* 41, 776–778. doi: 10.1093/schbul/sbv031

Soundy, A., Stubbs, B., Probst, M., Hemmings, L., and Vancampfort, D. (2014). Barriers to and facilitators of physical activity among persons with schizophrenia: a survey of physical therapists. *Psychiatr. Services* 65, 693–696. doi: 10.1176/appi.ps.201300276

Spalding, K. L., Bergmann, O., Alkass, K., Bernard, S., Salehpour, M., Huttner, H. B., et al. (2013). Dynamics of hippocampal neurogenesis in adult humans. *Cell* 153, 1219–1227.

Stanton, R., and Happell, B. (2014). A systematic review of the aerobic exercise program variables for people with schizophrenia. *Curr. Sports Med. Rep.* 13, 260–266. doi: 10.1249/JSR.0000000000000069

Stanton, R., and Reaburn, P. (2014). Exercise and the treatment of depression: a review of the exercise program variables. *J. Sci. Med. Sport* 17, 177–182. doi: 10.1016/j.jsams.2013.03.010

Stewart, R., Prince, M., and Mann, A. (2003). Age, vascular risk, and cognitive decline in an older, British, African-Caribbean population. *J. Am. Geriatr. Soc.* 51, 1547–1553. doi: 10.1046/j.1532-5415.2003.51504.x

Stranahan, A. M., Khalil, D., and Gould, E. (2007). Running induces widespread structural alterations in the hippocampus and entorhinal cortex. *Hippocampus* 17, 1017–1022. doi: 10.1002/hipo.20348

Stroth, S., Hille, K., Spitzer, M., and Reinhardt, R. (2009). Aerobic endurance exercise benefits memory and affect in young adults. *Neuropsychol. Rehabil.* 19, 223–243. doi: 10.1080/09602010802091183

Stubbs, B., Vancampfort, D., Rosenbaum, S., Ward, P. B., Richards, J., Soundy, A., et al. (2016). Dropout from exercise randomized controlled trials among people with depression: a meta-analysis and meta regression. *J. Affect. Disord.* 190, 457–466. doi: 10.1016/j.jad.2015.10.019

Suo, C., Singh, M. F., Gates, N., Wen, W., Sachdev, P., Brodaty, H., et al. (2016). Therapeutically relevant structural and functional mechanisms triggered by physical and cognitive exercise. *Mol. Psychiatry* doi: 10.1038/mp.2016.19 [Epub ahead of print].

Svatkova, A., Mandl, R. C. W., Scheewe, T. W., Cahn, W., Kahn, R. S., and Hulshoff Pol, H. E. (2015). Physical exercise keeps the brain connected: biking increases white matter integrity in patients with schizophrenia and healthy controls. *Schizophr. Bull.* 41, 869–878. doi: 10.1093/schbul/sbv033

Szabo, A. N., McAuley, E., Erickson, K. I., Voss, M., Prakash, R. S., Mailey, E. L., et al. (2011). Cardiorespiratory fitness, hippocampal volume, and frequency of forgetting in older adults. *Neuropsychology* 25, 545–553. doi: 10.1037/a0022733

Szeszko, P. R., Strous, R. D., Goldman, R. S., Ashtari, M., Knuth, K. H., Lieberman, J. A., et al. (2002). Neuropsychological correlates of hippocampal volumes in patients experiencing a first episode of schizophrenia. *Am. J. Psychiatry* 159, 217–226. doi: 10.1176/appi.ajp.159.2.217

Tamminga, C. A., Stan, A. D., and Wagner, A. D. (2010). The hippocampal formation in schizophrenia. *Am. J. Psychiatry* 167, 1178–1193. doi: 10.1176/appi.ajp.2010.09081187

Tandon, R. (2011). Antipsychotics in the treatment of schizophrenia: an overview. *J. Clin. Psychiatry* 72(Suppl. 1), 4–8. doi: 10.4088/JCP.10075su1.01

Tang, Y., Hojatkashani, C., Dinov, I. D., Sun, B., Fan, L., Lin, X., et al. (2010). The construction of a Chinese MRI brain atlas: a morphometric comparison study between Chinese and Caucasian cohorts. *Neuroimage* 51, 33–41. doi: 10.1016/j.neuroimage.2010.01.111

Teixeira, A. M., Pase, C. S., Boufleur, N., Roversi, K., Barcelos, R. C. S., Benvegnú, D. M., et al. (2011). Exercise affects memory acquisition, anxiety-like symptoms and activity of membrane-bound enzyme in brain of rats fed with different dietary fats: impairments of trans fat. *Neuroscience* 195, 80–88. doi: 10.1016/j.neuroscience.2011.08.055

Templer, V. L., and Hampton, R. R. (2013). Episodic memory in nonhuman animals. *Curr. Biol.* 23, R801–R806. doi: 10.1016/j.cub.2013.07.016

ten Brinke, L. F., Bolandzadeh, N., Nagamatsu, L. S., Hsu, C. L., Davis, J. C., Miran-Khan, K., et al. (2015). Aerobic exercise increases hippocampal volume in older women with probable mild cognitive impairment: a 6-month randomised controlled trial. *Br. J. Sports Med.* 49, 248–254. doi: 10.1136/bjsports-2013-093184

Thomas, A. G., Dennis, A., Bandettini, P. A., and Johansen-Berg, H. (2012). The effects of aerobic activity on brain structure. *Front. Psychol.* 3:86. doi: 10.3389/fpsyg.2012.00086

Thomas, A. G., Dennis, A., Rawlings, N. B., Stagg, C. J., Matthews, L., Morris, M., et al. (2016). Multi-modal characterization of rapid anterior hippocampal volume increase associated with aerobic exercise. *Neuroimage* 131, 162–170. doi: 10.1016/j.neuroimage.2015.10.090

Tomporowski, P. D., Davis, C. L., Miller, P. H., and Naglieri, J. A. (2008). Exercise and children's intelligence, cognition, and academic achievement. *Educ. Psychol. Rev.* 20, 111–131. doi: 10.1007/s10648-007-9057-0

Tomporowski, P. D., McCullick, B., Pendleton, D. M., and Pesce, C. (2014). Exercise and children's cognition: the role of exercise characteristics and a place for metacognition. *J. Sport Health Sci.* 4, 47–55. doi: 10.1016/j.jshs.2014.09.003

Toups, M. S. P., Greer, T. L., Kurian, B. T., Grannemann, B. D., Carmody, T. J., Huebinger, R., et al. (2011). Effects of serum brain derived neurotrophic factor on exercise augmentation treatment of depression. *J. Psychiatr. Res.* 45, 1301–1306. doi: 10.1016/j.jpsychires.2011.05.002

Travis, S., Coupland, N. J., Silversone, P. H., Huang, Y., Fujiwara, E., Carter, R., et al. (2015). Dentate gyrus volume and memory performance in major depressive disorder. *J. Affect. Disord.* 172, 159–164. doi: 10.1016/j.jad.2014.09.048

Trejo, J. L., Carro, E., and Torres-Aleman, I. (2001). Circulating insulin-like growth factor i mediates exercise-induced increases in the number of new neurons in the adult hippocampus. *J. Neurosci.* 21, 1628–1634.

Tseng, B. Y., Gundapuneedi, T., Khan, M. A., Diaz-Arrastia, R., Levine, B. D., Lu, H., et al. (2013). White matter integrity in physically fit older adults. *Neuroimage* 82, 510–516. doi: 10.1016/j.neuroimage.2013.06.011

Tulving, E. (1993). What is episodic memory? *Curr. Perspect. Psychol. Sci.* 2, 67–70.

Turner, A. D., Furey, M. L., Drevets, W. C., Zarate, C., and Nugent, A. C. (2012). Association between subcortical volumes and verbal memory in unmedicated depressed patients and healthy controls. *Neuropsychologia* 50, 2348–2355. doi: 10.1016/j.neuropsychologia.2012.06.003

Tybura, P., Mak, M., Samochowiec, A., Pełka-Wysiecka, J., Grzywacz, A., Grochans, E., et al. (2013). Wpływ leków przeciwpsychotycznych na funkcje poznawcze u pacjentów ze schizofrenią. *Psychiatr. Polska* 47, 567–578.

Undurraga, J., and Baldessarini, R. J. (2012). Randomized, placebo-controlled trials of antidepressants for acute major depression: thirty-year meta-analytic review. *Neuropsychopharmacology* 37, 851–864. doi: 10.1038/npp.2011.306

Uysal, N., Kiray, M., Sisman, A. R., Camsari, U. M., Gencoglu, C., Baykara, B., et al. (2015). Effects of voluntary and involuntary exercise on cognitive functions, and VEGF and BDNF levels in adolescent rats. *Biotech. Histochem.* 90, 55–68. doi: 10.3109/10520295.2014.946968

Vadodaria, K. C., and Jessberger, S. (2014). Functional neurogenesis in the adult hippocampus: then and now. *Front. Neurosci.* 8:55. doi: 10.3389/fnins.2014.00055

Vakhrusheva, J., Marino, B., Stroup, T. S., and Kimhy, D. (2016). Aerobic exercise in people with schizophrenia: neural and neurocognitive benefits. *Curr. Behav. Neurosci. Rep.* 3, 165–175. doi: 10.1007/s40473-016-0077-2

Van der Borght, K., Kóbor-Nyakas, D. E., Klauke, K., Eggen, B. J. L., Nyakas, C., Van der Zee, E. A., et al. (2009). Physical exercise leads to rapid adaptations in hippocampal vasculature: temporal dynamics and relationship to cell proliferation and neurogenesis. *Hippocampus* 19, 928–936. doi: 10.1002/hipo.20545

van Praag, H. (2008). Neurogenesis and exercise: past and future directions. *Neuromol. Med.* 10, 128–140. doi: 10.1007/s12017-008-8028-z

van Praag, H. (2009). Exercise and the brain: something to chew on. *Trends Neurosci.* 32, 283–290. doi: 10.1016/j.tins.2008.12.007

van Praag, H., Lucero, M. J., Yeo, G. W., Stecker, K., Heivand, N., Zhao, C., et al. (2007). Plant-derived flavanol (-)epicatechin enhances angiogenesis and retention of spatial memory in mice. *J. Neurosci.* 27, 5869–5878. doi: 10.1523/JNEUROSCI.0914-07.2007

van Praag, H., Shubert, T., Zhao, C., and Gage, F. H. (2005). Exercise enhances learning and hippocampal neurogenesis in aged mice. *J. Neurosci.* 25, 8680–8685. doi: 10.1523/JNEUROSCI.1731-05.2005

van Uffelen, J. G. Z., Chin, A., Paw, M. J. M., Hopman-Rock, M., and van Mechelen, W. (2008). The effects of exercise on cognition in older adults with and without cognitive decline: a systematic review. *Clin. J. Sport Med.* 18, 486–500. doi: 10.1097/JSM.0b013e3181845f0b

Vancampfort, D., Probst, M., De Hert, M., Soundy, A., Stubbs, B., Stroobants, M., et al. (2014). Neurobiological effects of physical exercise in schizophrenia: a systematic review. *Disabil. Rehabil.* 36, 1749–1754. doi: 10.3109/09638288.2013.874505

Vancampfort, D., Probst, M., Helvik Skjaerven, L., Catalán-Matamoros, D., Lundvik-Gyllensten, A., Gómez-Conesa, A., et al. (2012). Systematic review of the benefits of physical therapy within a multidisciplinary care approach for people with schizophrenia. *Phys. Ther.* 92, 11–23. doi: 10.2522/ptj.20110218

Vancampfort, D., Probst, M., Scheewe, T., De Herdt, A., Sweers, K., Knapen, J., et al. (2013). Relationships between physical fitness, physical activity, smoking and metabolic and mental health parameters in people with schizophrenia. *Psychiatry Res.* 207, 25–32. doi: 10.1016/j.psychres.2012.09.026

Vancampfort, D., Rosenbaum, S., Schuch, F. B., Ward, P. B., Probst, M., and Stubbs, B. (2016). Prevalence and predictors of treatment dropout from physical activity interventions in schizophrenia: a meta-analysis. *Gen. Hosp. Psychiatry* 39, 15–23. doi: 10.1016/j.genhosppsych.2015.11.008

Vasques, P. E., Moraes, H., Silveira, H., Deslandes, A. C., and Laks, J. (2011). Acute exercise improves cognition in the depressed elderly: the effect of dual-tasks. *Clinics* 66, 1553–1557. doi: 10.1590/S1807-59322011000900008

Vaynman, S., Ying, Z., and Gomez-Pinilla, F. (2004). Hippocampal BDNF mediates the efficacy of exercise on synaptic plasticity and cognition. *Eur. J. Neurosci.* 20, 2580–2590. doi: 10.1111/j.1460-9568.2004.03720.x

Verburgh, L., Konigs, M., Scherder, E. J. A., and Oosterlaan, J. (2013). Physical exercise and executive functions in preadolescent children, adolescents and young adults: a meta-analysis. *Br. J. Sports Med.* 48, 973–979. doi: 10.1136/bjsports-2012-091441

Vernon, A. C., Natesan, S., Modo, M., and Kapur, S. (2011). Effect of chronic antipsychotic treatment on brain structure: a serial magnetic resonance imaging study with ex vivo and postmortem confirmation. *Biol. Psychiatry* 69, 936–944. doi: 10.1016/j.biopsych.2010.11.010

Vivar, C., Potter, M. C., and van Praag, H. (2013). All about running: synaptic plasticity, growth factors and adult hippocampal neurogenesis. *Curr. Topics Behav. Neurosci.* 15, 189–210. doi: 10.1007/7854_2012_220

Voss, M. W., Heo, S., Prakash, R. S., Erickson, K. I., Alves, H., Chaddock, L., et al. (2013a). The influence of aerobic fitness on cerebral white matter integrity and cognitive function in older adults: results of a one-year exercise intervention. *Hum. Brain Mapp.* 2985, 2972–2985. doi: 10.1002/hbm.22119

Voss, M. W., Vivar, C., Kramer, A. F., and van Praag, H. (2013b). Bridging animal and human models of exercise-induced brain plasticity. *Trends Cogn. Sci.* 17, 525–544. doi: 10.1016/j.tics.2013.08.001

Wagner, G., Herbsleb, M., de la Cruz, F., Schumann, A., Brünner, F., Schachtzabel, C., et al. (2015). Hippocampal structure, metabolism, and inflammatory response after a 6-week intense aerobic exercise in healthy young adults: a controlled trial. *J. Cereb. Blood Flow Metab.* 35, 1570–1578. doi: 10.1038/jcbfm.2015.125

Wallace, J., Marston, H. M., McQuade, R., and Gartside, S. E. (2014). Evidence that aetiological risk factors for psychiatric disorders cause distinct patterns of cognitive deficits. *Eur. Neuropsychopharmacol.* 24, 879–889. doi: 10.1016/j.euroneuro.2013.12.005

Wallace, T. L., Ballard, T. M., Pouzet, B., Riedel, W. J., and Wettstein, J. G. (2011). Drug targets for cognitive enhancement in neuropsychiatric disorders. *Pharmacol. Biochem. Behav.* 99, 130–145. doi: 10.1016/j.pbb.2011.03.022

Wendell, C. R., Gunstad, J., Waldstein, S. R., Wright, J. G., Ferrucci, L., and Zonderman, A. B. (2014). Cardiorespiratory fitness and accelerated cognitive decline with aging. *J. Gerontol. A Biol. Sci. Med. Sci.* 69, 455–462. doi: 10.1093/gerona/glt144

Wilson, C. A., Schade, R., and Terry, A. V. (2012). Variable prenatal stress results in impairments of sustained attention and inhibitory response control in a 5-choice serial reaction time task in rats. *Neuroscience* 218, 126–137. doi: 10.1016/j.neuroscience.2012.05.040

Wojtowicz, J. M., Askew, M. L., and Winocur, G. (2008). The effects of running and of inhibiting adult neurogenesis on learning and memory in rats. *Eur. J. Neurosci.* 27, 1494–1502. doi: 10.1111/j.1460-9568.2008.06128.x

Wolf, S. A., Melnik, A., and Kempermann, G. (2011). Physical exercise increases adult neurogenesis and telomerase activity, and improves behavioral deficits in a mouse model of schizophrenia. *Brain Behav. Immun.* 25, 971–980. doi: 10.1016/j.bbi.2010.10.014

Wykes, T., Huddy, V., Cellard, C., McGurk, S. R., and Czobor, P. (2011). A meta-analysis of cognitive remediation for schizophrenia: methodology and effect sizes. *Am. J. Psychiatry* 168, 472–485. doi: 10.1176/appi.ajp.2010.10060855

Yaffe, K., Barnes, D., Nevitt, M., Lui, L.-Y., and Covinsky, K. (2001). A prospective study of physical activity and cognitive decline in elderly women. *Arch. Intern. Med.* 161, 1703. doi: 10.1001/archinte.161.14.1703

Yassa, M. A., and Stark, C. E. L. (2011). Pattern separation in the hippocampus. *Trends Neurosci.* 34, 515–525. doi: 10.1016/j.tins.2011.06.006

Yau, S.-Y., Lau, B. W.-M., Zhang, E.-D., Lee, J. C.-D., Li, A., Lee, T. M. C., et al. (2012). Effects of voluntary running on plasma levels of neurotrophins, hippocampal cell proliferation and learning and memory in stressed rats. *Neuroscience* 222, 289–301. doi: 10.1016/j.neuroscience.2012.07.019

Young, J., Angevaren, M., Rusted, J., and Tabet, N. (2015). Aerobic exercise to improve cognitive function in older people without known cognitive impairment (Review). *Cochrane Database Syst. Rev.* 22:CD005381. doi: 10.1002/14651858.CD005381.pub4

Zhang, X. Y., Liang, J., Chen, D. C., Xiu, M. H., Yang, F., De Kosten, T. A., et al. (2012). Low BDNF is associated with cognitive impairment in chronic patients with schizophrenia. *Psychopharmacology* 222, 277–284. doi: 10.1007/s00213-012-2643-y

Zheng, H., Liu, Y., Li, W., Yang, B., Chen, D., Wang, X., et al. (2006). Beneficial effects of exercise and its molecular mechanisms on depression in rats. *Behav. Brain Res.* 168, 47–55. doi: 10.1016/j.bbr.2005.10.007

Zschucke, E., Heinz, A., and Ströhle, A. (2012). Exercise and physical activity in the therapy of substance use disorders. *Sci. World J.* 2012:901745. doi: 10.1100/2012/901741

6

The Do's and Don'ts of Neurofeedback Training

*Jacek Rogala *, Katarzyna Jurewicz, Katarzyna Paluch, Ewa Kublik, Ryszard Cetnarski and Andrzej Wróbel*

Laboratory of Visual System, Nencki Institute of Experimental Biology, Polish Academy of Sciences, Warsaw, Poland

Edited by:
Soledad Ballesteros, Universidad Nacional de Educación a Distancia, Spain

Reviewed by:
Christian Beste, Technische Universität Dresden (TUD), Germany
Carlos J. Gomez-Ariza, Universidad de Jaén, Spain

***Correspondence:**
Jacek Rogala
j.rogala@nencki.gov.pl

The goal of EEG neurofeedback (EEG-NFB) training is to induce changes in the power of targeted EEG bands to produce beneficial changes in cognitive or motor function. The effectiveness of different EEG-NFB protocols can be measured using two dependent variables: (1) changes in EEG activity and (2) behavioral changes of a targeted function (for therapeutic applications the desired changes should be long-lasting). To firmly establish a causal link between these variables and the selected protocol, similar changes should not be observed when appropriate control paradigms are used. The main objective of this review is to evaluate the evidence, reported in the scientific literature, which supports the validity of various EEG-NFB protocols. Our primary concern is to highlight the role that uncontrolled nonspecific factors can play in the results generated from EEG-NFB studies. Nonspecific factors are often ignored in EEG-NFB designs or the data are not presented, which means conclusions should be interpreted cautiously. As an outcome of this review we present a do's and don'ts list, which can be used to develop future EEG-NFB methodologies, based on the small set of experiments in which the proper control groups have excluded non-EEG-NFB related effects. We found two features which positively correlated with the expected changes in power of the trained EEG band(s): (1) protocols which focused on training a smaller number of frequency bands and (2) a bigger number of electrodes used for neurofeedback training. However, we did not find evidence in support of the positive relationship between power changes of a trained frequency band(s) and specific behavioral effects.

Keywords: neurofeedback training, EEG, replicability, protocol efficacy, methodology

INTRODUCTION

Electroencephalogram (EEG) based neurofeedback (NFB) is a method in which brain activity is modulated via self-induced increases or decreases in the power of selected EEG frequency bands. The subject's control over his or her EEG activity is typically mediated with visual or auditory feedback. EEG-NFB is widely used as a therapy for certain mental, cognitive, and behavioral disorders (e.g. ADHD, for review see Arns et al., 2009); or as supportive training to improve cognitive performance (e.g. attention or memory, for review see Gruzelier, 2013a). Since the pioneering work of Sterman and Friar (1972), the number of publications devoted to EEG-NFB has systematically increased. During the first two decades (1972-1990), 162 NFB-based studies were published, based on a search in Google Scholar for the keyword 'neurofeedback'. This number increased rapidly in the subsequent decades, reaching 1,260 in nineties and 6,100 between 2001 and 2010. Since 2011, there have been over 9000 publications devoted to various aspects of EEG-NFB. However, despite multiple promising case reports, reliable experimental research is scarce, and the methodologies and results inconsistent.

The validity of EEG-NFB protocols can be measured by unambiguous changes in EEG activity and by changes in the targeted cognitive function. Unfortunately, most of the work conducted in the EEG-NFB field has failed to satisfy the unambiguity criterion for both of the variables and the field itself has shown a big tolerance for violations of scientific methodology. Several reviews have been published which focused mainly on the clinical aspects of EEG-NFB training and summarized the protocols and their effects. One of the first reviews, published by Vernon et al. (2004), concerned the application of EEG-NFB for the treatment of attention deficit hyperactivity disorder (ADHD). The authors discussed various experimental variables (factors), namely, protocol, duration of the training, location of electrodes, signal modality and discussed their possible impact on treatment. The methodological findings of this review recommended visual rather than auditory feedback, with the best results obtained with visual and auditory modalities combined. In addition, the review suggested that at least 20 EEG-NFB sessions were necessary to achieve therapeutic effects, and that beta band/SMR protocols may play a role in successful ADHD treatment. However, studies examining EEG-NFB in the treatment of ADHD have raised important concerns about the validity of the treatment paradigm(s) mainly due to the lack of control groups or evidence of training specificity related to EEG changes (Vollebregt et al., 2014; Zuberer et al., 2015).

The first quantitative review of EEG-NFB methodology was reported by Arns et al. (2009) and focused on controlled ADHD studies. This review supported the view that positive therapeutic effects of EEG-NFB training could be achieved for all symptoms of ADHD. However, in contrast to Vernon's conclusions (Vernon et al., 2004), Arns concluded that inattention and hyperactivity were most sensitive to the non-specific treatment factors (e.g., therapist-patient interactions) and not the EEG feedback itself. Similarly, according to Logemann et al. (2010), non-specific factors may be responsible for the effects observed in healthy subjects. A more recent review by May et al. (2013) carried out on traumatic brain injury patients also concluded that positive therapeutic effects of the EEG-NFB could be achieved, however, all the reviewed studies were missing proper sham control groups (with pseudo-feedback based on an EEG signal recorded from another individual/another session, or an artificial signal generated by a computer) that would undergo fake EEG-NFB training. The same methodological weakness characterized the therapeutic-oriented ADHD studies analyzed in another review published recently by Arns group (Arns et al., 2014). The majority of the reviewed studies included a limited control group such as a semi-active control group (aiming to control non-specific effects like time spent interacting with a computer) or an active control group (comparison with a treatment with known therapeutic effects). Importantly, for all studies using proper sham-control groups the results of EEG-NFB training appeared to be negative. Controls for both clinical treatment and basic research of EEG-NFB training should include sham groups that account for factors such as spontaneous EEG changes, coach-subject interactions or attention effort that accompanies any EEG-NFB training. The effect of the independent variable (the specific EEG-NFB protocol) should be estimated as the measurement in the experimental group minus the same measurement in the sham-control group or alternatively in a group with a different protocol. Without such quantification the experimental results do not constitute evidence for the efficacy of the independent variable, i.e., feedback training.

Unfortunately, a sham-control for the positive effects is ethically challenging, since the use of placebo (which includes also sham groups), instead of clinical treatments, may lead to a deterioration of symptoms (Helsinki Declaration 1964). Thus, well-controlled EEG-NFB studies can only be carried out on treatment-resistant or healthy subjects.

The recent review series by Gruzelier (2013a,b, 2014) stemmed from the increasingly abundant number of studies devoted to EEG-NFB experiments performed on healthy participants. The author presented overwhelmingly positive interpretation concerning the state-of-the-art of EEG-NFB research, however these reviews included multiple studies which did not include proper controls for nonspecific training effects (as mentioned above).

Here, we selectively review only of those EEG-NFB studies which have included an appropriate control group(s) to quantitatively evaluate the effects of this type of training. The fundamental assumptions of EEG-NFB are based on the causal relationships between (1) the desired feedback signal and changes in brain activity, and (2) between induced EEG power changes and behavior. Therefore, we quantitatively assessed the efficacy of the protocols reported to induce changes in these two variables (EEG activity and behavior). We also examined any possible mutual relationship between these two measures. Our evaluation included quantitative estimations of the contribution of individual experimental factors to the final outcome. Each experiment that qualified for analysis was verified to determine whether EEG-NFB training induced a significant modulation of EEG and/or behavioral features, and whether the EEG modulation and behavioral changes occurred concomitantly.

METHODS

Inclusion Criteria

The research papers selected and reviewed in this study were identified by (i) a search of web resources (Google Scholar and PubMed) using the following keywords: biofeedback and EEG, neurofeedback and EEG, brain-computer interface and EEG, and EEG operant conditioning; and (ii) an examination of the reference lists of the retrieved articles. From the collected database we selected 86 articles that described experiments carried out using healthy adult participants.

Two Steps Selection Process

First, we selected articles which included separate control groups and those in which training was performed in two parallel groups, each group with a different EEG-NFB protocol. In latter case we assumed the two groups could serve as a control for one another (Bird et al., 1978; Allen et al., 2001; Keizer et al., 2010a). We included purely behavioral studies that lacked elaboration of the EEG data. In these studies the authors only used EEG for generating feedback signals, the EEG recordings obtained from within the training sessions or the pre- vs. post-training data were not analyzed and outcomes were only focused on the final behavioral effect of training.

This criterion identified eligible 40 publications that described 43 EEG-NFB experiments (a few articles described more than one experimental paradigm) that were performed on healthy volunteers (**Table 1**) and included different types of control groups: sham EEG-NFB, alternative type of activities (relaxation techniques, yoga), or no activity. We carefully evaluated all these experimental paradigms and in the second selection step we excluded studies in which control did not unequivocally address major nonspecific factors. In an illustrative example no activity was required from participants in the control group, not even attendance at the laboratory on a similar schedule. In this case, since the control group was not exposed to nonspecific factors that accompanied EEG-NFB training, it is not known whether the observed behavioral effects resulted from the treatment, or from factors such as regular tasks that require focused attention and/or trainer care. Similarly, the EEG spectrum could also depend on nonspecific behavioral training. Thus, for further analysis we only included experiments in which EEG's were recorded and analyzed in both EEG-NFB and control groups.

During this second selection step the following studies were excluded: (i) experiments that used EEG feedback but did not provide the results of the EEG analysis in the article; (ii) experiments that did not provide a description of the EEG results for the control group which precluded reliable analysis; (iii) experiments that did not engage the members of the control group in any type of activity ("non-intervention group") and/or did not describe the control group manipulation); (iv) experiments that used non-responders (subjects not showing expected changes due to neurofeedback training) identified after completion of the training as a control. The identification of "non-responders" has been reported in published EEG-NFB experiments and clinical applications. It is possible that susceptibility to EEG-NFB training differs greatly between individuals, which alone demands further investigation (Weber et al., 2011; Wan et al., 2014; Nan et al., 2015). However, at present, it is not appropriate to restrict the experimental group to the participants with clear effects and exclude non-responders from the analyses. The set of papers selected for final analysis was composed of 28 experiments described in 25 studies (listed in **Tables 1, 4**). Supplementary Table 1 lists the eliminated studies and reasons for exclusion.

Key Experimental Factors

Many factors may potentially influence the success or failure of EEG-NFB procedures. Some factors can be controlled in our experimental paradigms, other cannot. An example of the latter is low training susceptibility of a subgroup of participants frequently referred to as non-responders. In order to identify potential non-responders and exclude them at the initial stages of screening for NFB training a new line of research has emerged focused on individual factors that might predict training success (Weber et al., 2011; Nan et al., 2015). Here we concentrate on the neurofeedback methodology, in which important factors influencing training success may be: feedback modality, training intensity, choice of EEG band(s) used for the feedback signal, and the number and positions of electrodes from which feedback signal is recorded. Since the role of these factors has not yet been quantified, we attempted to evaluate their influence in NFB training in the selected studies. Several other factors may also be important for EEG-NFB training, such as the age of the trainees, their personal traits and beliefs regarding EEG-NFB training (e.g., Witte et al., 2013), and trainer behavior; however, they could not be analyzed due to either insufficient variability of the data (e.g., with respect to age - in most cases the participants were university students) or a lack of a sufficient number of reports regarding a specific factor across the investigated experiments. In this study, we identified five factors which were investigated in a sufficient number of studies and had appropriate variability for statistical analyses in order to determine their influence on the training results.

Definitions used for all the analyzed factors were as follows:

(i) Protocol-EEG band or band combination used as the feedback signal;
(ii) Number of bands-number of simultaneously manipulated EEG bands, i.e., amplitude of bands which were used to shape the feedback signal presented to the subject;
(iii) Training Intensity index-training intensity was defined as the total number of training days divided by the average interval between them (in days). A higher Training Intensity Index indicated more intense training. The duration of a single training session was not taken into account;
(vi) Feedback modality-modality of the sensory signal presented to the subject: visual, auditory, or visual and auditory;
(v) Number of EEG-NFB electrodes-number of electrodes used for feedback signal generation.

Since the factors listed above were differentially described in the individual studies, we applied common categorization scales for analyses. The range of these scales is presented in **Table 2**. The EEG bands, which were also differently specified in the reviewed publications, were grouped based on their frequency ranges to six unified categories defined in **Table 3**. **Table 4** summarizes the parameter values for the database of all 28 experiments.

Selection of Thematic Groups

To assess the effectiveness of various EEG-NFB protocols and address the issue of the large diversity of applied protocols and investigated putative behavioral effects, we divided the database into groups based on the (i) EEG features used for training purposes and (ii) the behavioral tasks administered to the subjects (**Figure 1**). We then analyzed the data to identify the correlations

TABLE 1 | List of the analyzed studies (references in the second column) with their characteristics, including raw values of the experimental factors used for the analysis.

	Study	Protocol	Training intensity index	Number of participants	Average age	Modality	Electrodes position
1	Allen et al., 2001	Alpha−	5.0	20	28	Auditory	T3, F7
2	Becerra et al., 2012	Theta−	15.0	7	65	Auditory	F4, C3, C3, P3, F7, F8
3	Berner et al., 2006	Beta1+	0.3	6	21	Auditory	Cz
4	Bird et al., 1978	Gamma+	8.0	11	23	Auditory	O1, O2
5	Bird et al., 1978	Gamma−	8.0	11	23	Auditory	O1, O2
6	Boxtel van et al., 2012	Alpha+	8.6	15	21	Auditory	C3 C4
7	Chisholm et al., 1977	Alpha+	1.0	12	21	Auditory	Oz
8	DeGood and Chisholm, 1977	Alpha+	1.0	10	20	Auditory	Pz
9	Egner et al., 2002	Alpha−/theta+	1.7	9	23	Auditory	Pz
10	Enriquez-Geppert et al., 2013	Theta+	10.0	16	25	Visual	Fz, FC1, FCz, FC2, Cz
11	Enriquez-Geppert et al., 2014	Theta+	8	19	24	Visual	Fz
12	Hoedlmoser et al., 2008	SMR+	10.0	16	24	Mixed	C3
13	Keizer et al., 2010a	Gamma+	7.0	8	23	Auditory	Oz, Fz
14	Keizer et al., 2010b	Gamma/beta−	6.1	7	22	Auditory	Oz
15	Kober et al., 2015	SMR+	7	10	24	Visual	Cz
16	Konareva, 2005	Alpha−/theta+	1.0	30	22	Auditory	C3/C4
17	Landers and Petruzzello, 1991	SCP+	0.2	8	no data	Visual	No data
18	Logemann et al., 2010	SMR+/theta−	5.3	14	21	Mixed	No data
19	Peeters et al., 2014	Alpha−	1	16	22	Visual	F3
20	Reichert et al., 2015	SMR+	10	28	45	Mixed	Cz
21	Reis et al., 2015	Alpha+	6	8	60	Visual	Fz
22	Reis et al., 2015	Theta+	6	8	60	Visual	Fz
23	Ring et al., 2015	Alpha−	1	12	23	Auditory	Fz
24	Ros et al., 2010	Alpha+	1.0	12	31	Visual	C3
25	Ros et al., 2010	Beta1+	1.0	12	31	Visual	C3
26	Ros et al., 2013	Alpha−	0.2	17	33	Visual	C4
27	Wang and Hsieh, 2013	Theta+	6.0	16	65	Mixed	Fz
28	Witte et al., 2013	SMR+/theta−	2.7	10	24	Visual	Cz

In a few articles the authors did not supply sufficient information regarding the experimental paradigm (denoted as 'no data' in the table). The "+" and "−" signs in the "Protocol" column denote the enhancement or suppression of particular frequency bands.

TABLE 2 | Assignment of the factors' row values to the categories used for $X^2$and Kendall's T analyses.

Training intensity index		Feedback modality		Number of EEG-NFB electrodes		EEG-NFB electrode position	
Raw value	Category value	Raw value	Category value	Raw value	Category value	Raw value	Category value
0–5	1	Auditory	1	1	1	Other than Cz	1
5–10	2	Visual	2	>1	2	Cz	2
>10	3	Visual and auditory	3				

between training factors (defined in paragraph 2.2.) and the observed EEG modulation and/or behavioral changes.

(i) We selected three groups based on the frequency bands–theta (4–8 Hz), alpha (8–12 Hz) and beta1 (12–20 Hz), with a minimum of $n = 5$ experiments. Both, the up- or down-regulation of the band (as defined in **Table 3**) or its fraction were included in the same protocol group (i.e., the up-regulation of "low alpha" and the down-regulation of "high alpha" were both considered alpha protocols aimed at the assessment of the alpha band protocol effectiveness). This approach enables the estimation of whether training based on a particular frequency band induces the desired changes in the EEG or behavioral domains. For other single and multi-band protocols, we did not find a sufficient number of experiments for statistical evaluation.

(ii) Within the behavior-oriented experiments, we also identified two groups (based on the behavioral tests described): An Attention Group: experiments targeted to change

TABLE 3 | Definition of the EEG frequency bands used in this review.

Band Name	Band width (Hz)	Comments
SCP	0.5–2	Slow Cortical Potentials
Delta	2–4	
Theta	4–7	
Alpha	8–12	Also includes μ-rhythm (9–11 Hz)
Beta	12–30	Also includes SMR (12–15 Hz)
Gamma	31–100	

TABLE 4 | Success/Failure scores for studies (references in the second column) that qualified for analysis.

Number	Study	Protocol	EEG	Behavior		
				G	A	M
1	Allen et al., 2001	Alpha	1	1		
2	Becerra et al., 2012	Theta−	0	1	0	0
3	Berner et al., 2006	Beta1+	0	0		0
4	Bird et al., 1978	Gamma+	1			
5	Bird et al., 1978	Gamma−	0			
6	Boxtel van et al., 2012	Alpha+	1	0		
7	Chisholm et al., 1977	Alpha+	1	0		
8	DeGood and Chisholm, 1977	Alpha+	0			
9	Egner et al., 2002	Alpha-/theta+	0	0		
10	Enriquez-Geppert et al., 2013	Theta+	1	0	0	0
11	Enriquez-Geppert et al., 2014	Theta+	1	1		1
12	Hoedlmoser et al., 2008	SMR+	1	1		1
13	Keizer et al., 2010a	Gamma+	1	1	1	
14	Keizer et al., 2010b	Gamma/beta−	1			
15	Kober et al., 2015	SMR+	1	1	1	1
16	Konareva, 2005	Alpha-/theta+	0			
17	Landers and Petruzzello, 1991	SCP+	0	1		
18	Logemann et al., 2010	SMR+/theta−	0	0	0	
19	Peeters et al., 2014	SMR+	0			
20	Reichert et al., 2015	Alpha−	1	0		
21	Reis et al., 2015	Alpha+	1	1		1
22	Reis et al., 2015	Theta+	1	1		1
23	Ring et al., 2015	Alpha−	1	0		
24	Ros et al., 2010	Alpha−	1	0		
25	Ros et al., 2010	Beta1+	0	0		
26	Ros et al., 2013	Alpha−	1			
27	Wang and Hsieh, 2013	Theta+	1	1	1	1
28	Witte et al., 2013	SMR+/theta−	0			

Training results: 1, training success; 0, training failure. "EEG" column lists the results on the modulation of EEG features, "Behavior" column contains the list results in the behavioral domain, G, general effects of the training obtained in any of the investigated behaviors; A, attention; M, memory. Values in column G may also include effects not classified to attention (A) and memory (M) groups.

performance measured by attention tests (e.g., TOVA–Test of Variables of Attention, SSRT–Stop Signal Reaction Times, CPT–Continuous Performance Test or others) and a Memory Group: studies aimed at the identification of any type of memory improvement (estimated by different types of recall and recognition tasks; **Figure 2**).

Definition of Successful Training

In the reviewed articles, the efficacy of EEG-NFB training in the induction of EEG modulation was typically evaluated by comparing the amplitudes (absolute or relative) of the monitored EEG bands (in the case of single band protocols) or the amplitude ratios between the manipulated bands (in the case of multi-band protocols, i.e., theta/alpha or SMR/theta ratios) recorded before and after the whole training (interpreted as delayed effects of neurofeedback or, more general, brain plasticity [50]) or within/between training sessions. Significant differences of these parameters between the experimental and control groups indicated successful training in the EEG domain. The changes in behavioral performance were evaluated based on tests or measures typical for the given type of activity.

We reviewed each article and individually qualified the training results as a failure (0) or success (1) based on the statistical measures used by authors. Training was considered as being a success:

(i) If the measured effect (EEG or behavioral) was significantly different (at the level of $p < 0.05$ for any type of statistics) from the result achieved in the control group;

(ii) If the group effect or interaction between the groups and time were significant in an ANOVA test;

(iii) In cases where direct statistical comparison of the experimental and control groups were not available in the original text, we qualified them (**Table 4**) as a success when the comparison between the pre- and post-training measurements provided a different outcome in the experimental and control groups (e.g., a significant change in the experimental group and no change in the control group).

If direct (i) or (ii) and indirect (iii) comparisons for EEG or behavior were not described in the articles, we qualified the outcome of the training as giving no results. We considered EEG-NFB training as successful if either EEG or behavioral change reached significance. Similarly, a study was defined as a success when one of several results available for one category (e.g., scores from several attention tests or an amplitude change of different EEG bands) was unambiguously described as significantly changed as a result of the training.

Methods of Statistical Analyses

We estimated the correlation of each training factor with the EEG and behavioral success scores for all experiments and specific groups (defined in the paragraph' Selection of thematic subgroups'). An analysis was performed only for groups that comprised five or more experiments. For consistent comparison of all factors between all experimental groups, we used two non-parametric tests: X^2 to test for independence of training outcome and the Kendall's T (tau) rank correlation coefficients to precisely assess the strength and direction of any significant association. Although Kendall's T coefficient is similar to the Spearman rank correlation statistic, which is used to measure rank correlation, the advantage of using Kendall's T is in the direct interpretation of the probability of observing concordant and discordant pairs (Hauke and Kossowski, 2011).

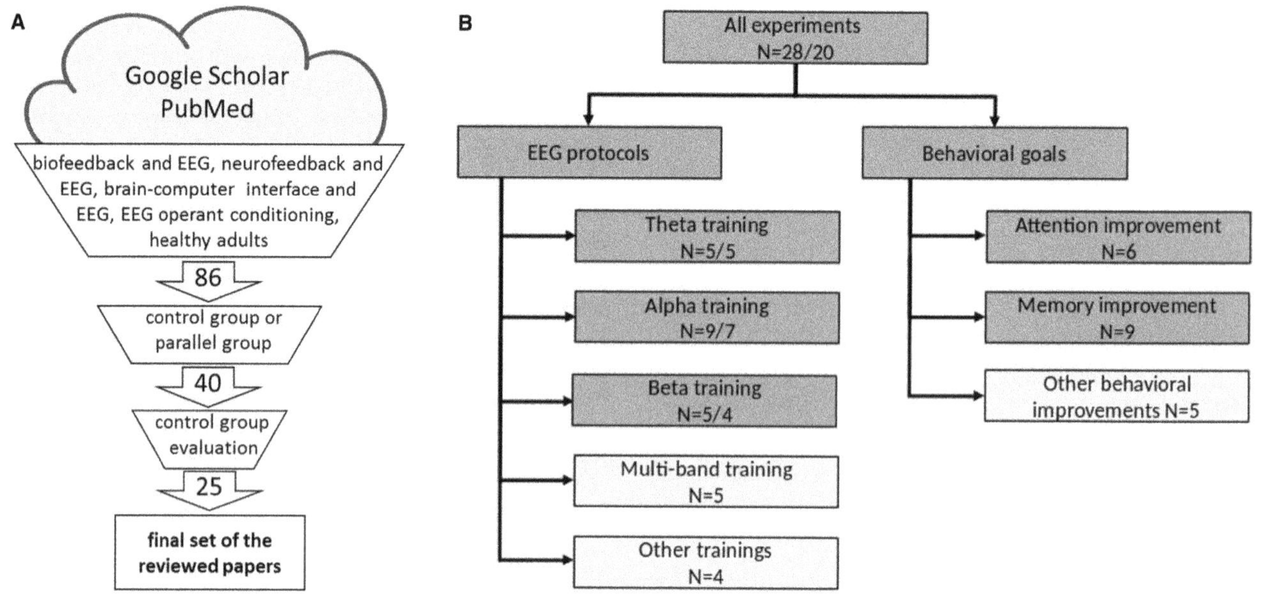

FIGURE 1 | (A) Schematic representation for article selection. **(B)** Schematic representation of the experiments used in the review. Dark gray boxes specify the experimental paradigms grouped for analytical studies according to EEG (left branch) or behavioral protocol (right), light gray boxes specify groups not included in the analyses. In the EEG protocols branch, N denotes the number of experiments included in each EEG and behavioral group (EEG/behavioral) where EEG effects (changes of the EEG spectrum) were analyzed. In the Behavioral goals branch N denotes the number of experiments in each behavioral or cognitive group. The 28 EEG-NFB experiments were used for analyses. Of these studies, smaller groups were defined according to their specific EEG training protocols or the expected behavioral/cognitive effects. The groups are not mutually exclusive; both types of data were often analyzed in the same study, which resulted in multiple classifications. Some experiments also investigated more than one behavioral goal (**Table 4**). Protocols that could not be attributed to any of the specific subgroups (lowermost boxes "Other") contributed only to the general analysis.

The partial η^2 (Bakeman, 2005; Lakens, 2013) can be used to estimate effect size from published studies using information about F statistic provided by the authors. It is suitable for the results extracted from multiple experiments with similar design and testing one (or equivalent) dependent variable. Unfortunately, the designs used in the reviewed papers did not meet these criteria. First of all, there was a great variety of EEG features (dependent variables) that underwent treatment. Next, within the same trained EEG feature, the statistics were available either for within group or between group analyses. Often, the statistics were incompletely described, which made calculation of effect size impossible. The details of statistical results provided in the reviewed articles are presented in the Supplementary Table 2.

After grouping the available effect sizes according to the training protocol and source of the effect (within group, between groups, interaction) the groups were not numerous enough for quantitative comparisons. We managed to construct only one group of 8 reports regarding alpha training from which we could extract F statistics for within subject effects which enabled evaluation of unspecific changes of this band.

Since the calculation of statistical power for all the other training factors was not possible, we used a more gross, binary approach. Instead of using F values we qualified experiments as a failure (0) or success (1, Section Definition of successful training) and calculated a success ratio (SR) defined as the percentage of successful studies within the total number of studies of the given set.

RESULTS

General Characteristics of the Participants

The average age of the participants ranged from 20 to 65 years, with median = 24 (most participants were students) and mean = 30 ± 14. The difference between the mean and median age was caused by two experiments in which the participants' ages ranged between 55 and 75 years (6, 41 in **Table 1**, correspondingly).

The mean number of subjects who participated in a single experiment was 26 ± 10, with an average experimental group size of 13 ± 6 subjects. The diversity of the relatively small number of qualified experiments permitted selection of two behavioral groups: Attention (n = 6) and Memory (n = 9) and three EEG protocol groups: Theta (n = 5), Alpha (n = 9), and Beta (n = 5) fulfilling the criterion of minimum group size. Seven out of nine experiments in the Alpha Group, four out of five in Beta Group and all five Theta Group experiments included also behavioral tests.

EEG-NFB Training Methods (EEG Protocols, Training Intensity, and Signal Modality)

Most of the experiments (23 of 28) used single EEG band protocols for EEG-NFB training, and most of these (17) intended to up-regulate the amplitudes of the trained band: theta (n = 4), alpha (n = 5), beta (including SMR, n = 5), gamma (n = 2), or slow cortical potentials (SCP, n = 1). The remaining five experiments (18%) used multi-band protocols that aimed to change the ratio of the amplitudes of the employed bands (**Table 1**).

The Memory Group ($n = 9$) was composed of experiments using only single band protocols: five experiments had theta protocol, three beta and one alpha. In the Attention Group ($n = 6$), the majority of experiments used a theta protocol ($n = 3$), and the three remaining studies used beta, gamma and SMR/theta protocols.

The daily training sessions across all experiments typically consisted of multiple, few minutes long runs interrupted by short pauses. The average training was 7.7 ± 3.8 sessions with 3 ± 2.4 day intervals; thus, the training intensity was relatively low compared with EEG-NFB training arrangements in clinical practice [4]. The average Training Intensity Index was 5.5 ± 3.4 for all experiments. In 46% of the experiments the EEG-NFB modality was auditory, in 40%, it was visual, and in 14%, it was mixed (visual and auditory).

Location of Electrodes

In the two behaviorally oriented groups (Attention and Memory) we did not find any consistency in the placement of feedback electrodes. Out of six experiments, oriented on training of attention, five different electrode(s) locations were used. In the Memory Group in five experiments the electrodes were placed at Fz or included this location, in the remaining four experiments we did not note any consistency in the placement of electrodes.

Among the EEG protocols most consistent electrode placement was observed in the Theta Group where all single electrode setups used the Fz location and one of two multi-electrode setups used frontal locations including Fz. All experiments with training provided from Fz solely or together with other locations succeeded in evoking EEG modulation (seven experiments, four using theta protocol, two using alpha protocol and one using gamma protocol). In the Beta Group four experiments used mainly electrodes located over central sulcus (in the three experiments electrodes were positioned at Cz and in two in C3 locations according to the 10–20 international system) and one in the F3 position. In the Alpha Group the most commonly used locations were frontal (Fz, F3, F7) and central (C3, C4), one experiment used occipital (Oz) and one parietal (Pz) location.

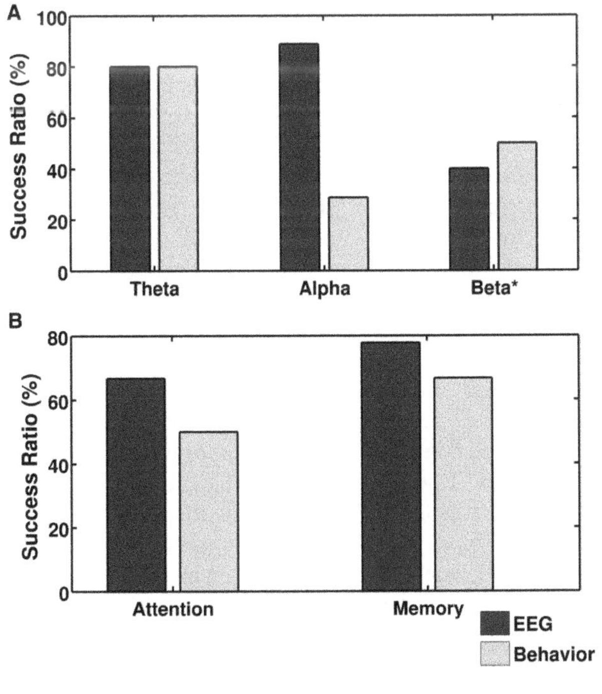

FIGURE 2 | Success ratio of the spectral EEG changes (dark gray bars) and behavioral improvement (light gray bars) calculated for: (A) experiments grouped according to training with particular frequency band protocols and (B) training aimed at different behavioral effects (i.e., improvement in attention and memory). Only protocols used in five or more experiments are included in the graphs with exception to four behavioral experiments in the Beta Group designated by *.

Dependence of Successful Training on the Analyzed Factors

According to the descriptions provided by the authors, EEG-NFB training yielded significant results in the EEG domain for 17 out of total 28 experiments which resulted in a 60.7% success ratio (SR) and in 10 out of 20 behaviorally-oriented experiments, which provided a SR of 50 %. SR values are given in **Table 4**. We did not find a significant relationship between behavioral or EEG success in general ($X^2 = 0.91, p = 0.33$) or any of the considered training factors (X^2 and T statistics for all analyzed factors are given in **Table 5**) except for number of bands which negatively correlated with the resulting EEG changes ($X^2 = 4.2303$, $p = 0.0397$; $T = -0.3887$, $p = 0.0472$). We also observed a tentative relation between SR and training intensity index (TI). In a sample of 6 studies, which had at least four training sessions completed on consecutive days (excluding weekends) SR was 100%.

In the consecutive steps of our review we analyzed the effectiveness of training for experiments classified to smaller groups specified by EEG or behavioral protocols.

Efficacy of Employed EEG Protocols

Theta and alpha EEG band appeared to be highly susceptible to EEG-NFB procedures resulting in SR's of 80 and 89% respectively,

TABLE 5 | Dependence (X^2) and correlation (T) values for EEG training success and analyzed factors.

	Number of bands	Training Intensity	Number of participants	Stimulus modality	Number of electrodes
X^2	4.2303	15.9216	10.9778	0.5865	2.9365
P for X^2 statistics	0.0397	0.2534	0.6878	0.7458	0.4015
T	−0.3887	0.3145	0.2932	0.1087	0.0304
P for T statistics	0.0472	0.0606	0.0902	0.5886	0.8966

Correlation was considered significant when $p < 0.05$ for both X^2 and Kendall T correlation.

trainings targeted at the beta band were less effective with a SR of 40%. The experiments using multi-band protocols were very diverse and only one of five yielded changes in EEG spectra, which is in line with our general conclusion of negative relation between number of bands used for training and induced EEG changes. In the behavioral domain out of three investigated protocols only theta was highly effective at inducing behavioral changes with a SR of 80%, the least effective was alpha protocol with a SR of 28% (**Figure 2**).

Efficacy of the Training Aimed at Specific Behavioral Effects

The SR of the desired behavioral effects in Attention and Memory Groups reached 50 and 67%, respectively (**Figure 2**). The effectiveness of inducing EEG changes was even higher with an SR of 67% (attention) and 78% (memory). A comparison of the chosen experiments that had positive results in the EEG domain and included behavioral tests before and after the training did not reveal any frequency band that was specifically effective for increased performance in attention or memory tests. In the Memory Group, of six experiments which yielded positive training results in both domains three experiments used theta, two SMR and one alpha protocol, additionally one theta protocol resulted with reported lack of significant results in the behavioral domain. In the Attention Group, there were four eligible experiments in which three cases had positive results in both EEG and behavioral domains, but each of them had a different protocol.

Summary of the Efficacy of Employed EEG Protocols

Our analysis demonstrated: (i) the effectiveness of the theta and alpha protocols at inducing EEG modulations; (ii) a negative correlation between the number of trained bands and success in evoking EEG modulations, (iii) a lack of specificity of the popular EEG-NFB protocols in obtaining desired behavioral changes.

DISCUSSION

The theoretical basis for EEG-NFB is that brain activity, modified according to the targeted changes of the EEG signal, can cause a plastic reorganization within the involved brain networks and lead to an expected improvement in a specific behavioral task (Anguera et al., 2013). The findings of this review cannot unambiguously disprove or support this hypothesis, since behavioral effects were not convincingly validated by any specific training protocol. This ambiguity may results from a limited number and high diversity of the available descriptions of well-controlled NFB studies.

The scientific community has produced a multitude of articles with enthusiastic case reports on EEG-NFB training. However, a rigorous scientific approach to EEG-NFB is rare, and experiments performed on healthy participants to study the effectiveness and/or mechanism of training are very limited; we identified only 86 relevant reports. From this list we selected 43 EEG-NFB experiments which described control groups. We next assessed the quality of the control paradigms and excluded all experiments that did not allow for unambiguous attribution of the results to the effects of EEG-NFB training.

The final, small number of accepted studies ($n = 28$) is alarming because it suggests that the field of EEG-NFB research is dominated by poorly controlled experiments. Analogous conclusions were drawn in other quantitative reviews of EEG-NFB research. In her review, Niv (2013) attempted to assess the efficacy of EEG-NFB applied to patients with neurological disorders (e.g., ADHD, autism, epilepsy) and identified only 22 well-controlled experiments. The review concluded that "only few controlled studies exist and more and better-organized research is necessary to confirm the efficacy and effectiveness of neurofeedback". The two meta-analyses of Arns et al. (2009) and Lofthouse et al. (2012), who investigated the efficacy of EEG-NFB treatment applied to children diagnosed with ADHD, included only 15 and 14 studies, respectively.

In our analysis of 28 well-controlled studies, we calculated the SR separately for EEG (60.7%) and behavioral (50%) effects. These numbers demonstrated that EEG-NFB training could influence both the amplitude of the chosen EEG signal and behavior. Because the effects were not consistent, it is essential to carefully evaluate all factors of experimental design to select those that promote successful training (see also review by Vernon et al., 2009). The fact that most of the investigated factors did not correlate with training success is worth consideration itself. The intuitively important factors such as feedback modality did not affect training results. SR for auditory and visual paradigms were similar (53% and 63%, respectively). Training success did show not dependency on the intensity of the stimuli ($X^2 = 15.9$, $p = 0.25$). High SR (75%) averaged from four experiments using mixed modality stimuli should be treated with caution, however Vernon et al. (2004) in his review suggested the optimal results with combined, auditory and visual feedback.

The assessment of the SR in the selected experiments was possible for theta, alpha and beta bands. From those three protocols the most effective in changing the EEG spectra were training involving the theta or alpha band. Alpha training calls for special attention for its popularity despite the low behavioral SR (out of nine well controlled EEG-NFB studies with alpha training, seven aimed to induce behavioral improvement, and only two were successful (Allen et al., 2001–reported mood increase and Reis et al., 2015–reported improvement of memory; comp. **Table 4**). It seems that the alpha band is highly susceptible to various manipulation. This notion is supported by Williams (1977) who used two sham-feedback groups (with no real experimental group) and reported that an increase in alpha band amplitude was achieved only in subjects who had been told that they were involved in the real alpha-inducing experiments. The subjects who were informed that they participated in the control group did not develop this change. Quandt et al. (2012) induced changes in the upper alpha and beta bands in subjects who observed actions performed by other individuals, further supporting the high susceptibility of the alpha band to nonspecific manipulations. Finally, Dempster and Vernon (2009) showed that an increase in alpha band amplitude often observed during EEG-NFB trainings might merely represent return to baseline level disturbed by training procedure. This rebound might be enhanced in EEG-NFB groups and impaired when subjects are engaged in e.g., sham feedback. Thus, inclusion of baseline measurements in scientific reports might be a valuable addition in studying inferences about EEG-NFB effects on EEG. In 4 out of 8 reviewed studies, alpha was found to be changing in both experimental and control conditions. In order to estimate non-specific alpha changes we pooled together increases and decreases of alpha over both sessions and epochs in all experimental conditions, resulting in average effect size 0.32 (STD = 0.15) (positions 6, 8, 9, 11, 31, 32, 34, 36 in Supplementary Table). The high susceptibility of the alpha band to neurofeedback manipulation, as resulting from our review, was, however, not accompanied by any specific behavioral effects.

There is an assumption behind NFB practice concerning specific protocols that target particular behavioral goals (Egner and Gruzelier, 2004; Keizer et al., 2010b; Gruzelier, 2013a,b; Enriquez-Geppert et al., 2014). However, our analysis of the training protocols that aimed to improve attention or memory performance does not enable such attribution of any of the frequency bands used for training to these two behavioral goals showing no privilege of any specific frequency band. A similar observation was reported by Arns et al. (2009) in conclusion of their meta-analysis: while EEG-NFB therapy provided, on average, positive therapeutic effects for children with ADHD, there was no difference in the effect size for different EEG-NFB protocols (SCP [0.5–2 Hz], SMR [12–15 Hz]/theta and beta/theta).

This lack of specificity between the frequency band of an EEG-NFB protocol and its behavioral effect does not necessarily discount the basic concept of behavioral correlates of specific EEG frequencies (Anguera et al., 2013). When investigating the roots of inconsistent EEG-NFB effects, a more careful examination of the old issue of spatial resolution and source localization in EEG recording is warranted (Zuberer et al., 2015). The recorded EEG signal can be generated by an infinite number of different sets of current sources, even with the assumption of an infinite number of recording electrodes (Fender, 1987). In the case of EEG-NFB, where it is expected to modify the activity of the local networks (Wood and Kober, 2014), the signal collected by a few EEG-NFB electrodes is generated also by other brain regions than those desired as a training target (Witte et al., 2013). A partial solution to this problem could be high resolution EEG combined with EEG source localization methods to enable training focused on specific regions. Although, results of preliminary studies, using multi-electrode EEG-NFB such as LORETA-EEG-NFB, Z-score-EEG-NFB, or blind source separation, seem promising (Cannon et al., 2006, 2009; Koberda et al., 2012; Bauer and Pllana, 2014; White et al., 2014) more experiments with sham control groups are necessary to verify this approach as a valuable EEG-NFB tool. The source localization problem worsens in experiments where a single EEG-NFB electrode is used. Unfortunately, a single electrode approach is the most common practice in EEG-NFB training and therapy. We argue that such a protocol would not be able to precisely affect the putative regions responsible for targeted behavior.

It is important to underline that several thoroughly prepared experiments clearly show positive effects of EEG-NFB training (Allen et al., 2001; Hoedlmoser et al., 2008; Keizer et al., 2010a). However, in other (equally thorough) studies, EEG-NFB was not found to be successful (Egner et al., 2002; Berner et al., 2006; Logemann et al., 2010). As noted above, this discrepancy might stem from the lack of optimal training paradigms. The presented quantitative review offers suggestions for concrete modifications of the used paradigms, which might improve the results of EEG-NFB training. We subsequently discuss two particular factors that originate from experiments collected in this review.

The Don'ts: The Number of EEG Bands Used for Training

One of our findings, is the negative correlation between the number of bands used to compose the feedback signal and the success of training, i.e., complicated protocols which promoted and/or inhibited several bands worsen the final results. This may be related to the interdependence of the EEG frequencies, i.e., their susceptibility to follow the modulation of the other, most often neighboring frequencies. Band interdependence has been reported by Ros et al. (2013) who demonstrated that training directed for up-regulation of the alpha band was accompanied by changes in the flanking frequencies (theta and beta bands). The interdependence of EEG frequencies may also affect the expected behavioral changes because the modulation of neighboring bands trained in opposite directions may cancel out the effects of up-regulation of the targeted band. Similarly, the observed behavioral change may result from an up-regulation of bands neighboring the band that was intentionally trained. This situation might at least partially explain why so many authors observed positive behavioral results despite the lack of noticeable modifications of the trained EEG band.

However, the issue requires deeper investigation as there is a contradictory example of theta band amplitude increase not accompanied by an increase in the flanking alpha frequency amplitude (Enriquez-Geppert et al., 2013).

The Do's: Location of EEG-NFB Electrodes

The analysis of experiments from the Theta Group showed that neurofeedback mediated by the electrodes positioned above well-identified sources of a given EEG frequency (e.g., frontal regions in case of frontal-middline theta training) might bring expected changes in the EEG spectrum (Keizer et al., 2010a; Boxtel van et al., 2012; Wang and Hsieh, 2013). In general, however, the targeted frequencies are generated by many structures of dispersed neural networks and the use of a one or two, arbitrarily located EEG-NFB electrodes (and they reference), does not allow for non-ambiguous estimation of the brain sources involved. A way to partially mitigate this issue might be the use of multiple electrodes located in the appropriate position for capturing activity of the brain regions associated with the targeted behavioral functions. Indeed, the rare experiments in which electrode location was justified for physiological reasons appeared to be successful (Enriquez-Geppert et al., 2013, 2014), which likely results from a substantial contribution of relevant sources into feedback signals.

Suitably positioned multiple electrodes increase the chances of collecting feedback signals from many regions engaged in the target activity. Attention is a cognitive function with relatively well-known networks of involved brain structures and a popular goal for improvement in many EEG-NFB paradigms. The fronto-parietal network (Buschman and Miller, 2007) is one of the brain systems that support attentional mechanisms and it is not surprising that most protocols that successfully increased attention used feedback signals from several EEG-NFB electrodes located at frontal and parietal locations (Allen et al., 2001; Becerra et al., 2012; Enriquez-Geppert et al., 2013), or from a single electrode located over frontal areas (Vernon et al., 2004). In contrast, an experiment with a similar goal, which used C3/C4 electrodes (Boxtel van et al., 2012) to record feedback signals did not achieve significant behavioral changes after EEG-NFB training. We posit that the locations of the EEG-NFB electrodes in many experiments reviewed in this analysis were non-optimally placed for an expected result. It is, therefore, important that future EEG-NFB experiments should identify optimal training electrode locations based on existing knowledge regarding the anatomical and functional substrates of various behavioral tasks. It appears feasible that for a dispersed target network new training paradigms should be developed in which the feedback signals would be weighed by a component analysis from many recording electrodes.

CONCLUSIONS

We posit that neurofeedback methodology used in the majority of the reviewed experiments did not enable proper targeting of the brain regions responsible for control over the desired behavioral changes. This may explain the lack of correlation between the changes induced in the trained EEG signal and the modification of the targeted behavior, as well as lack of correlation between the remaining analyzed factors and training success. We, therefore, recommend the following factors for improved EEG-NFB training efficacy:

- Use single band protocols.
- Localize brain regions functionally correlated with the targeted behavior for optimal electrode placement (if possible).
- Use of viable EEG source localization methods for the feedback signals used in the training (if possible).

AUTHOR CONTRIBUTIONS

JR Review concept, data analyses, main conclusions, article drafting. KJ Data analyses, verification of analytical methods, proof reading. KP Data analyses, proof reading. EK Conclusions verification, data analyses, proof reading. RC Data analyses, verification of analytical methods, proof reading. AW Verification of the review concept and of the conclusions.

ACKNOWLEDGMENTS

This work was supported by the Polish National Science Centre grant 2012/07/B/NZ7/04383.

REFERENCES

Allen, J. J. B., Harm-Jones, E., and Cavender, J. H. (2001). Manipulation of frontal EEG asymmetry through biofeedback alters self-reported emotional responses and facial EMG. *Psychophysiology* 38, 685–693. doi: 10.1111/1469-8986.3840685

Anguera, J. A., Boccanfuso, J., Rintoul, J. L., Al-Hashimi, O., Faraji, F., Janowich, J., et al. (2013). Video game training enhances cognitive control in older adults. *Nature* 501, 97–101. doi: 10.1038/nature12486

Arns, M., Heinrich, H., and Strehl, U. (2014). Evaluation of neurofeedback in ADHD: the long and winding road. *Biol. Psychol.* 95, 108–115. doi: 10.1016/j.biopsycho.2013.11.013

Arns, M., Ridder de, S., Strehl, U., Breteler, M., and Coenen, A. (2009). Efficacy of neurofeedback treatment in ADHD: the effects on inattention, impulsivity and hyperactivity: a meta-analysis. *Clin. EEG Neurosci.* 40, 180–189. doi: 10.1177/155005940904000311

Bakeman, R. (2005). Recommended effect size statistics for repeated measures designs. *Behav. Res. Methods* 37, 379–384. doi: 10.3758/BF03192707

Bauer, H., and Pllana, A. (2014). EEG-based local brain activity feedback training - tomographic neurofeedback. *Front. Hum. Neurosci.* 8:1005. doi: 10.3389/fnhum.2014.01005

Becerra, J., Fernández, T., Roca-Stappung, M., Díaz-Comas, L., Galán, L., Bosch, J., et al. (2012). Neurofeedback in healthy elderly human subjects with electroencephalographic risk for cognitive disorder. *J. Alzheimer's Dis.* 28, 357–367. doi: 10.3233/JAD-2011-111055

Berner, I., Schabus, M., Wienerroither, T., and Klimesch, W. (2006). The significance of sigma neurofeedback training on sleep spindles and aspects of declarative memory. *Appl. Psychophysiol. Biofeedb.* 31, 97–114. doi: 10.1007/s10484-006-9013-7

Bird, B. L., Newton, F. A., Sheer, D. E., and Ford, M. (1978). Biofeedback training of 40-Hz EEG in humans. *Biofeedb. Self Regul.* 3, 1–11.

Boxtel van, G. J. M., Denissen, A. J. M., Jäger, M., Vernon, D., Dekker, M. K. J., Mihajlović, V., et al. (2012). A novel self-guided approach to alpha activity training. *Int. J. Psychophysiol.* 83, 282–294. doi: 10.1016/j.ijpsycho.2011.11.004

Buschman, and T. J., and Miller, E. K. (2007). Top-down versus bottom-up control of attention in the prefrontal and posterior parietal cortices. *Science* 315, 1860–1862. doi: 10.1126/science.1138071

Cannon, R., Congedo, M., Lubar, J., and Hutchens, T. (2009). Differentiating a network of executive attention: LORETA neurofeedback in anterior cingulate and dorsolateral prefrontal cortices. *Int. J. Neurosci.* 119, 404–441. doi: 10.1080/00207450802480325

Cannon, R., Lubar, J., Gerke, A., Thornton, K., Hutchens, T., and McCammon, V. (2006). EEG spectral-power and coherence: LORETA neurofeedback training in the anterior cingulate gyrus. *J. Neurother.* 10, 5–31. doi: 10.1300/J184v10n01_02

Chisholm, R., DeGood, D., and Hartz, M. (1977). Effects of alpha feedback training on occipital EEG, heart rate, and experiential reactivity to a laboratory stressor. *Psychophysiology* 14, 157–163.

DeGood, D. E., and Chisholm, R. C. (1977). Multiple response comparison of parietal EEG and frontalis EMG biofeedback. *Psychophysiology* 14, 258–265.

Dempster, T., and Vernon, D. (2009). Identifying indices of learning for Alpha neurofeedback training. *Appl. Psychophysiol. Biofeedb.* 34, 309–318. doi: 10.1007/s10484-009-9112-3

Egner, T., and Gruzelier, J. H. (2004). EEG Biofeedback of low beta band components: frequency-specific effects on variables of attention and event-related brain potentials. *Clin. Neurophysiol.* 115, 131–139. doi: 10.1016/S1388-2457(03)00353-5

Egner, T., Strawson, E., and Gruzelier, J. H. (2002). EEG signature and phenomenology of alpha/theta neurofeedback training versus mock feedback. *Appl. Psychophysiol. Biofeedb.* 27, 261–270. doi: 10.1023/A:1021063416558

Enriquez-Geppert, S., Huster, R. J., Figge, C., and Herrmann, C. S. (2014). Self-regulation of frontal-midline theta facilitates memory updating and mental set shifting. *Front. Behav. Neurosci.* 8:420. doi: 10.3389/fnbeh.2014.00420

Enriquez-Geppert, S., Huster, R. J., Scharfenort, R., Mokom, Z. N., Vosskuhl, J., Figge, C., et al. (2013). The morphology of midcingulate cortex predicts frontal-midline theta neurofeedback success. *Front. Hum. Neurosci.* 7:453. doi: 10.3389/fnhum.2013.00453

Escolano, C., Aguilar, M., and Minguez, J. (2011). "EEG-based upper alpha neurofeedback training improves working memory performance" in *Conference Proceedings: Annual International Conference of the IEEE Engineering in Medicine and Biology Society* (Boston, MA: IEEE Engineering in Medicine and Biology Society. Conference), 2327–2330.

Fender, D. H. (1987). "Source localization of brain electrical activity," in *Methods of Analysis of Brain Electrical and Magnetic Signals*, eds A. Gevins and A. Rémond (Amsterdam: Elsevier Science Publication), 355–403.

Ghaziri, J., Tucholka, A., Larue, V., Blanchette-Sylvestre, M., Reyburn, G., Gilbert, G., et al. (2013). Neurofeedback training induces changes in white and gray matter. *Clin. EEG Neurosci.* 44, 265–272. doi: 10.1177/1550059413476031

Gruzelier, J. H. (2013a). EEG-neurofeedback for optimising performance. I: a review of cognitive and affective outcome in healthy participants. *Neurosci. Biobehav. Rev.* 44, 124–141. doi: 10.1016/j.neubiorev.2013.09.015

Gruzelier, J. H. (2013b). EEG-neurofeedback for optimising performance. II: Creativity, the performing arts and ecological validity. *Neurosci. Biobehav. Rev.* 44, 142–158. doi: 10.1016/j.neubiorev.2013.11.004

Gruzelier, J. H. (2014). EEG-neurofeedback for optimising performance. III: a review of methodological and theoretical considerations. *Neurosci. Biobehav. Rev.* 44, 159–182. doi: 10.1016/j.neubiorev.2014.03.015

Gruzelier, J. H., Holmes, P., Hirst, L., Bulpin, K., Rahman, S., van Run, C., et al. (2014a). Replication of elite music performance enhancement following alpha/theta neurofeedback and application to novice performance and improvisation with SMR benefits. *Biol. Psychol.* 95, 96–107. doi: 10.1016/j.biopsycho.2013.11.001

Gruzelier, J. H., Thompson, T., Redding, E., Brandt, R., and Steffert, T. (2014b). Application of alpha/theta neurofeedback and heart rate variability training to young contemporary dancers: State anxiety and creativity. *Int. J. Psychophysiol.* 93, 105–111. doi: 10.1016/j.ijpsycho.2013.05.004

Hanslmayr, S., Sauseng, P., Doppelmayr, M., Schabus, M., and Klimesch, W. (2005). Increasing individual upper Alpha power by neurofeedback improves cognitive performance in human subjects. *Appl. Psychophysiol. Biofeedb.* 30, 1–10. doi: 10.1007/s10484-005-2169-8

Hauke, J., and Kossowski, T. (2011). Comparison of values of Pearson's and Spearman's correlation coefficients on the same sets of data. *Quaestion. Geograph.* 30, 87–93. doi: 10.2478/v10117-011-0021-1

Hoedlmoser, K., Pecherstorfer, T., Gruber, G., Anderer, P., Doppelmayr, M., Klimesch, W., et al. (2008). Instrumental conditioning of human sensorimotor rhythm (12-15 Hz) and its impact on sleep as well as declarative learning. *Sleep* 31, 1401–1408.

Keizer, A. W., Verment, R. S., and Hommel, B. (2010b). Enhancing cognitive control through neurofeedback: a role of gamma-band activity in managing episodic retrieval. *Neuroimage* 49, 3404–3413. doi: 10.1016/j.neuroimage.2009.11.023

Keizer, A. W., Verschoor, M., Verment, R. S., and Hommel, B. (2010a). The effect of gamma enhancing neurofeedback on the control of feature bindings and intelligence measures. *Int. J. Psychophysiol.* 75, 25–32. doi: 10.1016/j.ijpsycho.2009.10.011

Kober, S. E., Witte, M., Stangl, M., Väljamäe, A., Neuper, C., and Wood, G. (2015). Shutting down sensorimotor interference unblocks the networks for stimulus processing: an SMR neurofeedback training study. *Clin. Neurophysiol.* 126, 82–95. doi: 10.1016/j.clinph.2014.03.031

Koberda, J. L., Mosesa, A., Koberda, L., and Koberda, P. (2012). Cognitive enhancement using 19-electrode Z-score neurofeedback. *J. Neurother.* 16, 3404–3413. doi: 10.1016/j.neuroimage.2009.11.023

Konareva, I. N. (2005). Modifications of the EEG frequency pattern in humans related to a single neurofeedback session. *Neurophysiology* 37, 388–395. doi: 10.1007/s11062-006-0015-0

Lakens, D. (2013). Calculating and reporting effect sizes to facilitate cumulative science: A practical primer for t-tests and ANOVAs. *Front. Psychol.* 4:863. doi: 10.3389/fpsyg.2013.00863

Landers, D., and Petruzzello, S. (1991). The influence of electrocortical biofeedback on performance in pre-elite archers. *Med. Sci. Sports Exerc.* 23, 123–130.

Lecomte, G. (2011). The effects of neurofeedback training on memory performance in elderly subjects. *Psychology* 02, 846–852. doi: 10.4236/psych.2011.28129

Lofthouse, N., Arnold, L. E., Hersch, S., Hurt, E., and DeBeus, R. (2012). A review of neurofeedback treatment for pediatric ADHD. *J. Atten. Disord.* 16, 351–372. doi: 10.1177/1087054711427530

Logemann, H. N. A., Lansbergen, M. M., Van Os, T. W. D. P., Böcker, K. B. E., and Kenemans, J. L. (2010). The effectiveness of EEG-feedback on attention, impulsivity and EEG: a sham feedback controlled study. *Neurosci. Lett.* 479, 49–53. doi: 10.1016/j.neulet.2010.05.026

May, G., Benson, R., Balon, R., and Boutros, N. (2013). Neurofeedback and traumatic brain injury: a literature review. *Ann. Clin. Psychiatry* 25, 289–296. doi: 10.5298/1081-5937-43.1.05

Mohr, B., Pulvermüller, F., and Schleichert, H. (1998). Learned changes of brain states alter cognitive processing in humans. *Neurosci. Lett.* 253, 159–162.

Nan, W., Rodrigues, J. P., Ma, J., Qu, X., Wan, F., Mak, P. I., et al. (2012). Individual alpha neurofeedback training effect on short term memory. *Int. J. Psychophysiol.* 86, 83–87. doi: 10.1016/j.ijpsycho.2012.07.182

Nan, W., Wan, F., Vai, M. I., and Da Rosa, A. C. (2015). Resting and initial beta amplitudes predict learning ability in beta/theta ratio neurofeedback training in healthy young adults. *Front. Hum. Neurosci.* 9:677. doi: 10.3389/fnhum.2015.00677

Niv, S. (2013). Clinical efficacy and potential mechanisms of neurofeedback. *Person. Indiv. Differ.* 54, 676–686. doi: 10.1016/j.paid.2012.11.037

Paul, M., Ganesan, S., and Sandhu, J. S., Simon, J. V. (2011). Effect of sensory motor rhythm neurofeedback on psycho-physiological, electro-encephalographic measures and performance of archery players. *Ibnosina J. Med. Biomed. Sci.* 32–39.

Peeters, F., Ronner, J., Bodar, L., van Os, J., and Lousberg, R. (2014). Validation of a neurofeedback paradigm: manipulating frontal EEG alpha-activity and its impact on mood. *Int. J. Psychophysiol.* 93, 116–120. doi: 10.1016/j.ijpsycho.2013.06.010

Quandt, L. C., Marshall, P. J., Shipley, T. F., Beilock, S. L., and Goldin-Meadow, S. (2012). Sensitivity of alpha and beta oscillations to sensorimotor characteristics of action: an EEG study of action production and gesture observation. *Neuropsychologia* 50, 2745–2751. doi: 10.1016/j.neuropsychologia.2012.08.005

Raymond, J., Varney, C., Parkinson, L. A., and Gruzelier, J. H. (2005). The effects of alpha/theta neurofeedback on personality and mood. *Cogn. Brain Res.* 23, 287–292. doi: 10.1016/j.cogbrainres.2004.10.023

Reichert, J. L., Kober, S. E., Neuper, C., and Wood, G. (2015). Resting-state sensorimotor rhythm (SMR) power predicts the ability to up-regulate SMR in an EEG-instrumental conditioning paradigm. *Clini. Neurophysiol.* 126, 2068–2077. doi: 10.1016/j.clinph.2014.09.032

Reiner, M., Rozengurt, R., and Barnea, A. (2014). Better than sleep: theta neurofeedback training accelerates memory consolidation. *Biol. Psychol.* 95, 45–53. doi: 10.1016/j.biopsycho.2013.10.010

Reis, J., Pereira, M. R., and Dias, N. (2015). "Alpha and theta intensive neurofeedback protocol for age - related cognitive deficits," in *7th Annual International IEEE EMBS Conference on Neural Engineering, (APRIL)* (Montpelier, VT), 715–718.

Ring, C., Cooke, A., Kavussanu, M., McIntyre, D., and Masters, R. (2015). Investigating the efficacy of neurofeedback training for expediting expertise and excellence in sport. *Psychol. Sport Exerc.* 16, 118–127. doi: 10.1016/j.psychsport.2014.08.005

Ros, T., Munneke, M. A. M., Ruge, D., Gruzelier, J. H., and Rothwell, J. C. (2010). Endogenous control of waking brain rhythms induces neuroplasticity in humans. *Eur. J. Neurosci.* 31, 770–778. doi: 10.1111/j.1460-9568.2010.07100

Ros, T., Théberge, J., Frewen, P. A., Kluetsch, R., Densmore, M., Calhoun, V., et al. (2013). Mind over chatter: plastic up-regulation of the fMRI salience network directly after EEG neurofeedback. *Neuroimage* 65, 324–335. doi: 10.1016/j.neuroimage.2012.09.046

Rostami, R., Sadeghi, H., Karami, K. A., Abadi, M. N., and Salamati, P. (2012). The effects of neurofeedback on the improvement of rifle shooters' performance. *J. Neurother.* 16, 264–269. doi: 10.1080/10874208.2012.730388

Sterman, M. B., and Friar, L. (1972). Suppression of seizures in an epileptic following sensorimotor EEG feedback training. *Electroencephalogr. Clin. Neurophysiol.* 33, 89–95. doi: 10.1016/0013-4694(72)90028-4

Strizhkova, O., Cherapkina, L., and Strizhkova, T. (2012). Neurofeedback course applying of high skilled gymnasts in competitive period. *J. Hum. Sport Exerc.* 7, S185–S193. doi: 10.4100/jhse.2012.7.Proc1.21

Vernon, D., Dempster, T., Bazanova, O., Rutterford, N., Pasqualini, M., and Andersen, S. (2009). Alpha neurofeedback training for performance enhancement: reviewing the methodology. *J. Neurother.* 13, 214–227. doi: 10.1080/10874200903334397

Vernon, D., Egner, T., Cooper, N., Compton, T., Neilands, C., Sheri, A., et al. (2003). The effect of training distinct neurofeedback protocols on aspects of cognitive performance. *Int. J. Psychophysiol.* 47, 75–85. doi: 10.1016/S0167-8760(02)00091-0

Vernon, D., Frick, A., and Gruzelier, J. H. (2004). Neurofeedback as a treatment for ADHD: a methodological review with implications for future research. *J. Neurother.* 8, 53–82. doi: 10.1300/J184v08n02_04

Vollebregt, M. A., van Dongen-Boomsma, M., Buitelaar, J. K., and Slaats-Willemse, D. (2014). Does EEG-neurofeedback improve neurocognitive functioning in children with attention-deficit/hyperactivity disorder? A systematic review and a double-blind placebo-controlled study. *J. Child Psychol. Psychiatry* 55, 460–472. doi: 10.1111/jcpp.12143

Wan, F., Nan, W., Vai, M. I., and Rosa, A. (2014). Resting alpha activity predicts learning ability in alpha neurofeedback. *Front. Hum. Neurosci.* 8:500. doi: 10.3389/fnhum.2014.00500

Wang, J.-R., and Hsieh, S. (2013). Neurofeedback training improves attention and working memory performance. *Clin. Neurophysiol.* 124, 2406–2420. doi: 10.1016/j.clinph.2013.05.020

Weber, E., Köberl, A., Frank, S., and Doppelmayr, M. (2011). Predicting successful learning of SMR neurofeedback in healthy participants: methodological considerations. *Appl. Psychophysiol. Biofeedback* 36, 37–45. doi: 10.1007/s10484-010-9142-x

White, D. J., Congedo, M., and Ciorciari, J. (2014). Source-based neurofeedback methods using EEG recordings: training altered brain activity in a functional brain source derived from blind source separation. *Front. Behav. Neurosci.* 8:373. doi: 10.3389/fnbeh.2014.00373

Williams, P. (1977). EEG alpha feedback–a comparison of two control groups. *Psychosom. Med.* 39, 44–47.

Witte, M., Kober, S. E., Ninaus, M., Neuper, C., and Wood, G. (2013). Control beliefs can predict the ability to up-regulate sensorimotor rhythm during neurofeedback training. *Front. Hum. Neurosci.* 7:478. doi: 10.3389/fnhum.2013.00478

Wood, G., and Kober, S. (2014). On the need to better specify the concept of "control" in brain-computer-interfaces/neurofeedback research. *Front. Syst. Neurosci.* 8:171. doi: 10.3389/fnsys.2014.00171

Zoefel, B., Huster, R. J., and Herrmann, C. S. (2011). Neurofeedback training of the upper alpha frequency band in EEG improves cognitive performance. *Neuroimage* 54, 1427–1431. doi: 10.1016/j.neuroimage.2010.08.078

Zuberer, A., Brandeis, D., and Drechsler, R. (2015). Are treatment effects of neurofeedback training in children with ADHD related to the successful regulation of brain activity? A review on the learning of regulation of brain activity and a contribution to the discussion on specificity. *Front. Hum. Neurosci.* 9:135. doi: 10.3389/fnhum.2015.00135

7

Exercise-Induced Fitness Changes Correlate with Changes in Neural Specificity in Older Adults

Maike M. Kleemeyer[1], Thad A. Polk[2], Sabine Schaefer[3], Nils C. Bodammer[1], Lars Brechtel[4] and Ulman Lindenberger[1,5]*

[1]Center for Lifespan Psychology, Max Planck Institute for Human Development, Berlin, Germany, [2]Computational and Cognitive Neuroscience Laboratory, Department of Psychology, University of Michigan, Ann Arbor, MI, USA, [3]Institute of Sport Science, Saarland University, Saarbruecken, Germany, [4]Berlin Academy of Sports Medicine, Berlin, Germany, [5]European University Institute, San Domenico di Fiesole (FI), Italy

Edited by:
Soledad Ballesteros,
National University of Distance Education, Spain

Reviewed by:
Jonas Kaplan,
University of Southern California, USA
Pietro Pietrini,
IMT School for Advanced Studies, Italy
Eduard Kraft,
Ludwig Maximilian University of Munich, Germany

***Correspondence:**
Maike M. Kleemeyer
kleemeyer@mpib-berlin.mpg.de

Neural specificity refers to the degree to which neural representations of different stimuli can be distinguished. Evidence suggests that neural specificity, operationally defined as stimulus-related differences in functional magnetic resonance imaging (fMRI) activation patterns, declines with advancing adult age, and that individual differences in neural specificity are associated with individual differences in fluid intelligence. A growing body of literature also suggests that regular physical activity may help preserve cognitive abilities in old age. Based on this literature, we hypothesized that exercise-induced improvements in fitness would be associated with greater neural specificity among older adults. A total of 52 adults aged 59–74 years were randomly assigned to one of two aerobic-fitness training regimens, which differed in intensity. Participants in both groups trained three times a week on stationary bicycles. In the low-intensity (LI) group, the resistance was kept constant at a low level (10 Watts). In the high-intensity (HI) group, the resistance depended on participants' heart rate and therefore typically increased with increasing fitness. Before and after the 6-month training phase, participants took part in a functional MRI experiment in which they viewed pictures of faces and buildings. We used multivariate pattern analysis (MVPA) to estimate the distinctiveness of neural activation patterns in ventral visual cortex (VVC) evoked by face or building stimuli. Fitness was also assessed before and after training. In line with our hypothesis, training-induced changes in fitness were positively associated with changes in neural specificity. We conclude that physical activity may protect against age-related declines in neural specificity.

Keywords: aging, fitness, physical exercise, neural specificity, multivariate pattern analysis

INTRODUCTION

Pictures of faces, houses, and many other stimulus categories elicit distinguishable patterns of neural response in ventral visual cortex (VVC). For example, using functional magnetic resonance imaging (fMRI), Haxby et al. (2001) found distinct neural activation patterns in response to eight stimulus categories within ventral temporal cortex. After being trained on a subset of activation patterns, machine learning classifiers can often decode the stimulus category associated with novel patterns (Haynes and Rees, 2006; Norman et al., 2006). And the more distinctive, or specific, the patterns are, the more accurately a classifier will be able to predict the stimulus category from neural activity, so classifier accuracy is a natural way to estimate neural specificity.

Evidence suggests that neural specificity declines with increasing age (Grady et al., 1994; Park et al., 2004) and reduced neural specificity is associated with lower cognitive performance in a variety of cognitive tasks in older adults (Park et al., 2010). But why does neural specificity decline with age? Age-related declines in neurotransmitter function and neuromodulation have been suggested as underlying mechanisms. For example, the number of dopamine (DA) neurons (Bäckman et al., 2006), as well as DA receptor levels (Inoue et al., 2001) show pronounced and widespread decrements with advancing adult age. Neurocomputational models predict that attenuated neuromodulation lowers a cell's responsivity and leads to less differentiated neural responses to different stimuli (i.e., less distinct neural representations), which in turn would explain age-related deficits across a wide range of cognitive domains (Li and Sikström, 2002).

On the other hand, regular physical activity has repeatedly been shown to preserve cognitive abilities in old age (for reviews see Bherer et al., 2013; Voss et al., 2013). Evidence from animal research suggests that exercise induces an upregulation of DA (Sutoo and Akiyama, 2003; Poulton and Muir, 2005; Foley and Fleshner, 2008), possibly by stimulating DA synthesis through a calcium/calmodulin-dependent system. Consistent with this hypothesis, Ruscheweyh et al. (2011) found increased plasma concentrations of DA after 6 months of physical training in older humans. Moreover, Stroth et al. (2010) showed that young adults with a genotype associated with lower DA levels (val/val COMT gene homozygotes) exhibited greater cognitive improvements after a 4-month exercise intervention compared with other genotypes (met carriers). Since the relationship between DA and cognitive performance seems to follow an inverted U-shape, Stroth et al. (2010) hypothesized that exercise may optimize central DA availability. This especially benefits those individuals with suboptimal initial levels, as it moves them further up the curve. Similarly, a cross-sectional study with older adults showed that val/val homozygotes benefitted most from better fitness in terms of Flanker task performance. The latter result suggests that high fitness levels may compensate for being a COMT val/val homozygote (Voelcker-Rehage et al., 2015).

Taken together, the two lines of research suggest that neural specificity may provide a potential mechanism for beneficial effects of exercise in preserving cognitive functions in older adulthood. If so, improvements in exercise-induced fitness should be associated with more positive changes in neural specificity.

We are aware of four previous intervention studies that looked at exercise-related changes in BOLD activation (Colcombe et al., 2004; Voss et al., 2010; Voelcker-Rehage et al., 2011; Maffei et al., 2017). All four of them focused on changes in *neural efficiency*, that is, more efficient usage of brain networks, which is typically reflected in a reduced BOLD signal, and in greater functional connectivity with increasing cognitive load. The results of these studies suggest that an aerobic fitness training as opposed to an anaerobic fitness training or a passive control improves neural efficiency during task performance, as reflected by maintained (Maffei et al., 2017) or even reduced (Colcombe et al., 2004; Voelcker-Rehage et al., 2011) BOLD activation in task-relevant areas, as well as by strengthened functional connections within the default mode and frontal executive networks (Voss et al., 2010). In contrast to these former studies, which focused on exercise-induced changes in neural efficiency, the present study investigates exercise-induced changes in *neural specificity*, that is, the distinctiveness of specific stimulus-evoked neural activation patterns, irrespective of BOLD signal strength. Note that it is possible to observe changes in neural efficiency without changes in neural specificity, such as when two different stimuli elicit smaller, more efficient activation after the intervention that are not accompanied by reductions in activation overlap. Likewise, one may observe changes in neural specificity without changes in neural efficiency, such as when two stimuli elicit more distinct activation patterns after the intervention that are not accompanied by reductions in BOLD signal strength.

To test whether exercise-induced fitness improvements translate to neural specificity we used fMRI and multivariate pattern analysis (MVPA) within an exercise-dose-response paradigm. Elderly participants were randomly assigned to training regimens with differing levels of intensity. Before and after the 6-month training phase, participants performed a graded maximal exercise test to assess their training-related fitness improvements as well as a passive viewing task while functional brain images were acquired. As in earlier work (see Carp et al., 2011), the distinctiveness of neural activation patterns in response to different stimulus categories served as an index of neural specificity. To examine the hypothesized association between fitness and neural specificity, we correlated changes in fitness with changes in neural specificity.

MATERIALS AND METHODS

Participants

The total sample consisted of 52 community-dwelling older adults aged 59–74 (mean 65.95 ± 4.36, 20 males). All participants met the following inclusion criteria: (1) age range in years between 59 and 75; (2) physical inactivity prior to study enrollment (MET < 40 based on the German version of the compendium of physical activities); (3) MMSE score ≥ 26; (4) free of neurological, psychiatric, and cardiovascular diseases; (5) right-handed; (6) no contraindication for heart-rate controlled exercise training (e.g., no medication with beta blockers); (7) suitability for MR assessment (e.g., no magnetic implants, no claustrophobia). This study was carried out in accordance with the recommendations of the ethics committee of the German Psychological Society (DGP). All participants gave written informed consent in accordance with the Declaration of Helsinki and participated voluntarily. They were paid for study completion; training adherence was reinforced through a bonus system. Details on the recruitment can be found in previously published work based on the same study (Kleemeyer et al., 2016). Five participants were excluded from the MVPA analyses, four due to incomplete fMRI data, and one due to improper slice positioning at pretest. One participant was excluded from the fitness analyses due to problems in VO_2max detection. Thus, correlation analyses were based on data from 46 participants.

Design

Participants completed a 6-month fitness intervention with a comprehensive test battery before (pre) and after (post) the training. Please note that we confine ourselves to describing only those methods relevant for the scope of this article, that is, training, fitness assessment, and imaging procedures. Additional information can be found in Kleemeyer et al. (2016).

Training

Participants were randomly assigned to a high-intensity (HI) or low-intensity (LI) training regimen subsequent to the pretest assessment. Groups were counterbalanced for age, sex, years of education, digit-symbol performance, and MMSE scores.

Participants in each of the two groups exercised in our lab on stationary bikes, three times a week for 55 min in each session, with a gradual increase during the first 3 weeks. Over the 6-month period, a total of 75 training sessions could be achieved. For the HI group, training intensity was calibrated to result in a heart rate at 80% of the individual's ventilatory anaerobic threshold (Wasserman et al., 1990). In contrast, the LI group exercised at a constant resistance of 10 W. For the last 21 sessions, five intervals of 2 min each were integrated after 20 min of training in order to further increase variance in fitness gains. During these 2-min time windows, the LI group only increased the cadence from 60–70 to 80–90 cycles/min, while the HI group also increased the intensity to a resistance corresponding to 110% of the individual's ventilatory anaerobic threshold. Training intensity was automatically controlled using the software custo cardio concept (custo med GmbH, Ottobrunn, Germany), with a staff member supervising compliance for each participant and each training session. Up to six participants exercised simultaneously, irrespective of intensity levels (e.g., HI and LI participants exercised together). The existence of different training regimens was conveyed only after termination of the study.

Cardiovascular Fitness Assessment

Participants performed a graded maximal exercise test on a cycle ergometer to assess their cardiovascular fitness. The test started at 10 W, increased to 25 W after 2 min followed by 25 W increments every 2 min until total exhaustion or signs of cardiac or respiratory distress. A sports physician continuously monitored the cardiogram, oxygen uptake, heart rate, and blood pressure. We computed an aggregate measure of the maximum oxygen consumption at exhaustion (VO_2max) and the oxygen consumption at the ventilatory anaerobic threshold (VO_2AT) to obtain a more robust fitness measure. Therefore, data were z-transformed in a way that preserves mean differences between time points, namely by subtracting the common mean from pretest and posttest data. The aggregate fitness measure VO_2 served as the outcome of the fitness assessment.

MRI Data Acquisition and Preprocessing

During functional imaging, participants passively viewed face, house, or phase-scrambled images, following the procedures of Park et al. (2010). They completed two runs, each of which consisted of four blocks per stimulus category. During every block 15 images were shown for 2 s each, resulting in 30 s per block and 6 min per run. Stimuli were presented via *E*-prime (Psychology Software Tools, Pittsburgh, PA, USA) and displayed by a projection system.

Brain images were acquired on a Siemens TIM Trio 3T MRI scanner (Siemens, Erlangen, Germany). A conventional echo-planar MR sequence was used for functional acquisitions (TR = 2000 ms, TE = 30 ms, flip angle = 80°, FOV = 216 mm) encompassing 192 volumes per run and 36 slices per volume (slice thickness 3 mm). Slices were 72 × 72 matrices acquired parallel to the Corpus Callosum. A high-resolution T1-weighted MPRAGE (TR = 2500 ms, TE = 4.76 ms, TI = 1100 ms, flip angle = 7°, acquisition matrix = 256 × 256 × 176, 1 mm isotropic voxels) was also acquired to facilitate warping masks from MNI to individual subject space. Data were preprocessed using SPM12 (Wellcome Department of Cognitive Neurology, London, UK[1]). Functional images were realigned to the mean volume. The T1-weighted image was normalized to MNI space. The inverse normalization parameters were then applied to an AAL atlas based mask of VVC (including bilateral occipital cortices, inferior temporal cortices, and fusiform gyri). As a last step, the T1-weighted image was co-registered to the mean functional image, and the same parameters were applied to the mask such that all images mapped into the subject's native space. No normalization, spatial smoothing or other transformation was applied to the functional images.

To obtain activation maps, we setup a General Linear Model (GLM) to estimate the response to each category relative to phase-scrambled control images. We defined a separate regressor for each experimental block, resulting in eight estimates of face-evoked activation and eight estimates of house-evoked activation. We also included six nuisance covariates per run in the GLM, modeling head translation and rotation.

Multivariate Pattern Analysis

Since we were interested in the responses to face and house stimuli, we restricted the analysis to voxels within VVC. We applied MVPA using correlation analysis (see Haxby et al., 2001) on individual subject data separately for pretest and posttest. More precisely, we used the 16 coefficient estimates for faces and houses vs. phase-scrambled images from the GLM and extracted the activation pattern for voxels within

[1]http://www.fil.ion.ucl.ac.uk/spm/

VVC. Next, we computed the Pearson correlation within categories (i.e., correlating the face-evoked activation patterns from odd blocks pairwise with the face-evoked activation patterns from even blocks and the same for house-evoked activation patterns) and the Pearson correlation between categories (i.e., correlating the face-evoked activation patterns from odd blocks pairwise with the house-evoked activation patterns from even blocks and vice versa). To ensure a more normal distribution, correlation coefficients were transformed into Fisher's z-values. Neural specificity was then defined as the difference between the mean within-category and between-category correlations.

Statistical Analyses

Statistical analyses were performed using SPSS (IBMCorp., IBM SPSS Statistics, V22, Armonk, NY, USA). To assess effects on fitness and neural specificity, we used repeated-measures analysis of variance (ANOVA) with time point as a within-subject factor and training group as a between-subject factor. To examine whether changes in fitness were associated with changes in neural specificity, we performed a two-tailed Pearson correlation analysis across participants from both groups using the absolute difference (post-training minus pre-training) in fitness and the absolute difference (post-training minus pre-training) in neural specificity. The alpha level for all analyses was set to $p = 0.05$.

RESULTS

There were no baseline differences between participants in the two training groups with respect to age, years of education, MMSE, BMI, fitness, hormone replacement therapy, and treated hypertension (see **Table 1** for means and standard deviations (SD) or proportion of participants, respectively). Also, training adherence did not differ reliably between the two groups (mean HI = 71.14, mean LI = 69.12, $t_{(44)} = -1.088, p = 0.282$).

The intervention was associated with increasing fitness levels ($F_{(1,49)} = 5.637$; $p = 0.022$; $\eta_p^2 = 0.103$). However, HI and LI groups did not differ in mean fitness changes ($F_{(1,49)} = 0.997$; $p = 0.323$; $\eta_p^2 = 0.020$). Consequently, data were collapsed across treatment conditions when investigating exercise effects on neural specificity.

As predicted, greater changes in fitness were associated with greater changes in neural specificity ($r_{(46)} = 0.310$, $p = 0.036$, $R^2 = 0.096$), irrespective of the training regimen's intensity (see **Figure 1**). Similar to changes in fitness, neural specificity increased from pretest to posttest in some participants, and decreased in others, especially among those whose fitness did not improve. Overall there was no significant change in neural specificity with training ($F_{(1,45)} = 1.891$; $p = 0.176$; $\eta_p^2 = 0.040$) and no reliable interaction of neural specificity changes with group ($F_{(1,45)} = 0.006$; $p = 0.936$; $\eta_p^2 = 0.000$). **Figure 2** displays mean changes in fitness and neural specificity.

To differentiate training-induced changes in neural specificity from changes in neural efficiency, we also tested whether training affected mean BOLD activation in stimulus-relevant regions, that is, the fusiform face area (FFA) for faces and parahippocampal place area (PPA) for buildings. We extracted the % BOLD signal change from four spherical ROIs (FFA left and right, PPA left and right, with 5 mm radius around center coordinates adapted from Ishai et al., 1999) for the appropriate condition (in FFA for faces, and in PPA for houses) using MarsBaR. We found a negative but non-significant relationship between change in fitness and change in BOLD activation in both the FFA ($r_{(46)} = -0.201$, $p = 0.18$, $R^2 = 0.040$) and the PPA ($r_{(46)} = -0.181$, $p = 0.23$, $R^2 = 0.033$). The average effect across both regions was also negative, but not significant ($r_{(46)} = -0.234, p = 0.12, R^2 = 0.055$). For neither region alone, nor for the average, did we observe significant training-induced changes in % BOLD signal change (all $p > 0.3$), nor were there significant interactions with training group (all $p > 0.2$). All means and SD are provided in **Table 2**.

DISCUSSION

In this study we investigated whether exercise-induced fitness improvements would be associated with enhanced neural specificity. We found a positive correlation between changes in fitness induced by a 6-month exercise intervention and changes in neural specificity, in the sense that participants whose physical fitness improved more also showed more positive changes in

TABLE 1 | Sample characteristics as a function of training group.

Characteristic	High intensity (N = 21)		Low intensity (N = 25)		p
	M	SD	M	SD	
Age (years)	66.56	4.33	65.93	4.50	0.631
Education (years)	11.05	1.63	11.36	1.63	0.520
MMSE	29.48	1.08	28.88	1.48	0.132
BMI	26.12	4.21	25.18	4.05	0.444
VO_2max (ml/min × kg)	21.39	5.14	22.06	5.79	0.683
	N	%	N	%	
Female	13	62	15	60	
Hormone replacement therapy	5	38	6	40	
Treated hypertension	3	14	2	8	

Values are means (M) and standard deviations (SD), or number of participants (N) and percentage within group (%), respectively. Abbreviations: MMSE, Mini-Mental State examination; BMI, Body mass index.

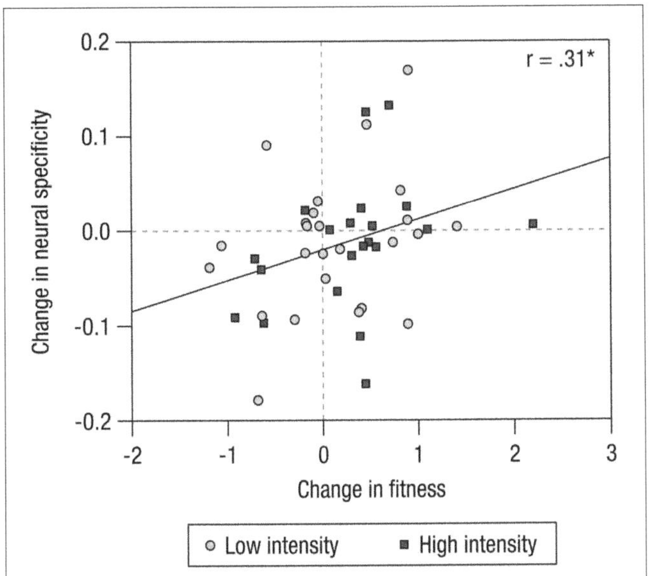

FIGURE 1 | Changes in fitness (aggregate measure of VO_2max and VO_2AT) are positively associated with changes in neural specificity. Circles represent participants from the low-intensity (LI) exercise group, and squares represent participants from the high-intensity (HI) exercise group. Change scores refer to post-training minus pre-training differences; a score of zero signifies no change. *$p < 0.05$.

neural specificity. These data suggest that regular physical activity may reduce or even reverse aging-related declines in neural specificity that have been reported in earlier studies (Park et al., 2004, 2010; Payer et al., 2006).

In terms of mechanisms, we propose that regular exercise may counteract the age-related weakening of dopaminergic neuromodulation (Bäckman et al., 2006). Neurocomputational models predict that adequate DA availability helps to keep the sigmoidal gain function within ranges that optimize signal transmission (Li et al., 2001). Optimized signaling reduces the detrimental effects of neural noise, and leads to the generation of more distinct internal representations (Li and Sikström, 2002). We note that this hypothesis could be tested more directly using Positron Emission Tomography (PET) to investigate DA binding and neural specificity before and after an exercise intervention.

Age-related losses in dopaminergic neuromodulation have more often been reported in frontal regions than in VVC. However, there is evidence for age-related losses of DA in the human temporal, parietal, and occipital cortices as well (Kaasinen and Rinne, 2002), closely resembling the dopaminergic decline repeatedly observed in the striatum. Recently, Garrett et al. (2015) found effects of d-amphetamine (boosting DA levels) on BOLD signal variability in regions beyond typical DA projections (e.g., primary visual cortices). Moreover, in a PET study with 181 healthy adults between 64 and 68 years of age, Nyberg et al. (2016) found that both caudate and hippocampal D2 DA receptor availability were positively associated with episodic memory. These findings provide further evidence for the functional significance of DA across many regions of the human brain.

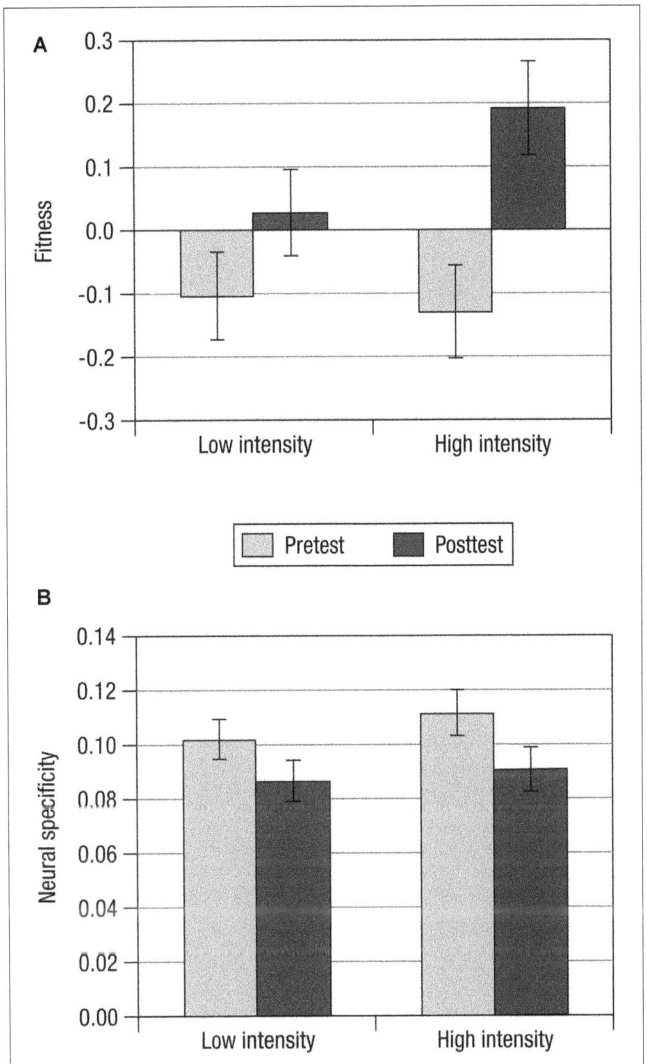

FIGURE 2 | Mean changes over the course of the training in (A) fitness (aggregate measure of VO_2max and VO_2AT) and **(B)** neural specificity. Whereas fitness increased reliably from pretest (light gray) to posttest (dark gray), changes in neural specificity were not significantly different from zero. For both measures, changes in the LI training group (left) were not reliably different from changes in the HI training group (right). Error bars depict the standard error after removing between-person variability (Cousineau and O'Brien, 2014).

It is also possible that other neurotransmitters are playing a role, instead of, or in addition to, DA. For example, in a proton magnetic resonance spectroscopy study, Maddock et al. (2016) observed increased signals for both glutamate and GABA in the visual cortex following vigorous exercise, indicating increased glutamate and GABA levels. Likewise, animal work showed an increased visual response in mouse visual cortex during running using *in vivo* calcium imaging. The suggested mechanism includes disinhibition of glutamatergic pyramidal neurons through the interaction of two different GABAergic interneurons (Fu et al., 2014). However, these results were obtained during running and there is only preliminary evidence to suggest that more exercise in the preceding week

TABLE 2 | Pre- and post-training values (mean ± SD) for fitness measures, multivariate pattern analysis, and % BOLD signal change.

	High intensity		Low intensity	
	Pre	Post	Pre	Post
VO_2max (ml/min × kg)*[1]	21.26 (± 4.76)	23.32 (± 5.06)	21.95 (± 5.70)	22.34 (± 5.29)
VO_2AT (ml/min × kg)*[2]	15.60 (± 3.18)	16.53 (± 3.49)	15.20 (± 4.25)	16.05 (± 3.57)
VO_2*[3]	−0.13 (± 0.84)	0.19 (± 0.92)	−0.10 (± 1.07)	0.03 (± 0.96)
MVPA	0.11 (± 0.07)	0.09 (± 0.06)	0.10 (± 0.07)	0.09 (± 0.07)
% Bold signal change FFA	0.18 (± 0.14)	0.15 (± 0.17)	0.20 (± 0.14)	0.18 (± 0.18)
% Bold signal change PPA	0.25 (± 0.20)	0.20 (± 0.19)	0.19 (± 0.17)	0.20 (± 0.20)

*Abbreviations: MVPA, Multivariate pattern analysis; FFA, fusiform face area; PPA, parahippocampal place area. *Indicates a significant main effect of time from the repeated measures ANOVA ($p < 0.05$). [1]$F_{(1,49)} = 4.805$; $p = 0.033$; $\eta_p^2 = 0.089$. [2]$F_{(1,50)} = 4.902$; $p = 0.031$; $\eta_p^2 = 0.089$. [3]$F_{(1,49)} = 5.637$; $p = 0.022$; $\eta_p^2 = 0.103$.*

also relates to higher resting glutamate (but not GABA) levels (Maddock et al., 2016). Furthermore, administration of GABA and a GABA agonist has been found to increase the orientation selectivity of individual visual neurons (increased neural specificity), while administration of a GABA antagonist has been found to decrease it (reduced neural specificity; Leventhal et al., 2003). Future work is needed to gauge the relative importance of different neurotransmitter systems, and their potential interactions, in mediating the effects of exercise on cognition.

Exercise has been shown to exert effects on other parameters of cerebral functioning, and these parameters may have contributed to our findings. Regarding fMRI, exercise-induced fitness changes were found to induce improved neural efficiency, that is, reductions (Colcombe et al., 2004; Voelcker-Rehage et al., 2011) or stability (Maffei et al., 2017) of BOLD activation in task-relevant areas as well as strengthened functional connections in relation to default mode and frontal executive networks (Voss et al., 2010). Though changes in neural efficiency, as investigated in these earlier studies, and changes in neural specificity, as investigated in the present study, can occur independently from each other, it seems worth exploring whether and in what way they are related empirically. Specifically, exercise training may lead to neural representations that achieve greater distinctiveness with a lower levels of neural activation.

Although our experimental task was not designed to look at neural efficiency, we were curious to see whether our training did affect mean BOLD activation in stimulus-relevant regions (FFA and PPA) and if so, in what way. Overall, we found negative, but non-significant, relationships between change in fitness and change in BOLD activation. These trends seem consistent with the hypothesis that improved fitness is associated with increased neural efficiency (i.e., less BOLD signal change). However, because we used a passive viewing task, there are no behavioral measures (e.g., reaction time, accuracy) from the scanning sessions that we could relate to the BOLD signal. We therefore acknowledge that the present study does not directly address neural efficiency, as this would require reduced BOLD activation in the absence of performance decrements.

At a more general level, exercise has been found to change brain perfusion (Pereira et al., 2007; Maass et al., 2015). Whereas Pereira et al. (2007) specifically looked at the hippocampus, Maass et al. (2015) also found fitness-related changes in perfusion to affect non-hippocampal cortical blood flow and blood volume. Changes in perfusion could potentially influence our results, as the fMRI BOLD signal measures a vascular response. Hence, we wondered whether the observed association might be due to changes in vascular response rather than changes in neural specificity. If so, one would expect to also observe an association between changes in mean activation level and changes in fitness. We therefore extracted mean activation values from VVC using MarsBaR, but found no reliable correlation with changes in fitness. Furthermore, vascular changes would not be expected to be limited to VVC, and so we tested whether associations between changes in fitness and changes in neural specificity were also present in brain regions that were not significantly activated by the task, such as medial orbitofrontal cortex, precentral gyrus, supramarginal gyrus, superior temporal gyrus, hippocampus, and parahippocampus. None of those regions, nor all of them combined, exhibited the change-change correlation observed in VVC. Each of these findings argues against a predominantly vascular interpretation of the observed effects. We note, however, that a calibrated fMRI approach would be needed to fully disentangle changes in neural activity from changes in vascular reactivity.

In contrast to Park et al. (2010), we did not observe associations between neural specificity and any of the cognitive tasks assessed in this study. One reason may be that Park et al. (2010) used a slightly different visual task in the fMRI scanner: Whereas our participants passively viewed single pictures, Park et al. (2010) presented two pictures side-by-side and asked their participants to make a same/different judgment, which may have introduced a demand characteristic that was absent in our task.

It is conceivable that exercise training as well as familiarization with the MR environment would alter participants' intention to lie quietly in the scanner. To minimize differences in head movement between pretest and posttest, all participants took part in a Mock-Scanner session before pretest. In addition, we used the FMRIB Software Library (Jenkinson et al., 2012) to check for head motion artifacts using the aggregated measures dvars as well as framewise displacement (implemented in fsl_motion_outlier). We found no evidence for significant session differences in head motion.

Also, sample size as well as sample selectivity may have influenced our results. In a study with similar sample selection criteria, Voelcker-Rehage et al. (2015) noticed a comparably high amount of COMT met/met allele carriers. Since our participants were inactive but healthy and willing to change their lifestyle, it is rather likely that they were even more selective. Given the absence of genetic information in this study, this conjecture cannot be tested.

As discussed in Kleemeyer et al. (2016), the absence of group differences in fitness changes between the HI and the LI groups may indicate that the level of challenge provided by LI training was already effective in boosting fitness in sedentary older adults, thereby rendering the two training regimes similar to one another. The observed absence of group differences in fitness changes also provides a reasonable explanation for the absence of group differences in neural specificity changes. As for neural specificity, we did not observe a mean increase over time, but rather stability, as the numerical decrease was not statistically different from zero. We interpret this finding in terms of two opposing forces, one related to normal aging and the other related to the fitness intervention. On the one hand, neural specificity tends to decline with age. Participants did not escape normal aging while taking part in our study, and for this reason alone one would expect that neural specificity measured later in time is lower than neural specificity measured earlier in time. On the other hand, the training-induced fitness improvements apparently counteracted aging-related decrements in neural specificity, and apparently reduced or, in some cases, actually offset the effects of aging. We conclude that the effects of fitness improvements on brain functioning were not strong enough to result in a mean positive trend in neural specificity. Nevertheless, and in full agreement with our hypothesis, participants whose fitness improved more showed smaller declines, or even improvements, in neural specificity. From a design perspective, it would have been preferable to also include a no-contact control group in the study in order to document changes in fitness and neural specificity that would take place in the absence of any intervention.

To conclude, we found that exercise-related changes in fitness are positively associated with changes in neural specificity. Greater neural specificity is related to better fluid processing ability, so these results may explain some of the beneficial effects of exercise on cognition. Future longitudinal and intervention work should include higher intensity levels, longer training durations, and no-contact control groups to replicate and extend these findings.

AUTHOR CONTRIBUTIONS

MMK designed and conducted the study, analyzed the data, interpreted the results, and wrote the manuscript. TAP assisted with MVPA analysis, interpreted the results, and revised the manuscript. SS designed the study and revised the manuscript. NCB designed the neuroimaging protocol and revised the manuscript. LB performed the cardiovascular fitness assessment and revised the manuscript. UL designed the study, interpreted the results, and revised the manuscript.

ACKNOWLEDGMENTS

We thank Timo Schmidt and Naftali Raz for helpful discussions.

REFERENCES

Bäckman, L., Nyberg, L., Lindenberger, U., Li, S. C., and Farde, L. (2006). The correlative triad among aging, dopamine, and cognition: current status and future prospects. *Neurosci. Biobehav. Rev.* 30, 791–807. doi: 10.1016/j.neubiorev.2006.06.005

Bherer, L., Erickson, K. I., and Liu-Ambrose, T. (2013). A review of the effects of physical activity and exercise on cognitive and brain functions in older adults. *J. Aging Res.* 2013:657508. doi: 10.1155/2013/657508

Carp, J., Park, J., Polk, T. A., and Park, D. C. (2011). Age differences in neural distinctiveness revealed by multi-voxel pattern analysis. *Neuroimage* 56, 736–743. doi: 10.1016/j.neuroimage.2010.04.267

Colcombe, S. J., Kramer, A. F., Erickson, K. I., Scalf, P., McAuley, E., Cohen, N. J., et al. (2004). Cardiovascular fitness, cortical plasticity, and aging. *Proc. Natl. Acad. Sci. U S A* 101, 3316–3321. doi: 10.1073/pnas.0400266101

Cousineau, D., and O'Brien, F. (2014). Error bars in within-subject designs: a comment on Baguley (2012). *Behav. Res. Methods* 46, 1149–1151. doi: 10.3758/s13428-013-0441-z

Foley, T. E., and Fleshner, M. (2008). Neuroplasticity of dopamine circuits after exercise: implications for central fatigue. *Neuromolecular Med.* 10, 67–80. doi: 10.1007/s12017-008-8032-3

Fu, Y., Tucciarone, J. M., Espinosa, J. S., Sheng, N., Darcy, D. P., Nicoll, R. A., et al. (2014). A cortical circuit for gain control by behavioral state. *Cell* 156, 1139–1152. doi: 10.1016/j.cell.2014.01.050

Garrett, D. D., Nagel, I. E., Preuschhof, C., Burzynska, A. Z., Marchner, J., Wiegert, S., et al. (2015). Amphetamine modulates brain signal variability and working memory in younger and older adults. *Proc. Natl. Acad. Sci. U S A* 112, 7593–7598. doi: 10.1073/pnas.1504090112

Grady, C. L., Maisog, J. M., Horwitz, B., Ungerleider, L. G., Mentis, M. J., Salerno, J. A., et al. (1994). Age-related changes in cortical blood flow activation during visual processing of faces and location. *J. Neurosci.* 14, 1450–1462.

Haxby, J. V., Gobbini, M. I., Furey, M. L., Ishai, A., Schouten, J. L., and Pietrini, P. (2001). Distributed and overlapping representations of faces and objects in ventral temporal cortex. *Science* 293, 2425–2430. doi: 10.1126/science.1063736

Haynes, J. D., and Rees, G. (2006). Decoding mental states from brain activity in humans. *Nat. Rev. Neurosci.* 7, 523–534. doi: 10.1038/nrn1931

Inoue, M., Suhara, T., Sudo, Y., Okubo, Y., Yasuno, F., Kishimoto, T., et al. (2001). Age-related reduction of extrastriatal dopamine D2 receptor measured by PET. *Life Sci.* 69, 1079–1084. doi: 10.1016/s0024-3205(01)01205-x

Ishai, A., Ungerleider, L. G., Martin, A., Schouten, J. L., and Haxby, J. V. (1999). Distributed representation of objects in the human ventral visual pathway. *Proc. Natl. Acad. Sci. U S A* 96, 9379–9384. doi: 10.1073/pnas.96.16.9379

Jenkinson, M., Beckmann, C. F., Behrens, T. E., Woolrich, M. W., and Smith, S. M. (2012). FSL. *Neuroimage* 62, 782–790. doi: 10.1016/j.neuroimage.2011.09.015

Kaasinen, V., and Rinne, J. O. (2002). Functional imaging studies of dopamine system and cognition in normal aging and Parkinson's disease. *Neurosci. Biobehav. Rev.* 26, 785–793. doi: 10.1016/s0149-7634(02)00065-9

Kleemeyer, M. M., Kühn, S., Prindle, J., Bodammer, N. C., Brechtel, L., Garthe, A., et al. (2016). Changes in fitness are associated with changes in hippocampal microstructure and hippocampal volume among older adults. *Neuroimage* 131, 155–161. doi: 10.1016/j.neuroimage.2015.11.026

Leventhal, A. G., Wang, Y., Pu, M., Zhou, Y., and Ma, Y. (2003). GABA and its agonists improved visual cortical function in senescent monkeys. *Science* 300, 812–815. doi: 10.1126/science.1082874

Li, S. C., Lindenberger, U., and Sikström, S. (2001). Aging cognition: from neuromodulation to representation. *Trends Cogn. Sci.* 5, 479–486. doi: 10.1016/s1364-6613(00)01769-1

Li, S. C., and Sikström, S. (2002). Integrative neurocomputational perspectives on cognitive aging, neuromodulation, and representation. *Neurosci. Biobehav. Rev.* 26, 795–808. doi: 10.1016/s0149-7634(02)00066-0

Maass, A., Düzel, S., Goerke, M., Becke, A., Sobieray, U., Neumann, K., et al. (2015). Vascular hippocampal plasticity after aerobic exercise in older adults. *Mol. Psychiatry* 20, 585–593. doi: 10.1038/mp.2014.114

Maddock, R. J., Casazza, G. A., Fernandez, D. H., and Maddock, M. I. (2016). Acute modulation of cortical glutamate and GABA content by physical activity. *J. Neurosci.* 36, 2449–2457. doi: 10.1523/JNEUROSCI.3455-15.2016

Maffei, L., Picano, E., Andreassi, M. G., Angelucci, A., Baldacci, F., Baroncelli, L., et al. (2017). Randomized trial on the effects of a combined physical/cognitive training in aged MCI subjects: the Train the Brain study. *Sci. Rep.* 7:39471. doi: 10.1038/srep39471

Norman, K. A., Polyn, S. M., Detre, G. J., and Haxby, J. V. (2006). Beyond mind-reading: multi-voxel pattern analysis of fMRI data. *Trends Cogn. Sci.* 10, 424–430. doi: 10.1016/j.tics.2006.07.005

Nyberg, L., Karalija, N., Salami, A., Andersson, M., Wåhlin, A., Kaboovand, N., et al. (2016). Dopamine D2 receptor availability is linked to hippocampal-caudate functional connectivity and episodic memory. *Proc. Natl. Acad. Sci. U S A* 113, 7918–7923. doi: 10.1073/pnas.1606309113

Park, J., Carp, J., Hebrank, A., Park, D. C., and Polk, T. A. (2010). Neural specificity predicts fluid processing ability in older adults. *J. Neurosci.* 30, 9253–9259. doi: 10.1523/JNEUROSCI.0853-10.2010

Park, D. C., Polk, T. A., Park, R., Minear, M., Savage, A., and Smith, M. R. (2004). Aging reduces neural specialization in ventral visual cortex. *Proc. Natl. Acad. Sci. U S A* 101, 13091–13095. doi: 10.1073/pnas.0405148101

Payer, D., Marshuetz, C., Sutton, B., Hebrank, A., Welsh, R. C., and Park, D. C. (2006). Decreased neural specialization in old adults on a working memory task. *Neuroreport* 17, 487–491. doi: 10.1097/01.WNR.0000209005.40481.31

Pereira, A. C., Huddleston, D. E., Brickman, A. M., Sosunov, A. A., Hen, R., McKhann, G. M., et al. (2007). An *in vivo* correlate of exercise-induced neurogenesis in the adult dentate gyrus. *Proc. Natl. Acad. Sci. U S A* 104, 5638–5643. doi: 10.1073/pnas.0611721104

Poulton, N. P., and Muir, G. D. (2005). Treadmill training ameliorates dopamine loss but not behavioral deficits in hemi-parkinsonian rats. *Exp. Neurol.* 193, 181–197. doi: 10.1016/j.expneurol.2004.12.006

Ruscheweyh, R., Willemer, C., Krüger, K., Duning, T., Warnecke, T., Sommer, J., et al. (2011). Physical activity and memory functions: an interventional study. *Neurobiol. Aging* 32, 1304–1319. doi: 10.1016/j.neurobiolaging.2009.08.001

Stroth, S., Reinhardt, R. K., Thone, J., Hille, K., Schneider, M., Hartel, S., et al. (2010). Impact of aerobic exercise training on cognitive functions and affect associated to the COMT polymorphism in young adults. *Neurobiol. Learn. Mem.* 94, 364–372. doi: 10.1016/j.nlm.2010.08.003

Sutoo, D., and Akiyama, K. (2003). Regulation of brain function by exercise. *Neurobiol. Dis.* 13, 1–14. doi: 10.1016/s0969-9961(03)00030-5

Voelcker-Rehage, C., Godde, B., and Staudinger, U. M. (2011). Cardiovascular and coordination training differentially improve cognitive performance and neural processing in older adults. *Front. Hum. Neurosci.* 5:26. doi: 10.3389/fnhum.2011.00026

Voelcker-Rehage, C., Jeltsch, A., Godde, B., Becker, S., and Staudinger, U. M. (2015). COMT gene polymorphisms, cognitive performance and physical fitness in older adults. *Psychol. Sport Exerc.* 20, 20–28. doi: 10.1016/j.psychsport.2015.04.001

Voss, M. W., Prakash, R. S., Erickson, K. I., Basak, C., Chaddock, L., Kim, J. S., et al. (2010). Plasticity of brain networks in a randomized intervention trial of exercise training in older adults. *Front. Aging Neurosci.* 2:32. doi: 10.3389/fnagi.2010.00032

Voss, M. W., Vivar, C., Kramer, A. F., and van Praag, H. (2013). Bridging animal and human models of exercise-induced brain plasticity. *Trends Cogn. Sci.* 17, 525–544. doi: 10.1016/j.tics.2013.08.001

Wasserman, K., Beaver, W. L., and Whipp, B. J. (1990). Gas exchange theory and the lactic acidosis (anaerobic) threshold. *Circulation* 81, II14–II30.

8

Pain Perception can be Modulated by Mindfulness Training: A Resting-State fMRI Study

*I-Wen Su[1,2,3], Fang-Wei Wu[4], Keng-Chen Liang[2,3,4], Kai-Yuan Cheng[5], Sung-Tsang Hsieh[2,3,6], Wei-Zen Sun[2,3,7] and Tai-Li Chou[2,4]**

[1] Graduate Institute of Linguistics, National Taiwan University, Taipei, Taiwan, [2] Neurobiology and Cognitive Science Center, National Taiwan University, Taipei, Taiwan, [3] Graduate Institute of Brain and Mind Sciences, National Taiwan University, Taipei, Taiwan, [4] Department of Psychology, National Taiwan University, Taipei, Taiwan, [5] Institute of Philosophy of Mind and Cognition, National Yang-Ming University, Taipei, Taiwan, [6] Department of Neurology, National Taiwan University Hospital, Taipei, Taiwan, [7] Department of Anesthesiology, National Taiwan University Hospital, Taipei, Taiwan

Edited by:
Louis Bherer,
Université de Montréal, Canada

Reviewed by:
Jeremy Hogeveen,
University of California, Davis, USA
Dhruman D. Goradia,
Banner Alzheimer's Institute, USA

***Correspondence:**
Tai-Li Chou
tlchou25@ntu.edu.tw

The multi-dimensional nature of pain renders difficult a holistic understanding of it. The conceptual framework of pain is said to be cognitive-evaluative, in addition to being sensory-discriminative and affective-motivational. To compare participants' brain-behavior response before and after a 6-week mindfulness-based stress reduction training course on mindfulness in relation to pain modulation, three questionnaires (the Dallas Pain Questionnaire, Short Form McGill Pain Questionnaire-SFMPQ, and Kentucky Inventory of Mindfulness) as well as resting-state functional magnetic resonance imaging were administered to participants, divided into a pain-afflicted group ($N = 18$) and a control group ($N = 16$). Our results showed that the pain-afflicted group experienced significantly less pain after the mindfulness treatment than before, as measured by the SFMPQ. In conjunction, an increased connection from the anterior insular cortex (AIC) to the dorsal anterior midcingulate cortex (daMCC) was observed in the post-training pain-afflicted group and a significant correlation was found between AIC-daMCC connectivity and SFMPQ scores. The results suggest that mindfulness training can modulate the brain network dynamics underlying the subjective experience of pain.

Keywords: pain, resting-state, connectivity, mindfulness, perspective shift

INTRODUCTION

Pain relates to a sensation that hurts. Pain is a very individual experience. Only the person experiencing it can be certain of its existence and even then may have great difficulty describing it with much accuracy. When it comes to measuring one's pain objectively, it is virtually impossible. The best way to find out how much pain a person is enduring depends at best on a subjective pain report.

Mindfulness-Based Stress Reduction (MBSR) and Pain Relief

A recent development in the study of pain indicates that mindfulness meditation brings pain relief rather than merely acting as a placebo (Zeidan et al., 2012). Mindfulness skills make it possible for participants to stay not only attentive but also clearly aware of what they are experiencing at the moment, suggesting that mindfulness meditation can be an effective way to reduce pain and deserves further investigation.

Kabat-Zinn's world-renowned Mindfulness-Based Stress Reduction (MBSR) Clinic, founded in 1979, provides training to participants so that they may develop the capacity to observe their own thoughts and feelings from a detached perspective (McCracken et al., 2013), and thus see themselves as if they were to "video-tape someone else" (Gallagher, 2000), and in turn to view their pain, together with their pain-elicited emotions and judgments, as transient passing events rather than as reflections of the self or reality (McCracken et al., 2013). MBSR's effect on chronic pain patients has been well established as an outpatient program in behavioral medicine (Kabat-Zinn, 1982). Inspired by such findings among populations of Westerners, we intend to explore in this study functional magnetic resonance imaging (fMRI) changes vis-à-vis behavioral changes in pain-afflicted Chinese subjects after a 6-week MBSR training intervention.

MBSR: Attention, Empathy, and Perspective Shift

Mindfulness is, according to Kabat-Zinn (2003), the "awareness that emerges through paying attention on purpose, in the present moment, and non-judgmentally to the unfolding of experience moment to moment." The role of awareness as a vital dimension of consciousness aiding in diverting one's sensational involvement with pain is not at all a new idea (Allport, 1988; Schmidt, 1994). Since "paying attention on purpose" to the very moment of existence is the basic skill and the ultimate outcome of MBSR training, we will focus mainly on attention in this study, and the word *awareness* will be included only as it pertains to our discussion of attention in this paper.

Mindfulness-based stress reduction training is in fact a means to cognitively "re-construct" participants' perception of pain, through developing their capacity to observe their own thoughts and feelings from a detached perspective (McCracken et al., 2013). The purpose of such a perspective shift is to place oneself in another's position, which is empathy, defined as the capacity to understand or feel what another person is experiencing from within the other being's frame of reference (Bellet and Maloney, 1991). It should be noted that the capacity to understand from another's frame of reference is a matter of perspective shifting. A speaker usually takes a stance from his own perspective, but to keep up with the true spirit of empathy, he will need to take the other's perspective in order to understand what the other is experiencing.

Brain Regions Related to Attention and Empathy

Mindfulness meditation is typically described as non-judgmental attention to experiences in the present moment, as reviewed in Tang et al. (2015). Their review has elucidated neural mechanisms as being an important topic of study in this domain since the complex mental state of mindfulness is supported by alterations in large-scale brain networks. The study of neural mechanisms is a crucial aspect of attempts to understand the mental state of mindfulness and includes analyses of complex networks such as those involved in resting-state connectivity. Also, Tang et al. (2015) considered exhaustively the current state of research on mindfulness meditation and discussed the methodological challenges the field now faces. Taking into account the several shortcomings discussed by Tang et al. (2015) in existing studies, we propose three methodological improvements in the present study. First, a longitudinal approach is designed to minimize pre-training differences that exist in cross-sectional studies. Using two time points allows us to contrast post-training with pre-training to tease apart differences that existed among participants before training. Second, a control group that receives the same mindfulness training as the experimental group is added. The control group enables us to reduce confounds such as practice, memory, or fatigue found in a one-group longitudinal design. Third, resting-state connectivity is utilized to observe changes in coordination among brain regions related to mindfulness training. The correlation of this functional connectivity with questionnaire performance is analyzed to strengthen our arguments by establishing brain-behavior relationships.

As for previous studies on emotional awareness, we are inspired by McRae et al. (2008) in their research of the role of arousal in the relationship between trait emotional awareness and dorsal anterior cingulate cortex (dACC) activity. The relationship between the dACC and emotional awareness is specific to highly arousing emotional stimuli, such as viewing highly arousing pictures. When this is considered in conjunction with the brain areas involved in pain processing, especially the "pain matrix" described by Tracey and Johns (2010), many findings (e.g., Apkarian et al., 2005) indicate that the dorsal anterior midcingulate cortex (daMCC) and the anterior insular cortex (AIC) are highly relevant to attention, with the former (see Bush, 2011; Fan et al., 2014) being involved in top-down attentional control. According to Brooks et al. (2002), paying attention to a pain stimulus results in activation of the AIC, an area of the brain which a later study (Schweinhardt et al., 2006) reports as being related to both acute and chronic pain. Craig (2002) further confirmed that the AIC contains interoceptive representations that substantialize feelings from the body and emotional awareness, especially the pain-related unpleasant ones (Medford and Critchley, 2010).

The AIC has been claimed to be necessary for empathetic pain perception (Gu et al., 2012). Singer et al. (2004) found that empathic feelings for close others experiencing painful stimuli were associated with bilateral activation of the AIC. All these studies have contributed to the present research in their design of experiments aimed at identifying brain regions responsible for attention control, with hopes to see its correlation with emotion regulation and self-awareness, the three core areas mentioned in Tang et al. (2015).

Our Working Hypotheses

The present study focuses on the change in signal intensity in areas anatomically related to the processing of nociceptive stimuli, as well as areas responsible for attention-related processes, and areas for empathic processes. Pain is a complex, multidimensional and subjective experience, which cannot be fully accounted for by any modality alone. It affects processes that are of a motor-integratory nature, as well as those that are deemed sensory–discriminative, affective–motivational, and cognitive–evaluative (Kupers, 2006). Based on what we have learned from MBSR training, we hypothesize that one may learn to shift one's subjective experiences via attention practices and we hope to verify such an effect via the participants' self-reported surveys and the results of the fMRI scans.

To observe changes related to mindfulness training, we use a two-group longitudinal design by taking pre- and post-training measurements with scans and questionnaires for both a pain-afflicted group and a control group. Thus, a 2 (group: low pain, high pain) × 2 (time: pre, post) mixed ANOVA design is used to explore the training effect on fMRI scans and three self-reported surveys, the Dallas Pain Questionnaire (DPQ), the Short Form McGill Pain Questionnaire (SFMPQ) and the Kentucky Inventory of Mindfulness (KIMS). Moreover, resting-state connectivity is also measured to explore changes in dynamic interactions among brain regions associated with mindfulness training. The changes in resting-state functional connectivity (rsFC) measurements are correlated with changes in the questionnaire measurements to elucidate the neural substrates of pain modulation.

Due to the multiple roles played by the AIC in attention, awareness and empathy networks, we hypothesize that the mindfulness training will influence pain perception by strengthening the AIC's connectivity with the dorsal ACC in meditators (Grant et al., 2011). The relationship between the AIC and the daMCC is crucial because these two regions are both involved in pain processing and in the attention salience network (Seeley et al., 2007), and therefore we hypothesize that the resting-state fMRI will display increased functional connectivity in brain regions associated with pain modulation, especially the AIC-daMCC connection, as a result of MBSR training.

MATERIALS AND METHODS

Thirty-four adult participants were recruited in Taiwan for the fMRI experiment. Eighteen participants were selected as the pain-afflicted group, those who both claimed to suffer from moderate or severe pain and scored greater than 1 on the present pain intensity (PPI) index of the standard McGill Pain questionnaire (Melzack, 1975). The remaining sixteen participants selected as the control group scored less than or equal to 1 on the PPI pain index, indicating mild or no pain. These 34 native speakers of Mandarin Chinese (mean age = 38.59, 25 females) were first given an informal interview to ensure that they met the following criteria: (1) right-handedness, (2) normal or corrected-to-normal vision, and (3) without a history of any language deficit or learning disability. After the interview, informed consent was obtained. Our study was approved by the Research Ethics Committee of National Taiwan University before the training and the experiments were administered.

The established model chosen for our mindfulness practices was a 6-week MBSR intervention developed by Kabat-Zinn (1982). The training consisted of six 2.5-h sessions per week and one 8-h non-speaking session in the 4th week. The participants were asked to learn and practice different kinds of mindfulness meditations during the training, including a body scan, sitting meditation, hatha yoga, walking meditation and other informal practices. The body scan was conducted under spoken directions, guiding the participants to progressively move their attention from their toes to head as they observed the physical sensations of different bodily regions. Sitting meditation involved concentration on one's own breath while remaining open-minded to thoughts, emotions, and other feelings. Hatha yoga contained gentle exercises and body stretching in order to improve the attentive awareness of one's physical situation in hopes of finding a balance of mind and body. Walking meditation involved walking with intense attention to changes in one's own gestures and movement. Lastly, the MBSR trainer demonstrates how to make use of the aforementioned methods so that the participants can use them for pain management and in other aspects of their daily life (Shapiro et al., 2007). During the training, the participants were encouraged to focus only on their own breathing, but had to remain aware of different sensations (e.g., sounds and thoughts), accepting the feelings without being responsive to them. All of these techniques were administered in order to encourage the participants to disengage from their personal thoughts and emotions.

In order to compare the differences between pre- and post-training, both the questionnaires and the resting-state fMRI were employed as our major instruments. The three questionnaires were meant to measure the mindfulness skills of the participants, the effects of pain on each individual's life, and their thoughts about pain, both before and after the training; the resting-state fMRI was used to measure brain functional connectivity before and after the 6-week training.

In order to understand the progression of pain perception and mindfulness skills, two questionnaires, the DPQ and the SFMPQ, were distributed. In addition, the KIMS was used to obtain the participants' subjective evaluation of their acquired mindfulness skills. All three questionnaires were translated into Mandarin Chinese for the participating subjects.

The DPQ is designed to assess how chronic pain affects different aspects of an individual's life, including daily activities, work and leisure activities, feelings of anxiety-depression, and social interest (Lawlis et al., 1989). Each of the DPQ's sixteen sections consists of a single item with a short question asking to what degree pain has adversely affected a particular aspect of life and a corresponding continuous rating scale divided into 5–8 equal sections on which respondents are asked to place a mark indicating the degree from 0 to 100% that expresses their answer. As suggested in Lawlis et al. (1989), the subjective evaluation of pain experience is an important factor in determining how motivated a person is to seek treatment. The self-reported outcome of the DPQ, on the other hand, is conducive to the understanding of chronic pain and, therefore, serves as one of our pain assessment tools.

The SFMPQ, a short version of the McGill pain questionnaire (MPQ) (Melzack, 1975), is commonly used in evaluating how chronic pain influences participants' sensory, affective, and present feelings. It consists of two subscales with adjectival pain descriptors, including eleven sensory ones and four affective ones. The PPI index of the standard MPQ is also included in the

SFMPQ, whose items are presented according to an intensity rating scale ranging from none, mild, moderate to severe, so designed in order to assess the participants' subjective pain experience (Melzack, 1987). Due to its accessibility and proven validity, the easy-to-follow SFMPQ was chosen as one of our pain assessment tools.

The KIMS is designed to assess whether or not people can exercise mindfulness skills in their daily lives with regard to four facets: observing, describing, acting with awareness, and accepting without judgment (Baer et al., 2004). Mindfulness practices in the KIMS focus on the participants' abilities to put their feelings, emotion, perceptions and thoughts into words (Bergomi et al., 2013). Based on the "thinking for speaking" hypothesis articulated by Slobin (1987) that one's language use may shape one's cognition and may further affect one's feelings (of pain), we used the KIMS to assess the connection between cognition (one's comprehension as well as communicative skills) and sensation (one's feelings).

A 2 (group: low pain, high pain) × 2 (time: pre, post) mixed ANOVA was conducted on the composite score of the DPQ, SFMPQ, and KIMS questionnaire, respectively. These analyses allowed us to assess the behavioral changes related to mindfulness training intervention.

In both groups, resting-state fMRI was used to detect differences in the functional connectivity in brain regions before and after the MBSR training. Such a comparison may help to discover how the training via linguistic instruction assists in regulating a participant's specific networks that are involved in the cognition of pain. Before fMRI scanning, participants were instructed to lie in the scanner with their head position secured. The head coil was then positioned over the participants' head. Scanning was conducted on the Bruker 3T S300 BIOSPEC/MEDSPEC MRI scanner, using a quadrature head coil. During the resting-state fMRI scans, participants were instructed to close their eyes and think about nothing, but had to remain awake (Raichle et al., 2001). Each resting scan lasted for 10 min. The data were collected using a gradient-echo planar pulse (EPI) sequence [repetition time (TR) = 3 s, echo time (TE) = 30 ms, 35 slices oriented to the AC-PC line, flip angle = 90°, matrix size = 64 × 64, voxel size = 3.75 × 3.75 × 3.75, slice gap = 0 mm, field of view (FOV) = 24 cm × 24 cm].

Image preprocessing was performed with the Resting-State fMRI Data Analysis Toolkit (REST) version 1.6 (Song et al., 2011) and SPM5 (Statistical Parametric Mapping). The images were corrected for differences in slice-acquisition time to the middle volume and were realigned to the first volume in the scanning session using affine transformations. No participant had more than 3 mm of movement in any plane according to the averages of the realignment parameters. Co-registered images were normalized to the ICBM EPI template, smoothed using a full-width at half-maximum (FWHM) kernel of 10 mm (Chou et al., 2009), detrended, and bandpass-filtered (0.01–0.1 HZ) to reduce non-neuronal contributions to BOLD fluctuations (Zang et al., 2007; Zou et al., 2008). Afterward, low frequency artifacts were removed with a high-pass filter (128-s cutoff period). The nuisance signals of the six head motion parameters, global mean signal, white matter, and cerebro-spinal fluid were regressed out from each voxel's time course.

The average BOLD signal time course within the seed of the AIC (radius = 8 mm), centered at [−34,16,6] based on a pain study (Tseng et al., 2010), was correlated to every voxel in the brain for each subject using Pearson's correlation coefficient. The threshold was set to $p < 0.01$ uncorrected at the voxel level. Before group comparisons, the correlation coefficients were converted to z-scores using the Fischer r-to-z transformation. These z-score images were entered into the statistical analysis. For each participant, the mean signal time course was computed from the seed (i.e., the AIC) and used as a regressor in a voxel-wise rsFC analysis with the functions of REST toolbox 1.6. For each participant, one whole-brain correlation map was obtained from the first-level analysis. Each map was then r-to-z-transformed in order to yield a normal distribution for parametric second-level group analysis. This level comprised a voxel-wise one-sample t-test for both the pre-training and post-training, examining whether the correlation coef?cient (z-value) indicates positive rsFC (Baur et al., 2013). Signi?cantly correlated voxels were determined at $p < 0.05$ corrected for FDR (false-discovery error rate) at the voxel level with a cluster size greater than or equal to 10 voxels with the use of the daMCC (radius = 10 mm) as our region of interest based on relevant studies (as reviewed in Bush, 2011).

In order to compare the changes in rsFC, we conducted a 2 (group: low pain, high pain) × 2 (time: pre, post) mixed ANOVA on the rsFC magnitudes as represented by the z-value. Finally, to explore the brain-behavior relationship, the rsFC magnitude was correlated to the composite score of the DPQ, SFMPQ, and KIMS questionnaire, respectively, with parametric (Pearson) correlation (Baur et al., 2013). All p-values were two-tailed. Correlations were assessed with SPSS (version 20).

RESULTS

Analysis of the scores on the questionnaires to assess the participants' pain perception and mindfulness skills showed that the participants' abilities improved after the 6-week training. A 2 (group) × 2 (time) mixed ANOVA on the SFMPQ revealed a main effect of time ($F = 8.91, p < 0.01$), a main effect of group ($F = 14.25, p < 0.01$), and an interaction of time × group ($F = 5.28, p < 0.05$). The *post hoc* comparisons showed that the change in the composite score of the SFMPQ was significant in the pain-afflicted group ($t = 3.05, p < 0.01$), but not in the control group ($t = 0.82$ $p = 0.42$). Moreover, the 2 (group) × 2 (time) mixed ANOVA on the DPQ indicated a main effect of time ($F = 6.45, p < 0.05$) and a main effect of group ($F = 6.23$, $p = 0.01$). In addition, the 2 (group) × 2 (time) mixed ANOVA on the KIMS showed that there was a main effect of time ($F = 75.25, p < 0.01$) and an interaction effect of group x time ($F = 5.12, p < 0.05$). Means and standard deviations for the three questionnaires are included in **Table 1**. The results of the 2 (group) × 2 (time) mixed ANOVAs performed on the scores of the three questionnaires are included in **Table 2**.

TABLE 1 | Mean and standard deviation (SD) for scores of the Dallas Pain Questionnaire (DPQ), the Short Form McGill Pain Questionnaire (SFMPQ), and the Kentucky Inventory of Mindfulness (KIMS) for pre- and post-training.

		High pain group ($n = 18$)		Low pain group ($n = 16$)	
		Pre Mean (SD)	Post Mean (SD)	Pre Mean (SD)	Post Mean (SD)
DPQ	Daily	38.83 (4.63)	29.04 (3.77)	19.73 (4.32)	14.4 (4.26)
	Working/Leisure	39.72 (4.62)	25.72 (3.62)	17.07 (5.74)	13.62 (5.71)
	Anxiety/Depression	39.44 (2.97)	37.96 (4.18)	32.72 (5.41)	30.1 (5.83)
	Social interests	25.28 (4.19)	19.84 (4.16)	12.55 (3.72)	11.39 (4.05)
SFMPQ	Sensation	12.61 (1.4)	7.78 (0.94)	5.59 (1.7)	3.65 (1.64)
	Affective	4.72 (0.56)	2.86 (0.54)	3.06 (0.87)	2.18 (0.68)
	PPI	2.5 (0.17)	1.52 (0.22)	0.41 (0.12)	0.53 (0.23)
KIMS	Observing	34.53 (2.01)	43.34 (1.43)	32.38 (1.82)	36.06 (2.44)
	Describing	21.88 (1.54)	27.93 (1.44)	25.59 (1.43)	29.12 (1.22)
	Acting with awareness	24.87 (1.66)	31.68 (2.05)	27.24 (1.59)	31.06 (1.44)
	Accepting without judgment	17.78 (1.47)	28.06 (1.11)	22.65 (1.7)	29.83 (1.37)

TABLE 2 | 2 (group: low pain, high pain) × 2 (time: pre, post) mixed ANOVA on the Dallas Pain Questionnaire (DPQ), the Short Form McGill Pain Questionnaire (SFMPQ), and the Kentucky Inventory of Mindfulness (KIMS).

		F	*p*
DPQ	Group	6.727	0.014*
	Time	6.453	0.016*
	Group × time	1.159	0.29
SFMPQ	Group	14.264	0.001*
	Time	8.913	0.005*
	Group × time	5.277	0.028*
KIMS	Group	0.054	0.817
	Time	75.254	<0.001*
	Group × time	5.124	0.031*

**indicates a significant difference.*

In the fMRI data analysis, a 2 (group) × 2 (time) mixed ANOVA on the rsFC magnitudes revealed an interaction between AIC activity and daMCC activity (the daMCC coordinates [−20,−6,21], $z = 3.07$, $p = 0.001$ uncorrected, **Figure 1**). The correlated voxels were also significant at $p < 0.05$ corrected for familywise errors (FWE), using a sphere of 10 mm radius based on relevant studies (Bush, 2011). The *post hoc* comparisons showed a significant increase in post vs. pre-training rsFC magnitudes in the pain-afflicted group ($t = 2.68$, $p < 0.01$), but not in the control group ($t = 1.08$ $p = 0.30$). Correlation analysis was also conducted between the AIC-daMCC connection strength and the composite score of the DPQ, SFMPQ, and KIMS questionnaire, respectively. The results showed a significant negative correlation between the AIC-daMCC connection strength for the pain-afflicted group, when measured against the composite score of the SFMPQ ($r = -0.48$, $p < 0.05$). There was no significant correlation for the DPQ ($r = -0.05$, $p = 0.79$) or KIMS ($r = -0.07$, $p = 0.68$) questionnaire.

DISCUSSION

We used a two-group longitudinal design as a methodological improvement over previous studies and found that, according to the SFMPQ questionnaire results, pain was reduced in the pain-afflicted group but not in the control group after MBSR training. Increased connectivity between the AIC and the daMCC was also found in the pain-afflicted group, but not in the control group. Furthermore, a negative correlation was found between the SFMPQ measure and the AIC-daMCC connection strength for the pain-afflicted group. We will center our discussion on how one's perception of pain may be different as a result of attention training, an MBSR-induced cognitive effect. We will also touch briefly on attention-triggered reappraisal.

Cognition-Based Attention and Perception of Pain

Based on the results of the questionnaires, significant reduction of pain was observed after the 6-week training course. With the reduction in emotional discomfort and somatic problems, the participants' quality of life was enhanced, which indicates a positive impact from such attention training.

Clinically, mindfulness-based cognitive training has been found to be effective in regulating the participants' attention to stressor stimuli, i.e., their pain and the associated self-evaluation of pain, by successfully distracting them from the physical feeling of pain and its related associations using the trained decentering techniques (Garland et al., 2009). For example, to report a stimulus of pain, the participants need to be attentive enough to become alert, to orient themselves toward the source of pain and lastly to detect how they may be affected by it. Decentering allows the participants to become more aware of the experience "from some distance" (McCracken et al., 2013).

During the 6-week training period, we observed that attention plays a pivotal role in shifting our perceptions away from pain, by transforming our associative responses to it, and eventually

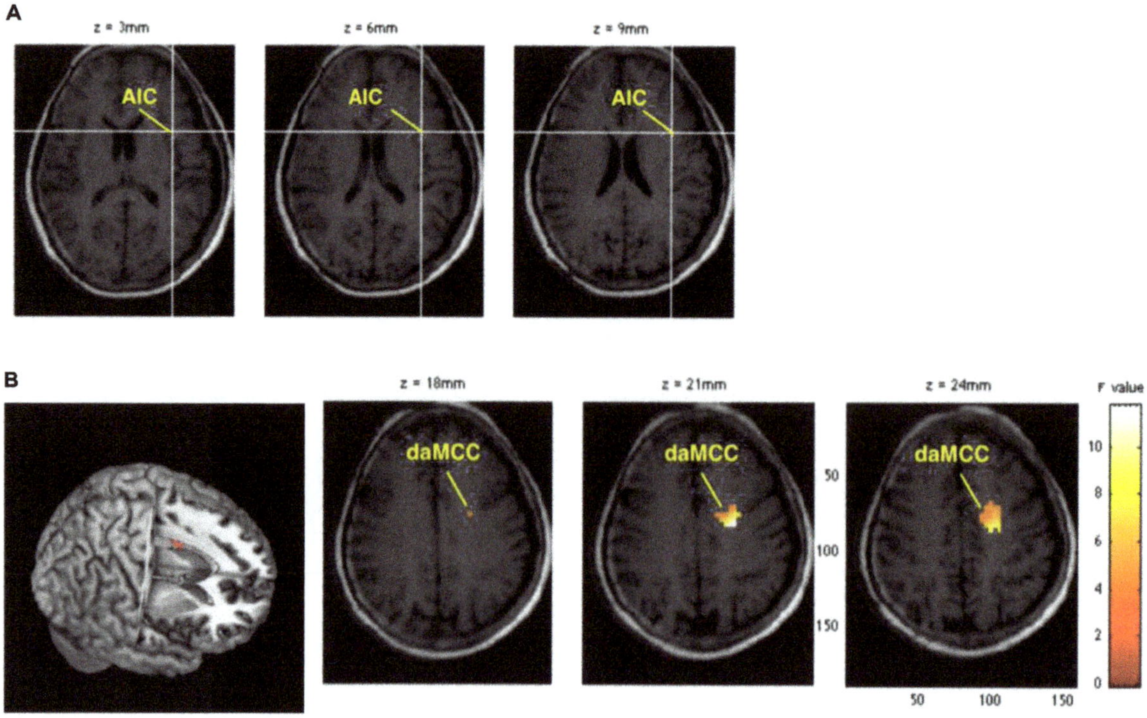

FIGURE 1 | (A) The seed region, the anterior insular cortex (AIC). **(B)** The significant increase in functional connectivity of the AIC-dorsal anterior midcingulate cortex (daMCC) after the 6-week training in the pain-afflicted group.

alleviating it. But, what enables the participants to report the stimuli of pain and the associated evaluation of it?

Our study does hint that one's application of attention enables a change in one's neural connections, which leads to the shift of pain sensation, as evidenced by the fMRI scans. By shifting their attention, the participants become detached observers who do not focus on being confronted with pain, but remain in a state of mindfulness; that is, they remain attentive. Their past experience of pain, often associated with negative emotions, is now viewed differently as a result of decentering. This may well expand into a new experience where one learns to be unaffected by obsession with one's own pain. The natural outcome of such perspective shifting may help reduce pain-related stress, mitigate emotional discomfort, or even yield positive emotions via pain modulation. Thus, by comparing the questionnaires conducted before and after the mindfulness-training course, we observed pain-reduction-induced emotional changes.

Mindfulness and Cognitive Reappraisal

When it comes to the results of the fMRI imaging, the increased connection strength observed between the AIC and the daMCC can be viewed as a result of the MBSR training in the pain-afflicted group. The AIC plays a pivotal role in deactivating the default mode network (DMN), which consists of brain areas that are activated during mind-wandering or resting states (Menon and Uddin, 2010). The DMN, most notably in the ventral medial prefrontal cortex (vmPFC) and the PCC, is deactivated during meditation—a state requiring constant focus on attention (Brewer et al., 2011). However, the DMN deactivation patterns that occur during meditation may vary from patient to patient (Buckner et al., 2008; Tagliazucchi et al., 2010).

We thus infer that the practice of MBSR may trigger AIC activation, which in turn may inhibit vmPFC activity, a signal reflecting emotional suffering (Apkarian et al., 2011). When receiving nociceptive stimuli, the AIC and the daMCC are both activated, and such co-activation is considered to be responsible for autonomic and emotional processes (Sterzer and Kleinschmidt, 2010). Both the AIC and the daMCC could very well be specific regions of the "salience network" (Sterzer and Kleinschmidt, 2010; Harsay et al., 2012), which "forms the fundamental neuroanatomical basis for all human emotions" (Decety, 2011). This significant difference between the experimental group and the control group indicates that the increased AIC-daMCC connectivity observed could be specifically related to pain perception.

The daMCC is said to take part in cognitive control and emotional regulation (Modinos et al., 2010; Kanske et al., 2011). Also, the daMCC is involved in attentional control (as reviewed in Bush, 2011). Together with the pain matrix proposed by Decety (2011), the strengthened connectivity associated with the participants' ability to modulate their perception of pain, based on a perspective shift, suggests that this strengthened connectivity is the underlying mechanism for such change in pain perception.

Alternatively, the AIC and the daMCC are often jointly activated, which appears consistent with the idea that both of them serve as complementary limbic sensory and motor regions

(Craig, 2009). These two regions work together to form a link between self-recognition and self-control. In the present study, the observed increase in AIC-daMCC connectivity may be related to enhanced self-recognition and self-control due to the MBSR training. The participants' perception of pain differed after the 6-week training program. We contend that the difference is a result of cognitive re-evaluation made possible via MBSR attention training, in keeping with the contention that a positive shift in perspective is an effective means of coping with stressful events and a good predictor of increased mindfulness, which is well supported by Garland et al. (2009, 2011). In the model advanced by Garland et al. (2011), there exists an upward-spiraling relationship between positive perspective shift and mindfulness: The more mindful one becomes, the more likely one is to use a positive perspective shift as a coping strategy in dealing with previously stressful or painful experiences.

CONCLUSION

Our resting-state fMRI results suggest that people can modify their cognition of pain through attention training. The results based on the resting-state fMRIs and questionnaires indicate that a possible mechanism, perspective shift, may be at work during the cognitive regulation of pain perception during the mindfulness training. Regardless, we need to admit that several confounding factors may limit the findings presented so far. One is that we should have investigated the importance of quantity and quality on the effect of MBSR skill training. We also are aware that we should have included a scanning of participants engaged in a cognitive task to further reveal the function and meaning of increased connection strength.

FUTURE STUDIES

Although recent studies, especially those involving neuroimaging, have started to identify brain areas and networks that mediate the correlation between mindfulness and attention, the underlying neural mechanisms remain unclear. To gain a better understanding of the neural basis of the changes in the brain, we would like to consider other mechanisms in our future study. For instance, is it via language that pain can be noticed, constructed, and assessed, notwithstanding the fact that it is hard to come by much pain-describing language (Dyer, 2011)? The notion that labeling emotional states can help to regulate negative emotional states is hardly new, as can often be seen in talk therapies which involve individuals instructed to put their feelings into words in hopes of managing or transforming their feelings. Lieberman (2011) further confirms that putting feelings into verbal language activates a region of the brain that is capable of inhibiting various kinds of immediate experience, including affective distress. Perspective-taking is clearly not foreign to language, and empathy (i.e., taking the perspective of someone else) is partially mediated by language (Izard et al., 1988).

AUTHOR CONTRIBUTIONS

I-WS, K-CL, K-YC, S-TH, and T-LC designed this study. I-WS, F-WW, W-ZS, and T-LC collected and analyzed data. I-WS, F-WW, K-CL, and T-LC wrote the paper.

ACKNOWLEDGMENTS

This work was supported by the Ministry of Science and Technology (formerly the National Science Council of Taiwan) (MOST 102-2420-H-002-011-MY3, MOST 104-2410-H-002-151, and NSC 101-2410-H-002-093-MY2). We thank the MOST-supported Imaging Center for Integrated Body, Mind and Culture Research, National Taiwan University for technical and facility supports. We also want to thank Mr. Roy Te-Chung Chen for conducting the MBSR training sessions.

REFERENCES

Allport, A. (1988). "What concept of consciousness?," in *Consciousness in Contemporary Science*, eds A. J. Marcel and E. Bisiach (London: Clarendon Press), 159–182.

Apkarian, A. V., Bushnell, M. C., Treede, R., and Zubieta, J. (2005). Human brain mechanisms of pain perception and regulation in health and disease. *Eur. J. Pain* 9, 463–484. doi: 10.1016/j.ejpain.2004.11.001

Apkarian, A. V., Hashmi, J. A., and Baliki, M. N. (2011). Pain and the brain: specificity and plasticity of the brain in clinical chronic pain. *Pain* 152, 49–64. doi: 10.1016/j.pain.2010.11.010

Baer, R. A., Gregory, T. S., and Kristin, B. A. (2004). Assessment of mindfulness by self-report the Kentucky inventory of mindfulness skills. *Assessment* 11, 191–206. doi: 10.1177/1073191104268029

Baur, V., Hänggi, J., Langer, N., and Jäncke, L. (2013). Resting-state functional and structural connectivity with an insula-amygdala route specifically index state and trait anxiety. *Biol. Psychiatry* 73, 85–92. doi: 10.1016/j.biopsych.2012.06.003

Bellet, P. S., and Maloney, M. (1991). The importance of empathy as an interviewing skill in medicine. *JAMA* 226, 1831–1832. doi: 10.1001/jama.1991.03470130111039

Bergomi, C., Tschacher, W., and Kupper, Z. (2013). Measuring mindfulness: first steps towards the development of a comprehensive mindfulness scale. *Mindfulness* 4, 18–32. doi: 10.1007/s12671-012-0102-9

Brewer, J. A., Worhunsky, P. D., Gray, J. R., Tang, Y. Y., Weber, J., and Kober, H. (2011). Meditation experience is associated with differences in default mode network activity and connectivity. *Proc. Natl. Acad. Sci. U.S.A.* 108, 20254–20259. doi: 10.1073/pnas.1112029108

Brooks, J. C. W., Nurmikko, T. J., Bimson, W. E., Singh, K. D., and Roberts, N. (2002). fMRI of thermal pain: effects of stimulus laterality and attention. *Neuroimage* 15, 293–301. doi: 10.1006/nimg.2001.0974

Buckner, R. L., Andrews-Hanna, J. R., and Schacter, D. L. (2008). The brain's default network: anatomy, function, and relevance to disease. *Ann. N. Y. Acad. Sci.* 1124, 1–38. doi: 10.1196/annals.1440.011

Bush, G. (2011). Cingulate, frontal, and parietal cortical dysfunction in attention-deficit/hyperactivity disorder. *Biol. Psychiatry* 69, 1160–1167. doi: 10.1016/j.biopsych.2011.01.022

Chou, T. L., Chen, C. W., Wu, M. Y., and Booth, J. R. (2009). The role of inferior frontal gyrus and inferior parietal lobule in semantic processing of Chinese characters. *Exp. Brain Res.* 198, 465–475. doi: 10.1007/s00221-009-1942-y

Craig, A. D. (2002). How do you feel? Interoception: the sense of the physiological condition of the body. *Nat. Rev. Neurosci.* 3, 655–666. doi: 10.1038/nrn894

Craig, A. D. (2009). How do you feel – now? The anterior insula and human awareness. *Nat. Rev. Neurosci.* 10, 59–70. doi: 10.1038/nrn2555

Decety, J. (2011). Dissecting the neural mechanisms mediating empathy. *Emot. Rev.* 3, 92–108. doi: 10.1177/1754073910374662

Dyer, B. L. (2011). *Learning Mindfulness: Dialogue and Inquiry from an Action-Theoretical Perspective.* Doctoral dissertation, University of British Columbia, Vancouver, BC.

Fan, L. Y., Gau, S. S., and Chou, T. L. (2014). Neural correlates of inhibitory control and visual processing in youths with attention-deficit/hyperactivity disorder: a counting Stroop functional MRI study. *Psychol. Med.* 44, 2661–2671. doi: 10.1017/S0033291714000038

Gallagher, S. (2000). Philosophical conceptions of the self: implications for cognitive science. *Trends Cogn. Sci.* 4, 14–21. doi: 10.1016/S1364-6613(99)01417-5

Garland, E., Gaylord, S., and Park, J. (2009). The role of mindfulness in positive reappraisal. *Explore (NY)* 5, 37–44. doi: 10.1016/j.explore.2008.10.001

Garland, E. L., Gaylord, S. A., and Fredrickson, B. L. (2011). Positive reappraisal mediates the stress-reductive effects of mindfulness: an upward spiral process. *Mindfulness* 2, 59–67. doi: 10.1007/s12671-011-0043-8

Grant, J. A., Courtemanche, J., and Rainville, P. (2011). A non-elaborative mental stance and decoupling of executive and pain-related cortices predicts low pain sensitivity in Zen meditators. *Pain* 152, 150–156. doi: 10.1016/j.pain.2010.10.006

Gu, X., Gao, Z., Wang, X., Liu, X., Knight, R. T., Hof, P. R., et al. (2012). Anterior insular cortex is necessary for empathetic pain perception. *Brain* 135(Pt 9), 2726–2735. doi: 10.1093/brain/aws199

Harsay, H. A., Spaan, M., Wijnen, J. G., and Ridderinkhof, K. R. (2012). Error awareness and salience processing in the oddball task: shared neural mechanisms. *Front. Hum. Neurosci.* 6:246. doi: 10.3389/fnhum.2012.00246

Izard, C. E., Kagan, J., and Zajonc, R. B. (1988). *Emotion, Cognition, and Behavior.* Cambridge: Cambridge University Press.

Kabat-Zinn, J. (1982). An outpatient program in behavioral medicine for chronic pain patients based on the practice of mindfulness meditation: theoretical considerations and preliminary results. *Gen. Hosp. Psychiatry* 4, 33–47. doi: 10.1016/0163-8343(82)90026-3

Kabat-Zinn, J. (2003). Mindfulness-based interventions in context: past, present, and future. *Clin. Psychol. Sci. Pract.* 10, 144–156.

Kanske, P., Heissler, J., Schonfelder, S., Bongers, A., and Wessa, M. (2011). How to regulate emotion? Neural networks for reappraisal and distraction. *Cereb. Cortex* 21, 1379–1388. doi: 10.1093/cercor/bhq216

Kupers, R. (2006). "Brain imaging of pain," in *Handbook of Clinical Neurology*, eds M. Hallett, J. Stone and A. Carson (Amsterdam: Elsevier).

Lawlis, G. F., Ramon, C., David, S., and McCoy, C. E. (1989). The development of the Dallas Pain Questionnaire: an assessment of the impact of spinal pain on behavior. *Spine* 14, 511–516. doi: 10.1097/00007632-198905000-00007

Lieberman, M. D. (2011). "Why symbolic processing of affect can disrupt negative affect," in *Social Neuroscience: Toward Understanding the Underpinnings of the Social Mind*, eds A. Todorov, S. Fiske, and D. Prentice (Oxford: Oxford Scholarship Online).

McCracken, L. M., Gutiérrez-Martínez, O., and Smyth, C. (2013). "Decentering" reflects psychological flexibility in people with chronic pain and correlates with their quality of functioning. *Health Psychol.* 32, 820–823. doi: 10.1037/a0028093

McRae, K., Reiman, E. M., Fort, C. L., Chen, K., and Lane, R. D. (2008). Association between trait emotional awareness and dorsal anterior cingulate activity during emotion is arousal-dependent. *Neuroimage* 41, 648–655. doi: 10.1016/j.neuroimage.2008.02.030

Medford, N., and Critchley, H. D. (2010). Conjoint activity of anterior insular and anterior cingulate cortex: awareness and response. *Brain Struct. Funct.* 214, 535–549. doi: 10.1007/s00429-010-0265-x

Melzack, R. (1975). The McGill Pain Questionnaire: major properties and scoring methods. *Pain* 1, 277–299. doi: 10.1016/0304-3959(75)90044-5

Melzack, R. (1987). The short-form McGill pain questionnaire. *Pain* 30, 191–197. doi: 10.1016/0304-3959(87)91074-8

Menon, V., and Uddin, L. Q. (2010). Saliency, switching, attention and control: a network model of insula function. *Brain Struct. Funct.* 214, 655–667. doi: 10.1007/s00429-010-0262-0

Modinos, G., Ormel, J., and Aleman, A. (2010). Individual differences in dispositional mindfulness and brain activity involved in reappraisal of emotion. *Soc. Cogn. Affect. Neurosci.* 5, 369–377. doi: 10.1093/scan/nsq006

Raichle, M. E., MacLeod, A. M., Snyder, A. Z., Powers, W. J., Gusnard, D. A., and Shulman, G. L. (2001). A default mode of brain function. *Proc. Natl. Acad. Sci. U.S.A.* 98, 676–682. doi: 10.1073/pnas.98.2.676

Schmidt, R. (1994). "Deconstructing consciousness in search of useful definitions for applied linguistics," in *Consciousness and Second Language Learning: Conceptual, Methodological and Practical Issues in Language Learning and Teaching, Thematic Issue of AILA Review*, Vol. 11, eds J. H. Hulstijn and R. Schmidt (Dubai: AILA Review), 11–26.

Schweinhardt, P., Glynn, C., Brooks, J., McQuay, H., Jack, T., Chessell, I., et al. (2006). An fMRI study of cerebral processing of brush-evoked allodynia in neuropathic pain patients. *Neuroimage* 32, 256–265. doi: 10.1016/j.neuroimage.2006.03.024

Seeley, W. W., Menon, V., Schatzberg, A. F., Keller, J., Glover, G. H., Kenna, H., et al. (2007). Dissociable intrinsic connectivity networks for salience processing and executive control. *J. Neurosci.* 27, 2349–2356. doi: 10.1523/JNEUROSCI.5587-06.2007

Shapiro, S. L., Brown, K. W., and Biegel, G. M. (2007). Teaching self-care to caregivers: effects of mindfulness-based stress reduction on the mental health of therapists in training. *Train. Educ. Prof. Psychol.* 1, 105–115. doi: 10.1037/1931-3918.1.2.105

Singer, T., Seymour, B., O'Doherty, J., Kaube, H., Dolan, R. J., and Frith, C. D. (2004). Empathy for pain involves the affective but not sensory components of pain. *Science* 303, 1157–1162. doi: 10.1126/science.1093535

Slobin, D. I. (1987). Thinking for speaking. *Paper Presented at the 13th Annual Meeting of the Berkeley Linguistic Society*, Berkeley, CA.

Song, X. W., Dong, Z. Y., Long, X. Y., Li, S. F., Zuo, X. N., Zhu, C. Z., et al. (2011). REST: a toolkit for resting-state functional magnetic resonance imaging data processing. *PLoS ONE* 6:e25031. doi: 10.1371/journal.pone.0025031

Sterzer, P., and Kleinschmidt, A. (2010). Anterior insula activations in perceptual paradigms: often observed but barely understood. *Brain Struct. Funct.* 214, 611–622. doi: 10.1007/s00429-010-0252-2

Tagliazucchi, E., Balenzuela, P., Fraiman, D., and Chialvo, D. R. (2010). Brain resting state is disrupted in chronic back pain patients. *Neurosci. Lett.* 485, 26–31. doi: 10.1016/j.neulet.2010.08.053

Tang, Y. Y., Holzel, B. K., and Posner, M. I. (2015). The neuroscience of mindfulness meditation. *Nat. Rev. Neurosci.* 16, 213–225. doi: 10.1038/nrn3916

Tracey, I., and Johns, E. (2010). The pain matrix: reloaded or reborn as we image tonic pain using arterial spin labeling. *Pain* 148, 359–360. doi: 10.1016/j.pain.2009.11.009

Tseng, M. T., Tseng, W. Y. I., Chao, C. C., Lin, H. E., and Hsieh, S. T. (2010). Distinct and shared cerebral activations in processing innocuous versus noxious contact heat revealed by functional magnetic resonance imaging. *Hum. Brain Mapp.* 31, 743–757. doi: 10.1002/hbm.20902

Zang, Y. F., He, Y., Zhu, C. Z., Cao, Q. J., Sui, M. Q., Liang, M., et al. (2007). Altered baseline brain activity in children with ADHD revealed by resting-state functional MRI. *Brain Dev.* 29, 83–91. doi: 10.1016/j.braindev.2006.07.002

Zeidan, F., Grant, J. A., Brown, C. A., McHaffie, J. G., and Coghill, R. C. (2012). Mindfulness meditation-related pain relief: evidence for unique brain mechanisms in the regulation of pain. *Neurosci. Lett.* 520, 165–173. doi: 10.1016/j.neulet.2012.03.082

Zou, Q. H., Zhu, C. Z., Yang, Y., Zuo, X. N., Long, X. Y., Cao, Q. J., et al. (2008). An improved approach to detection of amplitude of low-frequency fluctuation (ALFF) for resting-state fMRI: fractional ALFF. *J. Neurosci. Methods* 172, 137–141. doi: 10.1016/j.jneumeth.2008.04.012

9

Comparing Aging and Fitness Effects on Brain Anatomy

*Mark A. Fletcher[1,2], Kathy A. Low[1], Rachel Boyd[1,3], Benjamin Zimmerman[1,2], Brian A. Gordon[4], Chin H. Tan[1,3], Nils Schneider-Garces[1,3], Bradley P. Sutton[1,2,5], Gabriele Gratton[1,2,3,5] and Monica Fabiani[1,2,3,5]**

[1] Beckman Institute, University of Illinois, Urbana, IL, USA, [2] Neuroscience Program, University of Illinois, Urbana, Illinois, USA, [3] Department of Psychology, University of Illinois, Urbana, IL, USA, [4] Department of Radiology, Washington University in St. Louis, Saint Louis, MO, USA, [5] Department of Bioengineering, University of Illinois at Urbana–Champaign, Urbana, IL, USA

Edited by:
Soledad Ballesteros, Universidad Nacional de Educación a Distancia, Spain

Reviewed by:
Bonnie J. Nagel, Oregon Health & Science University
Keita Kamijo, Waseda University, Japan

***Correspondence:**
Monica Fabiani
mfabiani@illinois.edu

Recent studies suggest that cardiorespiratory fitness (CRF) mitigates the brain's atrophy typically associated with aging, via a variety of beneficial mechanisms. One could argue that if CRF is generally counteracting the negative effects of aging, the same regions that display the greatest age-related volumetric loss should also show the largest beneficial effects of fitness. To test this hypothesis we examined structural MRI data from 54 healthy older adults (ages 55–87), to determine the overlap, across brain regions, of the profiles of age and fitness effects. Results showed that lower fitness and older age are associated with atrophy in several brain regions, replicating past studies. However, when the profiles of age and fitness effects were compared using a number of statistical approaches, the effects were not entirely overlapping. Interestingly, some of the regions that were most influenced by age were among those not influenced by fitness. Presumably, the age-related atrophy occurring in these regions is due to factors that are more impervious to the beneficial effects of fitness. Possible mechanisms supporting regional heterogeneity may include differential involvement in motor function, the presence of adult neurogenesis, and differential sensitivity to cerebrovascular, neurotrophic and metabolic factors.

Keywords: aging, cardiorespiratory fitness, exercise, brain anatomy, FreeSurfer

INTRODUCTION

The brains of seemingly healthy individuals undergo various degrees of cortical and subcortical atrophy with aging (Raz et al., 2005, 2010; Gordon et al., 2008). The exact mechanisms underlying these changes are not completely known, although vascular (Brown and Thore, 2011; Davenport et al., 2012; Lähteenvuo and Rosenzweig, 2012; Fabiani et al., 2014), genetic (McGue and Johnson, 2008; Papenberg et al., 2015), oxidative stress (Muller et al., 2007; Dai et al., 2014; Thorin and Thorin-Trescases, 2014) and hormonal (Morrison and Baxter, 2012) factors may all contribute significantly. These anatomical changes are considered to have important functional consequences, and to influence some of the cognitive decline that accompanies aging (e.g., Salthouse, 2011; Fabiani, 2012; Nyberg et al., 2012).

In an attempt to delay or possibly even reverse some of these structural changes, investigators have focused on lifestyle factors as potential mitigators of the effects of aging.

Abbreviations: CRF, cardiorespiratory fitness; eCRF, estimated cardiorespiratory fitness; eTIV, estimated total intracranial volume; VO_{2max}, maximal oxygen uptake.

One such factor that has received particular attention is CRF. Higher CRF is correlated with a number of systemic benefits, including lower blood pressure (Blair et al., 1996; Barlow et al., 2006), decreased stress (Jackson and Dishman, 2006), and better lipid profiles (Dunn et al., 1999; Park et al., 2015). Extensive research has also demonstrated that higher CRF is correlated with improved brain tissue preservation and higher performance in neuropsychological tests (e.g., Colcombe and Kramer, 2003; Gordon et al., 2008; Voss et al., 2011, 2013; Verstynen et al., 2012; Weinstein et al., 2012; McAuley et al., 2013). It has also been shown that CRF mediates age-related changes in some structural (e.g., frontal cortex volume, Weinstein et al., 2012; caudate nucleus, Verstynen et al., 2012) and functional measures (e.g., cerebral blood flow; Zimmerman et al., 2014), and that these changes are relevant for cognitive function (Verstynen et al., 2012; Weinstein et al., 2012). Beneficial effects of CRF on the preservation of regional brain volumes have been reported for a number of brain regions in cross-sectional comparisons of age and fitness groups (Gordon et al., 2008; Bugg and Head, 2011; Verstynen et al., 2012), as well as in response to fitness intervention (Colcombe et al., 2003, 2006; Erickson et al., 2011; Voss et al., 2011). Most of the research conducted thus far, however, has not examined the regional specificity of CRF effects on brain anatomy in a systematic manner, but has instead focused on specific brain areas (such as the hippocampus and prefrontal cortex) that are known to be affected by aging (e.g., Bugg and Head, 2011; Erickson et al., 2011; McAuley et al., 2011).

In this study, we are proposing a strategy to investigate the extent to which the effects of CRF on volumetric brain measures are generalized or regional, and their overlap with the effects of aging. In other words, are the profiles of the effects of CRF and of aging similar throughout the brain or does CRF preferentially influence only some of the brain regions that are affected by aging and not others? To address these questions we report a direct comparison of the profiles of the effects of aging and fitness on volumetric measures obtained throughout the brain (including both cortical and subcortical structures) in older adults between the ages of 55 and 87.

In vivo volumetric measurement of brain areas based on structural magnetic resonance imaging (sMRI) allows for researchers to study the influence of demographic and lifestyle factors on different patterns of volumetric decline in aging. Further, measurements of brain structures throughout the whole brain are critical to provide the comprehensive data required for a profile analysis. Although manual tracing remains the gold standard for *in vivo* anatomical studies based on structural MR images (Raz et al., 2003; Kennedy et al., 2009), a number of semi-automated methods have become available in the last two decades. These methods, allowing for the parallel measurement of multiple structures, permit a more complete examination of brain anatomy in large groups of individuals without requiring extensive training. One of the first automatic methods used for investigating the effects of CRF on brain anatomy was voxel-based morphometry (VBM; Ashburner and Friston, 2000), which allows for probabilistic brain mapping across populations. VBM studies of the effects of aging on brain anatomy have demonstrated significant gray and white matter loss in a wide range of areas, including most of the frontal and parietal cortex, as well as most subcortical gray matter regions (e.g., Good et al., 2002; Gordon et al., 2008). VBM studies have also examined the effects of CRF. For example, in a cross-sectional study including younger (ages 20–28) and older adults (ages 65–81) Gordon et al. (2008) showed that higher CRF was associated with volumetric preservation in the inferior frontal, anterior parietal, and medial temporal regions, even when education, age and gender were controlled for. One of the first fitness intervention studies to use VBM (Colcombe et al., 2006) demonstrated that a 6-month aerobic fitness intervention in low-fit older adults (ages 60–79) led to significant volumetric increases in the dorsal anterior cingulate, supplementary motor area, middle frontal gyrus, left superior temporal lobe, and anterior third of the corpus callosum (CC). Other VBM studies examining subcortical regions have shown that higher CRF is associated with larger hippocampal volumes, and that exercise interventions may even lead to an increase in hippocampal size (Erickson et al., 2011; McAuley et al., 2011).

Although VBM can provide a useful estimate of anatomical effects, it also has several limitations, including the fact that coregistration of different structures across individuals relies on group templates, which may introduce biases in the comparison process (Bookstein, 2001; Salmond et al., 2002; Davatzikos, 2004; Ridgway et al., 2008; Kennedy et al., 2009; Whitwell, 2009). FreeSurfer© provides an alternative approach: It offers a way of coregistering anatomical structures across individuals using a semi-automatic parcellation of the cortex based on surface and border features, and the possibility of separating cortical volume from cortical thickness (Dale and Sereno, 1993; Dale et al., 1999; Fischl et al., 2001). Using FreeSurfer, Bugg and Head (2011) examined the correlation between the amount of running, jogging, and walking (as indexed by a questionnaire looking at the previous 10 years) and loss in a few regions of interest (ROIs) in older adults (ages 55–79). Although only some regions were examined, they showed that exercise mitigated age-related atrophy in the medial temporal lobe (MTL), but failed to show an interaction between age and exercise in other ROIs (including areas of the prefrontal cortex and parietal lobes). In the current study, we used FreeSurfer to derive volumetric brain measurements in a sample of middle-aged and older adults. We also used multiple statistical methodologies in an attempt to provide a more comprehensive description of the effects of fitness and age across brain regions to evaluate their profile overlap. We believe that an improved understanding of the overlap between these variables will help design more effective intervention programs (see for example Bherer et al., 2013; Voss et al., 2013).

MATERIALS AND METHODS

Participants

Fifty-six healthy adults (29 females, age range = 55–87) from the Champaign-Urbana community were recruited through local advertisements, mass emailing, and flyers. The study was approved by the University of Illinois Institutional Review Board, and all participants signed documents of informed consent in accordance with the Declaration of Helsinki. All participants were right-handed and fluent English speakers. Information about the participants' demographics is reported in **Table 1**.

Phone interviews were conducted to screen individuals for inclusion/exclusion. Exclusion criteria included a history of drug abuse, major psychiatric or neurological disease, or other serious chronic medical conditions. Those who passed the phone screening were invited into the lab and were given two additional screening measures, the Beck's Depression Inventory (Beck and Steer, 1987) and the modified Mini-Mental Status Exam (Mayeux et al., 1981). Individuals scoring above 14 on the BDI or 51 or less on the mMMSE were excluded from the study. Two male participants were excluded from analysis due to incomplete fitness estimates or missing neuropsychological data. Our final sample consisted of 54 participants.

The anatomical MRIs of 8 college students (age range = 19–22, Mean Age: = 21.53, *SD* = 0.99, five Females) were also used for head-size normalization but were excluded from all other analyses (see below for rationale). These younger participants reported themselves to be healthy, right-handed, fluent in English and also underwent a screening similar to the one described above.

Fitness Estimation

Estimated cardiorespiratory fitness (eCRF) scores were obtained for each participant using the regression model proposed by Jurca et al. (2005). The eCRF measures have been validated with a large sample of older adults (Mailey et al., 2010; McAuley et al., 2011). They are highly correlated (≈0.7) with VO_{2max}, which is obtained through a graded exercise protocol and is considered the gold standard for assessing CRF. Specifically, Mailey et al. (2010) found that within a population of older adults, eCRF was significantly correlated with metabolic equivalents (METs) ($r = 0.66$) and with estimates based on submaximal field testing ($r = 0.67$). Crucially, eCRF allowed us to include participants that may be at risk during standard VO_{2max} testing.

The regression model used for eCRF estimation is based on weighted data including gender, age, body mass index (BMI), resting heart rate, and a physical activity score. Height and weight were measured to calculate the BMI. Resting heart rate was recorded on three separate days, after participants had been sitting for a minimum of 5 min, and these measurements were then averaged. The activity score was derived from the Physical Activity Scale for the Elderly (PASE, Washburn et al., 1993). The PASE contains specific questions to determine the type and frequency (minutes per session and number of sessions per week) of exercise activities a participant does on an average week. Specifically, the total minutes per week of exercises requiring low exertion (i.e., activities that produce only a slight increase in heart rate) and those classified as aerobic exercise (jogging, swimming, cycling etc.) were quantified. These totals were used to categorize each participant into one of the five self-reported activity scores defined by Jurca et al. (2005), and then combined with the other weighted data to obtain an eCRF value for each participant. The eCRF score is expressed in METs, which are defined as the amount of oxygen consumed while sitting at rest (see Jetté et al., 1990). To estimate VO_{2max} from the METs values, the eCRF score needs to be multiplied by 3.5 (Masley, 2009). To facilitate cross-referencing with studies measuring VO_{2max}, **Table 1** also reports the VO_{2max} values estimated from eCRF. The means of the fitness estimates for each group, when compared to existing norms, indicate that they correspond to meaningful differences, with the low-fitness group classified as "poor prognosis in coronary patients; highly deconditioned individuals" (Jurca et al., 2005; see also McArdle et al., 2006).

TABLE 1 | Basic demographic, neuropsychological, and physiological characteristics.

	All (*N* = 54)		Low-fit (*N* = 27)		High-fit (*N* = 27)		*t*-test (2-tailed)	
Females: Males	29:25		15:12		14:13			
	Mean	*SD*	Mean	*SD*	Mean	*SD*	*p*	
Age (years)	69.48	8.46	70.20	8.51	68.75	8.51	0.533	
eCRF (MET)	6.58	2.47	5.28	1.97	7.88	2.25	0.000	**
Est. VO_{2max} (ml/min/Kg)	23.03	8.64	18.47	6.88	27.58	7.86	0.000	**
Education (years)	16.73	2.96	15.63	3.03	17.83	2.48	0.005	**
Weight (Kg)	79.05	16.88	84.28	15.69	73.82	16.66	0.021	*
BMI (Kg/m^2)	27.46	5.27	30.06	4.59	24.87	4.64	0.000	**
BDI score	2.91	3.34	3.63	3.64	2.19	2.91	0.114	
mMMS score	55.28	1.42	55.26	1.35	55.30	1.51	0.925	
Heart rate (bpm)	72.90	10.62	76.96	10.91	68.83	8.74	0.004	**
Systolic (mmHg)	136.90	15.66	139.33	16.59	134.48	14.58	0.258	
Diastolic (mmHg)	79.28	8.16	79.84	8.95	78.72	7.41	0.618	
Pulse pressure (mmHg)	57.63	14.01	59.49	14.26	55.76	13.77	0.332	

*eCRF, Estimated Cardiorespiratory Fitness; MET, Metabolic Equivalent; Estimated VO_{2max}, milliliters of oxygen per minute per kilogram of body weight; Kg, Kilograms; BMI, Body Mass Index – weight in Kg over height in meters squared (m^2); bpm, beats per minute; BDI, Beck's Depression Inventory; mMMS, Modified Mini-Mental Status Examination; Systolic and diastolic blood pressure: mmHg (millimeters of mercury). *$p < 0.05$, **$p < 0.01$.*

Sample Stratification and Analytic Strategies

The purpose of the present study is to *independently* assess the effects of age and fitness on brain anatomy. A critical step is to "orthogonalize" these two variables, which are typically highly correlated. To do so, participants were sorted into high- and low-fit groups using the following strategy. To control for the effects of age and gender on fitness, group membership was determined by first separating participants by age, split by the average age of the entire participant pool (mean = 69.56 years). Within each age group participants were then divided by gender and then split by eCRF scores using a median split for each age by gender group. In groups with uneven numbers of members, median participants were designated as high- or low-fit based on whether their eCRF scores were above or below the average eCRF scores of their peer group. Next, participants were combined into high-fit and low-fit categories collapsing across all other categorizations. Fitness designation was done in this way to account for the heavy weighting that gender and age receive in the CRF estimate, and to control for the gender bias known to exist within VO_{2max} scores (Jurca et al., 2005). Thus, each individual was classified as high- or low-fit based on a comparison with their similarly aged peers within the same gender group. As a result of this grouping strategy (see **Table 1**) the low-fit and high-fit groups had an almost equivalent number of males and females (14F, 13M), statistically similar average age (70.30 versus 68.75, $t = 0.63$, $p > 0.10$), but significantly different average eCRF scores (5.28 versus 7.88, $t = 4.53$, $p < 0.01$), thus effectively stratifying the sample and eliminating the inherent correlation between age and fitness.

Collection and Processing of Structural MRI Data

High-resolution T1-weighted images were acquired with a 3T Siemens Trio full body scanner using a 3D MPRAGE protocol. MPRAGE pulse parameters were: flip angle = 9, TR = 1900 ms, TE = 2.32 ms, and inversion time = 900 ms. Slices were acquired in the sagittal plane (192 slices, 0.9 mm slice thickness, voxel size 0.9 mm × 0.9 mm × 0.9 mm) with matrix dimensions of 192 × 256 × 256 (in-plane interpolated at acquisition to 192 × 512 × 512) and field of view of 172.8 mm × 230 mm × 230 mm. These parameters allowed for a clear delineation of gray–white matter boundaries upon visual inspection. Structural MRI images were processed with FreeSurfer© 5.0 (for technical details see Dale and Sereno, 1993; Dale et al., 1999; Fischl et al., 1999a,b, 2001, 2002, 2004; Fischl and Dale, 2000; Segonne et al., 2004; Desikan et al., 2006; Han et al., 2006; Jovicich et al., 2006). The FreeSurfer output was thoroughly inspected for errors through extensive visual screening performed by three trained individuals, and corrected according to the methods recommended on the FreeSurfer web site[1]. Finally, estimates of cortical and subcortical volumes were obtained, using an automated probabilistic labeling procedure based on the Desikan–Killiany anatomical atlas (Desikan et al., 2006).

Subcortical and cortical regions were then normalized by intracranial volume (see equation below) to account for volumetric differences in head size (Jack et al., 1989; Buckner et al., 2004). The anatomical data from eight college-aged students were also included in the normalization process in order to frame the results obtained from our 55–87 years-old sample into a broader age-related perspective. In other words, we included the young adults as a reference point, so that the normalized values can be more easily compared to those obtained from samples that, unlike this one, do include younger adults. Mathematically normalization consists of a scaling factor that operates equally for all subjects and groups and therefore does not introduce any bias. Every volume for each participant was corrected for head size with the following formula proposed by Buckner et al. (2004):

$$V_{adj} = V_{nat} - b(eTIV_{fs} - \overline{eTIV_{fs}})$$

where V_{adj} is the covariance-corrected (adjusted) volume, V_{nat} is the original volume calculated by FreeSurfer in native space, b is the slope of the regression of V_{nat} over $eTIV_{fs}$, which is the participant's eTIV produced by FreeSurfer, and $\overline{eTIV_{fs}}$ is the average eTIV of the group. Although several other normalization methods have been proposed, this particular one has been widely utilized throughout the field.

Statistical Analyses

The processed and corrected data were analyzed using two approaches: (a) a standard analysis evaluating all the cortical and subcortical ROIs included in the Desikan–Killiany atlas (Desikan et al., 2006); and (b) groupings of different cortical and subcortical regions showing similar effects based on a principal component analysis/VARIMAX decomposition (see Alexander-Bloch et al., 2013), in order to reduce the problem of multiple comparisons present in (a). The choice of an empirical, data-driven (rather than a theory-driven) approach for grouping the different regions was motivated by the following logic: (a) At present, the factors leading some regions more than others to be affected by aging or fitness are not yet known, and this study is, in fact, one of the first addressing this issue; and (b) the factor-analytic approach employed here allows for the data to reveal emergent groupings, which may be useful to drive future research aimed at understanding the mechanisms underlying regional variations in sensitivity to age and fitness. For all these analyses, left and right hemispheres were combined, as we had no specific hemispheric-based hypotheses.

To dissociate the effects of age and fitness we used a data-driven stratification approach, in which participants were given an "age-score" equal to the deviation of their age from the overall mean age (yielding two groups of participants above and below the overall mean age, respectively), and a "fitness-score" with a value of +1 for "high-fit-for-their-age" individuals (defined as above) and −1 for "low-fit-for-their-age individuals. This approach allowed also for the examination of age × fitness interactions, testing whether age effects were similar for high- and low-fit individuals (i.e., whether fitness moderates the effect of age), a pattern of results that is not typically examined by studies using a more traditional multiple regression approach.

[1] http://surfer.nmr.mgh.harvard.edu/fswiki/FsTutorial/TroubleshootingData

Pearson's correlation coefficients (r) were calculated to determine the associations of age, fitness and the age × fitness interaction with neuroanatomical measurements. Also, a multiple regression analysis was performed to determine the unique variance explained by these three variables. For this analysis, given the directional nature of the hypotheses (i.e., younger and more fit individuals should have larger brain volumes than older and less fit individuals), we used unidirectional tests.

The main purpose of this study is to compare the profiles of anatomical effects associated with aging and fitness. For this analysis we selected data from the ROI approach. For each of the 48 Desikan–Killiany areas, the effect sizes associated with age and fitness were calculated using Cohen's d. The similarity of the effect sizes of age and fitness across anatomical areas was estimated using a Pearson's correlation coefficient. A consistency-based two-way mixed intra-class correlation coefficient was also calculated to estimate the consistency of the profiles of regional volumetric changes with age and fitness.

RESULTS

Age and Fitness Effects: Demographics

Age, fitness, and various physiological and neuropsychological measures are reported in **Table 1**. Several variables demonstrated negative correlations with age including BMI [$r(52) = -0.48$, $p < 0.01$] and diastolic pressure [$r(52) = 0.39$, $p < 0.01$]. Pulse pressure (the difference between systolic and diastolic pressure, indexing arterial stiffness) was positively correlated with age [$r(52) = 0.36$, $p < 0.01$].

Regional Analyses of Age and Fitness Effects

To determine that the lack of correlation or consistency between the effect of age and fitness on brain volume is not merely due to lack of power, it is important to show that regional volumetric measures are sensitive to each of these two independent variables. To this end, we performed a set of multiple regressions investigating the effects of age, fitness, and their interaction on each individual area. A problem with this analysis is that it is based on a large number of comparisons, which are only partially independent of each other. Therefore, we also performed a second analysis in which we first grouped the different areas using a factor analysis (i.e., PCA followed by Varimax rotation).

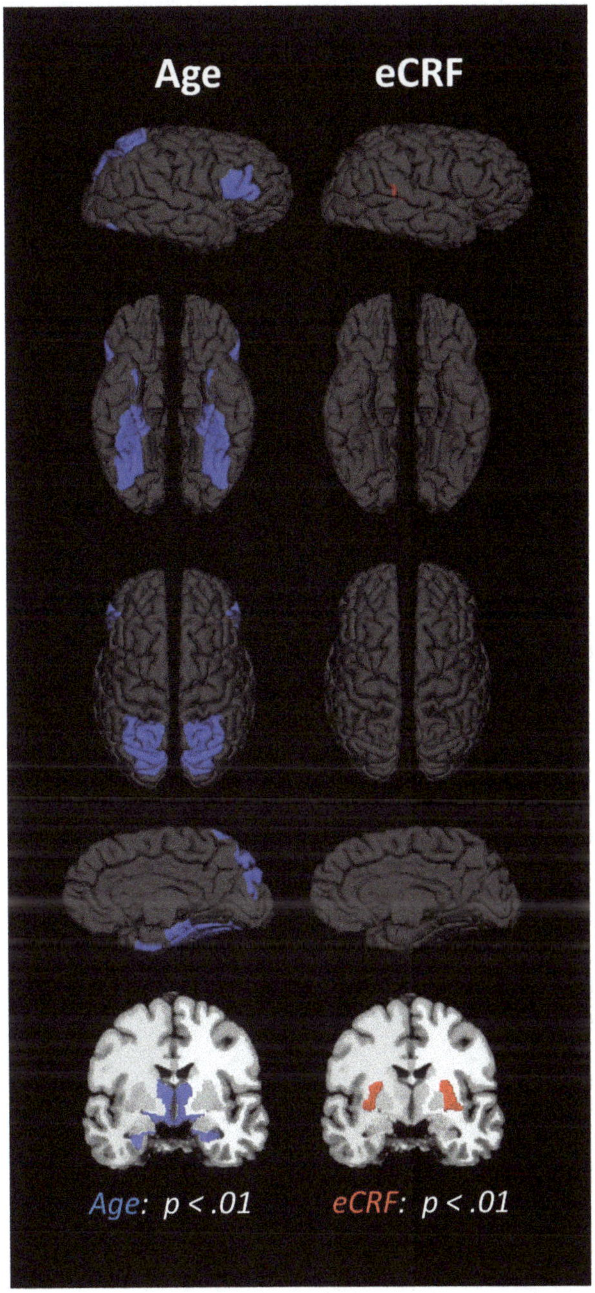

FIGURE 1 | Schematic representation of the results of the regression analysis for all of the ROIs. Colored areas indicate ROIs where age (blue) or eCRF (red) show strong partial correlations ($p < 0.01$) with the volume of the corresponding region. Although left and right volumes were not examined separately, for illustration purposes both hemispheres are included in the figure. Note that no ROI was significantly affected by both variables in this analysis.

Region by Region Analysis

The BERT template provided by FreeSurfer was colored (**Figure 1**) to provide a visual summary of cortical and subcortical regions of the Desikin–Killiany atlas that were most strongly ($p < 0.01$) associated with age and fitness. The correlations between age, fitness and the volumes of cortical ROIs are found in **Table 2**. Within the frontal lobe, only the pars opercularis, pars triangularis and precentral regions were found to be significantly negatively associated with age. However, the superior frontal and precentral regions were positively associated with fitness. In the temporal lobe, most of the regions were negatively associated with age. Furthermore, the superior temporal sulcus was positively associated with fitness, whereas superior temporal and middle temporal areas showed a similar, but not significant, trend ($p < 0.10$). The only region showing a modest interaction effect between age and fitness was the fusiform gyrus, with larger volumes in high-fit younger adults, but smaller volumes

TABLE 2 | Raw and partial correlations between anatomical ROIs and age, eCRF, and eCRF by age interaction (centered age multiplied by dichotomized fitness scores).

	Raw Correlations			Partial Correlations		
	Age (r)	eCRF (r)	Age × eCRF (r)	Age (β)	eCRF (β)	Age × eCRF (β)
Frontal Lobe						
Superior Frontal	−0.18	0.23 +	0.13	−0.17	0.22	0.13
Rostral Middle Frontal	−0.09	−0.09	−0.05	−0.10	−0.09	−0.05
Caudal Middle Frontal	−0.22	−0.01	0.21	−0.23	−0.03	0.21
Pars opercularis	−0.34 *	0.11	0.18	−0.34 *	0.08	0.20
Pars triangularis	−0.42 **	0.12	0.00	−0.42 **	0.09	0.00
Pars orbitalis	−0.18	0.09	0.13	−0.18	0.08	0.13
Lateral Orbitofrontal	−0.13	−0.07	0.06	−0.14	−0.09	0.06
Medial Orbitofrontal	−0.12	0.19	0.14	−0.11	0.18	0.14
Frontal Pole	0.10	−0.07	−0.05	0.09	−0.06	−0.05
Precentral	−0.32 *	0.28 *	0.10	−0.31 *	0.26 +	0.11
Paracentral	−0.20	0.16	−0.13	−0.19	0.15	−0.14
Temporal Lobe						
Superior Temporal	−0.33 *	0.22	0.21	−0.33 *	0.21	0.23
Middle Temporal	−0.23 +	0.22	0.12	−0.22	0.21	0.13
Inferior Temporal	−0.14	−0.12	0.03	−0.15	−0.13	0.03
Banks of the STS	−0.31 *	0.41 **	0.01	−0.30 *	0.41 **	0.01
Fusiform	−0.36 **	0.09	−0.24 +	−0.37 **	0.06	−0.25 +
Transverse Temporal	−0.13	0.22	0.09	−0.12	0.21	0.09
Entorhinal	−0.25 +	0.19	−0.01	−0.24 +	0.18	−0.02
Temporal Pole	−0.35 **	0.06	0.20	−0.35 *	0.03	0.21
Parahippocampal	−0.48 **	0.07	0.08	−0.47 **	0.03	0.09
Parietal Lobe						
Superior Parietal	−0.45 **	0.02	0.02	−0.45 **	−0.02	0.02
Inferior Parietal	−0.33 *	0.15	0.06	−0.32 *	0.13	0.06
Supramarginal	−0.25 +	0.14	−0.05	−0.24 +	0.12	−0.05
Postcentral	−0.29 *	0.08	−0.11	−0.29 *	0.06	−0.11
Precuneus	−0.30 *	0.08	0.06	−0.30 *	0.06	0.06
Occipital Lobe						
Lateral Occipital	−0.33 *	−0.05	−0.03	−0.34 *	−0.09	−0.03
Lingual	−0.34 *	0.17	−0.08	−0.34 *	0.15	−0.08
Cuneus	−0.26 +	0.02	−0.01	−0.26 +	0.00	−0.01
Pericalcarine	−0.26 +	0.14	0.00	−0.25 +	0.13	0.00
Insula						
Insula	−0.18	0.14	0.02	−0.17	0.13	0.02
Cingulate						
Rostral Anterior	−0.04	0.07	−0.01	−0.03	0.07	−0.01
Caudal Anterior	−0.06	0.23 +	0.12	−0.04	0.23 +	0.12
Posterior	−0.29 *	0.28 *	0.05	−0.28 *	0.27 +	0.06
Isthmus	−0.22	0.02	0.11	−0.22	0.00	0.11
Corpus Callosum (CC)						
Posterior	−0.35 **	0.06	0.10	−0.35 *	0.03	0.11
Mid-Posterior	−0.59 **	0.07	0.01	−0.59 **	0.03	0.02
Central	−0.59 **	0.13	0.01	−0.59 **	0.10	0.02
Mid-Anterior	−0.58 **	0.10	0.03	−0.57 **	0.06	0.04
Anterior	−0.62 **	−0.08	0.13	−0.63 **	−0.17	0.17
Subcortical						
Hippocampus	−0.47 **	0.23 +	0.00	−0.46 **	0.22	0.00
Amygdala	−0.36 **	0.34 *	−0.13	−0.35 *	0.34 *	−0.14

(Continued)

TABLE 2 | Continued

	Raw Correlations			Partial Correlations		
	Age (r)	**eCRF (r)**	**Age × eCRF (r)**	**Age (β)**	**eCRF (β)**	**Age × eCRF (β)**
Caudate	0.21	0.21	−0.08	0.24 +	0.24 +	−0.08
Putamen	−0.31 *	0.37 **	0.21	−0.31 *	0.37 **	0.23 +
Pallidum	−0.19	0.08	0.15	−0.19	0.07	0.15
Accumbens	−0.30 *	0.21	−0.20	−0.29 *	0.20	−0.21
Thalamus Proper	−0.46 **	0.24 +	0.19	−0.46 **	0.23 +	0.22
Brain-Stem	−0.31 *	0.10	0.18	−0.30 *	0.08	0.19
Ventral Diencephalon	−0.44 **	0.17	0.13	−0.44 **	0.15	0.15
Ventricle						
Lateral Ventricle	0.69 **	−0.20	−0.02	0.69 **	−0.19	−0.03
Inferior Lateral Ventricle	0.63 **	−0.05	0.05	0.63 **	0.00	0.06
3rd Ventricle	0.62 **	−0.06	0.08	0.62 **	−0.01	0.10
4th Ventricle	0.35 **	−0.10	−0.06	0.35 *	−0.07	−0.07

$N = 54$ $^{+}p < 0.05$, $^{*}p < 0.025$, $^{**}p < 0.005$ (one-tailed).

in high-fit older adults. All the sub-regions of the parietal lobe were negatively associated with age, but none were positively associated with eCRF. The insula was not associated with either age or eCRF. The posterior cingulate was associated with both age and eCRF, whereas the caudal anterior cingulate was associated only with eCRF.

The effects of age and fitness on the subcortical ROIs are reported in **Table 2**. The volumes of the hippocampus, amygdala, putamen, and thalamus were associated with both age and fitness. The nucleus accumbens, brain-stem and ventral diencephalon were associated with age but not eCRF. Lastly, age was positively associated with all ventricle measurements, with no corresponding association with fitness.

Anatomical Factor Analysis

A lack of overlap between age and CRF effects would be best demonstrated by a double-dissociation, in which some areas show effects of one independent variable and not the other, and some show the opposite effect. However, such a demonstration may be obscured by the large number of comparisons, due to the many areas that are being considered. To better identify which regions tended to covary in volume, and to reduce the number of comparisons in the age and fitness analyses, the volumes of the cortical and subcortical ROIs from the Desikan–Killiany atlas (Jack et al., 1989; Desikan et al., 2006) were submitted to a PCA. Scree plots suggested five components, or factors, which were subjected to Varimax rotation. A visualization of the regions loading on each factor (Factor Loading Score >0.5) is presented in **Figure 2**. Factor loadings of 0.3 or higher after rotation for each of the five components are reported in **Table 3**. The component scores were then submitted to a multiple regression analysis, whose results are presented in **Table 4**, using age, eCRF and the age × CRF interaction term as predictors.

The first factor consists of areas that cover most of the medial and lateral cortex. It also contains subcortical regions including the thalamus, putamen and amygdala. Regression analyses revealed that variance in Factor 1 amplitude was associated with both age and eCRF. The second factor (not shown in **Figure 2**) included the CC and ventricles, which were strongly associated with age, but not with eCRF. The third factor was made up almost exclusively of the basal ganglia with an additional contribution by the superior parietal cortex. This factor was positively associated with eCRF, but not age. The fourth factor was comprised of inferior frontal and occipital regions. This factor was associated with age, but was not associated with fitness. The fifth factor comprised regions around the dorsolateral prefrontal cortex, the anterior cingulate, and the inferior temporal lobe. Surprisingly, these regions were not associated with either age or fitness. Thus, we found one factor (Factor 1) that was affected by both aging and fitness, two factors (Factors 2 and 4) that were affected only by aging, one factor (Factor 3) that was affected only by fitness, and one factor (Factor 5) that was not affected by either variable.

Relationship between Age and Fitness Effects

The main purpose of this paper is to evaluate the overlap between the profiles of age and fitness effects across brain regions. The effect sizes (Cohen's *d*), across different anatomical areas, for high-fit and low-age participants are presented in **Figure 3** (a = cortical and b = subcortical regions). Positive values in this figure indicate age-related reductions in volume (black bars) or fitness-related increases in volume (gray bars), and vice-versa for negative values. Significant effects [$t(53) > 1.67$, $p < 0.05$, one-tailed] are denoted by bars crossing the horizontal dashed line. Nine (out of 48) regions showed significantly greater volumes in high- than in low-fit participants. Twenty-one (out of 48) regions showed significantly greater volumes in the younger than in the older participants.

The data presented in **Figure 3** suggest that age and fitness effects were especially different in regions that were most

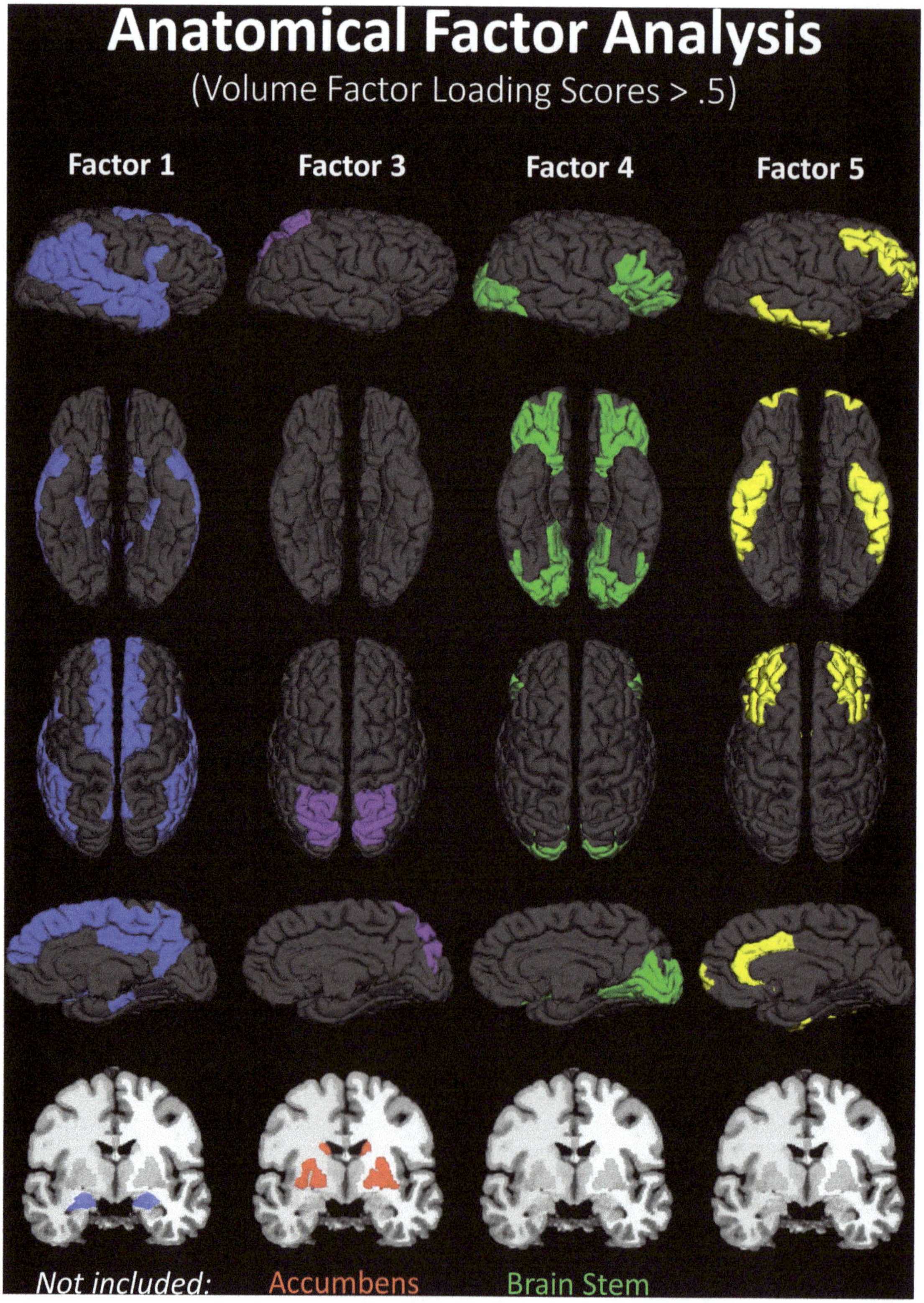

FIGURE 2 | Visualization of the ROIs loading highly (>0.5) on each factor of the PCA (from data presented in Table 3). Factor 2 (not represented here) is related to ventricles and corpus callosum size (for which loadings were positive and negative, respectively). For factor 3, significant and positive factor loadings were colored in red, with significant but negative factors colored in purple. Superior and inferior views are presented with the anterior portion of the brain pointing upward. Although left and right volumes were not examined separately, for illustration purposes both hemispheres are included in the figure. Anatomical ROIs that had high factor loadings but could not be displayed are listed at the bottom of each factor column.

TABLE 3 | Factor loadings for anatomical ROIs entered in the factor analysis.

Factor 1		Factor 2		Factor 3		Factor 4		Factor 5	
Supramarginal	**0.73**	CC Mid-Anterior	**0.83**	Putamen	**0.66**	Cuneus	**0.80**	Rostral Ant. C.	**0.67**
Sup. T.	**0.72**	CC Central	**0.80**	Pallidum	**0.62**	Pericalcarine	**0.77**	Rostral Mid. F.	**0.63**
Precuneus	**0.67**	CC Mid-Posterior	**0.79**	Caudate	0.55	Parorbitalis	**0.61**	F. Pole	**0.60**
Mid. T.	0.59	CC Anterior	**0.78**	Accumbens	0.55	Brain Stem	**0.61**	Caudal Ant. C.	0.56
Inferior P.	0.59	CC Posterior	**0.69**	Banks STS	0.32	Lat. Occipital	0.57	Inferior T.	0.54
Banks STS	0.58	Thal. Proper	0.48	Paracentral	0.32	Lingual	0.54	Isthmus C.	0.45
Pars opercularis	0.57	Parahippocampal	0.45	Thal. Proper	0.31	Insula	0.53	Med. Orbito F.	0.40
Paracentral	0.56	Hippocampus	0.44	Precuneus	−0.45	Pars triangularis	0.51	Entorhinal	0.36
Posterior C.	0.56	Precentral	0.36	Isthmus C.	−0.45	Lat. Orbito F.	0.51	Mid. T.	0.34
Insula	0.55	Brain Stem	0.33	Sup. Parietal	−0.55	Med. Orbito F.	0.48	Inferior Parietal	0.31
Parahippocampal	0.54	Postcentral	0.31			Sup. F.	0.46	Fusiform	0.30
Amygdala	0.53	CSF	−0.41			Accumbens	0.43		
Sup. F.	0.53	4th V.	−0.45			Precentral	0.33		
Transverse T.	0.49	Inferior Lat. V.	**−0.70**						
Postcentral	0.47	3rd V.	**−0.73**						
Fusiform	0.46	Lat. V.	**−0.73**						
Putamen	0.44								
Sup. Parietal	0.42								
Thal. Proper	0.41								
Caudal Mid. F.	0.40								
Med. OrbitoF.	0.37								
Caudal Ant. C.	0.37								
Lat. OrbitoF.	0.36								
Hippocampus	0.36								
Precentral	0.34								

Factors are ranked in descending order. Highlighted cells contain values greater than or less than 0.50. Bolded values are loading scores greater than 0.60. Values less than 0.30 are excluded for ease of presentation. F, Frontal; T, Temporal; C, Cingulate; V., Ventricle; P, Parietal; CC, Corpus Callosum; Thal, Thalamus; Lat, Lateral; Sup, Superior; Mid, Middle; Med, Medial.

TABLE 4 | Raw and partial correlations between anatomical factor loadings with age, eCRF, and eCRF by age interaction (centered age multiplied by centered fitness scores).

	Raw correlation			Partial correlation		
	Age (r)	eCRF (r)	Age × eCRF (r)	Age (β)	eCRF (β)	Age × eCRF (β)
Anatomical Factors						
Factor 1:	−0.31 *	0.31 *	0.04	−0.29 *	0.29 *	0.05
Factor 2:	−0.70 **	0.08	0.03	−0.70 **	0.03	0.05
Factor 3:	−0.01	0.26 +	0.00	0.01	0.26 +	0.00
Factor 4:	−0.24 +	0.04	0.03	−0.24 +	0.02	0.03
Factor 5:	0.03	−0.02	−0.03	0.03	−0.02	−0.03

N = 54 $^{+}p < 0.05$, $^{*}p < 0.025$, $^{**}p < 0.005$ *(one-tailed).*

impacted by age (left side of **Figures 3A,B**). This was especially true for the CC and ventral frontal regions. To characterize the relationship (or lack thereof) between the two types of effects, a scatter-plot displaying group-level age effects against group-level fitness effects across brain regions is presented in **Figure 4**. Overall, the correlation between these average *t*-scores was not significant, $r(46) = 0.078, p = 0.597$.

To quantify the relationship between the two profiles, we computed a consistency-based two-way mixed intra-class correlation coefficient. The result of this analysis indicate that there is little consistency between the profile of age effects and the profile of fitness effects on brain volumes, $r_{ic} = 0.078$, $p = 0.298$. Although this analysis failed to reach significance when examining all regions, a median split on the effect sizes of age effects revealed interesting differences. For those regions most significantly impacted by age (blue circles in **Figure 4**), a marginal, but *negative* association was found between age and fitness effects [$N = 24$, $r(22) = 0.380$, $p = 0.067$]. For regions

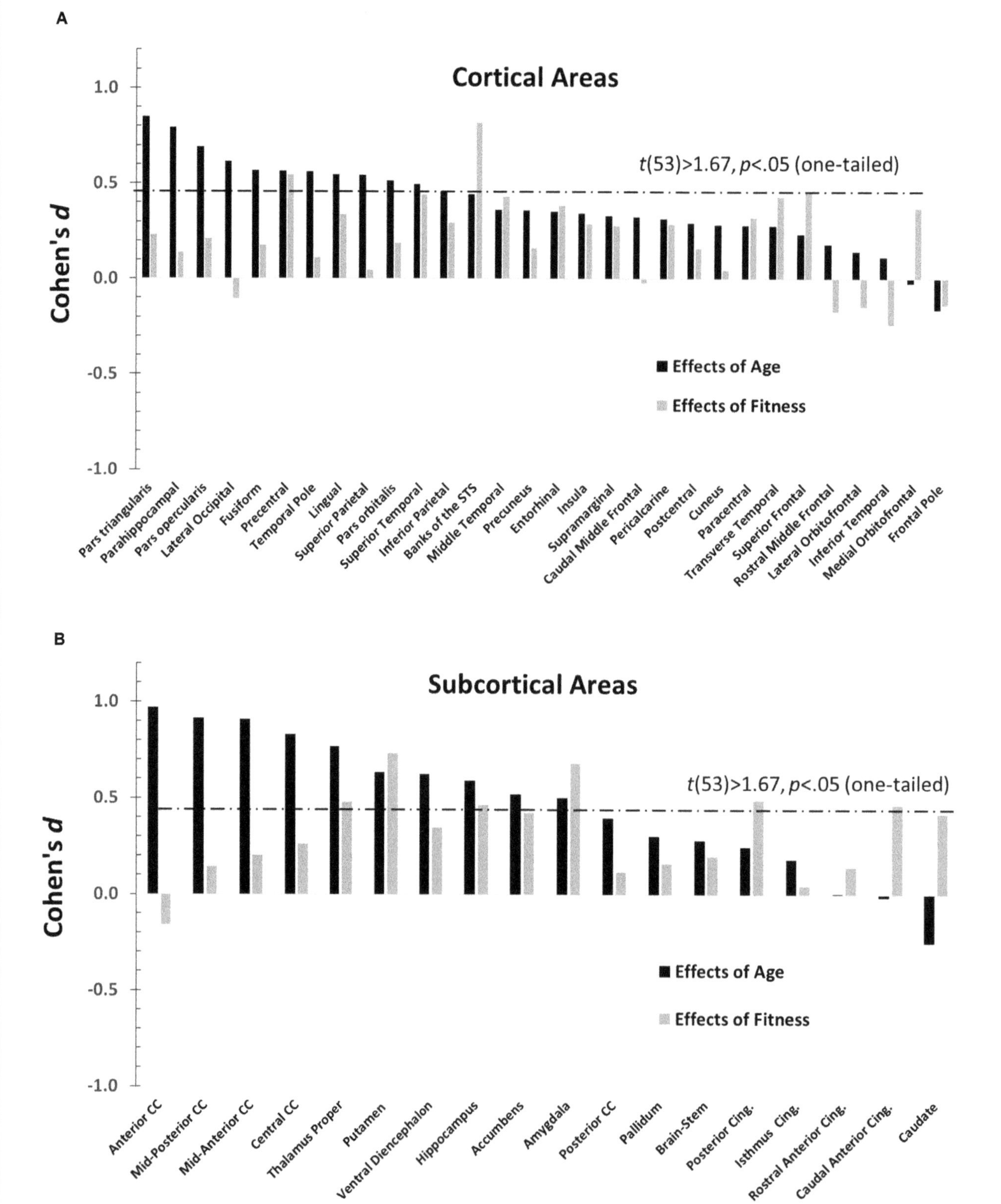

FIGURE 3 | Bar graphs depicting the Cohen's *d* (effect sizes) as a function of age (black), and CRF (gray) for all the ROIs examined (defined by the Desikan–Killiany atlas). For each graph, regions are separately arranged according to decreasing age effects, with regions most impacted by age on the far left. The horizontal dashed line represents the significance threshold for a one-tailed t-test, $t(53) = 1.67$, $p = 0.05$. **(A)** Cohen's d's for normalized cortical regions. **(B)** Cohen's d's for normalized subcortical gray and white matter regions.

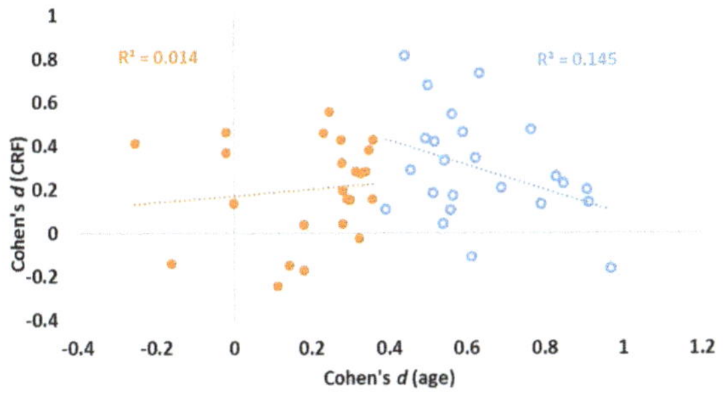

FIGURE 4 | Scatter plot reporting effect sizes (Cohen's *d*) for age (abscissa) and CRF (ordinate) for each of the 48 ROIs. Linear regression lines and coefficients of determination (R^2) computed across regions are also displayed separately for areas with high (blue) and low (orange) aging effect sizes (as determined by a median split of age effect sizes).

less impacted by age (orange circles in **Figure 4**), no association was found between age and fitness effects [$N = 24$, $r(22) = 0.117$, $p = 0.586$].

DISCUSSION

The main goal of this study was to determine the overlap between the profiles of the effects of fitness and age on the volumes of different brain areas in adults aged 55 and older. This may have theoretical and practical importance: If age and fitness were found to be related to similar (albeit opposite) volumetric profiles, it could be argued that fitness (or lack thereof) may be an important global mediator of the effects of aging, and a fitness-based intervention could be used to halt, delay or reverse the effects of aging on brain volumes. Although a large number of studies have investigated the effects of aging and those of fitness on the volumes of various brain regions (see Voss et al., 2013 for a detailed review), a determination of the degree of overlap between these two sets of effects is still lacking.

As found previously in several other studies, our results indicate that both age and fitness have effects on brain volumes. As in previous work (Raz, 2005; Raz and Rodrigue, 2006; Raz et al., 2007; Fjell et al., 2013), the effects of age were particularly evident for the ventricles, the CC, some subcortical gray structures such as the hippocampus and portions of the basal ganglia, as well as a number of cortical regions. Also confirming previous work (Gordon et al., 2008; Erickson et al., 2009, 2011; Chaddock et al., 2010; Bugg and Head, 2011; Verstynen et al., 2012), eCRF was associated with larger volumes in a small set of brain structures, including some cortical (precentral gyrus and superior temporal sulcus) and subcortical (amygdala and some portions of the basal ganglia) structures.

Importantly, however, three findings from our study suggest that the profiles of the effects of aging and fitness are not entirely overlapping. First, an intraclass correlation analysis failed to show a significant association between the two types of effects. Second, the multiple regression analysis of the anatomical PCA factor scores showed that age and fitness were by and large correlated with different components. Specifically, although factor 1 was associated with both variables, factors 2 and 4 were associated with age and not with fitness, and factor 3 (comprised mainly of the basal ganglia) was associated with fitness but not age. The results of the PCA, together with the multiple regression analysis, suggest that age has broad effects on much of the cortex. These are, however, at times separable from the effects of fitness, which are more localized to regions such as the basal ganglia and MTL. Third, very few interactions (no more than could be predicted on the basis of chance) were observed between age and fitness, suggesting that fitness did not moderate the age effects. In other words, according to an additive factor logic, this suggests that age and fitness contribute independent, additive effects to brain anatomy.

It is also interesting to note that those regions that are most impacted by age (blue circles on the right of **Figure 4**) are among those not significantly impacted by fitness. As mentioned previously, when considering only the 24 regions showing the largest age effects (top half), a marginally significant negative association between age and fitness effects is revealed. Although it is not entirely clear why this happens, it is possible that, when the effects of age become too prominent, then the effects of fitness can no longer counteract them. An alternative explanation is that, in some cases, area volume may not be the best measure of tissue preservation, and that other indices of anatomical reserve (such as cortical thinning or measures of myelination) may be more sensitive. This may account for the lack of correlation between CC volume and fitness obtained in our sample, while an association between fitness and white matter integrity (as measured by fractional anisotropy) has been reported in previous studies (e.g., Johnson et al., 2012; Chaddock-Heyman et al., 2014). It should be noted, however, that neither of these studies directly compared the effects of age and fitness on white matter integrity. In addition, the sensitivity explanation does not account for the fact that we still find a strong relationship between age and white matter preservation in our study.

There is of course ample evidence of both physiological (Burdette et al., 2010; Fabiani et al., 2014; Zimmerman et al., 2014) and cognitive (Colcombe and Kramer, 2003; Kashihara et al., 2009; Erickson et al., 2011; Weinstein et al., 2012) benefits of physical fitness in older adults. Further, the brain structures that we (as well as others) find to be associated with CRF actually support important functional phenomena (Gordon et al., 2008; Erickson et al., 2009, 2010; Chaddock et al., 2010; Bugg and Head, 2011; Verstynen et al., 2012; Weinstein et al., 2012).

A number of mechanisms might help explain why some regions seem to be more "fitness sensitive" compared to others. First, many of these "fitness sensitive" regions play unique roles in the planning, coordination, and execution of movements required during aerobic exercise. Indeed, many of the fitness-sensitive regions found in this study are related to motor functions including the precentral gyrus (primary motor cortex), basal ganglia (regulation of movement and motor control), superior temporal sulcus (perception of biological motion), and anterior cingulate (coordination of motor behavior) (DeLong et al., 1984; Grossman and Blake, 2001; Wenderoth et al., 2005; Colcombe et al., 2006; Gordon et al., 2008; Chaddock et al., 2010; Verstynen et al., 2012). Thus, it is possible that for those older adults who exercise, increased use of these regions might preserve them from age-related atrophy, contributing to regional variations.

A second possible contributor to this regional specificity is the fact that neurogenesis is restricted to just a few regions within the brain. Animal studies have shown that CRF induces neurogenesis in rodents, although this phenomenon seems to be restricted to the hippocampus (e.g., Altman, 1969; Brown et al., 2003; Farmer et al., 2004; van Praag, 2008). In humans adult neurogenesis has also been shown within the hippocampus and regions of the basal ganglia (Eriksson et al., 1998; Spalding et al., 2013; Ernst et al., 2014). In the current study and a number of prior investigations, the effects of fitness on the hippocampus and the basal ganglia are particularly pronounced (e.g., Erickson et al., 2009; Chaddock et al., 2010; Ahlskog, 2011; Bugg and Head, 2011; Erickson et al., 2011; McAuley et al., 2011; Nagamatsu et al., 2016). In fact, our study showed that regions of the basal ganglia (particularly the putamen) demonstrated the strongest association with eCRF, after partialing out the effects of age and gender.

Several other mechanisms could further explain the variations in fitness sensitivity of certain regions including: differences in cerebral blood flow and arterial stiffness across the cortex (e.g., Fabiani et al., 2014; Zimmerman et al., 2014); variations in the sensitivity to various neurotrophic factors (e.g., Voss et al., 2013); and differential oxygen requirements across regions (Kreisman et al., 2000). Indeed, it is likely that these mechanisms might work synergistically to prevent atrophy in some regions, while providing minimum influence on other areas. Our study, however, points out that fitness cannot completely offset the declines associated with normal aging, and illustrates a possible approach for future studies to examine the interactions between fitness and age on volumes across different brain structures.

Within this context, it is important to note that our study, by and large, replicates most of the major findings that have been reported both in the literature on anatomical brain aging as well as in the effects of fitness on brain volumes. This indicates that the results of our study are not outliers with respect to the extant literature. What is novel here is the profile approach used, and the consequent types of analyses that were carried out to examine it. A critical requirement for these analyses is the inclusion of a large number of areas distributed across the whole brain. Another feature of the current study is the dichotomization of the most critical independent variables (age, fitness, and gender), which permits their orthogonalization. This allows for a comprehensive and independent examination of the profiles of the effects of these variables (and of their interactions) across areas. Finally, another important feature of the analytic strategy employed in this study is the use of a factor-analysis approach to identify the brain structures that covary as a function of age and fitness. Although this is a data-driven (rather than theoretically based) approach, and therefore it is inherently exploratory, it does help reduce multiple comparisons. It could also help guide future research aimed at understanding the factors underlying the emergent grouping (as well as the stability of the grouping across different samples).

A possible limitation of the current work is the relatively small sample size ($N = 54$), which could diminish the power of the analysis. Since some of the findings depend on tests of the null hypothesis (such as the lack of a significant intra-class correlation), this lack of power may potentially be an important problem. However, it should be noted that the statistical power of a study depends not only on sample size but also on the extent to which experimental error can be controlled or minimized. In this study we used a very rigorous process of data quality control, as well as methods for orthogonalizing the variance due to age and CRF. The effectiveness of these procedures is demonstrated by our replication of the main significant effects for both age and fitness normally reported in the literature.

CONCLUSION

The current study presents an analytic approach to investigate the degree of overlap of the effects of critical variables on brain anatomy. A crucial aspect of this work is the orthogonalization of the effects of these two variables. This allows for the separate study of the profiles of the effects associated with age and fitness, and demonstrates that they are only partially overlapping. While some areas (such as the precentral gyrus, the banks of the superior temporal sulcus, and some subdivisions of the MTL) are affected by both age and fitness, there are a number of areas (including extensive regions of the frontal, parietal, and temporal cortex, as well as the CC) that are only affected by aging, and some structures (mostly in the basal ganglia) that are uniquely affected by fitness.

These findings support the idea that aging and fitness (or lack thereof) have differential effects on the brain. Understanding that fitness cannot revert all of the effects of aging is important for many reasons. First, it may lend support to the hypothesis that a comprehensive preventive approach to brain aging focusing on other lifestyle factors (such as diet or cognitive training) in addition to fitness may be more effective than fitness interventions alone, as these other factors may potentially help protect those brain regions not responsive to fitness. Second, the limited overlap of these effects in many regions may help explain the differential effects of fitness on the various domains of cognition found in previous studies. Finally, these differences may also help guide neurobiological research examining, in an area-specific way, the mechanisms by which fitness could impact the brain.

AUTHOR CONTRIBUTIONS

MF and GG designed the study and directed all aspects of the project, and helped write and edit the manuscript. MAF with the help of RB conducted all anatomical analyses, and MAF wrote the first version of this manuscript. KAL, BZ, HT, and NS-G carried out the data collection. AG and BPS provided consulting on FreeSurfer. Everyone commented on the paper.

ACKNOWLEDGMENT

This work was supported by NIA grant 1RC1AG035927 to FM.

REFERENCES

Ahlskog, J. E. (2011). Does vigorous exercise have a neuroprotective effect in Parkinson disease? *Neurology* 77, 288–294. doi: 10.1212/WNL.0b013e318225ab66

Alexander-Bloch, A., Giedd, J. N., and Bullmore, E. (2013). Imaging structural co-variance between human brain regions. *Nat. Rev. Neurosci.* 14, 322–336. doi: 10.1038/nrn3465

Altman, J. (1969). Autoradiographic and histological studies of postnatal neurogenesis. IV. Cell proliferation and migration in the anterior forebrain, with special reference to persisting neurogenesis in the olfactory bulb. *J. Comp. Neurol.* 137, 433–457. doi: 10.1002/cne.901370404

Ashburner, J., and Friston, K. J. (2000). Voxel-based morphometry: the methods. *Neuroimage* 11, 805–821. doi: 10.1006/nimg.2000.0582

Barlow, C. E., Lamonte, M. J., Fitzgerald, S. J., Kampert, J. B., Perrin, J. L., and Blair, S. N. (2006). Cardiorespiratory fitness is an independent predictor of hypertension incidence among initially normotensive healthy women. *Am. J. Epidemiol.* 163, 142–150. doi: 10.1093/aje/kwj019

Beck, A. T., and Steer, R. A. (1987). *BDI, Beck Depression Inventory: Manual.* New York, NY: Psychological Corporation.

Bherer, L., Erickson, K. I., and Liu-Ambrose, T. (2013). A review of the effects of physical activity and exercise on cognitive and brain functions in older adults. *J. Aging Res.* 2013, 657508. doi: 10.1155/2013/657508

Blair, S. N., Kampert, J. B., Kohl, H. W. III, Barlow, C. E., Macera, C. A., Paffenbarger, R. S. Jr. et al. (1996). INfluences of cardiorespiratory fitness and other precursors on cardiovascular disease and all-cause mortality in men and women. *JAMA* 276, 205–210. doi: 10.1001/jama.276.3.205

Bookstein, F. L. (2001). "Voxel-based morphometry" should not be used with imperfectly registered images. *Neuroimage* 14, 1454–1462. doi: 10.1006/nimg.2001.0770

Brown, J., Cooper-Kuhn, C. M., Kempermann, G., Van Praag, H., Winkler, J., Gage, F. H., et al. (2003). Enriched environment and physical activity stimulate hippocampal but not olfactory bulb neurogenesis. *Eur. J. Neurosci.* 17, 2042–2046. doi: 10.1046/j.1460-9568.2003.02647.x

Brown, W. R., and Thore, C. R. (2011). Review: cerebral microvascular pathology in ageing and neurodegeneration. *Neuropathol. Appl. Neurobiol.* 37, 56–74. doi: 10.1111/j.1365-2990.2010.01139.x

Buckner, R. L., Head, D., Parker, J., Fotenos, A. F., Marcus, D., Morris, J. C., et al. (2004). A unified approach for morphometric and functional data analysis in young, old, and demented adults using automated atlas-based head size normalization: reliability and validation against manual measurement of total intracranial volume. *Neuroimage* 23, 724–738. doi: 10.1016/j.neuroimage.2004.06.018

Bugg, J. M., and Head, D. (2011). Exercise moderates age-related atrophy of the medial temporal lobe. *Neurobiol. Aging* 32, 506–514. doi: 10.1016/j.neurobiolaging.2009.03.008

Burdette, J. H., Laurienti, P. J., Espeland, M. A., Morgan, A., Telesford, Q., Vechlekar, C. D., et al. (2010). Using network science to evaluate exercise-associated brain changes in older adults. *Front. Aging Neurosci.* 2:23. doi: 10.3389/fnagi.2010.00023

Chaddock, L., Erickson, K. I., Prakash, R. S., Vanpatter, M., Voss, M. W., Pontifex, M. B., et al. (2010). Basal ganglia volume is associated with aerobic fitness in preadolescent children. *Dev. Neurosci.* 32, 249–256. doi: 10.1159/000316648

Chaddock-Heyman, L., Erickson, K. I., Holtrop, J. L., Voss, M. W., Pontifex, M. B., Raine, L. B., et al. (2014). Aerobic fitness is associated with greater white matter integrity in children. *Front. Hum. Neurosci.* 8:584. doi: 10.3389/fnhum.2014.00584

Colcombe, S. J., Erickson, K. I., Raz, N., Webb, A. G., Cohen, N. J., Mcauley, E., et al. (2003). Aerobic fitness reduces brain tissue loss in aging humans. *J. Gerontol. A Biol. Sci. Med. Sci.* 58, 176–180. doi: 10.1093/gerona/58.2.M176

Colcombe, S. J., Erickson, K. I., Scalf, P. E., Kim, J. S., Prakash, R., Mcauley, E., et al. (2006). Aerobic exercise training increases brain volume in aging humans. *J. Gerontol. A Biol. Sci. Med. Sci.* 61, 1166–1170. doi: 10.1093/gerona/61.11.1166

Colcombe, S. J., and Kramer, A. F. (2003). Fitness effects on the cognitive function of older adults: a meta-analytic study. *Psychol. Sci.* 14, 125–130.

Dai, D.-F., Chiao, Y. A., Marcinek, D. J., Szeto, H. H., and Rabinovitch, P. S. (2014). Mitochondrial oxidative stress in aging and healthspan. *Longev. Healthspan* 3, 6. doi: 10.1186/2046-2395-3-6

Dale, A. M., Fischl, B., and Sereno, M. I. (1999). Cortical surface-based analysis. I. Segmentation and surface reconstruction. *Neuroimage* 9, 179–194. doi: 10.1006/nimg.1998.0395

Dale, A. M., and Sereno, M. I. (1993). Improved localizadon of cortical activity by combining eeg and meg with mri cortical surface reconstruction: a linear approach. *J. Cogn. Neurosci.* 5, 162–176. doi: 10.1162/jocn.1993.5.2.162

Davatzikos, C. (2004). Why voxel-based morphometric analysis should be used with great caution when characterizing group differences. *Neuroimage* 23, 17–20. doi: 10.1016/j.neuroimage.2004.05.010

Davenport, M. H., Hogan, D. B., Eskes, G. A., Longman, R. S., and Poulin, M. J. (2012). Cerebrovascular reserve: the link between fitness and cognitive function? *Exerc. Sport Sci. Rev.* 40, 153–158. doi: 10.1097/JES.0b013e3182553430

DeLong, M. R., Alexander, G. E., Georgopoulos, A. P., Crutcher, M. D., Mitchell, S. J., and Richardson, R. T. (1984). Role of basal ganglia in limb movements. *Hum. Neurobiol.* 2, 235–244.

Desikan, R. S., Segonne, F., Fischl, B., Quinn, B. T., Dickerson, B. C., Blacker, D., et al. (2006). An automated labeling system for subdividing the human cerebral cortex on MRI scans into gyral based regions of interest. *Neuroimage* 31, 968–980. doi: 10.1016/j.neuroimage.2006.01.021

Dunn, A. L., Marcus, B. H., Kampert, J. B., Garcia, M. E., Kohl, I. H., and Blair, S. N. (1999). Comparison of lifestyle and structured interventions to increase physical activity and cardiorespiratory fitness: a randomized trial. *JAMA* 281, 327–334. doi: 10.1001/jama.281.4.327

Erickson, K. I., Prakash, R. S., Voss, M. W., Chaddock, L., Hu, L., Morris, K. S., et al. (2009). Aerobic fitness is associated with hippocampal volume in elderly humans. *Hippocampus* 19, 1030–1039. doi: 10.1002/hipo.20547

Erickson, K. I., Raji, C. A., Lopez, O. L., Becker, J. T., Rosano, C., Newman, A. B., et al. (2010). Physical activity predicts gray matter volume in late adulthood: the Cardiovascular Health Study. *Neurology* 75, 1415–1422. doi: 10.1212/WNL.0b013e3181f88359

Erickson, K. I., Voss, M. W., Prakash, R. S., Basak, C., Szabo, A., Chaddock, L., et al. (2011). Exercise training increases size of hippocampus and improves memory. *Proc. Natl. Acad. Sci. U.S.A.* 108, 3017–3022. doi: 10.1073/pnas.1015950108

Eriksson, P. S., Perfilieva, E., Björk-Eriksson, T., Alborn, A.-M., Nordborg, C., Peterson, D. A., et al. (1998). Neurogenesis in the adult human hippocampus. *Nat. Med.* 4, 1313–1317. doi: 10.1038/3305

Ernst, A., Alkass, K., Bernard, S., Salehpour, M., Perl, S., Tisdale, J., et al. (2014). Neurogenesis in the striatum of the adult human brain. *Cell* 156, 1072–1083. doi: 10.1016/j.cell.2014.01.044

Fabiani, M. (2012). It was the best of times, it was the worst of times: a psychophysiologist's view of cognitive aging. *Psychophysiology* 49, 283–304. doi: 10.1111/j.1469-8986.2011.01331.x

Fabiani, M., Low, K. A., Tan, C.-H., Zimmerman, B., Fletcher, M. A., Schneider-Garces, N., et al. (2014). Taking the pulse of aging: mapping pulse pressure and elasticity in cerebral arteries with optical methods. *Psychophysiology* 51, 1072–1088. doi: 10.1111/psyp.12288

Farmer, J., Zhao, X., Van Praag, H., Wodtke, K., Gage, F. H., and Christie, B. R. (2004). Effects of voluntary exercise on synaptic plasticity and gene expression in the dentate gyrus of adult male sprague–dawley rats in vivo. *Neuroscience* 124, 71–79. doi: 10.1016/j.neuroscience.2003.09.029

Fischl, B., and Dale, A. M. (2000). Measuring the thickness of the human cerebral cortex from magnetic resonance images. *Proc. Natl. Acad. Sci. U.S.A.* 97, 11050–11055. doi: 10.1073/pnas.200033797

Fischl, B., Liu, A., and Dale, A. M. (2001). Automated manifold surgery: constructing geometrically accurate and topologically correct models of the human cerebral cortex. *IEEE Trans. Med. Imaging* 20, 70–80. doi: 10.1109/42.906426

Fischl, B., Salat, D. H., Busa, E., Albert, M., Dieterich, M., Haselgrove, C., et al. (2002). Whole brain segmentation: automated labeling of neuroanatomical structures in the human brain. *Neuron* 33, 341–355. doi: 10.1016/S0896-6273(02)00569-X

Fischl, B., Salat, D. H., Van Der Kouwe, A. J., Makris, N., Segonne, F., Quinn, B. T., et al. (2004). Sequence-independent segmentation of magnetic resonance images. *Neuroimage* 23(Suppl. 1), S69–S84. doi: 10.1016/j.neuroimage.2004.07.016

Fischl, B., Sereno, M. I., and Dale, A. M. (1999a). Cortical surface-based analysis. II: inflation, flattening, and a surface-based coordinate system. *Neuroimage* 9, 195–207. doi: 10.1006/nimg.1998.0396

Fischl, B., Sereno, M. I., Tootell, R. B., and Dale, A. M. (1999b). High-resolution intersubject averaging and a coordinate system for the cortical surface. *Hum. Brain Mapp.* 8, 272–284. doi: 10.1002/(SICI)1097-0193(1999)8:4<272::AID-HBM10>3.0.CO;2-4

Fjell, A. M., Westlye, L. T., Grydeland, H., Amlien, I., Espeseth, T., Reinvang, I., et al. (2013). Critical ages in the life course of the adult brain: nonlinear subcortical aging. *Neurobiol. Aging* 34, 2239–2247. doi: 10.1016/j.neurobiolaging.2013.04.006

Good, C. D., Johnsrude, I. S., Ashburner, J., Henson, R. N., Fristen, K., and Frackowiak, R. S. (2002). "A voxel-based morphometric study of ageing in 465 normal adult human brains," in *Proceedings of the 5th IEEE EMBS International Summer School on: Biomedical Imaging* (Rome: IEEE), 16.

Gordon, B. A., Rykhlevskaia, E. I., Brumback, C. R., Lee, Y., Elavsky, S., Konopack, J. F., et al. (2008). Neuroanatomical correlates of aging, cardiopulmonary fitness level, and education. *Psychophysiology* 45, 825–838. doi: 10.1111/j.1469-8986.2008.00676.x

Grossman, E. D., and Blake, R. (2001). Brain activity evoked by inverted and imagined biological motion. *Vision Res.* 41, 1475–1482. doi: 10.1016/S0042-6989(00)00317-5

Han, X., Jovicich, J., Salat, D., Van Der Kouwe, A., Quinn, B., Czanner, S., et al. (2006). Reliability of MRI-derived measurements of human cerebral cortical thickness: the effects of field strength, scanner upgrade and manufacturer. *Neuroimage* 32, 180–194. doi: 10.1016/j.neuroimage.2006.02.051

Jack, C. R. Jr., Twomey, C. K., Zinsmeister, A. R., Sharbrough, F. W., Petersen, R. C., and Cascino, G. D. (1989). Anterior temporal lobes and hippocampal formations: normative volumetric measurements from MR images in young adults. *Radiology* 172, 549–554. doi: 10.1148/radiology.172.2.2748838

Jackson, E. M., and Dishman, R. K. (2006). Cardiorespiratory fitness and laboratory stress: a meta-regression analysis. *Psychophysiology* 43, 57–72. doi: 10.1111/j.1469-8986.2006.00373.x

Jetté, M., Sidney, K., and Blümchen, G. (1990). Metabolic equivalents (METS) in exercise testing, exercise prescription, and evaluation of functional capacity. *Clin. Cardiol.* 13, 555–565. doi: 10.1002/clc.4960130809

Johnson, N. F., Kim, C., Clasey, J. L., Bailey, A., and Gold, B. T. (2012). Cardiorespiratory fitness is positively correlated with cerebral white matter integrity in healthy seniors. *Neuroimage* 59, 1514–1523. doi: 10.1016/j.neuroimage.2011.08.032

Jovicich, J., Czanner, S., Greve, D., Haley, E., Van Der Kouwe, A., Gollub, R., et al. (2006). Reliability in multi-site structural MRI studies: effects of gradient non-linearity correction on phantom and human data. *Neuroimage* 30, 436–443. doi: 10.1016/j.neuroimage.2005.09.046

Jurca, R., Jackson, A. S., Lamonte, M. J., Morrow, J. R., Blair, S. N., Wareham, N. J., et al. (2005). Assessing cardiorespiratory fitness without performing exercise testing. *Am. J. Prev. Med.* 29, 185–193. doi: 10.1016/j.amepre.2005.06.004

Kashihara, K., Maruyama, T., Murota, M., and Nakahara, Y. (2009). Positive effects of acute and moderate physical exercise on cognitive function. *J. Physiol. Anthropol.* 28, 155–164. doi: 10.2114/jpa2.28.155

Kennedy, K. M., Erickson, K. I., Rodrigue, K. M., Voss, M. W., Colcombe, S. J., Kramer, A. F., et al. (2009). Age-related differences in regional brain volumes: a comparison of optimized voxel-based morphometry to manual volumetry. *Neurobiol. Aging* 30, 1657–1676. doi: 10.1016/j.neurobiolaging.2007.12.020

Kreisman, N. R., Soliman, S., and Gozal, D. (2000). Regional differences in hypoxic depolarization and swelling in hippocampal slices. *J. Neurophysiol.* 83, 1031–1038.

Lähteenvuo, J., and Rosenzweig, A. (2012). Effects of aging on angiogenesis. *Circ. Res.* 110, 1252–1264. doi: 10.1161/CIRCRESAHA.111.246116

Mailey, E. L., White, S. M., Wojcicki, T. R., Szabo, A. N., Kramer, A. F., and Mcauley, E. (2010). Construct validation of a non-exercise measure of cardiorespiratory fitness in older adults. *BMC Public Health* 10:59. doi: 10.1186/1471-2458-10-59

Masley, S. C. (2009). "Measuring physical fitness," in *Exercise Stress Testing for Primary Care and Sports Medicine*, eds C. H. Evans and R. D. White (New York, NY: Springer), 275–288.

Mayeux, R., Stern, Y., Rosen, J., and Leventhal, J. (1981). Depression, intellectual impairment, and Parkinson disease. *Neurology* 31, 645–650. doi: 10.1212/WNL.31.6.645

McAuley, E., Mullen, S., and Hillman, C. (2013). "Physical activity, cardiorespiratory fitness, and cognition across the lifespan," in *Social Neuroscience and Public Health*, ed. P. A. Hall (New York, NY: Springer), 235–252.

McAuley, E., Szabo, A. N., Mailey, E. L., Erickson, K. I., Voss, M., White, S. M., et al. (2011). Non-exercise estimated cardiorespiratory fitness: associations with brain structure, cognition, and memory complaints in older adults. *Ment. Health Phys. Act.* 4, 5–11. doi: 10.1016/j.mhpa.2011.01.001

McArdle, W. D., Katch, F. I., and Katch, V. L. (2006). *Exercise Physiology: Energy, Nutrition, and Human Performance*, 6th Edn. Baltimore: Lippincott Williams & Wilkins.

McGue, M., and Johnson, W. (2008). "Genetics of cognitive aging," in *Handbook of Aging and Cognition*, 3rd Edn, eds F. I. M. Craik and T. A. Salthouse (New York, NY: Psychology Press).

Morrison, J. H., and Baxter, M. G. (2012). The ageing cortical synapse: hallmarks and implications for cognitive decline. *Nat. Rev. Neurosci.* 13, 240–250. doi: 10.1038/nrn3200

Muller, F. L., Lustgarten, M. S., Jang, Y., Richardson, A., and Van Remmen, H. (2007). Trends in oxidative aging theories. *Free Radic. Biol. Med.* 43, 477–503. doi: 10.1016/j.freeradbiomed.2007.03.034

Nagamatsu, L. S., Weinstein, A. M., Erickson, K. I., Fanning, J., Awick, E. A., Kramer, A. F., et al. (2016). Exercise mode moderates the relationship between mobility and basal ganglia volume in healthy older adults. *J. Am. Geriatr. Soc.* 64, 102–108. doi: 10.1111/jgs.13882

Nyberg, L., Lövdén, M., Riklund, K., Lindenberger, U., and Bäckman, L. (2012). Memory aging and brain maintenance. *Trends Cogn. Sci. (Regul. Ed.)* 16, 292–305. doi: 10.1016/j.tics.2012.04.005

Papenberg, G., Salami, A., Persson, J., Lindenberger, U., and Bäckman, L. (2015). Genetics and functional imaging: effects of APOE, BDNF, COMT, and KIBRA in aging. *Neuropsychol. Rev.* 25, 47–62. doi: 10.1007/s11065-015-9279-8

Park, Y.-M. M., Sui, X., Liu, J., Zhou, H., Kokkinos, P. F., Lavie, C. J., et al. (2015). The effect of cardiorespiratory fitness on age-related lipids and lipoproteins. *J. Am. Coll. Cardiol.* 65, 2091–2100. doi: 10.1016/j.jacc.2015.03.517

Raz, N. (2005). "The aging brain observed in vivo: differential changes and their modifiers," in *Cognitive Neuroscience of AGING: LINKING COGNITIVE and Cerebral Aging*, eds R. Cabeza, L. Nyberg, and D. C. Park (New York, NY: Oxford University Press), 19–57.

Raz, N., Ghisletta, P., Rodrigue, K. M., Kennedy, K. M., and Lindenberger, U. (2010). Trajectories of brain aging in middle-aged and older adults: regional and individual differences. *Neuroimage* 51, 501–511. doi: 10.1016/j.neuroimage.2010.03.020

Raz, N., Lindenberger, U., Rodrigue, K. M., Kennedy, K. M., Head, D., Williamson, A., et al. (2005). Regional brain changes in aging healthy adults: general trends, individual differences and modifiers. *Cereb. Cortex* 15, 1676–1689. doi: 10.1093/cercor/bhi044

Raz, N., and Rodrigue, K. M. (2006). Differential aging of the brain: patterns, cognitive correlates and modifiers. *Neurosci. Biobehav. Rev.* 30, 730–748. doi: 10.1016/j.neubiorev.2006.07.001

Raz, N., Rodrigue, K. M., and Haacke, E. M. (2007). Brain aging and its modifiers: insights from in vivo neuromorphometry and susceptibility weighted imaging. *Ann. N. Y. Acad. Sci.* 1097, 84–93. doi: 10.1196/annals.1379.018

Raz, N., Rodrigue, K. M., Kennedy, K. M., Dahle, C., Head, D., and Acker, J. D. (2003). Differential age-related changes in the regional metencephalic volumes in humans: a 5-year follow-up. *Neurosci. Lett.* 349, 163–166. doi: 10.1016/S0304-3940(03)00820-6

Ridgway, G. R., Henley, S. M. D., Rohrer, J. D., Scahill, R. I., Warren, J. D., and Fox, N. C. (2008). Ten simple rules for reporting voxel-based morphometry studies. *Neuroimage* 40, 1429–1435. doi: 10.1016/j.neuroimage.2008.01.003

Salmond, C. H., Ashburner, J., Vargha-Khadem, F., Connelly, A., Gadian, D. G., and Friston, K. J. (2002). Distributional assumptions in voxel-based morphometry. *Neuroimage* 17, 1027–1030. doi: 10.1006/nimg.2002.1153

Salthouse, T. A. (2011). Neuroanatomical substrates of age-related cognitive decline. *Psychol. Bull.* 137, 753–784. doi: 10.1037/a0023262

Segonne, F., Dale, A. M., Busa, E., Glessner, M., Salat, D., Hahn, H. K., et al. (2004). A hybrid approach to the skull stripping problem in MRI. *Neuroimage* 22, 1060–1075. doi: 10.1016/j.neuroimage.2004.03.032

Spalding, K. L., Bergmann, O., Alkass, K., Bernard, S., Salehpour, M., Huttner, H. B., et al. (2013). Dynamics of hippocampal neurogenesis in adult humans. *Cell* 153, 1219–1227. doi: 10.1016/j.cell.2013.05.002

Thorin, E., and Thorin-Trescases, N. (2014). "Role of oxidative stress in vascular endothelial cells through aging–a double-edged sword," in *Systems Biology of Free Radicals and Antioxidants*, ed. I. Laher (Heidelberg: Springer), 1383–1403.

van Praag, H. (2008). Neurogenesis and exercise: past and future directions. *Neuromol. Med.* 10, 128–140. doi: 10.1007/s12017-008-8028-z

Verstynen, T. D., Lynch, B., Miller, D. L., Voss, M. W., Prakash, R. S., Chaddock, L., et al. (2012). Caudate nucleus volume mediates the link between cardiorespiratory fitness and cognitive flexibility in older adults. *J. Aging Res.* 2012, 939285. doi: 10.1155/2012/939285

Voss, M. W., Nagamatsu, L. S., Liu-Ambrose, T., and Kramer, A. F. (2011). Exercise, brain, and cognition across the life span. *J. Appl. Physiol. (1985)* 111, 1505–1513. doi: 10.1152/japplphysiol.00210.2011

Voss, M. W., Vivar, C., Kramer, A. F., and Van Praag, H. (2013). Bridging animal and human models of exercise-induced brain plasticity. *Trends Cogn. Sci. (Regul. Ed.)* 17, 525–544. doi: 10.1016/j.tics.2013.08.001

Washburn, R. A., Smith, K. W., Jette, A. M., and Janney, C. A. (1993). The Physical Activity Scale for the Elderly (PASE): development and evaluation. *J. Clin. Epidemiol.* 46, 153–162. doi: 10.1016/0895-4356(93)90053-4

Weinstein, A. M., Voss, M. W., Prakash, R. S., Chaddock, L., Szabo, A., White, S. M., et al. (2012). The association between aerobic fitness and executive function is mediated by prefrontal cortex volume. *Brain Behav. Immun.* 26, 811–819. doi: 10.1016/j.bbi.2011.11.008

Wenderoth, N., Debaere, F., Sunaert, S., and Swinnen, S. P. (2005). The role of anterior cingulate cortex and precuneus in the coordination of motor behaviour. *Eur. J. Neurosci.* 22, 235–246. doi: 10.1111/j.1460-9568.2005.04176.x

Whitwell, J. L. (2009). Voxel-based morphometry: an automated technique for assessing structural changes in the brain. *J. Neurosci.* 29, 9661–9664. doi: 10.1523/JNEUROSCI.2160-09.2009

Zimmerman, B., Sutton, B. P., Low, K. A., Fletcher, M. A., Tan, C. H., Schneider-Garces, N., et al. (2014). Cardiorespiratory fitness mediates the effects of aging on cerebral blood flow. *Front. Aging Neurosci.* 6:59. doi: 10.3389/fnagi.2014.00059

10

Improvements in Orientation and Balancing Abilities in Response to One Month of Intensive Slackline-Training: A Randomized Controlled Feasibility Study

Milos Dordevic[1,2]*, Anita Hökelmann[2], Patrick Müller[1], Kathrin Rehfeld[2] and Notger G. Müller[1,3]

[1] Department of Neuroprotection, German Center for Neurodegenerative Diseases, Magdeburg, Germany, [2] Institute of Sports Science, Otto von Guericke University, Magdeburg, Germany, [3] Center for Behavioral Brain Sciences, Magdeburg, Germany

Edited by:
Claudia Voelcker-Rehage, Chemnitz University of Technology, Germany

Reviewed by:
Oliver Faude, University of Basel, Switzerland
Astrid Zech, Jena University, Germany

****Correspondence:***
Milos Dordevic
milos.dordevic@dzne.de

Background: Slackline-training has been shown to improve mainly task-specific balancing skills. Non-task specific effects were assessed for tandem stance and preferred one-leg stance on stable and perturbed force platforms with open eyes. It is unclear whether transfer effects exist for other balancing conditions and which component of the balancing ability is affected. Also, it is not known whether slackline-training can improve non-visual-dependent spatial orientation abilities, a function mainly supported by the hippocampus.

Objective: To assess the effect of one-month of slackline-training on different components of balancing ability and its transfer effects on non-visual-dependent spatial orientation abilities.

Materials and Methods: Fifty subjects aged 18–30 were randomly assigned to the training group (T) (n = 25, 23.2 ± 2.5 years; 12 females) and the control group (C) (n = 25, 24.4 ± 2.8 years; 11 females). Professional instructors taught the intervention group to slackline over four consecutive weeks with three 60-min-trainings in each week. Data acquisition was performed (within 2 days) by blinded investigators at the baseline and after the training. Main outcomes Improvement in the score of a 30-item clinical balance test (CBT) developed at our institute (max. score = 90 points) and in the average error distance (in centimeters) in an orientation test (OT), a triangle completion task with walking and wheelchair conditions for 60°, 90°, and 120°.

Results: Training group performed significantly better on the closed-eyes conditions of the CBT (1.6 points, 95% CI: 0.6 to 2.6 points vs. 0.1 points, 95% CI: −1 to 1.1 points; $p = 0.011$, $\eta_p^2 = 0.128$) and in the wheelchair (vestibular) condition of the OT (21 cm, 95% CI: 8–34 cm vs. 1 cm, 95% CI: −14–16 cm; $p = 0.049$, $\eta_p^2 = 0.013$).

Conclusion: Our results indicate that one month of intensive slackline training is a novel approach for enhancing clinically relevant balancing abilities in conditions with closed eyes as well as for improving the vestibular-dependent spatial orientation capability; both of the benefits are likely caused by positive influence of slackline-training on the vestibular system function.

Keywords: balance, slackline-training, orientation, vestibular system, hippocampus

INTRODUCTION

Intact balance control is required not only to maintain postural stability but also to assure safe mobility-related activities during daily life (Mancini and Horak, 2010). Approximately 1.5% of healthcare expenditures in European countries are caused by falls, which mainly occur because of impaired balance, aging and cognitive decline (Ambrose et al., 2013); this large number does not take into account any additional indirect costs. Prevention in the earliest stages, already at young age, is hence justified. Balance and strength training is considered to be by far the most efficient intervention for fall prevention (Karlsson et al., 2013) and it can be effective for postural and neuromuscular control improvements; in addition, balance training is considered to be an effective intervention for improvement in static postural sway and dynamic balance in both athletes and non-athletes (Zech et al., 2010). Moreover, both gray and white matter alterations have been reported in young people in response to only six weeks of balance training (Taubert et al., 2010). The optimal interaction between visual, vestibular and somatosensory systems is the key to stability of the body. While the visual factor can be corrected in many different ways, the other two can be best enhanced through optimal training interventions.

Several recent studies have demonstrated particularly beneficial effect of slacklining on balancing abilities in both younger and older populations (Pfusterschmied et al., 2013; Thomas and Kalicinski, 2016), through enhancement in postural control and functional knee joint stability. Although in other studies mainly task-specific effects were found in response to six weeks of slackline training, larger non-task specific effects on postural control could not be found in these studies for only several relatively simple testing assignments, such as one-leg and tandem stance on stable force platform surface (Donath et al., 2013, 2016b); moreover, the amount of training in these studies was limited to approximately only one hour per week. Slackline length in previous studies was set to between 5 and over 15 m, which proportionally decreases the rate of turns per training, limiting thereby the stimulation of the vestibular system and its output pathways mainly to the otolith organs; in other words, important function of semicircular canals and related brain regions might have been underemployed and an additional potential effect overseen (Highstein, 1991; Cullen and Minor, 2002). Earlier research using several other types of balance-training interventions found transfer effects of training on performance in clinical tests of balance, and these tests are considered very important for both diagnostic and therapeutic purposes (Mancini and Horak, 2010). Some questions remain, however, still unanswered: (1) can slackline-training cause such non-specific transfer effects on performance in a comprehensive clinical balance test clinical balance test (CBT) and (2) what component of balancing ability, as assessed by this test, is mainly affected by slackline-training, with the vestibular component being of particular interest here.

The hippocampus and neighboring cortical regions are the main loci where the onset of Alzheimer's disease pathology occurs (Raskin et al., 2015), followed by their progressive degeneration, and early prevention treatments (in younger age) concerning this problem are strongly encouraged (Brookmeyer et al., 2007). Several previous animal and human studies have pointed towards a strong link between the vestibular system and orientation centers of the brain, considered to be located in the hippocampus and neighboring regions (Stackman et al., 2002; Russell et al., 2003; Brandt et al., 2005; Jahn et al., 2009). These studies found serious deficits in the orientation function of the temporal lobe as a result of disturbed or lost vestibular input. Many other studies also suggested that the vestibular system provides self-motion information which is important for the hippocampus and related brain regions to develop spatial memories; when this input is lost, spatial memory becomes impaired (Smith et al., 2010). Moreover, professionals who intensively make use of their vestibular system during their daily artistic performances, such as ballet/ice(Pfusterschmied et al., 2011) dancers and slackliners, have differently structured temporal brain regions, including the hippocampus, compared to non-professionals (Hüfner et al., 2011). A study by Allen et al. (2004) clearly demonstrated a reduction in vestibular-kinesthetic dependent orientation abilities with aging, by comparing performance of younger and older adults on the triangle completion task; the older adults performed particularly worse on this task when their input was restricted to the vestibular system only (passively pushed in a wheelchair), implying deterioration of this system with aging. A question that remains unanswered here is if an intensive slackline-training can lead to significant improvement in the vestibular system's function, which can then be beneficial for spatial orientation abilities in a trained person. Therefore, here we wanted to find out whether an especially challenging balance training program (learning to slackline) can also induce transfer effects on cognitive function, namely spatial orientation. The idea behind this assumption was that a) a strong connection between the vestibular system (which is important for balancing) and the hippocampus has been suggested and b) that spatial orientation is a function that is to a great extent supported by the hippocampus (Hitier et al., 2014). We chose intensive slacklining in young adults as an intervention measure under the assumption that if this training is not capable of inducing transfer effects then other, less demanding regimen (such as those typically used to enhance balancing skills in elderly, sick patients) will surely not be able to do so either. In other words, this was a feasibility pilot study, using a young population.

Thus, having in mind the close connection between the vestibular and orientation systems, we asked whether intensive slackline training can improve not only one's ability to maintain balance but also has transfer effects on the capability to successfully orientate in space. Up to this point we are not aware of any longitudinal studies that investigated whether the vestibular-dependent temporal lobe orientation function can be enhanced through an intervention aimed towards improvements in balancing skills. The goal of this study was to find out whether learning how to slackline over a period of one month can be of benefit for both stability and orientation skills.

MATERIALS AND METHODS

Ethics Statement

This study was carried out in accordance with the recommendations of and was approved by the Medical Faculty Ethics Committee at the Otto von Guericke University (approval number: 156/14). Each participant signed a document of informed consent before the beginning of the study.

Subjects

Fifty healthy young (18 to 30 years old) subjects were recruited for this study and randomly assigned (without stratification) into two groups, control (12 females and 13 males; mean age = 23.2 years; *SD* = 2.6 years) and training (11 females and 14 males; mean age = 24.4 years; SD = 2.7 years) (**Table 1**). The two groups did not significantly differ in any of the recorded demographic and other characteristics, including age, height, weight, years of education, handedness etc. Physical activity was assessed by asking subjects how many hours they spend on sports weekly on average; all sports were taken into consideration, including jogging, various team sports, cycling etc., but not walking. Participants of both groups were paid the same amount of money for their participation in the study. Sample size and characteristics, as well as the balance-training duration have been justified by several previous slackline- and other balance-training studies (Zech et al., 2010; Pfusterschmied et al., 2013).

Eligible subjects for this study were all those aged from 18 to 30 years who had no previous experience in slacklining or similar activity (i.e., highly demanding balancing activities, such as ballet dancing, rhythmic gymnastics etc.) and normal or corrected to normal vision. Exclusion criteria were injuries to the musculoskeletal system and systemic diseases (e.g., cardiovascular, metabolic, nervous system diseases etc.). Participants were recruited through advertisement in the buildings of Otto von Guericke University in Magdeburg, both at the main and medical campus.

TABLE 1 | Characteristics of participants.

Characteristic	Training (n = 25)	Control (n = 25)
Age (years)	24.5 ± 2.7	23.2 ± 2.6
Sex (females)	11 (44%)	12 (48%)
Weight (kg)	69.1 ± 12.5	65.0 ± 10.0
Height (cm)	173.4 ± 9.2	170.3 ± 8.4
Hours of activity (per week)	3.0 ± 1.8	3.2 ± 2.5
Handedness (right)	24 (96%)	23 (92%)
Profession (student)	22 (88%)	23 (92%)
Suffered a small injury (e.g., ankle sprain)	5 (20%)	5 (20%)
Ethnic origin		
• European	20 (80%)	19 (76%)
• Asian (Indian)	5 (20%)	5 (20%)
• Arabic	0 (0%)	1 (4%)

Study Design

Flow diagram of the study is shown in the **Figure 1**. This study was planned and organized as a randomized controlled single-blinded trial with factorial design (factors: time and group). Participants were randomly assigned to the training and control groups using computer-based randomization procedure[1]. The computer-based randomization and assignment of participants to groups were performed by MD (not involved in data collection), with all other investigators blinded to the outcome of the randomization.

The study consisted of measurements at two time points: baseline and one month (±2 days) after baseline. All trainings took place in the movement lab of our institute (German Center for Neurodegenerative Diseases) from February to April 2015.

Intervention

During this one month period the training group underwent intensive balance training consisting of 12 trainings (three trainings/week with each training lasting 1 h; max. 2 consecutive non-training days) on a 3-m long slackline ("Power-wave 2.0" slackline rack), whilst the control group was instructed to abstain from any type of similar activity; the abstinence from this type of activity was confirmed by control group participants at the post-test.

Trainings were led and supervised by an experienced instructor, whose assignment was to achieve the best possible skill level in the training group participants; content of teaching is shown in the **Table 2**. Minimum requirement to be achieved was set to walking forward two slackline lengths with turn at the end of the first length; each participant must have achieved this minimum requirement to be considered for the analysis, and all participants were successful in achieving this. Each training unit consisted of a 10-min warm up session and 50-min training session. Maximum group size allowed was four participants, so the instructor could dedicate enough time to each trainee. Moreover, the trainings were highly individualized, according to the skill and progression levels of each of the participant. At the end of each training session the instructor collected the information about skill progression, by writing down the achieved skill level of each participant. To do so, the amount of time every participant needed to walk up to four slackline lengths forward, backward, sideways, and turn in between was recorded.

The slackline tension was also individualized, so that when standing in the middle and applying a light vertical force (as during walking) the slackline would not get more than several centimeters away from the metal bar located 15 cm underneath. Our goal here was to increase difficulty of training by keeping the slackline slack and thus more unstable, rather than tight and stable, which would otherwise resemble walking on a firm surface. The length of the slackline was also intentionally set to 3 meters; in this way we wanted to achieve a higher rate of turns on the slackline, and thus a higher rate of semicircular canal stimulation. This is in contrast to earlier studies which used moderately to much longer slacklines (5 to over 15 m in length) (Granacher et al., 2010; Pfusterschmied et al., 2013; Donath et al., 2016b),

[1] www.randomizer.org

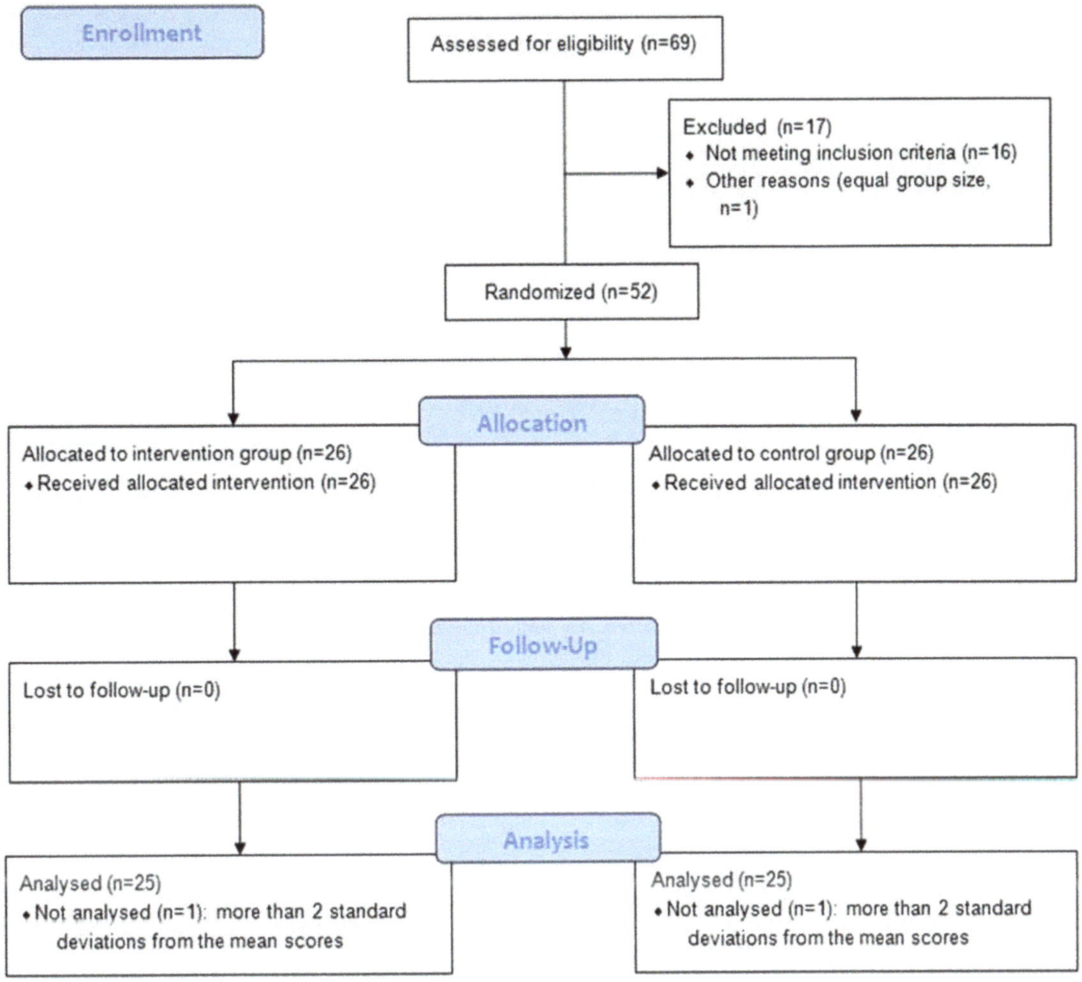

FIGURE 1 | Study flow diagram.

stimulating thereby mainly otolith organs and related central vestibular pathways.

Tests

All tests were performed by two trained members of our institute and the results of the following sets of measurements were recorded before and after the training:

TABLE 2 | Contents participants were taught during slackline-trainings; the minimum difficulty level they had to achieve in order to be considered for the final analysis is also presented.

Task	Difficulty levels/Minimum to be achieved
Stable tandem stance	5–10 s/5 s
Stable one-leg stance	5–10 s/5 s
Turn	1–4 times/2 times
Walk forward (with turn for ≥2)	1–4 lengths/2 lengths
Walk backward (with turn for ≥2)	1–4 lengths/1 length
Walk sideways (with turn for ≥2)	1–4 lengths/1 length

Clinical Balance Test

Considering that every CBT has its advantages and disadvantages (Mancini and Horak, 2010), this comprehensive test was developed by experts in our institute (DZNE) with the goal to assess different components of patients' ability to maintain equilibrium, in both standing and gait conditions. Many of the test conditions are consistent with similar comprehensive CBTs (Mancini and Horak, 2010) used in other clinics. The inter-rater reliability of the test (determined with ICC coefficient) is 0.98 ± 0.04 (SEM $= 0.003$), and its validity is still to be evaluated. The conditions can be briefly divided into standing and walking (**Figure 2**), both of which further contain sub-conditions with open and closed eyes (for detailed list of conditions see the **Table 3**).

Standing conditions include:

- two- and one-leg stance on both stable (floor) and unstable (soft pad) surfaces, with both open and closed eyes

Walking conditions included:

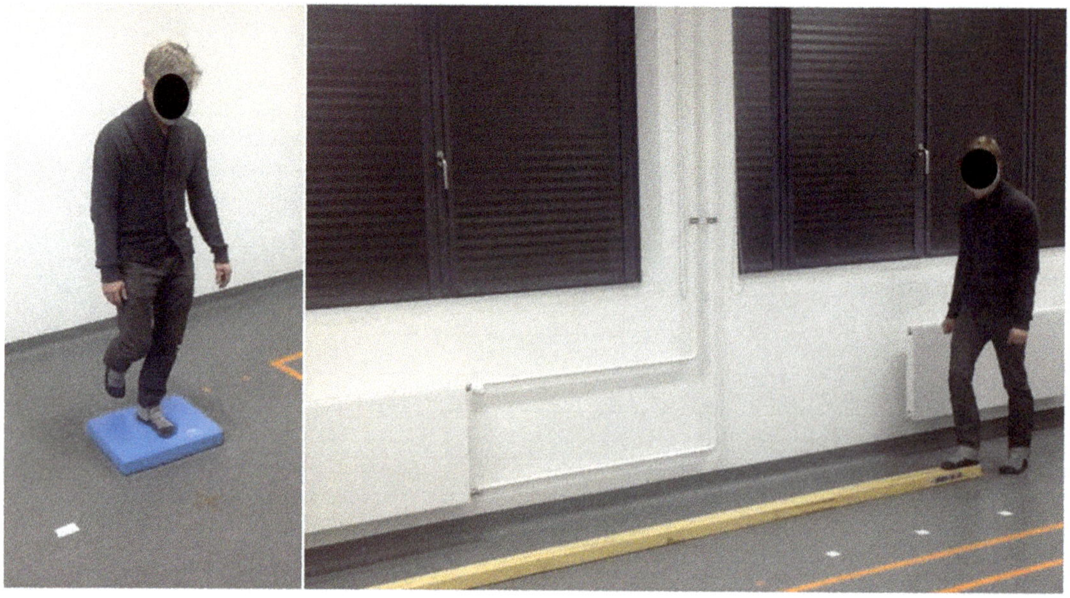

FIGURE 2 | Examples of clinical balance test (CBT) conditions: unstable surface one-leg stand (left) and balance beam walking (right) conditions.

- Walking forwards, backwards, and turning inside a 30 cm wide and 4 m long polygon with open eyes, followed by the same test on a 5 cm wide line as well as on 10 cm wide balance beam.
- Walking forward on 5 cm line with closed eyes.

In total, there are 30 assessment items within this test, 14 of which assess standing and 16 walking; 8 of all measurements are performed with closed eyes. The maximum amount of points that could be collected on the test was 90, with each condition carrying the minimum of 0 and the maximum of 3 points, similar to other comprehensive CBT batteries (Horak et al., 2009). Assessment was based on the subjective opinion of trained assessor who graded postural sway during each of the conditions; to avoid potential differences in subjective opinion between the assessors, each participant was tested by only one assessor at both pre- and post-test. In each of the standing conditions participants were instructed to maintain the required position for 15 s, whereas in walking conditions there was no time requirement and participants were asked to walk at their own pace.

Orientation Test (OT)

Orientation test was a modified version of the test described by (Allen et al., 2004), whereby the only modification was the inclusion of only three conditions (turning angles) from this study, due to time and space limitations. In brief, six triangular paths were marked on the floor of a room, three in the left and three in the right direction, giving thus three pairs of triangular paths. Lengths of the segments of each triangular path as well as the turn angles between the segments of the triangles are presented in the **Table 4**, with examples of the polygon and test conditions shown in the **Figures 3** and **4**. The test consisted of two conditions: active-walking and passive-wheelchair.

In the active-walking condition, while being guided on foot, the participant's movement was controlled by leading him or her along two sides of the triangular path as he or she held onto a wooden bar. The passive-wheelchair condition included transport along the same routes with the use of a standard wheelchair with attached footpads.

Each participant was walked (active) and pushed (passive) only once along each of the paths, giving thus 12 trials per participant in total (3 to the left and 3 to the right, times 2 conditions).

Once the participant was walked/pushed in the wheelchair along two sides of each triangle, his or her task was to walk along the third one, back to the starting point, using thus the shortest possible way back; that is, the participants were instructed not to walk back along the two sides that were used to bring them to the drop-off point, but to use the shortest possible way back to the starting point instead, which is actually always the third side of the respective triangle.

The main outcome variable was the distance error on each trial, which was assessed by marking the participant's stopping point with adhesive dots on the floor and later measuring the distance from that stopping point to the starting point, from which the respective movement was initiated. The dots were placed on the floor exactly between the feet, aiming thus for the center of pressure, by second assessor, so that the first assessor could focus on giving instructions and guiding participants. After each trial participants were led or pushed back from the stopping point to the starting point, which was for the whole test at the same location, so the next trial could begin.

For the whole duration of the test participants were blindfolded in a quiet room and thereby could not use any visual nor auditory cues that might help them in finding their way back to the starting point. It can thus be assumed that the only cues

TABLE 3 | Test conditions of the clinical balance test (CBT).

No.	Condition	Task		Points (min = 0, max = 3)			
				0	1	2	3
1.	Static – stable surface (floor)	Stand with feet together – open eyes					
2.		Stand with feet together – closed eyes					
3.		One leg stance – left – open eyes					
4.		One leg stance – right – open eyes					
5.		One leg stance – left – closed eyes					
6.		One leg stance – right – closed eyes					
7.	Static – unstable surface (pad)	Stand normally (hip width stance) – open eyes					
8.		Stand with feet together – open eyes					
9.		Stand normally (hip width stance) – closed eyes					
10.		Stand with feet together – closed eyes					
11.		One leg stance – left – open eyes					
12.		One leg stance – right – open eyes					
13.		One leg stance – left – closed eyes					
14.		One leg stance – right – closed eyes					
15.	Dynamic	Walk inside the zone (4 m × 30 cm)	Forward				
16.			Turn (90°)				
17.			Backward				
18.		Walk on the line (4 m × 5 cm)	Forward				
19.			Turn (90°)				
20.			Backward				
21.		Walk on the line with feet one after the other (4 m × 5 cm)	Forward				
22.			Turn (90°)				
23.			Backward				
24.		Walk on the beam (4 m × 10 cm)	Forward				
25.			Turn (90°)				
26.			Backward				
27.		Walk on the beam sideways (4 m × 10 cm)	Rightward				
28.			Turn (90°)				
29.			Leftward				
30.		Walk on the line with closed eyes(4 m × 5 cm)	Forward				

they could use were somatosensory and vestibular in the active-walking condition and vestibular only in the passive-wheelchair condition.

Outcome Variables and Data Analysis

Pre-specified primary outcomes were improvement in score (in points) on the CBT and decrement in average error distance (in cm) on the orientation test (OT).

TABLE 4 | Length of segments and turning angles of triangular paths in the orientation test (OT).

Direction	Turning angle (°)	Segment 1 (cm)	Segment 2 (cm)	Segment 3 (cm)
Right	60		203	201
	90	203	196	286
	120		250	377
Left	60		203	201
	90	203	196	286
	120		250	377

Data were analyzed with MatLab (Mathworks, USA) and SPSS (IBM, USA) software. Statistical analysis included paired *t*-tests for within group analyses and repeated-measures-ANOVAs with time and group as factors for between group and interaction effects analyses. The significance level was set to $\alpha = 0.05$. The descriptive results are shown as mean $\pm$ standard deviation; in addition, effect sizes (η_p^2) and 95% confidence intervals of change are reported; the effect size magnitude of $\geq$0.01 indicated small, $\geq$0.059 medium and $\geq$0.138 large effects(Cohen, 1988; Donath et al., 2013). All of the datasets were checked for normal distribution and homogeneity of variance before running parametric tests.

RESULTS

Final analysis included 25 participants in each group. Two participants (one from each group) were not considered for the analysis because of major outliers, reaching more than 2 standard deviations away from the mean score of all participants. All subjects were recruited from December 2014 until March 2015 and their characteristics are shown in the **Table 1**.

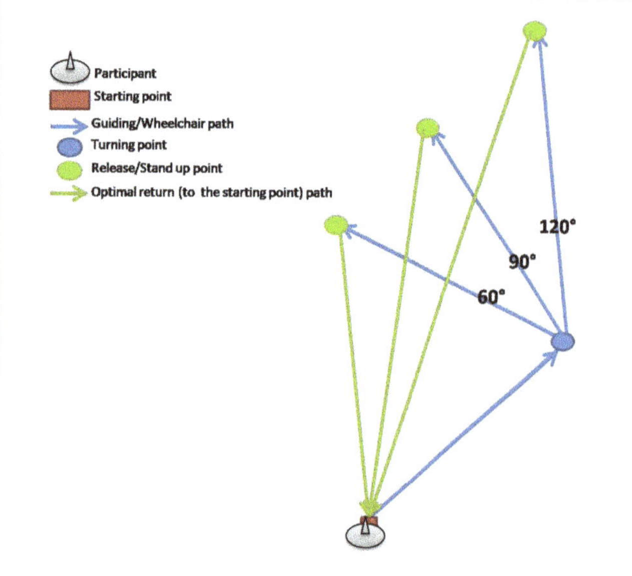

FIGURE 3 | Example of three triangular paths in right direction used for the orientation test (OT); blue arrows mark two sides of respective triangular paths along which participants where guided or pushed in a wheelchair, whereas green arrows show the optimal route for walking back to the starting point from the respective release/stand up point.

Clinical Balance Test

Figure 5 shows both results of the overall test as well as the results for closed eyes condition of the CBT; the respective significance levels are summarized in the **Table 5**.

When overall results are considered, both of the groups demonstrated pre- to post-training improvements. In the training group this improvement was on average 5.1 points (71.8 ± 5.2 to 77.0 ± 4.5) whereas in the control group it amounted to 2.4 points on average (71.1 ± 6.4 to 73.50 ± 4.4). The interaction effect here was not large enough to reach our preset significance level and the effect size was small ($p = 0.166$, $\eta_p^2 = 0.039$) (**Figure 5**; **Table 5**).

In contrast to the overall test results, when only those conditions were analyzed in which the participants had their eyes closed, a significant interaction effect with medium to large effect size was observed ($p = 0.011$, $\eta_p^2 = 0.128$), as can be seen from the **Figure 5** and **Table 5**. In these conditions the training group improved (13.7 ± 1.8 to 15.4 ± 2.2) while the control group performed slightly worse on the post-test (13.7 ± 2.6 to 13.6 ± 2.4).

The results from test conditions where participants had their eyes open did not reach significant interaction effect ($p = 0.594$). A learning effect could be observed here, with very similar improvements of about 3 points in both the training and control group (**Table 5**).

Orientation Test

Overall OT results gave a non-significant interaction effect with very small effect size ($p = 0.063$, $\eta_p^2 = 0.006$) (**Figure 6**; **Table 5**). Errors in the training group decreased by 11 cm (114 ± 68 to 103 ± 62) whereas the error in the control group increased slightly by 2 cm (111 ± 74 to 113 ± 75) (**Figure 6**; **Table 5**).

Further analysis of the wheelchair condition results revealed a much larger improvement in the training group compared to the control group; the training group improved by about 21 cm (131 ± 75 to 110 ± 63) in comparison to a very small 1 cm (121 ± 68 to 120 ± 79) improvement in the control group. This difference in improvements between the two groups that occurred over time led also to a significant interaction effect with small effect size ($p = 0.049$, $\eta_p^2 = 0.013$) (**Figure 6**; **Table 5**).

Lastly, the condition where participants were walking while actively guided over the polygon did not reveal a significant time x group interaction effect ($p = 0.591$). Within this condition of the OT the training group remained at about the same level of

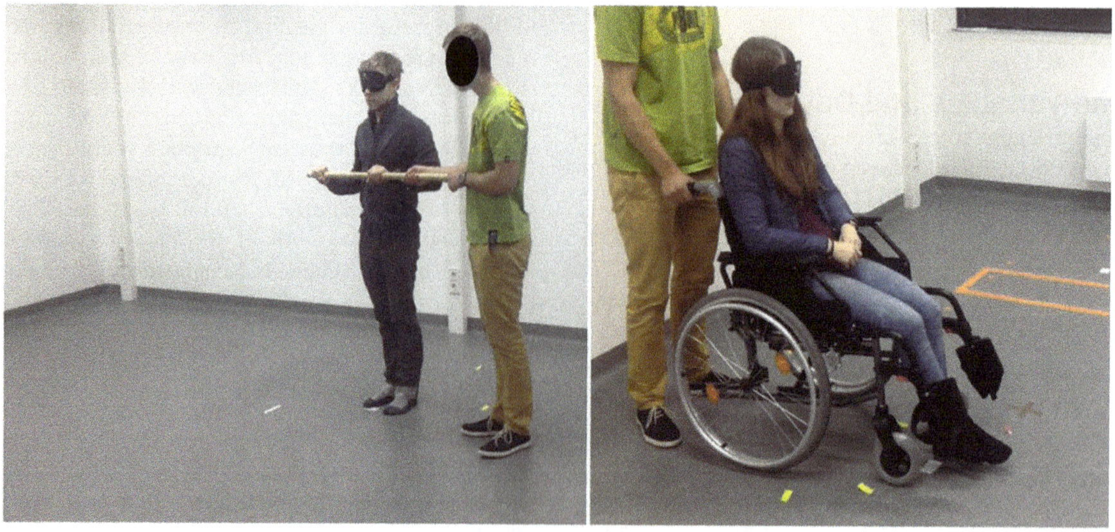

FIGURE 4 | Examples of OT conditions: guided walking (left) and wheelchair sitting (right) conditions.

TABLE 5 | Summary of mean improvements over time, interaction effects and effect sizes on CBT and OT; cm – centimeters, pts – points, *–$p < \alpha$.

Test	Condition	Mean improvements over time (95% CI)		F	p	η_p^2
		Training	Control			
CBT	All conditions	5.1pts (2.5, 7.7pts)	2.4pts (0.4, 5.3pts)	1.93	0.171	0.039
	Closed eyes	1.7pts (0.6, 2.7pts)	0.1pts (–1, 1.1pts)	7.06	0.011*	0.128
	Open eyes	3.5pts (0.9, 6.0pts)	2.5pts (0, 5.1pts)	0.20	0.594	0.004
OT	All conditions	11 cm (2, 19 cm)	–2 cm (–11, 8 cm)	3.46	0.063	0.006
	Wheelchair	21 cm (8, 34 cm)	1 cm (–14, 16 cm)	3.91	0.049*	0.013
	Walking	0 cm (–10, 10 cm)	–4cm (–16, 8 cm)	0.29	0.591	0.001

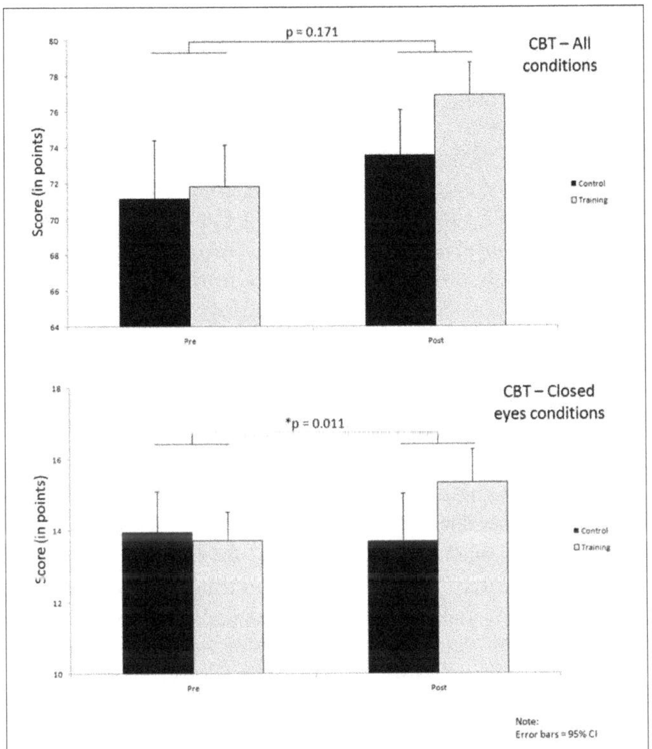

FIGURE 5 | Improvements over time in both groups on CBT, for all conditions together and closed eyes conditions only; significance levels (*p*) indicate time*group interaction effects.

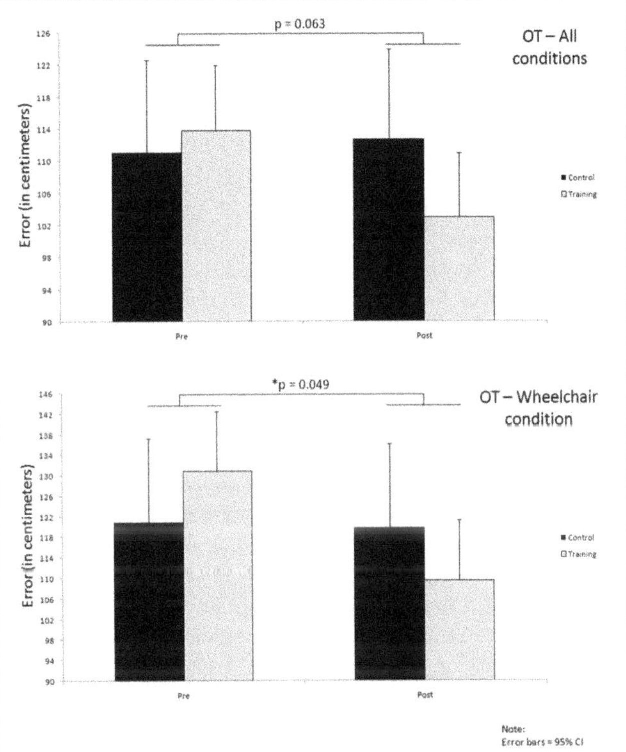

FIGURE 6 | Improvements over time in both groups on OT, for all conditions together and wheelchair condition only; significance levels (*p*) indicate time*group interaction effects.

error while the control group performed worse at the post test by about 4 cm (**Table 5**).

DISCUSSION

The main findings of this study are twofold, both of which are supportive of the a priori hypothesized improvements of vestibular system function in response to intensive balance training.

Firstly, 1 month of intensive balance training during which participants learned how to slackline, led to significantly better performance of our training group participants on the CBT compared to their control counterparts, but only on those measurements where their visual input was blocked, i.e., where they had to balance with eyes closed. The magnitude of the effect of slackline-training here was medium to large. In contrast, on tasks where visual input was not blocked, both groups improved about the same, thus revealing a potential practice effect which might have taken place between pre- and post-test. Considering that the input from three systems involved in balance maintenance is present normally in a moving person (visual, vestibular and somatosensory) (Horak, 2006), it appears from our test results that the vestibular and somatosensory systems were particularly affected by the slackline-training. Secondly and similarly to the previous finding, the training group performed significantly better on the OT compared to the control group, but again only in one condition, namely the passive-wheelchair condition (passively pushed along the designated routes). In this condition the input was intentionally limited to the vestibular system, and the performance thus depended solely on the function of the vestibular system and related brain regions which process this input. Many connections have been proposed to exist between the vestibular system and temporal lobe, in particular the hippocampus, for the purpose of processing these spatial and orientation inputs (Hitier et al., 2014). Once more, the results of the OT used in our study allow us to speculate that vestibulo-hippocampal spatial orientation function has been positively affected by the slackline-training, with a small effect size.

Many earlier studies used numerous diverse approaches to enhance balancing skills in various target groups (Zech et al., 2010; Sherrington et al., 2011). The majority of balance trainings were reported to be successful in improving outcome variables in healthy young (Zech et al., 2010) and elderly (Sherrington et al., 2011; Cadore et al., 2013; El-Khoury et al., 2015) participants, athletes (Hubscher et al., 2010; Boccolini et al., 2013), as well as patients suffering from Alzheimer's (Ries et al., 2015) and Parkinson's disease (Sehm et al., 2014), post-stroke patients (Lubetzky-Vilnai and Kartin, 2010) and patients with vestibular disorders (Porciuncula et al., 2012). A literature review pertained to our first finding (stability improvement in closed-eyes conditions of CBT) revealed that similar studies (involving slackline-training) published before suggested large task-specific improvements (standing on slackline) in response to training but only small to moderate non-task specific improvements (for meta-analytical review see (Donath et al., 2016a)). However, these studies used different training and evaluation methodologies; that is, the only non-task specific transfer effects evaluated were postural sway displacement and velocity changes, while participants stood with open eyes on a firm or suddenly perturbed flat surface of a force platform, mostly in one-leg and tandem stance modes. In contrast to these studies, for our analysis outcome from comprehensive clinical balance assessment was used, in which the standing conditions included standing on both and each leg separately (not only one by own choice) in open and closed eyes conditions, on a firm flat but also on a soft, unstable surface. In fact, our main finding here was related to the larger improvement in the closed eyes conditions, which was not even assessed by these studies; for the open-eyes conditions we could also not find any significant effects. Furthermore, our training methodology differed from that applied in previous studies in at least two points: (a) it involved more hours spent on the slackline (around 600 min vs. an average of 380 min in other studies) and was implemented on slacklines of shorter length (3 m vs. 5 to over 15 m in other studies). As we already mentioned earlier, this slackline length was intentionally chosen for the purpose of stimulating semicircular canal function, in addition to that of otolith organs; this important input (Highstein, 1991; Cullen and Minor, 2002) might have been neglected in other training interventions and its effects could hence have been overlooked. Regarding the training intensity, variation in intensity of motor training has already been shown to differentially affect the skill learning and brain structure (Sampaio-Baptista et al., 2014), an effect which could have also contributed to our results. One of previous studies investigated improvements in balancing skills with both open and closed eyes in response to 6 weeks of balance training (Strang et al., 2011). Their results from postural movement measurement were, interestingly, very similar to our results; in the eyes closed condition they noticed a significant improvement while in the eyes open condition no significant change could be observed. The authors argued that this finding was to be expected, because only imposing a constraint during test, such as blockading visual input, would allow the effects of training to emerge. Another study on basketball players also reported improvements in tests with closed eyes in response to a 6-week balance training (Zemkova and Hamar, 2010). Whereas in that study improvements were seen mainly in dynamic balance tests we found them in the static balance tests only, consisting of various conditions on stable and unstable surfaces, which might be due to methodological differences between the studies; that is, the training methods differed and only one dynamic test condition was performed with closed eyes in our CBT, whereas all the other closed eyes conditions of the CBT belonged to the static group. Since the participants improved significantly on the closed eyes conditions, this had to be to the greatest extent within the static conditions. Had, however, our test involved more dynamic conditions with closed eyes, it appears from our results that it would have been reasonable to expect a significant difference in the amount of improvement between groups there as well.

The importance of stimulating both the rotational (semicircular canal function) and the translational (otolith organs) component of the vestibular system becomes obvious and is also crucial for our second finding. Namely, this was to show that the link between the vestibular system and its central vestibular-dependent spatial-orientation brain regions, primarily hippocampal regions (Hitier et al., 2014), can be affected by an adequately designed slackline-training. No previous studies investigated this possibility, making consequently our results novel in that sense. After learning how to slackline, our participants were able to return to the starting position more precisely after being taken away from it in a wheelchair along three different triangular paths. The triangle completion task was already used by many previous studies, mainly to examine the difference between younger and older persons in their ability to navigate in space (Allen et al., 2004; Adamo et al., 2012) or to investigate functions of the medial temporal lobe (Wolbers et al., 2007; Wiener et al., 2011). Consequently, the design of these studies was cross-sectional and no particular treatment was used to improve this ability over time. Our study is the first one to our knowledge to show transfer effects of slackline-training on orientation abilities in young people assessed with this task. Several authors studied rats to demonstrate the importance of the vestibular system for successful orientating in space (Stackman and Herbert, 2002; Russell et al., 2003; Smith et al., 2005). It has been shown that peripheral vestibular deficiency leads to impairments in functioning of the medial temporal lobe in spatial orientation tasks as well as in spatial learning. These impairments are due to alterations in electrophysiological and neurochemical signaling between the two systems. Other previous studies went on further to investigate the importance of the vestibular system for orientation in humans (Brandt et al., 2005; Hüfner et al., 2011; Previc et al., 2014), thereby confirming the findings of animal studies. The structure of the hippocampal formation has been found to be altered in persons who suffer from vestibular deficiency, but also in persons who need to rely heavily on their vestibular system because of their profession, for example ballet dancers. It has even been proposed that vestibular system degeneration might be a significant contributor to development of the Alzheimer's disease (Previc, 2013). Although our study sample consisted of young and healthy subjects, considering neuroplasticity principles in response to motor task learning over the entire lifespan (Dayan and Cohen, 2011), it is legitimate to hypothesize that similar results could be expected in older populations, particularly as a prevention strategy in those at early stages of dementia. Some studies could not find significant relevant transfer effects of slackline-training in this population (Donath et al., 2016b), but, as discussed earlier, the methodological issues might have contributed to such findings; in our opinion additional research on this topic is required to answer this question.

Therefore, as far as the external validity or generalizability of our findings is concerned, our sample consisted of young and healthy (18–30 years old) subjects, and the results are thus mostly applicable to the same population. Considering, however, that many balance-training interventions can benefit both healthy and diseased populations of various ages in their original form (Taubert et al., 2010; Sehm et al., 2014), it is reasonable to assume that similar interventions to that used in our study could be beneficial for healthy older or even non-healthy older populations, in the direction obtained with our younger sample. It would be of a particular interest for us to see if similar interventions would demonstrate a significant gain in patients suffering from various stages of neurodegeneration, from those with mild cognitive impairment to those with Alzheimer's disease, in whom the spatial orientation capabilities are considerably reduced (Allen et al., 2004).

There are several limitations of our study which we would like to list here. First, our CBT has not yet been validated; however, many of its items resemble those applied in other validated CBTs and its inter-rater reliability is very high. Another argument against could be that the subjective nature of our postural sway assessment is less accurate than the quantitative assessments at force platforms; most CBTs, however, are subjective opinion-based tests, but are comprehensive and specifically designed to assess various components of balancing abilities, and remain important and valid assessment tools for this purpose (Mancini and Horak, 2010). Our OT comes from the extensively used triangle completion test that assesses orientation abilities; still, only a subset of conditions was applied in our study, in accordance with availability of facilities at our institute; although the error distance measurement has been performed thoroughly, reliability data is still to be provided. Secondly, we did not report any follow up results which would signify a potential of this training to cause eventual retention of the achieved effects over a longer period of subsequent inactivity. Third limitation can be considered the fact that we yet have to show neural correlates of our behavioral improvements, by analyzing pre/post MR data. Finally, our participants performed the training with open eyes; it would be interesting to know whether the same training performed with closed eyes would bring any different results, compared to both the control group and the actual training group, since in this third group visual input would be blocked. We will attempt to successfully deal with these limitations in our future work.

CONCLUSION

Our results indicate that 1 month of intensive balance training, through learning how to slackline, is a successful novel approach for enhancing clinically relevant balancing abilities in conditions with closed eyes and simultaneous improvements in vestibular-dependent spatial orientation capability; both of the benefits are possibly caused by positive influence of slackline-training on vestibular system function, and possibly its connectivity with temporal lobe regions responsible for orienting in space, such as the hippocampus. We can highly recommend this method, both its intensity and type, to all young persons who need to improve functioning of their vestibular system, either for the purpose of increasing stability, upgrading spatial orientation abilities or both. Modifying the training protocol could be also potentially of advantage for healthy elderly and those at risk of neurodegeneration of the medial temporal lobe orientation-system, such as in AD, but this is yet to be proven by future studies.

AUTHOR CONTRIBUTIONS

MD: Study planning and organization, data collection, data analysis, paper writing, paper revision, paper submission. AH: Study planning and organization, paper revision. PM: Data collection, paper revision. KR: Study planning and organization, paper revision. NM: Study planning and organization, data analysis, paper writing, paper revision.

REFERENCES

Adamo, D. E., Briceño, E. M., Sindone, J. A., Alexander, N. B., and Moffat, S. D. (2012). Age differences in virtual environment and real world path integration. *Front. Aging Neurosci* 4:26. doi: 10.3389/fnagi.2012.00026

Allen, G. L., Kirasic, K. C., Rashotte, M. A., and Haun, D. B. M. (2004). Aging and path integration skill: kinesthetic and vestibular contributions to wayfinding. *Percept. Psychophys.* 66, 170–179. doi: 10.3758/BF0319 4870

Ambrose, A. F., Paul, G., and Hausdorff, J. M. (2013). Risk factors for falls among older adults: a review of the literature. *Maturitas* 75, 51–61. doi: 10.1016/j.maturitas.2013.02.009

Boccolini, G., Brazzit, A., Bonfanti, L., and Alberti, G. (2013). Using balance training to improve the performance of youth basketball players. *Sport Sci. Health* 9, 37–42. doi: 10.1007/s11332-013-0143-z

Brandt, T., Schautzer, F., Hamilton, D. A., Brüning, R., Markowitsch, H. J., Kalla, R., et al. (2005). Vestibular loss causes hippocampal atrophy and impaired spatial memory in humans. *Brain* 128, 2732–2741. doi: 10.1093/brain/awh617

Brookmeyer, R., Johnson, E., Ziegler-Graham, K., and Arrighi, H. M. (2007). Forecasting the global burden of Alzheimer's disease. *Alzheimers Dement.* 3, 186–191. doi: 10.1016/j.jalz.2007.04.381

Cadore, E. L., Rodríguez-Mañas, L., Sinclair, A., and Izquierdo, M. (2013). Effects of different exercise interventions on risk of falls, gait ability, and balance in physically frail older adults: a systematic review. *Rejuvenation Res.* 16, 105–114. doi: 10.1089/rej.2012.1397

Cohen, J. (1988). *Statistical Power Analysis for the Behavioral Sciences*, 2nd Edn. Cambridge, MA: Academic Press, doi: 10.1234/12345678

Cullen, K. E., and Minor, L. B. (2002). Semicircular canal afferents similarly encode active and passive head-on-body rotations: implications for the role of vestibular efference. *J. Neurosci.* 22:RC226.

Dayan, E., and Cohen, L. G. (2011). Neuroplasticity subserving motor skill learning. *Neuron* 72, 443–454. doi: 10.1016/j.neuron.2011.10.008

Donath, L., Roth, R., Rueegge, A., Groppa, M., Zahner, L., and Faude, O. (2013). Effects of slackline training on balance, jump performance & muscle activity in young children. *Int. J. Sports Med.* 34, 1093–1098. doi: 10.1055/s-0033-1337949

Donath, L., Roth, R., Zahner, L., and Faude, O. (2016a). Slackline training (Balancing Over Narrow Nylon Ribbons) and balance performance: a meta-analytical review. *Sports Med.* doi: 10.1007/s40279-016-0631-9 [Epub ahead of print].

Donath, L., Roth, R., Zahner, L., and Faude, O. (2016b). Slackline training and neuromuscular performance in seniors: a randomized controlled trial. *Scand. J. Med. Sci. Sports* 26, 275–283. doi: 10.1111/sms.12423

El-Khoury, F., Cassou, B., Latouche, A., Aegerter, P., Charles, M.-A., and Dargent-Molina, P. (2015). Effectiveness of two year balance training programme on prevention of fall induced injuries in at risk women aged 75-85 living in community: ossébo randomised controlled trial. *BMJ* 351:h3830. doi: 10.1136/bmj.h3830

Granacher, U., Iten, N., Roth, R., and Gollhofer, A. (2010). Slackline training for balance and strength promotion. *Int. J. Sports Med.* 31, 717–723. doi: 10.1055/s-0030-1261936

Highstein, S. M. (1991). The central nervous system efferent control of the organs of balance and equilibrium. *Neurosci. Res.* 12, 13–30. doi: 10.1016/0168-0102(91)90096-H

Hitier, M., Besnard, S., and Smith, P. F. (2014). Vestibular pathways involved in cognition. *Front. Integr. Neurosci.* 8:59. doi: 10.3389/fnint.2014.00059

Horak, F. B. (2006). Postural orientation and equilibriumL What do we need to know about neural control of balance to prevent falls? *Age Ageing* 35, (Suppl. 2), ii7–ii11.

Horak, F. B., Wrisley, D. M., Frank, J., Horak, F. B., and Wrisley, D. M. (2009). The balance evaluation systems test (BESTest) to differentiate balance deficits. *Phys. Ther.* 89, 484–498. doi: 10.2522/ptj.20080071

Hubscher, M., Zech, A., Pfeifer, K., Hansel, F., Vogt, L., and Banzer, W. (2010). Neuromuscular training for sports injury prevention: a systematic review. *Med. Sci. Sports Exerc.* 42, 413–421. doi: 10.1249/MSS.0b013e3181b88d37

Hüfner, K., Binetti, C., Hamilton, D. A., Stephan, T., Flanagin, V. L., Linn, J., et al. (2011). Structural and functional plasticity of the hippocampal formation in professional dancers and slackliners. *Hippocampus* 21, 855–865. doi: 10.1002/hipo.20801

Jahn, K., Wagner, J., Deutschländer, A., Kalla, R., Hüfner, K., Stephan, T., et al. (2009). Human hippocampal activation during stance and locomotion: FMRI study on healthy, blind, and vestibular-loss subjects. *Ann. N. Y. Acad. Sci.* 1164, 229–235. doi: 10.1111/j.1749-6632.2009.03770.x

Karlsson, M. K., Vonschewelov, T., Karlsson, C., Cöster, M., and Rosengen, B. E. (2013). Prevention of falls in the elderly: a review. *Scand. J. Public Health* 41, 442–454. doi: 10.1177/1403494813483215

Lubetzky-Vilnai, A., and Kartin, D. (2010). The effect of balance training on balance performance in individuals poststroke: a systematic review. *J. Neurol. Phys. Ther.* 34, 127–137. doi: 10.1097/NPT.0b013e3181ef764d

Mancini, M., and Horak, F. B. (2010). The relevance of clinical balance assessment tools to differentiate balance deficits. *Eur. J. Phys. Rehabil. Med.* 46, 239–248.

Pfusterschmied, J., Buchecker, M., Keller, M., Wagner, H., Taube, W., and Müller, E. (2011). Supervised slackline training improves postural stability. *Eur. J. Sport Sci.* 13, 1–9. doi: 10.1080/17461391.2011.583991

Pfusterschmied, J., Stöggl, T., Buchecker, M., Lindinger, S., Wagner, H., and Müller, E. (2013). Effects of 4-week slackline training on lower limb joint motion and muscle activation. *J. Sci. Med. Sports* 16, 562–566. doi: 10.1016/j.jsams.2012.12.006

Porciuncula, F., Johnson, C. C., and Glickman, L. B. (2012). The effect of vestibular rehabilitation on adults with bilateral vestibular hypofunction: a systematic review. *J. Vestib. Res.* 22, 283–298. doi: 10.3233/VES-120464

Previc, F. H. (2013). Vestibular loss as a contributor to Alzheimer's disease. *Med. Hypotheses* 80, 360–367. doi: 10.1016/j.mehy.2012.12.023

Previc, F. H., Krueger, W. W., Ross, R. A., Roman, M. A., and Siegel, G. (2014). The relationship between vestibular function and topographical memory in older adults. *Front. Integr. Neurosci.* 8:46. doi: 10.3389/fnint.2014.00046

Raskin, J., Cummings, J., Hardy, J., Schuh, K., and Dean, R. A. (2015). Neurobiology of Alzheimer's Disease: integrated molecular, physiological, anatomical, biomarker, and cognitive dimensions. *Curr. Alzheimer Res.* 12, 712–722. doi: 10.2174/1567205012666150701103107

Ries, J. D., Hutson, J., Maralit, L. A., and Brown, M. B. (2015). Group balance training specifically designed for individuals with Alzheimer Disease : impact on berg balance scale, timed up and go, gait speed, and mini-mental status examination. *J. Geriatr. Phys. Ther.* 37, 1–11. doi: 10.1519/JPT.0000000000000030

Russell, N. A., Horii, A., Smith, P. F., Darlington, C. L., and Bilkey, D. K. (2003). Long-term effects of permanent vestibular lesions on hippocampal spatial firing. *J. Neurosci.* 23, 6490–6498.

Sampaio-Baptista, C., Scholz, J., Jenkinson, M., Thomas, A. G., Filippini, N., Smit, G., et al. (2014). Gray matter volume is associated with rate of subsequent skill learning after a long term training intervention. *Neuroimage* 96, 158–166. doi: 10.1016/j.neuroimage.2014.03.056

Sehm, B., Taubert, M., Conde, V., Weise, D., Classen, J., Dukart, J., et al. (2014). Structural brain plasticity in parkinson's disease induced by balance training. *Neurobiol. Aging* 35, 232–239. doi: 10.1016/j.neurobiolaging.2013.06.021

Sherrington, C., Tiedemann, A., Fairhall, N., Close, J. C. T., and Lord, S. R. (2011). Exercise to prevent falls in older adults: an updated meta-analysis and best practice recommendations. *N. S. W. Public Health Bull.* 22, 78–83. doi: 10.1071/NB10056

Smith, P. F., Darlington, C. L., and Zheng, Y. (2010). Move it or lose it–is stimulation of the vestibular system necessary for normal spatial memory? *Hippocampus* 20, 36–43. doi: 10.1002/hipo.20588

Smith, P. F., Horii, A., Russell, N., Bilkey, D. K., Zheng, Y., Liu, P., et al. (2005). The effects of vestibular lesions on hippocampal function in rats. *Prog. Neurobiol.* 75, 391–405. doi: 10.1016/j.pneurobio.2005.04.004

Stackman, R. W., Clark, A. S., and Taube, J. S. (2002). Hippocampal spatial representations require vestibular input. *Hippocampus* 12, 291–303. doi: 10.1002/hipo.1112

Stackman, R. W., and Herbert, A. M. (2002). Rats with lesions of the vestibular system require a visual landmark for spatial navigation. *Behav. Brain Res.* 128, 27–40. doi: 10.1016/S0166-4328(01)00270-4

Strang, A. J., Haworth, J., Hieronymus, M., Walsh, M., and Smart, L. J. (2011). Structural changes in postural sway lend insight into effects of balance training, vision, and support surface on postural control in a healthy population. *Eur. J. Appl. Physiol.* 111, 1485–1495. doi: 10.1007/s00421-010-1770-6

Taubert, M., Draganski, B., Anwander, A., Müller, K., Horstmann, A., Villringer, A., et al. (2010). Dynamic properties of human brain structure: learning-related changes in cortical areas and associated fiber connections. *J. Neurosci.* 30, 11670–11677. doi: 10.1523/JNEUROSCI.2567-10.2010

Thomas, M., and Kalicinski, M. (2016). The effects of slackline balance training on postural control in older adults. *J. Aging Phys. Act.* 24, 393–398. doi: 10.1123/japa.2015-0099

Wiener, J. M., Berthoz, A., and Wolbers, T. (2011). Dissociable cognitive mechanisms underlying human path integration. *Exp. Brain Res.* 208, 61–71. doi: 10.1007/s00221-010-2460-7

Wolbers, T., Wiener, J. M., Mallot, H. A., and Büchel, C. (2007). Differential recruitment of the hippocampus, medial prefrontal cortex, and the human motion complex during path integration in humans. *J. Neurosci.* 27, 9408–9416. doi: 10.1523/JNEUROSCI.2146-07.2007

Zech, A., Hübscher, M., Vogt, L., Banzer, W., Hänsel, F., and Pfeifer, K. (2010). Balance training for neuromuscular control and performance enhancement: a systematic review. *J. Athl. Train.* 45, 392–403. doi: 10.4085/1062-6050-45.4.392

Zemkova, E., and Hamar, D. (2010). The effect of 6-week combined agility-balance training on neuromuscular performance in basketball players. *J. Sports Med. Phys. Fitness* 50, 262–267.

11

Near-Infrared Spectroscopy-Based Frontal Lobe Neurofeedback Integrated in Virtual Reality Modulates Brain and Behavior in Highly Impulsive Adults

Justin Hudak[1]*, Friederike Blume[1], Thomas Dresler[1,2], Florian B. Haeussinger[2], Tobias J. Renner[3], Andreas J. Fallgatter[1,2,4], Caterina Gawrilow[1,5,6] and Ann-Christine Ehlis[1,2]

[1] LEAD Graduate School & Research Network, University of Tübingen, Tübingen, Germany, [2] Department of Psychiatry and Psychotherapy, University Hospital Tübingen, Tübingen, Germany, [3] Department of Child and Adolescence Psychiatry, University Hospital Tübingen, Tübingen, Germany, [4] Center for Integrative Neuroscience, University of Tübingen, Tübingen, Germany, [5] Department of Psychology, University of Tübingen, Tübingen, Germany, [6] Center for Individual Development and Adaptive Education of Children at Risk, Goethe University Frankfurt, Frankfurt, Germany

Edited by:
Soledad Ballesteros,
Universidad Nacional de Educación a Distancia (UNED), Spain

Reviewed by:
Sabrina Brigadoi,
University of Padua, Italy
Hasan Ayaz,
Drexel University, United States

***Correspondence:**
Justin Hudak
justin.hudak@lead.uni-tuebingen.de

Based on neurofeedback (NF) training as a neurocognitive treatment in attention-deficit/hyperactivity disorder (ADHD), we designed a randomized, controlled functional near-infrared spectroscopy (fNIRS) NF intervention embedded in an immersive virtual reality classroom in which participants learned to control overhead lighting with their dorsolateral prefrontal brain activation. We tested the efficacy of the intervention on healthy adults displaying high impulsivity as a sub-clinical population sharing common features with ADHD. Twenty participants, 10 in an experimental and 10 in a shoulder muscle-based electromyography control group, underwent eight training sessions across 2 weeks. Training was bookended by a pre- and post-test including go/no-go, n-back, and stop-signal tasks (SST). Results indicated a significant reduction in commission errors on the no-go task with a simultaneous increase in prefrontal oxygenated hemoglobin concentration for the experimental group, but not for the control group. Furthermore, the ability of the subjects to gain control over the feedback parameter correlated strongly with the reduction in commission errors for the experimental, but not for the control group, indicating the potential importance of learning feedback control in moderating behavioral outcomes. In addition, participants of the fNIRS group showed a reduction in reaction time variability on the SST. Results indicate a clear effect of our NF intervention in reducing impulsive behavior possibly via a strengthening of frontal lobe functioning. Virtual reality additions to conventional NF may be one way to improve the ecological validity and symptom-relevance of the training situation, hence positively affecting transfer of acquired skills to real life.

Keywords: NIRS, neurofeedback, virtual reality, impulsivity, ADHD

INTRODUCTION

Impulsivity refers to the inability to inhibit behavioral responses to urges created by external stimuli as well as internal desires, often brought about by the current environment. It is a ubiquitous behavioral trait found in healthy individuals as well as those with developmental disorders such as attention-deficit/hyperactivity disorder (ADHD), substance-use disorders, binge eating disorders, and others (Whiteside and Lynam, 2001; Bari and Robbins, 2013). Individual impulsive episodes, such as drunk driving, can negatively impact the lives of the impulsive individual, as well as the lives of others. On neuropsychological tasks, impulsive behavior is associated with certain types of errors, typically on conditions requiring inhibitory control. For example, the more impulsive an individual is, the more commission errors [i.e., false alarms (FA)] they make on go/no-go tasks (Aichert et al., 2012; Weidacker et al., 2016). Impulsive subgroups such as binge eaters (Hege et al., 2014) and binge drinkers (Henges and Marczinski, 2012) also make more FA than healthy controls.

From a neuroscientific perspective, impulsivity is strongly linked with dysfunctional frontal lobe activity and frontal lobe excisions (Fallgatter and Herrmann, 2001; Bari and Robbins, 2013). Development of impulse control is the result of maturation of the cognitive control network (CCN; Casey et al., 2008; Steinberg, 2008; in Shulman et al., 2016) which consists of the lateral prefrontal cortex and its connectivity with other frontal, striatal, motoric, and parietal regions (for comprehensive reviews see Cubillo et al., 2012; Rubia et al., 2013). Highly impulsive subgroups require a stronger activation of the CCN than healthy controls to achieve comparable response inhibition (Horn et al., 2003; Ding et al., 2014). Additionally, evidence for negative correlations between trait impulsiveness and activation as well as connectivity in prefrontal brain structures has been provided (Farr et al., 2012). Furthermore, there is evidence that the bilateral dorsolateral prefrontal cortex (dlPFC) may be involved in inhibitory control as transcranial direct current stimulation (tDCS) of the left dlPFC led to improved inhibitory control on a go/no-go task in participants with ADHD (Soltaninejad et al., 2015).

Neurofeedback (NF), a therapeutic technique in which participants are tasked with regulating their own brain activity, is used as a way to effect long-term change in abnormal brain activity (Arns et al., 2013). Thereby, electroencephalography (EEG)-based NF protocols have shown promise in reducing impulsive symptoms in ADHD (Gevensleben et al., 2012, 2014a). However, these protocols have had mixed effects, particularly as they are often based on brain-frequency imbalances that are highly heterogeneous within subjects (Holtmann et al., 2014). A recently emerging NF protocol for ADHD using functional near-infrared spectroscopy (fNIRS) to measure the blood oxygenation level dependent (BOLD) response within the dlPFC has several potential advantages over traditional EEG protocols (Marx et al., 2015).

Compared to EEG, fNIRS has improved spatial resolution and better correspondence of channel to underlying brain region, as well as reduced sensitivity to movement-based artifacts, making it ideal for NF training of circumscribed brain areas in motorically restless individuals (e.g., ADHD patients, children, etc.). Furthermore, evidence from BOLD-based NF paradigms suggest that they yield effects faster than their EEG-based counterparts. In a pilot study with children with ADHD, significant symptom improvements were found after only 12 sessions of fNIRS-based dlPFC training (Marx et al., 2015). Sherwood et al. (2016) found that – in healthy subjects – achieving control of the BOLD response in the dlPFC is possible after just five sessions of real-time functional magnetic resonance imaging (fMRI) NF training. Current EEG protocols, on the other hand, require between 25 and 50 sessions to realize significant effects (for a review and meta-analysis see Begemann et al., 2016). However, despite the promise of BOLD-based protocols as a potential treatment for impulsivity, such protocols still need to translate from laboratory to real-world settings.

Neurofeedback treatment is often criticized for its lack of ecological validity. Simply put, strategies of brain regulation learned in a lab setting may not translate well into the real world. Those with impulsivity struggle in the classroom where academic achievement is negatively correlated to impulsivity severity (Spinella and Miley, 2003). Therefore, any effective strategies developed in NF therapy should ultimately be applied in the classroom (or a similar real-world) setting, a concept known as transfer (e.g., Strehl, 2014). However, NF protocols – at this point – cannot be utilized in a real scholastic setting as they require large and delicate equipment, and students need to concentrate on the current lesson. An increasingly viable option, virtual reality (VR), has been used for assessment of clinical symptoms of ADHD in the classroom (Muhlberger et al., 2016) and with an EEG-based NF protocol designed to reduce inattentive and impulsive behavior in adolescents displaying behavioral problems (Cho et al., 2004). In the latter study, the VR group showed the greatest improvement following NF training on attention-related tasks relative to both a control group and a 2-D classroom group, but no difference in impulsivity. However, this study was controlled with a waiting group, thus not ruling out non-specific effects of NF training, such as continuous performance monitoring, reinforcement of compliance, and the idea that one is being treated by a sophisticated technology and professional (Gevensleben et al., 2012, 2014b). Furthermore, the NF was a separate module, not incorporated into the experience of the class itself.

Based on these findings, we developed a virtual classroom-based fNIRS NF protocol (for study design see Blume et al., 2017) in order to directly facilitate transfer of NF training effects to the classroom. Importantly, feedback is delivered in the form of gentle dimming or brightening of the overhead lighting which does not distract the participant from the experience of being in a classroom. In the present study, we implement a 2 week accelerated protocol in highly impulsive young adults, consisting of eight training sessions (one per day) which were bookended by a pre- and a post-test to assess behavioral changes during a go/no-go, n-back, and stop-signal task (SST). Changes in frontal lobe function were also assessed during the go/no-go and n-back tasks using fNIRS. To control for the previously mentioned non-specific effects of the NF training, we used bilateral musculi supraspinatus-based electromyography (EMG) biofeedback (BF) (see Marx et al., 2015; Mayer et al., 2015). This method has been successfully used in the aforementioned studies as a control for NIRS-based NF. Sham-based NF control groups (e.g., targeting putatively unrelated brain areas) invite ethical concerns, as training random areas may have unforeseeable negative effects on the participant, who is often recruited on the premise that the training will be helpful to their condition (Holtmann et al., 2014). Furthermore, participants sometimes become aware that they are part of some sham conditions (particularly if the sham feedback contains data completely unrelated to the current training situation, e.g., training data of another participant), or even assume they are part of one when they are not, leading to both drop-outs and reduced motivation, a critical aspect for any successful NF training (Birbaumer et al., 1991; Gevensleben et al., 2014a). As we did not explicitly inform participants that EMG BF was a control condition, they were less susceptible to this motivation loss.

We hypothesize that the fNIRS-based NF group will show an improvement in dlPFC activity during the cognitive tasks (go/no-go and n-back) relative to the EMG-based control group following the treatment program. We also expect the NF group to show a reduction in FA (go/no-go task) as well as reduced stop-signal reaction time (SSRT) on the SST from pre- to post-test measurement (as measures of response inhibition). As secondary outcomes, we expect reaction time (RT) and RT variability [standard deviation of the reaction time (SDRT)] to decrease for the NF group on all tasks, as the dlPFC plays a role in a multitude of executive functions. The expected neurocognitive improvements following frontal lobe focused fNIRS-based NF in a virtual training environment would confirm the general feasibility of a combination of NF with virtual training scenarios which could – in the long run – increase the ecological validity of NF interventions.

MATERIALS AND METHODS

Participants

We recruited 22 students from the University of Tübingen out of a larger group of potential participants who had completed the Barratt Impulsiveness Scale (BIS; Barratt, 1959) using an online format. Based on their high BIS scores (M_{BIS} = 85.75, SD_{BIS} = 9.36), these students were selected and invited to an in-person screening for ADHD [according to criteria from the Diagnostic and Statistical Manual of Mental Disorders (DSM-IV-TR; Sass et al., 2003)] using two subtests from the Homburger ADHD Scale for Adults (HASE; Rösler et al., 2008), the German versions of the Wender Utah Rating Scale (WURS-K) and the ADHD-Self Assessment Scale (ADHS-SB). Participants meeting the criteria for an indication of ADHD under this context (WURS-K > 30 and ADHS-SB > 18) were excluded from the study and informed about the outpatient ADHD program at the Department of Psychiatry and Psychotherapy at the University Hospital Tübingen ($n = 1$). The remaining participants ($n = 21$; nine female, $M_{Age} = 23.4$, $SD_{Age} = 2.8$) reported no history of serious or chronic illness, neurological, or psychiatric disorders.

This study was approved by the Ethics Committee of the Medical Faculty of the University and the University Hospital of Tübingen and all procedures were in accordance with the Helsinki Declaration of 1975, as revised in 2013. Participants provided written informed consent and were compensated with 100 Euros for completing the duration of the training including pre- and post-measurements (10 sessions, 1 h each, over 2 weeks). One participant dropped out of the study due to feeling ill from the VR and was payed pro-rata of 10 Euro per hour participated.

Study Design

The study followed a randomized, controlled experimental design. Participants were randomized (10 participants in each group) to either eight fNIRS-based NF (experimental) or eight EMG-based BF (control) sessions taking course daily over two weeks (Tuesday to Friday in the first week, Monday to Thursday in the second week). We randomized without stratifying for any other variables. Groups did not differ significantly in gender (NF: 4 female, 6 male; BF: 5 female, 5 male; Fisher's exact test, $p = 0.50$), or in age ($M_{BF} = 22.9$, $SD = 2.88$; $M_{NF} = 23.9$, $SD = 2.77$; $t(18) = 0.80$, $p = 0.44$). The pre-test and post-test were exactly the same and included a go/no-go task, an n-back task, and an SST. The pre-test took place on the Monday of the first week, while the post-test occurred on the Friday of the second week. Order of the pre- and post-test measures was counter-balanced between subjects.

Virtual Classroom Scenario

The participants were seated and wore the Oculus Rift (Oculus Rift, United States[1]) VR head-mounted display (HMD). The HMD rendered a virtual classroom developed by KatanaSim (KatanaSim, Germany[2]) with animated students and a teacher. The participants' point of view was seated first-person, facing the teacher (**Figure 1**). The participant had a full 360° view from the desk seat, with other students seated nearby. The task was to control the brightness of the lighting in the classroom. When an upward-pointing arrow was shown on the chalkboard, the participant was required to "activate" in order to make the light brighter. When the arrow pointed downward, the participant was required to "deactivate" in order to make the light darker. Briefly, activation requires higher output compared to baseline from the respective feedback source, while deactivation requires reduced output compared to baseline (see below for more details on fNIRS and EMG activation/deactivation protocols). Importantly, participants were not told, in either condition, how to regulate the lighting in the classroom, they were instructed simply to try to increase the lighting in the room when the arrow pointed upward and to decrease the lighting when the arrow pointed downward. In this way, only the positive or negative feedback they received from the scenario should have enforced their learning of the feedback parameter. The probability that a trial was activation (arrow up) was 50% in sessions 1–4 and 80% in sessions 5–8. More activation was encouraged in the second half of the scenario, as more upregulation of the prefrontal cortex is

[1] www.oculusvr.com

[2] www.katanasim.com

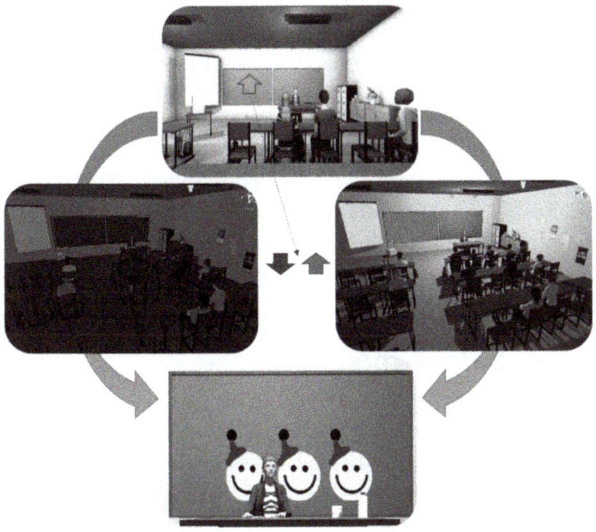

FIGURE 1 | The virtual reality classroom scenario. The top image depicts the view from the participant's head-mounted display (HMD). An arrow pointing either up or down was displayed on the chalkboard. If the arrow pointed downward, the participant should decrease the lighting in the classroom. If it pointed up, the participant should increase the lighting in the classroom. If the participant performed the task adequately, they would receive one to three smileys, presented on the chalkboard, based on the duration of success.

associated with stronger inhibitory control (Rubia et al., 2013; Soltaninejad et al., 2015). Participants were confronted with distractions within the scenario (e.g., students turning around or cell phones ringing) from the second half of each session until the end.

Before each trial, a baseline and threshold of light fluctuation were calculated to determine the point at which the classroom light was balanced between fully bright and fully dark and the range within which it could fluctuate. Following successful activation or deactivation – when the signal was 60, 70, or 80% of the time above or below the baseline, respectively – the participant was rewarded with one, two, or three smiley faces, respectively, on the chalkboard.

Each session was comprised of three blocks, the first and the last being 12 min in length while the second, the transfer block, was 8 min. In the transfer block, the light's brightness was fixed, meaning that the only feedback came at the end of each trial. Trial number and length varied depending on the feedback source and will be discussed in the following sections.

fNIRS

Functional near-infrared spectroscopy records change in oxygenated (O_2Hb) and deoxygenated (HHb) hemoglobin relative to a baseline; the amount of local O_2Hb infers the amount of local brain activation, via the process of hemodyamic coupling, wherein increases of cortical activation lead to increases in O_2Hb and decreases in HHb (Haeussinger et al., 2014). The ETG-4000 continuous Optical Topography System (Hitachi Medical Co., Japan) was used for pre- and post-tests as well as NF sessions.

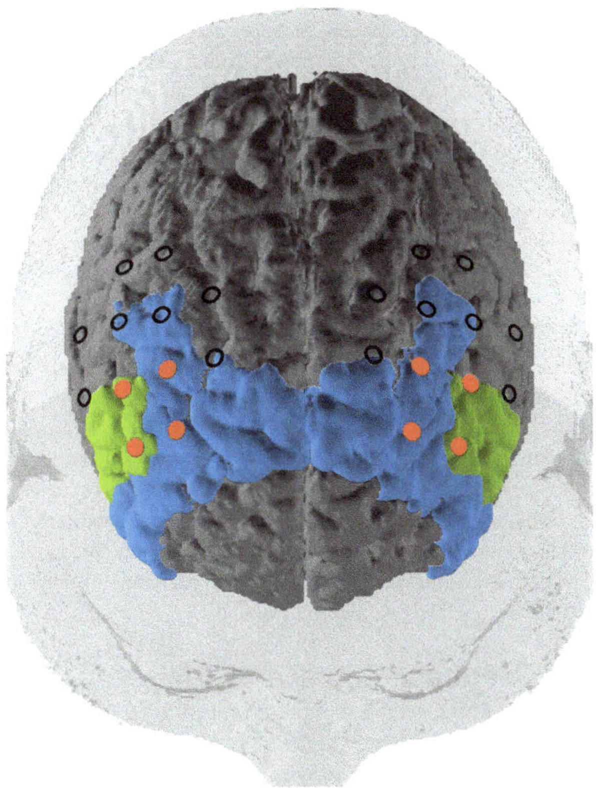

FIGURE 2 | Probeset. Depiction of the target regions of the neurofeedback training (in red) and the rest of the optode array. The optodes cover a space mostly located in the dlPFC (blue, Brodmann areas 9 and 46) but also extending to the inferior frontal gyrus (green, Brodmann area 45) according to a virtual registration method (see subsection Functional Near-Infrared Spectroscopy Data).

Our optode montage featured two 3 × 3 optode arrays centered with the innermost channel of the front row of each array placed on F3 (left hemisphere) and F4 (right hemisphere) of the international 10–20 EEG system (Jasper, 1958). Source–detector distances were kept at 3 cm. The optode arrays were rotated 45° laterally along the transversal plane so that the innermost four channels in the two frontal rows were oriented over the left and right dlPFC (**Figure 2**). The third optode array was a 3 × 5 arrangement where the most superior and lateral optode on the left and right of the array were oriented on P3 and P4, respectively. Subtending the parieto-occipital cortex, this probeset was used exclusively for common average (CA) reference, a signal correction method (see below).

fNIRS Feedback Signal and Trials

The feedback target was the average amplitude of O_2Hb within the bilateral dlPFC (see Marx et al., 2015). The raw fNIRS signal was sampled at 10 Hz and preprocessed in MATLAB version 9.0 (The MathWorks Inc., United States). A moving average Kalman filter with a 5 s sliding window was then applied to the data. Finally, we used a CA artifact removal method used in previous NF designs serving as a basis for this design (Marx et al., 2015; Mayer et al., 2015). This method was preferred because of its ability to remove probeset-wide effects from individual channels (Heinzel et al., 2013). For the CA, the raw average of all 46 channels was subtracted from the raw average of the eight emitter–detector channel pairings over the dlPFC in order to limit the influence of artifacts – e.g., superficial blood flow, head and jaw movements, and respiration – on the hemodynamic response in the feedback channels. All preprocessing occurred online.

The fNIRS trials were 30 s in duration with a 5 s baseline period. Relative O_2Hb concentration higher than baseline led to brightening of the lights; concentration lower than baseline led to dimming. Trials were divided into three blocks (**Figure 3**). The first and last blocks contained 12 trials and subsequent rests of 20 s duration. The middle block contained eight trials and rests and was used as the transfer block, wherein no continuous feedback was provided, though participants were still given feedback at the end of the trial. There was no jittering of intertrial intervals.

EMG Feedback Signal and Trials

Monopolar EMG, with a sampling rate of 1000 Hz, provided feedback from the bilateral *musculus supraspinatus* for the control group (see Mayer et al., 2015). The signal was referenced to the right mastoid and was grounded on the left mastoid. The data stream was bandpass filtered between 80 and 300 Hz. The resulting signal was then normalized via a maximum output and a resting output, for which the participant flexed both muscles maximally for 10 s and sat completely at rest for 10 s, respectively. At each time point, feedback was equivalent to:

$$\text{Feedback Index} = \text{R} - \text{L},$$

where R and L were the right and left normalized muscle outputs, respectively, given by:

$$\text{R(L)} = \frac{\text{Right (Left) EMG Signal} - \text{Average Resting Baseline Right (Left)}}{\text{Average Maximal Muscle Output Right (Left)}}.$$

Therefore, more tensing of right muscle led to brightening; more tensing of left muscle led to dimming. Baseline for each trial was an average of the last 2 s of the resting feedback signal.

The EMG trials were 15 s in duration with a 2 s baseline period. Relative muscular feedback index higher than baseline led to brightening of the lights; feedback index lower than baseline led to dimming. Trials were divided into three blocks (**Figure 3**). The first and last blocks contained 24 trials and subsequent rests of 10 s duration. The middle block contained 16 trials and rests and was used as the transfer block, wherein no contingent feedback was provided.

Pre- and Post-measures

Go/no-go and n-Back Task

The go/no-go and the n-back tasks were programmed in Presentation version 18.0 (Neuro Behavioral Systems, United States) following previously published protocols (Mayer et al., 2015; see also Ehlis et al., 2008). We recorded fNIRS during both tasks. Briefly, the go/no-go task consisted of alternating go and no-go blocks (four repetitions each) separated by rest blocks, each block lasting 30 s. In the "go" condition, participants were asked to respond as fast as possible to each stimulus. In the "no-go" condition, participants were instructed to withhold their response on no-go trials (here: presentation of the letter "N"; 25% of trials). Dependent variables were RT, SDRT, FA, and omission errors.

The n-back task consisted of three blocks each of 2-back (high working memory load), 1-back (low working memory load), and 0-back (control) (block length: 30 s; separated by 30 s rest periods). In the 2- (1-)back task, the participants were instructed to press the space bar as quickly as possible whenever the current letter was the same as the letter two letters (one letter) back. In the 0-back task, the participant was instructed to respond when the letter "O" appeared on the screen. Dependent variables were RT, SDRT, and correct hits.

Stop-Signal Task

The SST followed the protocol described in Verbruggen et al. (2008). The task consisted of one practice block and three 3-min verum blocks wherein the participant should respond to the direction of an arrow pointing on the screen as quickly as possible. In roughly 25% of trials, the arrow would turn blue,

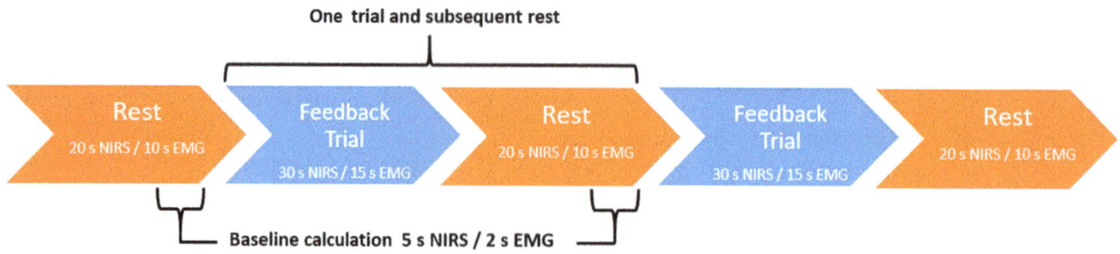

FIGURE 3 | Feedback block design. fNIRS-based NF blocks consisted of either 12 NF trials and subsequent rest trials (continuous feedback blocks one and three) or 8 NF trials and subsequent rests (transfer block two). EMG-based BF blocks consisted of either 24 BF trials and subsequent rests (continuous feedback blocks one and three) or 16 BF trials and subsequent rests (transfer block two). In both conditions, blocks always began with a rest trial.

indicating the participant should withhold their response, after a variable stop-signal delay (SSD) that started at 250 ms and increased or decreased by 50 ms depending on if they failed or succeeded to stop, respectively. Dependent variables in the SST included the SSRT - a measure of behavioral inhibition - RT, and SDRT. The SST was added as a secondary measure for behavior. We did not record simultaneous fNIRS with this measure.

Analysis

Functional Near-Infrared Spectroscopy Data

All analysis was performed using MATLAB. In order to analyze fNIRS data, we used subroutines programmed in our research group, adapted for fNIRS from the Statistics Parametrical Mapping toolbox for MATLAB (SPM8; Friston et al., 1994). Raw signals were bandpass filtered between 0.01 and 0.2 Hz to remove unwanted physiological artifacts such as heartbeat and respiration. Next, channels exceeding three times the within-subject standard deviation over the course of the measurement were interpolated (see Hagen et al., 2014) using a Gaussian distribution with the O_2Hb values of proximal channels given a higher weighting than distal ones; less than 10% of all channels were interpolated. We then applied a wavelet-based transform (Molavi and Dumont, 2012) to detect and correct motion artifacts that were still part of the data. We used the hmrMotionCorrectWavelet algorithm from the Homer2 fNIRS analysis package for MATLAB with the standard motion artifact detection threshold of 1.5 *SD* above the interquartile range of the data (Huppert et al., 2009). Finally, a block-related average amplitude was calculated for each channel using an interval of 0–60 s after block onset with a 10-s baseline correction. Linear detrending was applied to remove slow drifts in the data. Finally, average amplitudes over the duration of the task blocks (0–30 s) were calculated.

Region of Interest (ROI)

We mapped fNIRS channels to corresponding, underlying cortical areas based on a virtual registration method (Rorden and Brett, 2000; Singh et al., 2005; Tsuzuki et al., 2007). The left and right dlPFC regions of interest (ROIs) consisted of the channels that we used for the NF training. These channels are concentrated in Brodmann Areas 9, 45, and 46. This includes the dlPFC and also slightly expands into the inferior frontal gyrus (IGF; see **Figure 2**).

Rate of Learning and Correlation with Primary Outcome Variables

Additionally, we analyzed the success of the participants in obtaining control of the feedback parameter. Our success rate was calculated as the average percentage of time spent in the correct direction of the desired feedback (above or below the baseline, for activation vs. deactivation trials, respectively) for the duration of the trial. An average was calculated for all trials from the first week (four sessions) and the second week (four sessions). The rate of learning was calculated as the average of the second week minus the average of the first week. Rate of learning was then correlated with the primary outcome variables of FA rate in the no-go task and average amplitude of O_2Hb of the feedback channels during the no-go task. Similar metrics were created in order to compute the correlations: pre–post FA errors were computed for each subject, to give a metric of individual improvement. Similarly, a post–pre average amplitude of O_2Hb of the feedback channels was computed to reflect difference in activation after the training. In the event of significant correlations in one or more groups, we computed a pseudo-permutation test (n = 10,000 permutations), permuting the group assignment while keeping within-subject correlation pairs intact, to determine a significant difference between groups. The number of permutations in which the permuted group difference in ρ value was larger than the verum group difference in ρ value was divided by the total number of permutations to create a p-value.

Statistical Analysis

To evaluate the statistical significance of pre–post changes in O_2Hb and HHb in the go/no-go and n-back tasks, we conducted $2 \times 2 \times 2 \times 2(3)$ repeated measures analyses of variance (ANOVAs), with the between-subjects factor treatment group (NIRS vs. EMG) and the within-subject factors of time (pre vs. post), ROI (left dlPFC vs. right dlPFC), and condition (n-back (3): 2-, 1-, and 0-back; go/no-go (2): go and no-go). For behavioral data, repeated measures ANOVAs were performed using the same factors excluding ROI. When data violated the assumption of sphericity, Greenhouse-Geisser corrected values were reported. For significant main and interaction effects, two-tailed Student's t-tests were employed for *post hoc* analyses (paired or independent samples, as appropriate). In cases where the assumption of normality was violated, we used two-tailed Mann–Whitney U tests or Wilcoxon signed-rank tests, respectively.

ROI Specificity

In order to determine specificity of ROIs we used pseudo-permutations tests, wherein the mean difference in the average amplitudes from pre to post measurement for a given verum ROI (vROI) for all participants was compared to a pseudo-ROI (pROI) composed of an equal number of randomly chosen NIRS channels. $N = 10{,}000$ permutations of pROI were calculated and the resulting p-value was the sum of trials in which the resulting statistic from the vROI was greater than the permuted statistic from the pROI.

RESULTS

Behavioral Data

Only significant results related to the hypotheses are reported here. For a full summary of behavioral data, see **Table 1**.

Go/no-go

False alarm errors in the go/no-go task showed a trend with a large effect size for a measurement time*group interaction effect

TABLE 1 | Behavioral data from pre- and post-test in the two experimental groups.

	Pre-test		Post-test	
Task	**NIRS group means (±*SD*)**	**EMG group means (±*SD*)**	**NIRS group means (±*SD*)**	**EMG group means (±*SD*)**
Go/no-go				
Go RT (ms)	300.0 (20.3)	289.6 (47.1)	290.5 (18.5)	293.5 (43.3)
Go SDRT (ms)	90.9 (43.1)	90.4 (39.4)	77.7 (18.1)	144.5 (99.6)
Go omission errors	0.2 (0.4)	2.9 (5.7)	0.8 (0.9)	1.6 (2.5)
No-go FA errors	4.8 (2.4)	4.8 (2.7)	2.6 (1.3)	6.0 (5.2)
No-go RT (ms)	434.6 (30.4)	417.4 (30.4)	438.3 (48.3)	411.3 (38.0)
No-go SDRT (ms)	82.0 (37.6)	81.0 (38.8)	71.1 (23.6)	79.6 (30.3)
N-back				
2-back Hit rate	0.95 (0.06)	0.93 (0.11)	0.98 (0.04)	0.93 (0.11)
1-back Hit rate	1 (0)	0.99 (0.03)	0.98 (0.08)	0.97 (0.04)
0-back Hit rate	1 (0)	0.99 (0.03)	1 (0)	0.96 (0.06)
2-back RT (ms)	554.2 (65.8)	485.8 (77.8)	550.3 (74.0)	433.5 (66.4)
1-back RT (ms)	473.6 (61.0)	411.7 (46.8)	491.2 (78.8)	427.2 (76.2)
0-back RT (ms)	423.9 (48.3)	388.7 (35.1)	450.0 (49.2)	418.8 (83.6)
2-back SDRT (ms)	173.1 (57.5)	163.8 (50.2)	171.7 (69.5)	87.9 (25.9)
1-back SDRT (ms)	122.6 (58.1)	71.8 (19.1)	123.5 (81.5)	82.7 (36.9)
0-back SDRT (ms)	96.6 (18.3)	139.7 (50.1)	139.7 (50.4)	113.3 (55.1)
Stop-signal task				
SSRT (ms)	223.5 (36.8)	224.2 (53.9)	232.2 (55.8)	223.6 (55.7)
Go trial RT (ms)	659.2 (212.8)	543.4 (96.9)	605.1 (186.5)	568.9 (102.5)
Go trial SDRT (ms)	160.8 (64.9)	125.6 (46.1)	124.1 (60.6)	145.7 (61.0)

SD, standard deviation; RT, reaction time; SDRT, standard deviation of the reaction time; FA, false alarms; SSRT, stop-signal reaction time.

($F(1,18) = 4.08$, $p = 0.059$, $\eta^2 = 0.185$). *Post hoc* Wilcoxon signed-rank tests revealed a reduction of FA errors from pre to post measurement in the experimental group ($M_{pre} = 4.8$, $SD_{pre} = 2.4$; $M_{post} = 2.6$, $SD_{post} = 1.3$; $Z = -2.57$, $p = 0.01$), but not in the control group ($M_{pre} = 4.8$, $SD_{pre} = 2.7$; $M_{post} = 6.0$, $SD_{post} = 5.2$; $Z = -0.30$, $p = 0.77$) (**Figure 4A**). No other interaction effects were observed.

Rate of Learning

A one-sample Kolmogorov–Smirnov test rejected the null hypothesis that the learning rates for the first half and second half of the experimental and control groups, respectively, followed a normal distribution ($D = 0.65, 0.65, 0.64, 0.65$, $N = 10$ each, and $p < 0.05$ each). Therefore, Wilcoxon signed-rank tests and Spearman correlations were calculated. For the experimental group, there was no significant difference between first half and second half performance, but a medium effect size indicating better second half performance ($Z = 1.48$, $p = 0.13$, $r = 0.33$). There was, however, a significant difference between first and second half performance for the control group ($Z = 2.68$, $p = 0.013$, $r = 0.60$), indicating a significantly better performance in the second week with a large effect size.

The rate of learning of both groups failed to correlate significantly with post–pre changes in average O_2Hb concentration in feedback channels ($|\rho| < 0.224$, $p > 0.05$). The rate of learning in the experimental group, however, correlated strongly with size of pre–post reduction in FA ($\rho = 0.75$, $p = 0.013$; see **Figure 4B**). Rate of learning in the control group did not correlate with pre–post reduction in FA ($\rho = -0.24$, $p = 0.508$). The resulting pseudo-permutation test concluded that there was a significant group difference ($p = 0.015$).

N-Back Task

No significant behavioral interaction effects were observed. Hit rates for each condition were nearly 100% in the pre-test. Furthermore, no FA errors were made in this task. A ceiling effect was evident for this task.

Stop-Signal Task

Reaction time variability yielded a significant interaction effect of measurement time*group ($F(1,18) = 5.39$, $p = 0.03$, $\eta^2 = 0.231$), with the experimental group showing significantly reduced RT variability following the training ($M_{pre} = 160.78$ ms, $SD_{pre} = 64.88$; $M_{post} = 124.13$, $SD_{post} = 60.60$; $t(9) = 2.48$, $p = 0.035$). The control group showed no difference between measurements ($M_{pre} = 125.55$ ms, $SD_{pre} = 46.13$; $M_{post} = 145.70$, $SD_{post} = 61.04$; $t(9) = 1.04$, $p = 0.328$).

fNIRS Data

Go/no-go O_2Hb

We observed a main effect of task ($F(1,18) = 11.92$, $p = 0.003$, $\eta^2 = 0.398$, mean amplitudes: $M_{go} = 0.005$, $SD = 0.033$ mm*mol/l, $M_{no\text{-}go} = -0.005$, $SD = 0.029$ mm*mol/l) and an interaction effect of time*task*ROI*group ($F(1,18) = 5.63$, $p = 0.029$, $\eta^2 = 0.238$). This interaction was caused by a pre to post increase in O_2Hb amplitudes of the left dlPFC in the experimental group during the no-go task ($M_{pre} = -0.029$, $SD = 0.035$ mm*mol/l; $M_{post} = 0.010$,

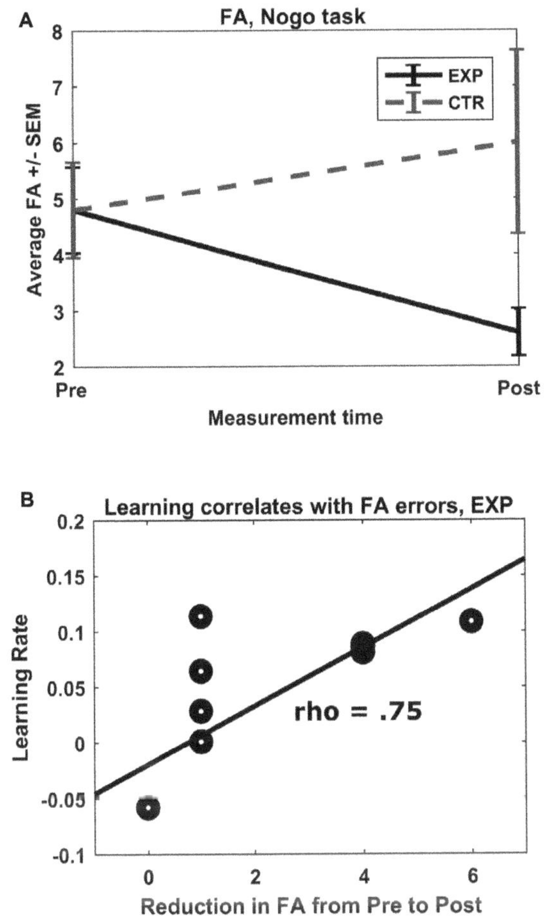

FIGURE 4 | (A) No-go FA errors. Mean total FA errors for the no-go condition shown for both groups for both pre- and post-test. *$p = 0.01$. **(B)** Rate of learning correlation with FA reduction. In the experimental group, there was a strong correlation between rate of learning of the feedback parameter (prefrontal oxygenation) and pre–post reduction in FA errors committed.

$SD = 0.040$ mm*mol/l; $t(9) = -3.63$, $p = 0.005$; see **Figure 5**). In the control group of the same condition, time, and ROI, there was no significant change ($M_{pre} = 0.006$, $SD = 0.017$ mm*mol/l; $M_{post} = -0.006$, $SD = 0.031$ mm*mol/l; $t(9) = 1.15$, $p = 0.281$). All other *post hoc* comparisons failed to reach significance ($|t(9)| < 1.837$, $p > 0.1$). The permutation test indicated that this ROI was indeed the focal point for the increase in brain activation. The resulting *p*-value was equal to $p = 0.003$, indicating that there is high spatial specificity to the activation, located in the left dlPFC.

Go/no-go HHb

We observed no main effects, only an interaction effect of task*hemisphere ($F(1,18) = 5.79$, $p = 0.027$, $\eta^2 = 0.243$). *Post hoc* testing indicated that there was a trend toward a significant difference in HHb activation between the left and right hemisphere in the "go" condition ($M_{left} = -0.005$, $SD = 0.023$; $M_{right} = -0.013$, $SD = 0.026$; $t(9) = 2.07$, $p = 0.052$).

N-Back O_2Hb

We observed no main effects or significant interaction effects (all $|F(2,36)| < 2.50$; all $p > 0.11$).

N-Back HHb

We observed a trend for a main effect of task ($F(1.39,24.93) = 3.75$, $p = 0.052$, $\eta^2 = 0.173$; mean amplitudes: $M_{2Back} = -0.011$, $SD = 0.023$; $M_{1Back} = -0.007$, $SD = 0.021$; $M_{0Back} = 0.001$, $SD = 0.024$). Again, the indication is a higher activation in tasks with a higher working load. We also observed a trend for a main effect of time ($F(1,18) = 3.26$, $p = 0.088$, $\eta^2 = 0.153$; $M_{Pre} = -0.008$, $SD = 0.026$; $M_{Post} = -0.003$, $SD = 0.021$), indicating a marginal decrease in activation across all tasks from pre to post measurement time. No other main effects or interaction effects were observed.

DISCUSSION

The present study was designed to test the efficacy of a novel neurofeedback intervention (fNIRS-based frontal lobe NF in a virtual classroom environment) with the ultimate aim of reducing ADHD symptoms in schoolchildren by increasing their ability to regulate prefrontal cortex activity (Blume et al., 2017). Here, we focused on the effects of this newly developed NF protocol in a sample of highly impulsive young adults, a sub-clinical risk population that exhibits many of the behavioral abnormalities also seen in patients with ADHD (e.g., Herrmann et al., 2009). In this proof-of-concept study, we were primarily interested in first, whether the fNIRS-based NF group would show increased cortical activation in feedback channels during frontal lobe/impulsivity-related tasks (go/no-go and n-back), following focused training of these channels and second, whether the fNIRS-based NF group would show a reduction in impulsive behaviors (go/no-go, n-back, SST).

During a go/no-go task, we observed a significant increase compared to a pre-training baseline in cortical O_2Hb concentration in the left dlPFC of the experimental (fNIRS) group only. During the same task, we observed a concurrent and significant reduction in FA errors of the same group. Importantly, this reduction in FA errors correlated significantly with the rate of learning of the experimental subjects but not the control subjects. Additionally, we observed a reduction in RT variability on the SST for the experimental group. We observed no group differences in either cortical activation or behavior on the n-back task. The lack of a group difference after training on this task is likely due to the study specifically focusing on the recruitment of highly impulsive students. There is no evidence to suggest that highly impulsive participants have explicit deficits in working memory. In fact, in a study examining the correlations between trait impulsivity (as measured by BIS self-report) and performance on various neurocognitive tasks, no significant correlation was found between trait impulsivity and working memory performance, while trait impulsivity correlated strongest with go/no-go errors (Keilp et al., 2005). Furthermore, task accuracy reflected a ceiling effect from the pre-test, indicating that the task was not difficult for these

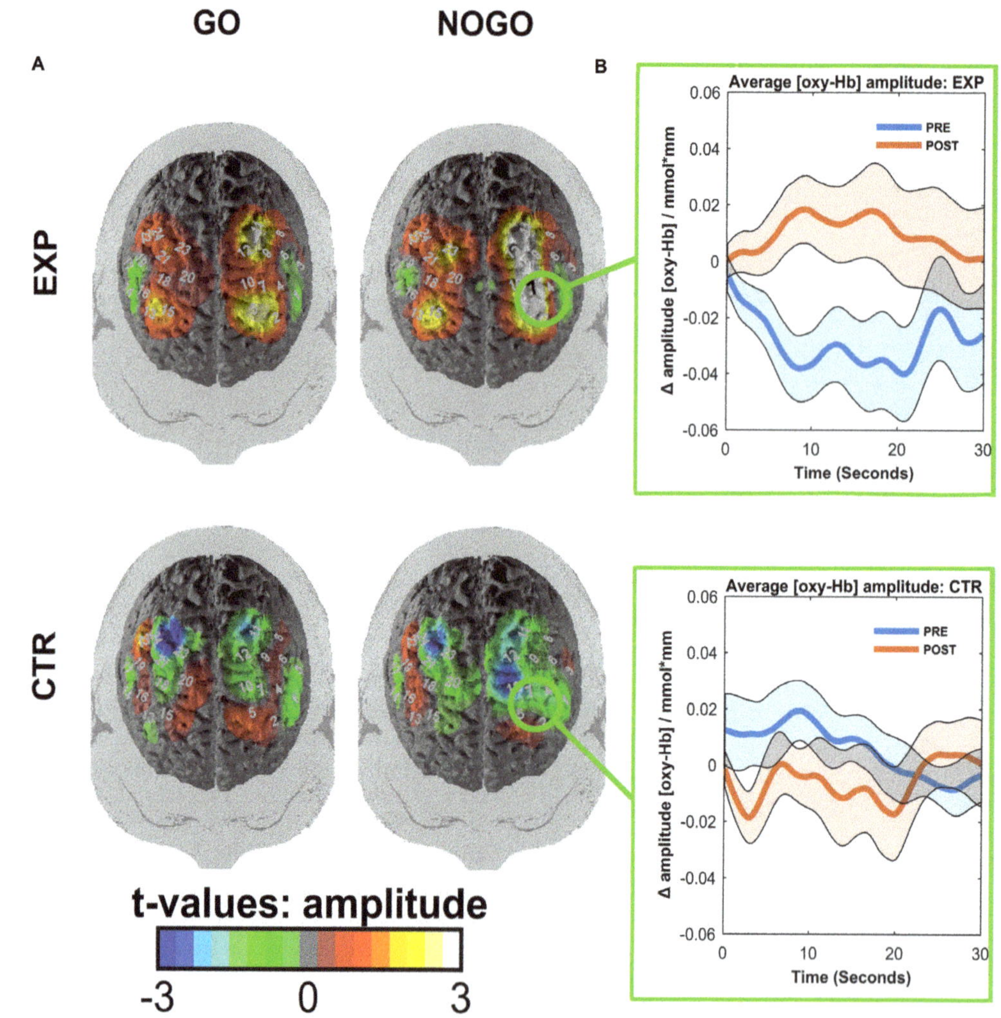

FIGURE 5 | (A) Contrasted t-maps of the average amplitudes of O_2Hb for different blocks of the go/no-go task. Contrasts represent post-test values minus pre-test values. CTR represents the EMG control group, while EXP represents the experimental fNIRS group. *T*-values were obtained by *t*-tests corrected for multiple comparisons with the Armitage–Parmar correction. Positive channels indicate stronger activation in the post-relative to the pre-test. Significant channels are depicted in black. **(B)** ROI event-related averages. Circled regions from **(A)** indicate the left dlPFC ROI for which the event-related average of $O_2Hb \pm$ standard error of the mean (SEM) is depicted for both pre-(blue) and post-(red) tests.

subjects. Therefore, despite the potential benefit to working memory that training the dlPFC might imbue, in our case there may have been no deficit to correct. Lastly, HHb data showed no differences in activation in either task. These results make sense in the context of the NF training; since O_2Hb was trained, the hypothesis would be that O_2Hb and not HHb would show the strongest pre–post effects. In addition, O_2Hb is more sensitive to detection of changes than HHb (Strangman et al., 2002).

False alarm errors, or incorrect go-responses to no-go stimuli, represent a failure to exhibit response inhibition (Aichert et al., 2012), an impulsive trait that subjects with ADHD share with highly impulsive participants. A reduction for the experimental group and not for the control group suggests that the fNIRS intervention was effective in reducing impulsive behavior as specified. The strong O_2Hb correlation observed between a reduction in FA errors and the rate of learning within the experimental group, but not within the control group, further illustrates the importance of specificity in NF training. The goal of actually learning to control the feedback parameter is often overlooked in NF studies, where the rate of obtained control is rarely reported (Zuberer et al., 2015). Interestingly, the control group showed a significant improvement between the first and second week in regulating the feedback parameter while the experimental group did not. This likely has to do with the comparable ease of the EMG feedback; once one learns the correct movement, it can relatively easily be replicated every trial. The fNIRS feedback is likely more complex, as there is no right or wrong way to achieve the feedback parameter, and sustaining oxygenation of the dlPFC over time is strenuous. Given this complexity, the medium effect size observed in the fNIRS learning rate is encouraging, and may simply mean that more sessions are needed to fully gain control. Moreover, for the specific sample investigated and trained here (i.e., highly impulsive subjects), frontal lobe alterations have been shown as a central neurophysiological correlate, so it is perhaps not surprising that improving control over this area of the brain seems to have been particularly difficult. However, this behavioral effort seems to pay dividends, as we see that the more control impulsive subjects were able to gain over the activation of their dlPFC, the fewer FA errors they made, whereas the successful learning of the EMG parameter had little effect. This result supports the findings of an fNIRS study that sought to differentiate the roles of the medial and lateral prefrontal cortex during a go/no-go task. The bilateral middle frontal gyrus (i.e., the dlPFC) was responsible for error monitoring during the motor inhibition segment of the go/no-go task (Rodrigo et al., 2014). Our results indicate that the combination of both correct feedback parameter (i.e., frontal lobe focused) and successful learning of that parameter, not one or the other in isolation, is important to the feedback's overall success.

The task-specific increase in prefrontal oxygenation coinciding with a reduction in FA errors suggests that – following the frontal fNIRS training – the highly impulsive participants were able to recruit more cognitive resources, particularly from the dlPFC, during this task, leading to improved performance. Whether or not this was intentional is a matter of debate, but the goal of NF interventions remains to train implicit activation of brain activity through operant and classical conditioning (Strehl, 2014). Therefore, it seems that the participants were able to transfer skills learned either implicitly or explicitly from the training into a performance situation. Furthermore, this increase in cortical activation was both task- (no-go) and region-specific (left dlPFC). While there was no increase in activation in the right dlPFC, the left-specific increase as well as the increase in inhibitory control are in line with the tDCS study of Soltaninejad et al. (2015) who used cathodal stimulation over the left dlPFC of adolescents with ADHD and observed a decrease in FA errors. While the literary consensus places the locus of inhibitory control within the right dlPFC, inferior prefrontal, premotoric, and striatal brain structures (Aron et al., 2004, 2014; Bari and Robbins, 2013; Obeso et al., 2013), the left dlPFC shares strong functional connectivity with the above-mentioned areas (Ridderinkhof et al., 2004; Aron et al., 2014). Moreover, the dlPFC does not seem to be directly responsible for inhibitory control, but rather functions as a higher order mechanism that organizes the relevant brain structures above when attention control or increased working memory capacity is needed, in particular for oddball or complex no-go tasks (Criaud and Boulinguez, 2013). Because our go/no-go paradigm could be considered oddball, with an occurrence of no-go stimuli in only 25% of trials, it may be that the extra dlPFC resources recruited were used for focusing attention, rather than inhibitory control *per se*. Indeed, the reduction in SDRT seen in the SST also indicates an increase in attentional resources, possibly also mediated by an increase in prefrontal brain activity, though NIRS data were not available for this task. Increases in SDRT are generally considered to be related to lapses in attention (Alderson et al., 2007), though Kirkeby and Robinson (2005) found SDRT to be inversely correlated with trait impulsivity. Still, this does not rule out the idea that our impulsive sample also suffered from inattentiveness.

Treatment effects for both impulsivity and possibly inattention are encouraging from a translational perspective regarding potential use of our NF design with an ADHD population. We chose the dlPFC as a NF site because of its involvement in general top-down cognitive control, and the realization of significant training effects in impulsivity and possible inattention suggests that the protocol may be useful for an ADHD population. Several reasons lead us to be hopeful of even greater effects in a current study in our lab with ADHD schoolchildren (Blume et al., 2017). First, the sample size of this study was small. Only large effects could be detected, and with a greater sample size, we would expect to see effects in a wide range of other cognitive and behavioral deficits. Secondly, the training was compact and about half the number of training sessions we would recommend (and currently use) for a clinical ADHD project. As far as we know, this is the shortest number of training sessions to produce effects in brain activation and behavior that was adequately controlled for specificity. Cho et al. (2004) also used a 2 week, eight session NF paradigm with EEG and found training effects for inattention and impulsivity, but they did not have an adequate control group (waiting group), and additionally, did not measure differences in brain activity pre and post. Lastly, but most importantly, children have a greater capacity for brain plasticity than adults (Kolb and Gibb, 2011). For children with ADHD, this capacity is even more pronounced within the dlPFC, a region that develops particularly late for them (Rubia et al., 2013). Given the current study's results, we would expect even greater improvements within a child population.

The current study was limited by several factors, which we hope to improve upon in a second study with children with an ADHD diagnosis (Blume et al., 2017). The sample size was small which limited data analysis. Our aim was to test the viability of an immersive VR NF paradigm, and it appears that the full classroom immersion did not detract from the ability of the participants to regulate their brain activity. There was a difference between experimental groups in pre-test no-go activation, with the experimental group showing less activation than the control group. Small groups, even with proper randomization, have a much greater chance of having differing baseline measurements simply due to sampling error (Marshall, 1996). The larger the group, the smaller the chance of pre-baseline differences due to a random sampling error. As NF studies require large time and monetary investments per participant, and the aim of our study was to ultimately test the efficacy of VR NF, we chose 10 participants per group as a balance between power and realism. For technical reasons, we did not have triggers to compare the extent to which participants were able to regulate their brain activity across sessions, something that will be improved in the next study. While we used distractors in the current study, there was no way to compare trials in which a distractor occurred to trials in which they did not. Furthermore, we lack a comparison of the effects of the immersive VR NF paradigm to a 2-D version. In an ongoing study with children with ADHD (Blume et al., 2017), we include a 2-D group that still uses lighting in the classroom as the feedback source, but the child sees the classroom on a normal computer monitor. In this way, we will be able to determine if immersive NF is actually more effective for the transfer of the learned regulation. Furthermore, the classroom itself is only one of many possible VR NF designs. Virtual reality scenarios coupled with NF are limited only to the imagination and relevance to a certain psychological disorder. Virtual reality NF with subjects with social phobias, for example, could be integrated within a potentially stressful social situation, like a bar or dinner party, furthering the ecological validity of the treatment while also avoiding an exposition-driven therapeutic approach that cannot be as easily controlled.

Considering these limitations and the relative ease with which they could be improved upon going forward, it seems that VR NF is a very promising modality for the treatment of behavioral disorders with known pathophysiological alterations.

ETHICS STATEMENT

This study was approved by the Ethics Committee of the Medical Faculty of the University and the University Hospital of Tübingen and all procedures were in accordance with the Helsinki Declaration of 1975, as revised in 2013.

AUTHOR CONTRIBUTIONS

All authors have approved of the final version of this manuscript. JH study design, data collection and analysis, and manuscript preparation; FB study design, data collection, and manuscript preparation; TD study design and manuscript preparation; FH data analysis; TR study design and manuscript preparation; AF study design and manuscript preparation; CG study design and manuscript preparation; and A-CE study design, data analysis, and manuscript preparation.

FUNDING

This research was funded by the LEAD Graduate School & Research Network (GSC1028), a project of the Excellence Initiative of the German federal and state governments. JH and FB are doctoral candidates and TD is a Junior Research Group Leader at the LEAD Graduate School & Research Network. A-CE was partly supported by the Interdisciplinary Center for Clinical Research (IZKF) Tübingen (Junior Research Group, grant 2115-0-0). We acknowledge support by the Deutsche Forschungsgemeinschaft and the Open Access Publishing Fund of the University of Tübingen.

ACKNOWLEDGMENTS

The authors would like to give additional thanks to those who contributed with measurements, in particular Marc Werth, Silke M. Bieck, and Nana Ambs. Sandru Razvan was influential in editing and structuring of the manuscript. Additionally, uncompromising support was given by Betti Schopp and Ramona Taeglich in coordinating measurements and training. They would also like to thank the participants for their participation and a very involved study.

REFERENCES

Aichert, D. S., Wöstmann, N. M., Costa, A., Macare, C., Wenig, J. R., Möller, H., et al. (2012). Associations between trait impulsivity and prepotent response inhibition. *J. Clin. Exp. Neuropsychol.* 34, 1016–1032. doi: 10.1080/13803395.2012.706261

Alderson, R. M., Rapport, M. D., and Kofler, M. J. (2007). Attention-deficit/hyperactivity disorder and behavioral inhibition: a meta-analytic review of the stop-signal paradigm. *J. Abnorm. Child Psychol.* 35, 745–758. doi: 10.1007/s10802-007-9131-6

Arns, M., Heinrich, H., and Strehl, U. (2013). Evaluation of neurofeedback in ADHD: the long and winding road. *Biol. Psychol.* 95, 108–115. doi: 10.1016/j.biopsycho.2013.11.013

Aron, A. R., Robbins, T. W., and Poldrack, R. A. (2004). Inhibition and the right inferior frontal cortex. *Trends Cogn. Sci.* 8, 170–177. doi: 10.1016/j.tics.2004.02.010

Aron, A. R., Robbins, T. W., and Poldrack, R. A. (2014). Inhibition and the right inferior frontal cortex: one decade on. *Trends Cogn. Sci.* 18, 177–185. doi: 10.1016/j.tics.2013.12.003

Bari, A., and Robbins, T. W. (2013). Inhibition and impulsivity: behavioral and neural basis of response control. *Prog. Neurobiol.* 108, 44–79. doi: 10.1016/j.pneurobio.2013.06.005

Barratt, E. S. (1959). Anxiety and impulsiveness related to psychomotor efficiency. *Percept. Mot. Skills* 9, 191–198. doi: 10.2466/pms.1959.9.3.191

Begemann, M. J. H., Florisse, E. J. R., Van Lutterveld, R., Kooyman, M., and Sommer, I. E. (2016). Efficacy of EEG neurofeedback in psychiatry: a comprehensive overview and meta-analysis. *Transl. Brain Rhythmicity* 1, 19–29. doi: 10.15761/TBR.1000105

Birbaumer, N., Elbert, T., Rockstroh, B., Daum, I., Wolf, P., and Canavan, A. (1991). "Clinical-psychological treatment of epileptic seizures: a controlled study," in *Perspectives and Promises in Clinical Psychology*, ed. A. Ehlers (New York, NY: Plenum Press), 81–96.

Blume, F., Hudak, J., Dresler, T., Ehlis, A.-C., Kühnhausen, J., Renner, T. J., et al. (2017). NIRS-based neurofeedback training in a virtual reality classroom for children with attention-deficit/hyperactivity disorder: study protocol for a randomized controlled trial. *Trials* 18, 41. doi: 10.1186/s13063-016-1769-3

Casey, B., Getz, S., and Galvan, A. (2008). The adolescent brain. *Dev. Rev.* 28, 62–77. doi: 10.1016/j.dr.2007.08.003

Cho, B.-H., Kim, S., Shin, D. I., Lee, J. H., Min Lee, S., Young Kim, I., et al. (2004). Neurofeedback training with virtual reality for inattention and impulsiveness. *Cyberpsychol. Behav.* 7, 519–526. doi: 10.1089/cpb.2004.7.519

Criaud, M., and Boulinguez, P. (2013). Have we been asking the right questions when assessing response inhibition in go/no-go tasks with fMRI? A meta-analysis and critical review. *Neurosci. Biobehav. Rev.* 37, 11–23. doi: 10.1016/j.neubiorev.2012.11.003

Cubillo, A., Halari, R., Smith, A., Taylor, E., and Rubia, K. (2012). A review of fronto-striatal and fronto-cortical brain abnormalities in children and adults with Attention Deficit Hyperactivity Disorder (ADHD) and new evidence for dysfunction in adults with ADHD during motivation and attention. *Cortex* 48, 194–215. doi: 10.1016/j.cortex.2011.04.007

Ding, W., Sun, J., Sun, Y.-W., Chen, X., Zhou, Y., Zhuang, Z., et al. (2014). Trait impulsivity and impaired prefrontal impulse inhibition function in adolescents with internet gaming addiction revealed by a Go/No-Go fMRI study. *Behav. Brain Funct.* 10:20. doi: 10.1186/1744-9081-10-20

Ehlis, A.-C., Bähne, C. G., Jacob, C. P., Herrmann, M. J., and Fallgatter, A. J. (2008). Reduced lateral prefrontal activation in adult patients with attention-deficit/hyperactivity disorder (ADHD) during a working memory task: a functional near-infrared spectroscopy (fNIRS) study. *J. Psychiatr. Res.* 42, 1060–1067. doi: 10.1016/j.jpsychires.2007.11.011

Fallgatter, A. J., and Herrmann, M. J. (2001). Electrophysiological assessment of impulsive behavior in healthy subjects. *Neuropsychologia* 39, 328–333. doi: 10.1016/S0028-3932(00)00115-9

Farr, O. M., Hu, S., Zhang, S., Li, C., and Shan, R. (2012). Decreased saliency processing as a neural measure of Barratt impulsivity in healthy adults. *Neuroimage* 63, 1070–1077. doi: 10.1016/j.neuroimage.2012.07.049

Friston, K. J., Holmes, A. P., Worsley, K. J., Poline, J.-P., Frith, C. D., and Frackowiak, R. S. J. (1994). Statistical parametric maps in functional imaging: a general linear approach. *Hum. Brain Mapp.* 2, 189–210. doi: 10.1002/hbm.460020402

Gevensleben, H., Kleemeyer, M., Rothenberger, L. G., Studer, P., Flaig-Röhr, A., Moll, G. H., et al. (2014a). Neurofeedback in ADHD: further pieces of the puzzle. *Brain Topogr.* 27, 20–32. doi: 10.1007/s10548-013-0285-y

Gevensleben, H., Moll, G. H., Rothenberger, A., and Heinrich, H. (2014b). Neurofeedback in attention-deficit/hyperactivity disorder – different models, different ways of application. *Front. Hum. Neurosci.* 8:846. doi: 10.3389/fnhum.2014.00846

Gevensleben, H., Rothenberger, A., Moll, G. H., and Heinrich, H. (2012). Neurofeedback in children with ADHD: validation and challenges. *Expert Rev. Neurother.* 12, 447–460. doi: 10.1586/ern.12.22

Haeussinger, F. B., Dresler, T., Heinzel, S., Schecklmann, M., Fallgatter, A. J., and Ehlis, A. C. (2014). Reconstructing functional near-infrared spectroscopy (fNIRS) signals impaired by extra-cranial confounds: an easy-to-use filter method. *Neuroimage* 95, 69–79. doi: 10.1016/j.neuroimage.2014.02.035

Hagen, K., Ehlis, A.-C., Haeussinger, F. B., Heinzel, S., Dresler, T., Mueller, L. D., et al. (2014). Activation during the Trail Making Test measured with functional near-infrared spectroscopy in healthy elderly subjects. *Neuroimage* 85(Pt 1), 583–591. doi: 10.1016/j.neuroimage.2013.09.014

Hege, M. A., Stingl, K. T., Kullmann, S., Schag, K., Giel, K. E., Zipfel, S., et al. (2014). Attentional impulsivity in binge eating disorder modulates response inhibition performance and frontal brain networks. *Int. J. Obes.* 39, 353–360. doi: 10.1038/ijo.2014.99

Heinzel, S., Metzger, F. G., Ehlis, A.-C., Korell, R., Alboji, A., Haeussinger, F. B., et al. (2013). Aging-related cortical reorganization of verbal fluency processing: a functional near-infrared spectroscopy study. *Neurobiol. Aging* 34, 439–450. doi: 10.1016/j.neurobiolaging.2012.05.021

Henges, A. L., and Marczinski, C. A. (2012). Impulsivity and alcohol consumption in young social drinkers. *Addict. Behav.* 2, 217–220. doi: 10.1016/j.addbeh.2011.09.013

Herrmann, M. J., Saathoff, C., Schreppel, T. J., Ehlis, A. C., Scheuerpflug, P., Pauli, P., et al. (2009). The effect of ADHD symptoms on performance monitoring in a non-clinical population. *Psychiatry Res.* 169, 144–148. doi: 10.1016/j.psychres.2008.06.015

Holtmann, M., Sonuga-Barke, E., Cortese, S., and Brandeis, D. (2014). Neurofeedback for ADHD: a review of current evidence. *Child Adolesc. Psychiatr. Clin. N. Am.* 23, 789–806. doi: 10.1016/j.chc.2014.05.006

Horn, N. R., Dolan, M., Elliott, R., Deakin, J. F. W., and Woodruff, P. W. R. (2003). Response inhibition and impulsivity: an fMRI study. *Neuropsychologia* 41, 1959–1966. doi: 10.1016/S0028-3932(03)00077-0

Huppert, T. J., Diamond, S. G., Franceschini, M. A., and Boas, D. A. (2009). HomER: a review of time-series analysis methods for near-infrared spectroscopy of the brain. *Appl. Opt.* 48, D280. doi: 10.1364/AO.48.00D280

Jasper, H. H. (1958). Report of the committee on methods of clinical examination in electroencephalography. *Electroencephalogr. Clin. Neurophysiol. Suppl.* 10, 370–375. doi: 10.1016/0013-4694(58)90053-1

Keilp, J. G., Sackeim, H. A., and Mann, J. J. (2005). Correlates of trait impulsiveness in performance measures and neuropsychological tests. *Psychiatry Res.* 135, 191–201. doi: 10.1016/j.psychres.2005.03.006

Kirkeby, B. S., and Robinson, M. D. (2005). Impulsive behavior and stimulus-response variability in choice reaction time. *J. Res. Pers.* 39, 263–277. doi: 10.1016/j.jrp.2004.04.001

Kolb, B., and Gibb, R. (2011). Brain plasticity and behaviour in the developing brain. *J. Can. Acad. Child Adolesc. Psychiatry* 20, 265–276.

Marshall, M. N. (1996). Sampling for qualitative research. *Fam. Pract.* 13, 522–526. doi: 10.1093/fampra/13.6.522

Marx, A.-M., Ehlis, A.-C., Furdea, A., Holtmann, M., Banaschewski, T., Brandeis, D., et al. (2015). Near-infrared spectroscopy (NIRS) neurofeedback as a treatment for children with attention deficit hyperactivity disorder (ADHD)—a pilot study. *Front. Hum. Neurosci.* 8:1038. doi: 10.3389/fnhum.2014.01038

Mayer, K., Wyckoff, S. N., Fallgatter, A. J., Ehlis, A.-C., and Strehl, U. (2015). Neurofeedback as a nonpharmacological treatment for adults with attention-deficit/hyperactivity disorder (ADHD): study protocol for a randomized controlled trial. *Trials* 16, 174. doi: 10.1186/s13063-015-0683-4

Molavi, B., and Dumont, G. A. (2012). Wavelet-based motion artifact removal for functional near-infrared spectroscopy. *Physiol. Meas.* 33, 259–270. doi: 10.1088/0967-3334/33/2/259

Muhlberger, A., Jekel, K., Probst, T., Schecklmann, M., Conzelmann, A., Andreatta, M., et al. (2016). The influence of methylphenidate on hyperactivity and attention deficits in children with ADHD: a virtual classroom test. *J. Atten. Disord.* doi: 10.1177/1087054716647480 [Epub ahead of print].

Obeso, I., Robles, N., Marron, E. M., and Redolar-Ripoll, D. (2013). Dissociating the role of the pre-SMA in response inhibition and switching: a combined online and offline TMS approach. *Front. Hum. Neurosci.* 7:150. doi: 10.3389/fnhum.2013.00150

Ridderinkhof, K. R., Van Den Wildenberg, W. P. M., Segalowitz, S. J., and Carter, C. S. (2004). Neurocognitive mechanisms of cognitive control: the role of prefrontal cortex in action selection, response inhibition, performance monitoring, and reward-based learning. *Brain Cogn.* 56, 129–140. doi: 10.1016/j.bandc.2004.09.016

Rodrigo, A. H., Di Domenico, S. I., Ayaz, H., Gulrajani, S., Lam, J., and Ruocco, A. C. (2014). Differentiating functions of the lateral and medial prefrontal cortex in motor response inhibition. *Neuroimage* 85, 423–431. doi: 10.1016/j.neuroimage.2013.01.059

Rorden, C., and Brett, M. (2000). Stereotaxic display of brain lesions. *Behav. Neurol.* 12, 191–200. doi: 10.1155/2000/421719

Rösler, M., Retz-Junginger, P., Retz, W. W., and Stieglitz, R. D. (2008). *Homburger ADHS Skalen für Erwachsene [Homburg's ADHD Scales for Adults (HASE)].* Gottingen: Hogrefe.

Rubia, K., Lim, L., Ecker, C., Halari, R., Giampietro, V., Simmons, A., et al. (2013). Effects of age and gender on neural networks of motor response inhibition: from adolescence to mid-adulthood. *Neuroimage* 83, 690–703. doi: 10.1016/j.neuroimage.2013.06.078

Sass, H., Wittchen, H. U., Zaudig, M., and Houben, I. (2003). *Diagnostisches und Statistisches Manual Psychischer Störungen DSM-IV-TR: Textrevision*, 1st Edn. Bern: Hogrefe Verlag.

Sherwood, M. S., Kane, J. H., Weisend, M. P., and Parker, J. G. (2016). Enhanced control of dorsolateral prefrontal cortex neurophysiology with real-time functional magnetic resonance imaging (rt-fMRI) neurofeedback training and working memory practice. *Neuroimage* 124, 214–223. doi: 10.1016/j.neuroimage.2015.08.074

Shulman, E. P., Smith, A. R., Silva, K., Icenogle, G., Duell, N., Chein, J., et al. (2016). The dual systems model: review, reappraisal, and reaffirmation. *Dev. Cogn. Neurosci.* 17, 103–117. doi: 10.1016/j.dcn.2015.12.010

Singh, A. K., Okamoto, M., Dan, H., Jurcak, V., and Dan, I. (2005). Spatial registration of multichannel multi-subject fNIRS data to MNI space without MRI. *Neuroimage* 27, 842–851. doi: 10.1016/j.neuroimage.2005.05.019

Soltaninejad, Z., Nejati, V., and Ekhtiari, H. (2015). Effect of anodal and cathodal transcranial direct current stimulation on DLPFC on modulation of inhibitory control in ADHD. *J. Atten. Disord.* doi: 10.1177/1087054715618792 [Epub ahead of print].

Spinella, M., and Miley, W. M. (2003). Impulsivity and academic achievement in college students. *Coll. Stud. J.* 37, 545–549.

Steinberg, L. (2008). A social neuroscience perspective on adolescent risk-taking. *Dev. Rev.* 28, 78–106. doi: 10.1016/j.dr.2007.08.002

Strangman, G., Culver, J. P., Thompson, J. H., and Boas, D. A. (2002). A quantitative comparison of simultaneous BOLD fMRI and NIRS recordings during functional brain activation. *Neuroimage* 17, 719–731. doi: 10.1016/S1053-8119(02)91227-9

Strehl, U. (2014). What learning theories can teach us in designing neurofeedback treatments. *Front. Hum. Neurosci.* 8:894. doi: 10.3389/fnhum.2014.00894

Tsuzuki, D., Jurcak, V., Singh, A. K., Okamoto, M., Watanabe, E., and Dan, I. (2007). Virtual spatial registration of stand-alone fNIRS data to MNI space. *Neuroimage* 34, 1506–1518. doi: 10.1016/j.neuroimage.2006.10.043

Verbruggen, F., Logan, G. D., and Stevens, M. A. (2008). STOP-IT: windows executable software for the stop-signal paradigm. *Behav. Res. Methods* 40, 479–483. doi: 10.3758/BRM.40.2.479

Weidacker, K., Whiteford, S., Boy, F., and Johnston, S. J. (2016). Response inhibition in the parametric Go/No-Go task and its relation to impulsivity and subclinical psychopathy. *Q. J. Exp. Psychol.* 70, 473–487. doi: 10.1080/17470218.2015.1135350

Whiteside, S. P., and Lynam, D. R. (2001). The five factor model and impulsivity: using a structural model of personality to understand impulsivity. *Pers. Individ. Dif.* 30, 669–689. doi: 10.1016/S0191-8869(00)00064-7

Zuberer, A., Brandeis, D., and Drechsler, R. (2015). Are treatment effects of neurofeedback training in children with ADHD related to the successful regulation of brain activity? A review on the learning of regulation of brain activity and a contribution to the discussion on specificity. *Front. Hum. Neurosci.* 9:135. doi: 10.3389/fnhum.2015.00135

12

Temporal Dynamics of the Default Mode Network Characterize Meditation-Induced Alterations in Consciousness

Rajanikant Panda[1,2†], Rose D. Bharath[1,2†], Neeraj Upadhyay[3], Sandhya Mangalore[2], Srivas Chennu[4,5] and Shobini L. Rao[1]*

[1] Cognitive Neuroscience Center, National Institute for Mental Health and Neurosciences, Bangalore, India, [2] Department of Neuroimaging and Interventional Radiology, National Institute for Mental Health and Neurosciences, Bangalore, India, [3] Department of Neurology and Psychiatry, Sapienza University of Rome, Rome, Italy, [4] School of Computing, University of Kent, Chatham Maritime, UK, [5] Department of Clinical Neurosciences, University of Cambridge, Cambridge, UK

Edited by:
Claudia Voelcker-Rehage,
Chemnitz University of Technology,
Germany

Reviewed by:
Tao Liu,
Zhejiang University, China
Márk Molnár,
Hungarian Academy of Sciences,
Hungary

***Correspondence:**
Rose D. Bharath
cns.researchers@gmail.com
drrosedawn@yahoo.com

†These authors have contributed equally to this work.

Current research suggests that human consciousness is associated with complex, synchronous interactions between multiple cortical networks. In particular, the default mode network (DMN) of the resting brain is thought to be altered by changes in consciousness, including the meditative state. However, it remains unclear how meditation alters the fast and ever-changing dynamics of brain activity within this network. Here we addressed this question using simultaneous electroencephalography (EEG) and functional magnetic resonance imaging (fMRI) to compare the spatial extents and temporal dynamics of the DMN during rest and meditation. Using fMRI, we identified key reductions in the posterior cingulate hub of the DMN, along with increases in right frontal and left temporal areas, in experienced meditators during rest and during meditation, in comparison to healthy controls (HCs). We employed the simultaneously recorded EEG data to identify the topographical microstate corresponding to activation of the DMN. Analysis of the temporal dynamics of this microstate revealed that the average duration and frequency of occurrence of DMN microstate was higher in meditators compared to HCs. Both these temporal parameters increased during meditation, reflecting the state effect of meditation. In particular, we found that the alteration in the duration of the DMN microstate when meditators entered the meditative state correlated negatively with their years of meditation experience. This reflected a trait effect of meditation, highlighting its role in producing durable changes in temporal dynamics of the DMN. Taken together, these findings shed new light on short and long-term consequences of meditation practice on this key brain network.

Keywords: default mode network, microstate, DMN-microstate, simultaneous EEG-fMRI, meditation

INTRODUCTION

The grand challenge of characterizing the dynamic neural substrate underlying human consciousness has captured the interest of many researchers cutting across disciplinary boundaries and covering altered states ranging from sleep, meditation, hypnosis, anesthesia, coma, disorders of consciousness, delirium tremens, psychoses, etc. Normal consciousness is thought to require both wakefulness and arousal, and several neuro scientifc studies conceptualize wakefulness as a continuum with different levels of awareness (Grill-Spektor et al., 2000; Bar et al., 2001; Kouider et al., 2010). Resting state functional magnetic resonance imaging (rsfMRI) has been used to study the neural correlates of conscious awareness in normal and altered states of consciousness. In particular, this research enterprise has highlighted and progressively refined our understanding of the so-called default mode network (DMN) of the brain, consisting of precuneus/posterior cingulate cortex (PCC), medial frontal cortex (mPFC), the temporoparietal junction (TPJ) and hipocampal formation including parahipocampal cortex, as a key neural correlate of consciousness (Buckner et al., 2008). In particular, researchers have studied changes in the DMN as a function of meditative and introspective cognitive states like day dreaming, mind wandering, and autobiographical memory retrieval (Baerentsen et al., 2010; Baron Short et al., 2010; Hasenkamp et al., 2012; Garrison et al., 2013). These investigations into the neurophenomenology of meditation have found PCC deactivation to be associated with "undistracted awareness" and "effortless doing", with PCC activation being linked to "distracted awareness" and "controlling" in experienced meditators (Garrison et al., 2013). This evidence is in line with the contrasting approaches in two major types of meditation, which either emphasize focused attention or open monitoring. Focused attention meditation aims to reduce mind wandering by concentrating on tasks like breath, sounds or mental imagery, while open monitoring meditation practice encourages mind wandering, and makes one aware of this process (Xu et al., 2014). Extensive study of the DMN in health and disease have also found correlations between DMN connectivity and sleep (Fukunaga et al., 2006; Horovitz et al., 2008; Picchioni et al., 2008), anesthesia (Vincent et al., 2007), disorders of consciousness (Fernández-Espejo et al., 2012; Guldenmund et al., 2012).

While rsfMRI has enabled us to have a fine-grained spatial understanding of the DMN in these states of consciousness, conventional analytical approaches are not best suited to measure the temporal dynamics of its activity, especially during meditation-induced alterations in the state of consciousness. To better understand the temporal dynamics of the DMN, researchers have developed a range of techniques, including time resolved resting fMRI analysis where DMN connectivity is assessed multiple times using sliding temporal windows (Chang and Glover, 2010; Hutchison et al., 2013; Leonardi et al., 2013; Allen et al., 2014; Zalesky et al., 2014). Alternative techniques to obtain temporal detail with fMRI include identification of temporal functional modes using temporal independent component analysis (ICA; Smith et al., 2012), modified seed to voxel based connectivity to define coactivation patterns (Liu and Duyn, 2013) and the recent innovation driven coactivation pattern (Karahanoglu and Van De Ville, 2015). While these methods have attempted to capture the temporal dynamics of the DMN, the time scales of the observed fluctuations in its activity vary from tens of seconds to few minutes in fMRI based studies (Chang and Glover, 2010; Handwerker et al., 2012; Hutchison et al., 2013). In contrast, modeling of electromagnetic brain dynamics using electroencephalography (EEG) and MEG suggest that these neuronal fluctuations called microstates have durations of 100–200 ms (Brandeis and Lehmann, 1989; Pascual-Marqui et al., 1995; Michel et al., 2004; Lehmann et al., 2010; Baker et al., 2014). The concept of microstates was first proposed and demonstrated by Lehmann et al. (1987) when they described brain states that remain stable for 80–120 ms before rapidly evolving into another quasi-stable microstate. The most common parameters used to quantify microstate dynamics are duration or lifespan, which is the average length of time each microstate remains stable whenever it appears. Another useful parameter is frequency of occurrence, which is the average number of times per second that the microstate becomes dominant (Lehmann et al., 1987). Most microstate studies reports four classic microstates which can explain more than 70% of the variation in the scalp topographies manifesting in EEG time series (Tei et al., 2009; Khanna et al., 2015), which have been found to be correlated with rsfMRI networks associated with phonological processing, visual processing, the salience network, and attentional switching (Mantini et al., 2007; Britz et al., 2010). Other studies have reported a higher number of microstates (10–13) with different analysis methods (Musso et al., 2010; Yuan et al., 2012), some of which correlate with the DMN. Here, we refer to the "DMN microstate" as the EEG microstate which correlated maximally with the DMN identified with fMRI. Such microstate analyses have been applied to the study of meditation, where increased duration of microstates has been reported in EEG-based studies in Chan-meditators and Ch'anMo'chao, or Vipassana meditators (Faber et al., 2005; Lo and Zhu, 2009; Tei et al., 2009). Microstate parameters have also been shown to be modulated by psychiatric disorders (Dierks et al., 1997; Lehmann et al., 2005; Kikuchi et al., 2011; Nishida et al., 2013) and even by personality type (Schlegel et al., 2012).

In this study, we analyzed the DMN microstate to understand the mechanisms of meditation-induced alterations in consciousness. By contrasting healthy controls (HCs) at rest against expert meditators at rest and during meditation, we explored both state and trait changes in DMN-microstate dynamics produced by meditation with a hypothesis that these could cause differential alterations in its duration and frequency. The state changes felt during meditation are usually described as a deep sense of calm peacefulness, cessation or slowing of mind's internal dialog and conscious awareness merging completely with the object of meditation (Brown, 1977; Wallace, 1999). Alongside, long-term expertise in meditation also produces durable changes in neural dynamics, with improvements in mental and physical health presumably due to its trait effects (Chiesa and Serretti, 2010, 2011; Hofmann et al., 2010). Here, we describe changes in the spatial configuration of the DMN as a function of meditation, and show that state and trait influences on the temporal dynamics of the DMN microstate can indeed be dissociated.

MATERIALS AND METHODS

Participants

This was a prospective study conducted at a tertiary neurological institute, the National Institute of Mental Health and

Neurosciences (NIMHANS) in Bangalore, India. The study was performed after obtaining informed written consent from the participants. They were recruited as healthy participants in the multi-institutional study on cognitive networks. Ethical approval was obtained from the institutional ethics committee for studies involving humans, convened by NIMHANS (No.NIMHANS/69th IES/2010). The meditator cohort included 20 Raja Yoga expert meditators (male; age: 35 ± 7.9 years, years of education: 15.4 ± 1.6 years, right handed) from the Brahma Kumaris Spiritual Organization, all of them with more than 10 years of Raja yoga meditation practice. Raja yoga meditation involves internally visualizing a glowing star as rays emerging between the eye brows and thus could be considered a type of focused attention type of meditation practice. All participants reported that they spent 1.68 ± 0.59 h in meditation per day in the last 10–22 years (15.2 ± 3.54). They also reported having a cumulative experience of 11332.5 ± 6009.86 h of meditation practice (cumulative experience calculated by combining the numbers of hours per day with years of meditation practice) in their life. Twenty HCs were also recruited for the study. The control participants were matched with the meditator cohort by age, gender, education and ethnicity (male; age: 29 ± 6.8 years, years of education: 16.1 ± 1.1 years, right handed) and both the groups were comparable. None of controls had experience in any type of regular meditative practices. Both meditators and control participants were multilingual (languages known 3.38 ± 0.58), with kannada as first language. None of the participants had any history of neurological or psychiatric illnesses, or prior trauma, and were not on any chronic medications that could affect the experiment.

Experiment Design

The study design was explained to the subjects and instructions were given before performing the EEG-fMRI data collection in the MRI scanner. The participants (both controls and meditators) were instructed to lie awake, with their eyes closed in a relaxed state within the MRI gantry. They were advised to refrain from any cognitive, language or motor tasks during the acquisition. Ear plugs were given to reduce scanner induced noise. Initially a 4.24 min structural MRI was recorded. This allowed them to get familiarized with the MRI environment before starting the rest and meditation session. A single resting EEG-fMRI was obtained in HCs (9.24 min). However in meditators two serial (9.24 min each) resting EEG-fMRI were recorded, one during resting wakefulness, followed immediately by one during meditation. During a *post hoc* interview, all meditators reported that they could satisfactorily achieve the meditative state inside the scanner. This was also subsequently confirmed with analysis of the EEG wave form, where we visually inspected the EEG time series in the time and spectral domains to identify an increase in alpha oscillations during meditation, consistent with previous studies which have reported this increase (Takahashi et al., 2005; Lagopoulos et al., 2009).

Data Acquisition

EEG Data Acquisitions

EEG data were recorded using a 32-channel MR-compatible EEG system (Brain Products GmbH, Gilching, Germany). The EEG cap (BrainCap MR, Brain Products) consisted of 31 scalp electrodes placed according to the international 10–20 system electrode placement and one additional electrode dedicated to the ECG which was placed on the back of the subject. Data were recorded relative to an FCz reference and a ground electrode (GND) according to 10–20 electrode system. Data was sampled at 5000 Hz to enable removal of MRI gradient artifact. The impedance between electrode and scalp was kept below 5 kΩ. EEG was recorded using the Brain Recorder software (Version 1.03, Brain Products). To prevent the movement of the subjects' head, we placed sufficient padding between the head and the head coil of the MRI scanner. Total time for each rest EEG recoding was same as rsfMRI recording (9.24 min), and time locked to each other.

fMRI Data Acquisition

rsfMRI was acquired using a 3T scanner (Skyra, Siemens, Erlangen, Germany). One hundred and eighty-five volumes of gradient-echo, Echo-Planar Images (EPI) were obtained using the following EPI parameters: 36 slices, 4 mm slice thickness in interleaved manner with an field of view (FOV) of 192 × 192 mm, matrix 64 × 64, repetition time (TR) 3000 ms, echo time (TE) 35 ms, re-focusing pulse 90°, matrix- 256 × 256 × 114, voxel size-3 × 3 × 4 mm. We also acquired a three dimensional magnetization prepared rapid acquisition gradient echo (3D MPRAGE) sequence for anatomical information (with the voxel size 1 × 1 × 1 mm, 192 × 192 × 256 matrix) for better registration and overlay of brain activity.

Data Analysis

EEG Artifact Removal and Preprocessing

Raw EEG data was processed offline using BrainVision Analyzer software version 2 (Brain Products GmbH, Gilching, Germany). The gradient artifacts were corrected according to Allen et al. (2000). A moving average width of 20 MR volumes (TRs) was used for gradient correction. Corrected EEG data were filtered using a high-pass filter at 0.03 Hz and a low-pass filter at 75 Hz. The data was then down-sampled to 250 Hz. Ballistocardiogram (BCG) artifacts were removed from the EEG using an averaged subtraction method using heartbeat events (R peaks; Allen et al., 1998, 2000; Goldman et al., 2000), implemented in BrainVision Analyzer 2. Once gradient and BCG artifacts were removed, the data were downsampled to 250 Hz. They were visually inspected for artifacts resulting from muscular sources or head movement artifact and any epoch containing any channel varying more than 150 μV was rejected. Finally, the signal was filtered with a band-pass of 0.01–45 Hz. To confirm that the meditators were in the meditative state during the second session, EEG spectral analysis was carried out for the entire 9.24 min for resting state and for the entire 9.24 min for meditative state. A fast fourier transform (FFT) was used to calculate spectral power density (μV^2).

EEG Feature Extraction

The EEG microstates were derived from the resting EEG data using sLORETA software. To compute microstates the local maxima of the global field power (GFP; Lehmann and Skrandies, 1980) were identified. Since scalp topography remains stable around peaks of GFP as a result of temporal smoothing in sLORETA, they are representative of the transient microstates (Pascual-Marqui et al., 1995; Koenig et al., 2002). The algorithm implemented for estimating microstates is based on a modified version of the classical k-means clustering method in which cluster orientations are estimated. An optimal number of 13 clusters for this method was determined by means of a cross-validation criterion (Pascual-Marqui et al., 1995). The entire EEG data at each time point was decomposed into a temporal sequence of one of these 13 EEG microstates. We used this EEG microstate decomposition to guide the analysis of the rsfMRI data at the single subject level.

rsfMRI Preprocessing

The rsfMRI analysis was performed using FSL software (FMRIB's Software Library[1]), in particular with the fMRI Expert Analysis Tool (FEAT) and multivariate exploratory linear decomposition into independent components (MELODIC) modules. The first five functional images (EPI volumes) were discarded from each of the subjects' rsfMRI data to allow for signal equilibration, giving a total of 180 volumes used in analysis. We conducted motion correction using MCFLIRT (Jenkinson et al., 2002), and non-brain tissue (Scalp, CSF, etc.) removal using the Brain Extraction Toolbox (Smith, 2002). The average head motion of the subjects was also not found to significantly differ between the groups. Spatial smoothing was performed using a Gaussian kernel of 5 mm full width at half maximum (FWHM), followed by a mean based intensity normalization of all volumes by the same factor, and then a high temporal band-pass filtering with sigma 180 s. These temporal filtering parameters were based on previously validated methodology employed by Beckmann and Smith (Smith et al., 2004; Beckmann and Smith, 2005; Beckmann et al., 2005). We co-registered the EPI volumes with the individual subject's high-resolution anatomical volume in MNI152 standard space template and re-sampled the filtered data into standard space, keeping the re-sampled resolution at the fMRI resolution (3 mm) using FNIRT, the FMRIB non-linear image registration tool (Klein et al., 2009). Two participants from each group were excluded due to uncorrectable cardio-ballistic and motion artifacts during data preprocessing.

Identification of DMN-Microstate

The spectral Z-stats maps of the EEG microstates were created by convolving all the 13 microstates with the gamma hemodynamic response function using customized three column format in FEAT Version 5.98, part of FSL (FMRIB's Software Library[2]). The GLM was modeled as an event related design, where EEG microstates were considered as explanatory variables (regressors) for rsfMRI analysis. This procedure, enabled us to combine EEG and fMRI time series despite their very different sampling rates. To do so, the onset time and the duration of each EEG microstate were provided as inputs to the GLM and convolved with a gamma hemodynamic response function (Musso et al., 2010). This rsfMRI, thus informed by the EEG microstates, was analyzed at the individual level to derive subject-wise Z-stats maps for each microstate. We examined the spatial correlation (R) between the spectral Z-stats map and the DMN component estimated by ICA of blood-oxygen-level dependent (BOLD) activity (see below). Using the FSL utility "fslcc", the Z-stats maps which correlated with BOLD ICA map of the DMN with a correlation of at least 0.3 were selected for further analysis (Kiviniemi et al., 2011). When more than one microstate Z-map correlated with the DMN the one with highest correlation was selected. This subject-wise spectral Z-stats map of the DMN microstate was included in further group analysis. Group level analysis was done using the higher level FEAT tool, where three group mean effects (controls at rest, meditators at rest and meditation state) were extracted by specifying the contrast (1 0 0; 0 1 0; 0 0 1) respectively.

Independent Components (ICs)

Functional connectivity was ascertained using ICA which decomposes the rsfMRI data into statistically independent spatial maps (and associated time series). This is a data driven approach by which we can extract the functional networks in a voxel-wise manner based on their spatial and temporal signal fluctuations. ICA of rsfMRI was carried out with the probabilistic independent components analysis (PICA) using FSL's MELODIC method. This single-subject ICA was carried out with FEAT MELODIC data exploration, in which the rsfMRI data was extracted into the independent components (ICs) during the preprocessing step. All extracted IC were visually inspected. Non-motion related noise sources such as eye related artifacts, field in homogeneity, high frequency noise, slice dropout and gradient instability were removed on the basis of existing literature (Smith et al., 2004; Beckmann and Smith, 2005; Beckmann et al., 2005). ICs that showed clearly identifiable patterns in both spatial and frequency domains, and activations in frequency plots below 0.1 Hz were removed to reduce respiration and heart rate related artifacts. The selected noise components were removed using the command "fsl_regfilt" defined in FSL MELODIC. Multivariate group PICA was then carried out using FSL MELODIC (Beckmann and Smith, 2005; Beckmann et al., 2005), to derive maximally spatially ICs across all datasets (18 control and 18 meditator × 2 sessions), which were temporally concatenated. The data set was decomposed into 15 sets of independent vectors which describe signal variation across the

[1]www.fmrib.ox.ac.uk/fsl

[2]http://fsl.fmrib.ox.ac.uk/fsl/fslwiki/

temporal (timecourses) and spatial (maps) domain by optimizing for non-Gaussian spatial source distributions using the Fast ICA algorithm. The resulting maps were threshold using an alternative hypothesis test with a significance level of $p > 0.5$ (i.e., an equal weight is placed on false positives and false negatives) by fitting a Gaussian/Gamma mixture model to the histogram of intensity values (Smith et al., 2004; Beckmann and Smith, 2005). Finally, the components representing the DMN were visually identified from the set of group IC maps by comparing their constituent cortical sources with the regions of the DMN reported in the literature (Beckmann and Smith, 2005; Beckmann et al., 2005; Damoiseaux et al., 2006).

DMN-Microstate Statistical Analysis

The mean duration and number of occurrences per second of the DMN microstates were calculated for each subject. The duration of the DMN-microstate was defined as a continuous time epoch (milliseconds) during which all EEG GFP maps were assigned to the the DMN-microstate class by the k-means clustering algorithm. The frequency of occurrence of the DMN-microstate is defined the number of such occurrences per second. Group differences were calculated for both the DMN-microstate duration and frequency of occurrence for all subjects. Independent samples *t*-tests were carried out to compare the difference between meditators and controls at rest, and a paired sample *t*-test was carried out between the meditator at rest and during meditation. At a 95% confidence interval (CI), a *p*-value of < 0.05 was considered significant. Furthermore, the number of years of meditation practice were correlated with the duration and occurrence of DMN microstates with a pearson correlation. Multiple comparisons were compensated for by FDR correction.

DMN Dual Regression Analysis

Groupwise comparison of rsfMRI ICs was performed using dual regression, which allows for voxel-wise comparisons[3]. The set of spatial maps from the group-mean analysis (GroupICs) was used to generate subject-specific-spatial maps and associated time series (Beckmann et al., 2009; Filippini et al., 2009). DMN component maps from all subjects were arranged into a single 4D file and voxel-wise differences were estimated. Statistical differences were assessed using randomized, on-parametric permutation, incorporating the threshold-free cluster enhancement (TFCE) technique (Smith et al., 2009). Separate null distributions of *t*-values were derived for the contrasts reflecting the inter-group effects by performing 5000 random permutations and testing the difference between groups or against zero for each iteration (Nichols and Holmes, 2002). To estimate group mean effects, HC > meditator, meditator > HCs, meditator > meditation and mediation > meditator contrasts were used and the resultant statistical maps were threshold at $p < 0.05$ (family-wise error (FWE) corrected). Following this, inter-group effects were threshold by at $p < 0.05$ (false discovery rate (FDR) corrected; Filippini et al., 2009). When the voxel wise differences between the groups were higher, the term "increased connectivity" was used and vice versa.

[3]http://fsl.fmrib.ox.ac.uk/fsl/fslwiki/DualRegression

RESULTS

Despite being in an MRI scanner with gradient acoustic noise, with a fixed head and body position, all meditators reported that they were able to stay awake in relaxed state and also enter into a meditative state as instructed. Visual inspection of the EEG for sleep spindles and K-complexes confirmed that none of the subjects fell asleep during rsfMRI data acquisition. In all the results presented below, three conditions are compared, controls at rest, meditators at rest, and the same meditators during meditation.

Group Level EEG Frequency Differences During Meditation

Significant changes were noted in spectral power of EEG frequency bands between the meditation and rest states in meditators. Meditators had increased power particularly in the alpha, theta and beta frequencies in the meditation state compared to rest state, which is depicted in the **Figure 1**. This also ascertained that the meditators did not go into meditative state during resting state and performed meditation in meditative state as instructed.

Spatial Analysis of DMN-Microstate and DMN During Meditation

Figure 2 depicts the average DMN-microstate, the corresponding Z-stats map and rsfMRI-derived DMN ICA component in HCs, meditators at rest (meditator) and during meditation.

Dual regression analysis (**Figure 3**) of the rsfMRI DMN revealed that meditators were different from HCs ($p < 0.05$) already at rest, as they had decreased posterior cingulate (number of voxels: 223, T-max: 0.987, coordinates: −4, −40, 26) connectivity, increased right middle frontal gyrus (MFG; number of voxels: 263, T-max: 0.956, coordinates: 42, 8, 46) and left middle temporal gyrus (MTG; number of voxels: 53, T-max: 0.963, coordinates: −52, −48, 6) connectivity. This

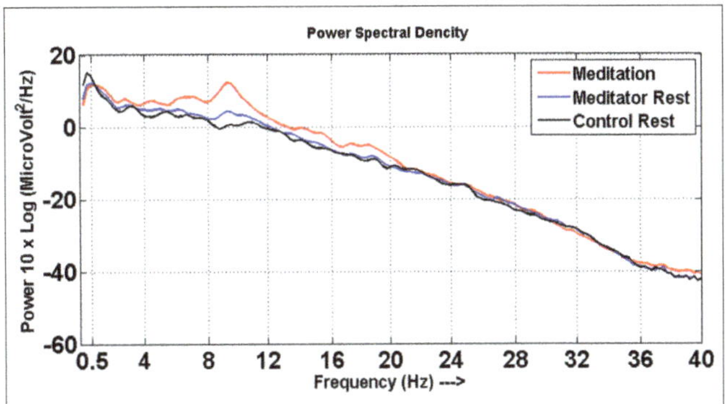

FIGURE 1 | Power spectra. Power spectral density distribution for meditators at meditative state (red line) and at rest (blue line), control at rest (black line).

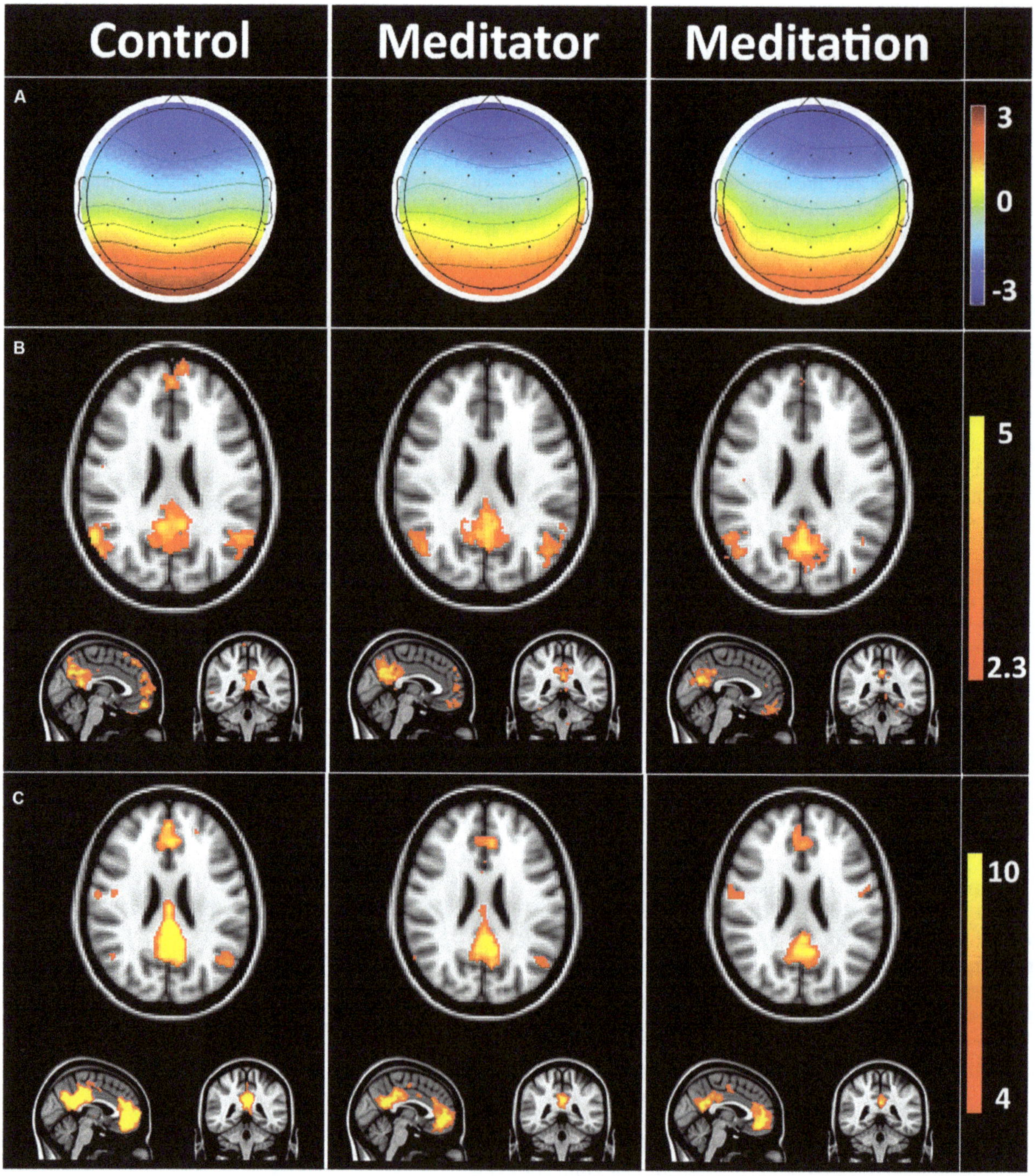

FIGURE 2 | Default mode network (DMN) microstates during rest and meditation. (A) Group averaged electroencephalography (EEG) microstate in controls at rest (control), meditator at rest state (meditator) and meditator during meditation (meditation). **(B)** Group averaged Z-stats maps corresponding to the DMN microstates. **(C)** Corresponding DMN components derived from resting state functional magnetic resonance imaging (rsfMRI) using independent components analysis (ICA). The striking spatial similarity between the EEG-derived DMN Z-stats map **(B)** and rsfMRI-derived DMN **(C)** is evident. Meditators showed evidence of decreased connectivity in precuneus/posterior cingulate cortex (PCC) and medial prefrontal cortex (mPFC) at rest, which decreased further during meditation **(C)**.

relatively lower cingulate connectivity was further significantly reduced relative to rest, when the meditators entered into the meditative state (number of voxels: 107, T-max: 0.998, coordinates: −2, −40, 26). Alongside this reduction, we also observed increased left MTG (number of voxels: 122, T-max: 0.992, coordinates: −58, −46, 8) and right MFG (number of voxels: 424, T-max: 0.998, coordinates: 40, 8, 46) connectivity during meditation.

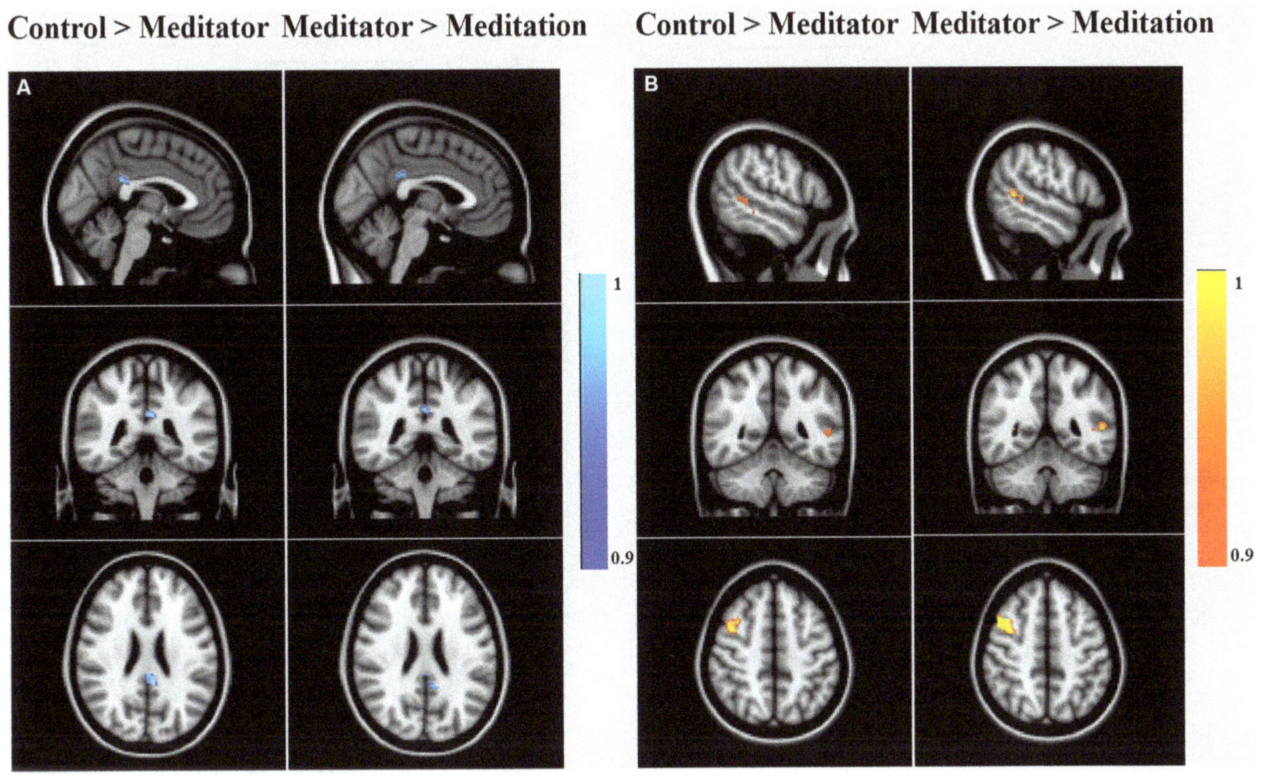

FIGURE 3 | Dual regression analysis of group main and between-group effects in the rsfMRI DMN component. Between-group effects showed significant ($p < 0.05$ false discovery rate (FDR) corrected) decreased PCC connectivity in meditators compared to controls, which further decreased during meditation. **(A)** Meditators had higher connectivity in right middle frontal gyrus (MFG) and left middle temporal gyrus (MTG) than controls, which again increased during meditation **(B)**.

Temporal Analysis of the DMN-Microstate

The meditators at rest had increased duration and higher frequency of occurrence of the DMN-microstate compared to controls (**Figure 4**).The mean duration of the DMN-microstate was 93.05 ± 15.18 ms in HCs and 118.88 ± 12.78 ms in meditators at rest (Unpaired t-test, $t = -3.55$; df = 34; $p = 3.6\text{E-}06$); the mean frequency of its occurrence was 3.15 ± 0.66/s in controls and 3.84 ± 0.48/s in meditators (Unpaired t-test, $t = -3.56$; df = 34; $p = 0.001$). During meditation the duration and frequency of occurrence increased significantly further. Specifically, during meditation, the mean duration of DMN-microstate was 134.27 ± 11.21 ms (Paired t-test, $t = -5.06$; df = 17; $p = 9.5\text{E-}05$) and the mean frequency of occurrence was 4.03 ± 0.46/s (Paired t-test, $t = -5.06$; df = 17; $p = 1.3\text{E-}06$; **Figure 4**).

Correlation of DMN-Microstate Dynamics With Years of Experience in Meditation

The observed differences in the temporal properties of the DMN-microstate suggested a combination of state and trait-based influencces. To further explicate the influence of long-term meditation experience in engendering trait differences between meditators and controls, we correlated the duration and frequency of occurrence of the DMN-microstate in individual meditators with their meditation experience in years. The results are summarized in **Figure 5**. There was a very strong, significant positive correlation in the duration of DMN-microstate in meditators at rest ($r = 0.96$, $p = 7.3\text{E-}11$) and in the meditative state ($r = 0.51$, $p = 0.03$) with years of meditation practice (**Figure 5A**). Interestingly, in each meditator, the net increase in the duration of the DMN-microstate during meditation relative to rest actually correlated negatively with the years of meditation practice (**Figure 5C**, $r = -0.549$, $p = 0.023$). This implied that the more experienced meditators had a DMN-microstate duration akin to being in a meditative state even at rest, highlighting how the state effect of meditation on DMN dynamics gradually transitions into a trait effect that potentially permanently alters it over many years of practice. However, this effect could potentially be explained away by the age of the meditators rather than their years of experience, as participants with longer years of experience were older than those with lesser experience. To address this potential confound, we regressed out this effect by including age of the meditator as a covariate in the correlation analysis. Having accounted for the influence of age, we still found a significant negative correlation between the state-induced change in DMN-microstate duration and years of mediation experience ($r = -0.549$, $p = 0.03$). This confirmed that there was indeed a trait-level modulation of the DMN's dynamics produced

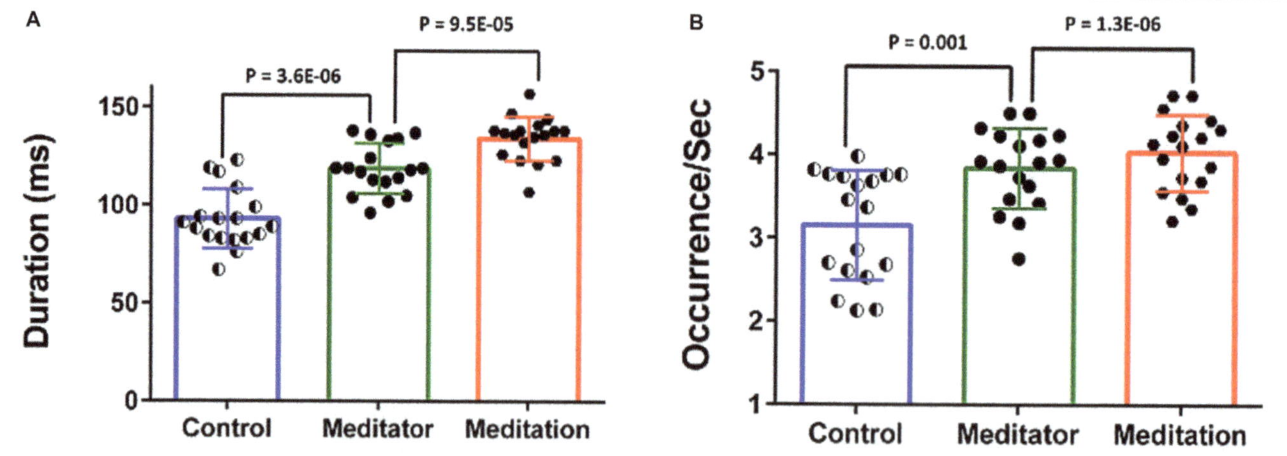

FIGURE 4 | Temporal dynamics of the DMN-microstate. Bar charts plot the duration **(A)** and occurence/s **(B)** of the DMN-microstate in healthy controls (HCs), meditators at rest and during meditation. Both measures were significantly higher in meditators than in controls, and increased further during meditation.

by meditation experience, that could not be explained away by aging.

Further, we found that this pattern of effects were specific to the duration of the DMN-microstate. Specifically, the effect of meditation experience on the frequency of occurrence of the DMN-microstate was not statistically significant, either at rest ($r = 0.43$, $p = 0.06$) or in the meditative state ($r = 0.46$, $p = 0.053$), though there was a trend towards increasing DMN-microstate occurrence with increasing years of meditation practice (**Figure 5B**). Further, the meditation state induced increase in the frequency of occurrence did not correlate with years of practice ($r = -0.004$, $p = 0.98$). As the frequency of occurrence of the DMN-microstate was unaffected by the years of experience, it was distinct from duration and is probably indicative of the state effect of meditation, as seen in **Figure 4B**.

DISCUSSION

We have investigated dynamic alterations of the DMN using simultaneous EEG-fMRI, with the aim of characterizing the spatial and temporal changes caused by meditation induced alterations of consciousness. Using spatial ICA analysis of our fMRI data, we found that the posterior cingulate hub of the DMN was less strongly connected in meditators, which became further reduced during meditation. In contrast, the right middle frontal and left middle temporal gyri were more active in meditators and during meditation. By linking the fMRI with EEG, we were able to identify the DMN microstate in all participants, by matching its spatial configuration to their respective DMN ICA components. The temporal properties of this DMN-microstate highlighted its significantly higher duration and frequency of occurrence, in meditators at rest and during meditation. Further, the relationship between these temporal properties and years of meditation experience enabled us to explore state and trait influences on DMN dynamics. This analysis suggested that in less experienced meditators, entering into a meditative state was associated with significant increases both in the duration and frequency of the DMN-microstate. As experience with meditation increased, there was a progressively higher duration of the DMN-microstate at rest and entering a state of meditation only brought about an increase in its frequency of occurrence. Taken together, these findings elucidate salient spatiotemporal mechanisms of meditation, and particularly highlight its role in altering the temporal dynamics of brain activity over short and long time scales.

Within the large body of fMRI literature on resting state networks, the DMN has been a particular focus of attention (Raichle et al., 2001; Buckner et al., 2008) as a key brain network that underlies awareness of the self within the environment. Our finding of decreased PCC connectivity and increased temporal and frontal connectivity within the DMN during meditation has been reported previously in seed to voxel connectivity studies (Farb et al., 2007; Brewer et al., 2011). Alongside, the significance of the temporo-frontal regions during meditation has been consistently highlighted in previous task based fMRI studies (Brefczynski-Lewis et al., 2007; Lagopoulos et al., 2009). Indeed, our findings mirror those from recent studies on fMRI of meditation (Baijal and Srinivasan, 2010; Cahn et al., 2010; Hasenkamp and Barsalou, 2012; Hasenkamp et al., 2012). In particular, Hasenkamp and Barsalou (2012) studied the effects of meditation experience on DMN functional connectivity, and demonstrated increased connectivity in frontal areas during meditation in meditators with more experience, which they interpreted as evidence of greater attentional control gained with such experience. In our meditator cohort, these attentional control networks could also be similarly more active in the expert meditators. This increased attentional control, along with decreased PCC connectivity, is hypothesized to undergo neuroplastic changes that enable them to gain better control of mind-wandering. Based on evidence of task positive networks being recruited at rest, it has been argued that continuous and regular meditation

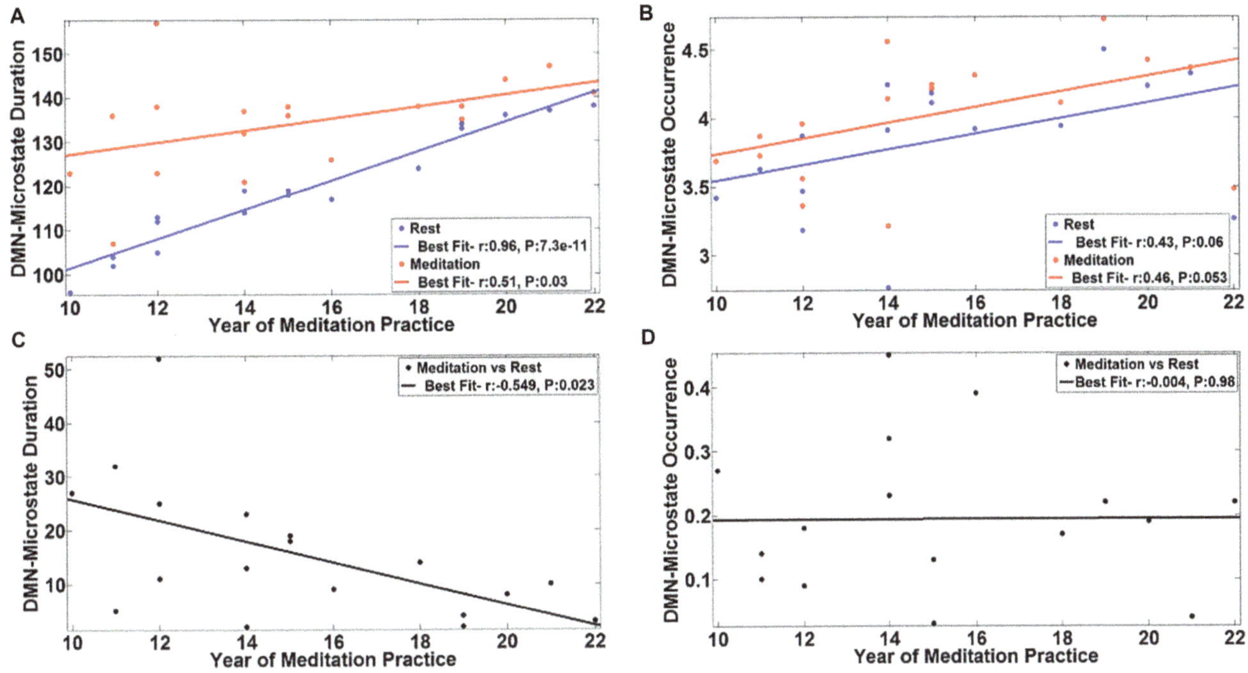

FIGURE 5 | Correlation of DMN-microstate dynamics with meditation experience. The duration **(A)** and frequency of occurrence **(B)** of the DMN-microstate were positively correlated with years of experience. The blue and red lines in dicate the linear fits of these DMN-microstate properties measured during meditation and rest, respectively. Duration was less altered as a function of state in more experienced meditators. Corroborating this trait effect, the difference in DMN-microstate duration between meditation and rest was negatively correlated with years of experience **(C)**. No such trait effect was observed in the frequency of occurrence of the DMN-microstate **(D)**.

practice transforms the rest state of experienced meditators (Brewer et al., 2011). However in the current study the right frontal and left temporal areas described are part of the DMN and do not represent task positive networks. However, it is possible that this neuroplasticity is mediated by task positive networks, and future research could elucidate how meditation modulates the relationship between these different brain networks.

Within this research context, our finding have generated new evidence delineating temporal changes in DMN activity that accompanies these spatial changes. Our finding of increasing frequency of occurrence of the DMN-microstate during meditiation implies that there is a decreased occurrence of other microstates, thus resulting in an overall decrease in variability in the temporal dynamics of brain activity. According to large scale dynamical models of consciousness (Deco et al., 2013), resting brain can be divided into three states, namely the spontaneous state, multistable attractor states and unstable spontaneous state, differing in their coupling strengths. The state with least coupling strength is the spontaneous state and that with highest coupling strength is the unstable spontaneous state often associated with a task. Human consciousness is postulated to be positioned at the verge of instability defined to lie between the multistable attractor state and the unstable spontaneous state. Within this framework, decreased variability within such a dynamical system is compatible with our finding of increased frequency of the DMN microstate during meditation. It is worth noting that the focus of the analysis here has been on the DMN-microstate, as that was the only microstate that was consistently present in all subjects. This is similar to findings reported by Musso et al. (2010), whose group analysis only revealed a fronto-occipital network that overlapped with visual networks and the DMN. This is despite the fact that all the subjects in their study had microstates which correlated with several other resting state networks. With the continual advancement in methodological tools for simultaneous EEG-fMRI analysis, we might be able parse spatiotemporal brain dynamics with the requisite detail and consistency for mapping all the resting state networks.

Our finding of experienced meditators having a higher duration of DMN microstate that did not change much in the meditative state is consistent with the philosophical perspective (Lutz et al., 2008), behavioral (Carter et al., 2005; Srinivasan and Baijal, 2007) and brain structural changes (Lazar et al., 2005) related to the trait effects of meditative practice. Because of the synergistic interaction between state and trait effects it has been largely difficult to design studies to separate these effects (Cahn and Polich, 2006) and hence relatively few studies that have exclusively looked at the state effect of meditation. In future research, the study of neurophenomenology of meditation, which correlates moment-to-moment first person reports of internal experience to guide neuroimaging analysis might be able to separate state effect from trait effects of meditation (Jack and Shallice, 2001; Jack and Roepstorff, 2002; Lutz et al., 2002).

CONCLUSION

Our investigation of the spatial configuration of the DMN in meditators and during meditation revealed a decrease in posterior cingulate connectivity, and a complementary increase in middle frontal and temporal connectivity. Using temporal microstate analysis applied to simultaneous EEG-fMRI data, we found that the duration and frequency of occurrence of the DMN-microstates are useful metrics of meditation-induced altered consciousness, and increase systematically across controls, meditators during rest and during meditation. We report complementary roles of these metrics, where duration primarily reflected the trait effect and occurrence represented the state effect of meditation. Our results shed new light on the neurobiology of meditation, and its effect on the spatiotemporal properties of the DMN in particular.

AUTHOR CONTRIBUTIONS

RP and RDB have contributed equally for this article. Contributions to the conception or design of the work by RP, RDB, SLR. Data acquisition done by RP and NU and analysis was carried out by RP, RDB, NU, SM. RDB, SC interpreted the results of the study. Manuscript drafted by RP followed by RDB, SC, NU revised the manuscript critically for important intellectual content. Final approval and agreement to be accountable for all aspects of the work in ensuring that questions related to the accuracy or integrity of any part of the work are appropriately investigated and resolved by all authors.

ACKNOWLEDGMENTS

We thank Dr. S. R. Chandra for ascertaining the quality of EEG (Department of Neurology, National Institute of Mental Health and Neurosciences (NIMHANS), India). We thank BK. Ambika, BK. Sneha, BK. Sushilchandra and BK. Srikant from Spiritual Application Research Center (SpARC), Prajapita Brahamakumari Iswariya Viswa Vidyalaya for facilitating the participation of expert meditators. We are grateful to the staff especially the radiographers, for their support. Finally, we thank all the participants for their time.

REFERENCES

Allen, E. A., Damaraju, E., Plis, S. M., Erhardt, E. B., Eichele, T., and Calhoun, V. D. (2014). Tracking whole-brain connectivity dynamics in the resting state. *Cereb. Cortex* 24, 663–676. doi: 10.1093/cercor/bhs352

Allen, P. J., Josephs, O., and Turner, R. (2000). A method for removing imaging artifact from continuous EEG recorded during functional MRI. *Neuroimage* 12, 230–239. doi: 10.1006/nimg.2000.0599

Allen, P. J., Polizzi, G., Krakow, K., Fish, D. R., and Lemieux, L. (1998). Identification of EEG events in the MR scanner: the problem of pulse artifact and a method for its subtraction. *Neuroimage* 8, 229–239. doi: 10.1006/nimg.1998.0361

Baerentsen, K. B., Stødkilde-Jørgensen, H., Sommerlund, B., Hartmann, T., Damsgaard-Madsen, J., Fosnaes, M., et al. (2010). An investigation of brain processes supporting meditation. *Cogn. Process.* 11, 57–84. doi: 10.1007/s10339-009-0342-3

Baijal, S., and Srinivasan, N. (2010). Theta activity and meditative states: spectral changes during concentrative meditation. *Cogn. Process.* 11, 31–38. doi: 10.1007/s10339-009-0272-0

Baker, A. P., Brookes, M. J., Rezek, I. A., Smith, S. M., Behrens, T., Smith, P. J. P., et al. (2014). Fast transient networks in spontaneous human brain activity. *Elife* 3:e01867. doi: 10.7554/elife.01867

Bar, M., Tootell, R. B. H., Schacter, D. L., Greve, D. N., Fischl, B., Mendola, J. D., et al. (2001). Cortical mechanisms specific to explicit visual object recognition. *Neuron* 29, 529–535. doi: 10.1016/s0896-6273(01)00224-0

Baron Short, E., Kose, S., Mu, Q., Borckardt, J., Newberg, A., George, M. S., et al. (2010). Regional brain activation during meditation shows time and practice effects: an exploratory FMRI study. *Evid Based Complement. Alternat. Med.* 7, 121–127. doi: 10.1093/ecam/nem163

Beckmann, C. F., DeLuca, M., Devlin, J. T., and Smith, S. M. (2005). Investigations into resting-state connectivity using independent component analysis. *Philos. Trans. R. Soc. Lond. B Biol. Sci.* 360, 1001–1013. doi: 10.1098/rstb.2005.1634

Beckmann, C. F., Mackay, C. E., Filippini, N., and Smith, S. M. (2009). Group comparison of resting-state fMRI data using multi-subject ICA and dual regression. *Neuroimage* 47:S148. doi: 10.1016/s1053-8119(09)71511-3

Beckmann, C. F., and Smith, S. M. (2005). Tensorial extensions of independent component analysis for multisubject fMRI analysis. *Neuroimage* 25, 294–311. doi: 10.1016/j.neuroimage.2004.10.043

Brandeis, D., and Lehmann, D. (1989). Segments of event-related potential map series reveal landscape changes with visual attention and subjective contours. *Electroencephalogr. Clin. Neurophysiol.* 73, 507–519. doi: 10.1016/0013-4694(89)90260-5

Brefczynski-Lewis, J. A., Lutz, A., Schaefer, H. S., Levinson, D. B., and Davidson, R. J. (2007). Neural correlates of attentional expertise in long-term meditation practitioners. *Proc. Natl. Acad. Sci. U S A* 104, 11483–11488. doi: 10.1073/pnas.0606552104

Brewer, J. A., Worhunsky, P. D., Gray, J. R., Tang, Y.-Y., Weber, J., and Kober, H. (2011). Meditation experience is associated with differences in default mode network activity and connectivity. *Proc. Natl. Acad. Sci. U S A* 108, 20254–20259. doi: 10.1073/pnas.1112029108

Britz, J., Van De Ville, D., and Michel, C. M. (2010). BOLD correlates of EEG topography reveal rapid resting-state network dynamics. *Neuroimage* 52, 1162–1170. doi: 10.1016/j.neuroimage.2010.02.052

Brown, D. P. (1977). A model for the levels of concentrative meditation. *Int. J. Clin. Exp. Hypn.* 25, 236–273. doi: 10.1080/00207147708415984

Buckner, R. L., Andrews-Hanna, J. R., and Schacter, D. L. (2008). The brain's default network: anatomy, function, and relevance to disease. *Ann. N Y Acad. Sci.* 1124, 1–38. doi: 10.1196/annals.1440.011

Cahn, B. R., Delorme, A., and Polich, J. (2010). Occipital gamma activation during Vipassana meditation. *Cogn. Process.* 11, 39–56. doi: 10.1007/s10339-009-0352-1

Cahn, B. R., and Polich, J. (2006). Meditation states and traits: EEG, ERP and neuroimaging studies. *Psychol. Bull.* 132, 180–211. doi: 10.1037/0033-2909.132.2.180

Carter, O. L., Presti, D. E., Callistemon, C., Ungerer, Y., Liu, G. B., and Pettigrew, J. D. (2005). Meditation alters perceptual rivalry in Tibetan Buddhist monks. *Curr. Biol.* 15, R412–R413. doi: 10.1016/j.cub.2005.05.043

Chang, C., and Glover, G. H. (2010). Time-frequency dynamics of resting-state brain connectivity measured with fMRI. *Neuroimage* 50, 81–98. doi: 10.1016/j.neuroimage.2009.12.011

Chiesa, A., and Serretti, A. (2010). A systematic review of neurobiological and clinical features of mindfulness meditations. *Psychol. Med.* 40, 1239–1252. doi: 10.1017/s0033291709991747

Chiesa, A., and Serretti, A. (2011). Mindfulness based cognitive therapy for psychiatric disorders: a systematic review and meta-analysis. *Psychiatry Res.* 187, 441–453. doi: 10.1016/j.psychres.2010.08.011

Damoiseaux, J. S., Rombouts, S. A. R. B., Barkhof, F., Scheltens, P., Stam, C. J., Smith, S. M., et al. (2006). Consistent resting-state networks across healthy subjects. *Proc. Natl. Acad. Sci. U S A* 103, 13848–13853. doi: 10.1073/pnas.0601417103

Deco, G., Jirsa, V. K., and McIntosh, A. R. (2013). Resting brains never rest: computational insights into potential cognitive architectures. *Trends Neurosci.* 36, 268–274. doi: 10.1016/j.tins.2013.03.001

Dierks, T., Jelic, V., Julin, P., Maurer, K., Wahlund, L. O., Almkvist, O., et al. (1997). EEG-microstates in mild memory impairment and Alzheimer's disease: possible association with disturbed information processing. *J. Neural. Transm. (Vienna)* 104, 483–495. doi: 10.1007/bf01277666

Faber, P. L., Lehmann, D., Barendregt, H., Kaelin, M., and Gianotti, L. R. R. (2005). Increased duration of EEG microstates during meditation. *Brain Topogr.* 18, 131.

Farb, N. A. S., Segal, Z. V., Mayberg, H., Bean, J., Mckeon, D., Fatima, Z., et al. (2007). Attending to the present: mindfulness meditation reveals distinct neural modes of self-reference. *Soc. Cogn. Affect. Neurosci.* 2, 313–322. doi: 10.1093/scan/nsm030

Fernández-Espejo, D., Soddu, A., Cruse, D., Palacios, E. M., Junque, C., Vanhaudenhuyse, A., et al. (2012). A role for the default mode network in the bases of disorders of consciousness. *Ann. Neurol.* 72, 335–343. doi: 10.1002/ana.23635

Filippini, N., MacIntosh, B. J., Hough, M. G., Goodwin, G. M., Frisoni, G. B., Smith, S. M., et al. (2009). Distinct patterns of brain activity in young carriers of the APOE-ϵ4 allele. *Proc. Natl. Acad. Sci. U S A* 106, 7209–7214. doi: 10.1016/s1053-8119(09)71381-3

Fukunaga, M., Horovitz, S. G., van Gelderen, P., de Zwart, J. A., Jansma, J. M., Ikonomidou, V. N., et al. (2006). Large-amplitude, spatially correlated fluctuations in BOLD fMRI signals during extended rest and early sleep stages. *Magn. Reson. Imaging* 24, 979–992. doi: 10.1016/j.mri.2006.04.018

Garrison, K. A., Santoyo, J. F., Davis, J. H., Thornhill, T. A., Kerr, C. E., and Brewer, J. A. (2013). Effortless awareness: using real time neurofeedback to investigate correlates of posterior cingulate cortex activity in meditators' self-report. *Front. Hum. Neurosci.* 7:440. doi: 10.3389/fnhum.2013.00440

Goldman, R. I., Stern, J. M., Engel, J., and Cohen, M. S. (2000). Acquiring simultaneous EEG and functional MRI. *Clin. Neurophysiol.* 111, 1974–1980. doi: 10.1016/s1388-2457(00)00456-9

Grill-Spektor, K., Kushnir, T., Hendler, T., and Malach, R. (2000). The dynamics of object-selective activation correlate with recogntion performance in human. *Nat. Neurosci.* 3, 837–843. doi: 10.1038/77754

Guldenmund, J. P., Vanhaudenhuyse, A., Boly, M., Laureys, S., and Soddu, A. (2012). A default mode of brain function in altered states of consciousness. *Arch. Ital. Biol.* 150, 107–121. doi: 10.4449/aib.v150i2.1373

Handwerker, D. A., Roopchansingh, V., Gonzalez-Castillo, J., and Bandettini, P. A. (2012). Periodic changes in fMRI connectivity. *Neuroimage* 63, 1712–1719. doi: 10.1016/j.neuroimage.2012.06.078

Hasenkamp, W., and Barsalou, L. W. (2012). Effects of meditation experience on functional connectivity of distributed brain networks. *Front. Hum. Neurosci.* 6:38. doi: 10.3389/fnhum.2012.00038

Hasenkamp, W., Wilson-Mendenhall, C. D., Duncan, E., and Barsalou, L. W. (2012). Mind wandering and attention during focused meditation: a fine-grained temporal analysis of fluctuating cognitive states. *Neuroimage* 59, 750–760. doi: 10.1016/j.neuroimage.2011.07.008

Hofmann, S. G., Sawyer, A. T., Witt, A. A., and Oh, D. (2010). The effect of mindfulness-based therapy on anxiety and depression: a meta-analytic review. *J. Consult. Clin. Psychol.* 78, 169–183. doi: 10.1037/a0018555

Horovitz, S. G., Fukunaga, M., de Zwart, J. A., van Gelderen, P., Fulton, S. C., Balkin, T. J., et al. (2008). Low frequency BOLD fluctuations during resting wakefulness and light sleep: a simultaneous EEG-fMRI study. *Hum. Brain Mapp.* 29, 671–682. doi: 10.1002/hbm.20428

Hutchison, R. M., Womelsdorf, T., Allen, E. A., Bandettini, P. A., Calhoun, V. D., Corbetta, M., et al. (2013). Dynamic functional connectivity: promise, issues and interpretations. *Neuroimage* 80, 360–378. doi: 10.1016/j.neuroimage.2013.05.079

Jack, A. I., and Shallice, T. (2001). Introspective physicalism as an approach to the science of consciousness. *Cognition* 79, 161–196. doi: 10.1016/s0010-0277(00)00128-1

Jack, A. I., and Roepstorff, A. (2002). Introspection and cognitive brain mapping: from stimulus-response to script-report. *Trends Cogn. Sci.* 6, 333–339. doi: 10.1016/s1364-6613(02)01941-1

Jenkinson, M., Bannister, P., Brady, M., and Smith, S. (2002). Improved optimization for the robust and accurate linear registration and motion correction of brain images. *Neuroimage* 17, 825–841. doi: 10.1006/nimg.2002.1132

Karahanoglu, F. I., and Van De Ville, D. (2015). Transient brain activity disentangles fMRI resting-state dynamics in terms of spatially and temporally overlapping networks. *Nat. Commun.* 6:7751. doi: 10.1038/ncomms8751

Khanna, A., Pascual-Leone, A., Michel, C. M., and Farzan, F. (2015). Microstates in resting-state EEG: current status and future directions. *Neurosci. Biobehav. Rev.* 49, 105–113. doi: 10.1016/j.neubiorev.2014.12.010

Kikuchi, M., Koenig, T., Munesue, T., Hanaoka, A., Strik, W., Dierks, T., et al. (2011). EEG microstate analysis in drug-naive patients with panic disorder. *PLoS One* 6:e22912. doi: 10.1371/journal.pone.0022912

Kiviniemi, V., Vire, T., Remes, J., Elseoud, A. A., Starck, T., Tervonen, O., et al. (2011). A sliding time-window ICA reveals spatial variability of the default mode network in time. *Brain Connect.* 1, 339–347. doi: 10.1089/brain.2011.0036

Klein, A., Andersson, J., Ardekani, B. A., Ashburner, J., Avants, B., Chiang, M. C., et al. (2009). Evaluation of 14 nonlinear deformation algorithms applied to human brain MRI registration. *Neuroimage* 46, 786–802. doi: 10.1016/j.neuroimage.2008.12.037

Koenig, T., Prichep, L., Lehmann, D., Sosa, P. V., Braeker, E., Kleinlogel, H., et al. (2002). Millisecond by millisecond, year by year: normative EEG microstates and developmental stages. *Neuroimage* 16, 41–48. doi: 10.1006/nimg.2002.1070

Kouider, S., de Gardelle, V., Sackur, J., and Dupoux, E. (2010). How rich is consciousness? The partial awareness hypothesis. *Trends Cogn. Sci.* 14, 301–307. doi: 10.1016/j.tics.2010.04.006

Lagopoulos, J., Xu, J., Rasmussen, I., Vik, A., Malhi, G. S., Eliassen, C. F., et al. (2009). Increased theta and alpha EEG activity during nondirective meditation. *J. Altern. Complement. Med.* 15, 1187–1192. doi: 10.1089/acm.2009.0113

Lazar, S. W., Kerr, C. E., Wasserman, R. H., Gray, J. R., Greve, D. N., Treadway, M. T., et al. (2005). Meditation experience is associated with increased cortical thickness. *Neuroreport* 16, 1893–1897. doi: 10.1097/01.wnr.0000186598.66243.19

Lehmann, D., and Skrandies, W. (1980). Reference-free identification of components of checkerboard-evoked multichannel potential fields. *Electroencephalogr. Clin. Neurophysiol.* 48, 609–621. doi: 10.1016/0013-4694(80)90419-8

Lehmann, D., Faber, P. L., Galderisi, S., Herrmann, W. M., Kinoshita, T., Koukkou, M., et al. (2005). EEG microstate duration and syntax in acute, medication-naïve, first-episode schizophrenia: a multi-center study. *Psychiatry Res.* 138, 141–156. doi: 10.1016/j.pscychresns.2004.05.007

Lehmann, D., Ozaki, H., and Pal, I. (1987). EEG alpha map series: brain micro-states by space-oriented adaptive segmentation. *Electroencephalogr. Clin. Neurophysiol.* 67, 271–288. doi: 10.1016/0013-4694(87)90025-3

Lehmann, D., Pascual-Marqui, R. D., Strik, W. K., and Koenig, T. (2010). Core networks for visual-concrete and abstract thought content: a brain electric microstate analysis. *Neuroimage* 49, 1073–1079. doi: 10.1016/j.neuroimage.2009.07.054

Leonardi, N., Richiardi, J., Gschwind, M., Simioni, S., Annoni, J. M., Schluep, M., et al. (2013). Principal components of functional connectivity: a new approach to study dynamic brain connectivity during rest. *Neuroimage* 83, 937–950. doi: 10.1016/j.neuroimage.2013.07.019

Liu, X., and Duyn, J. H. (2013). Time-varying functional network information extracted from brief instances of spontaneous brain activity. *Proc. Natl. Acad. Sci. U S A* 110, 4392–4397. doi: 10.1073/pnas.1216856110

Lo, P. C., and Zhu, Q. (2009). "Microstate analysis of alpha-event brain topography during chan meditation," in *Proceedings of the 2009 International Conference on Machine Learning and Cybernetics* (Baoding, China), Vol. 2, 717–721.

Lutz, A., Lachaux, J.-P., Martinerie, J., and Varela, F. J. (2002). Guiding the study of brain dynamics by using first-person data: synchrony patterns correlate with ongoing conscious states during a simple visual task. *Proc. Natl. Acad. Sci. U S A* 99, 1586–1591. doi: 10.1073/pnas.032658199

Lutz, A., Slagter, H. A., Dunne, J. D., and Davidson, R. J. (2008). Attention regulation and monitoring in meditation. *Trends Cogn. Sci.* 12, 163–169. doi: 10.1016/j.tics.2008.01.005

Mantini, D., Perrucci, M. G., Del Gratta, C., Romani, G. L., and Corbetta, M. (2007). Electrophysiological signatures of resting state networks in the human brain. *Proc. Natl. Acad. Sci. U S A* 104, 13170–13175. doi: 10.1073/pnas.0700668104

Michel, C. M., Murray, M. M., Lantz, G., Gonzalez, S., Spinelli, L., and Grave de Peralta, R. (2004). EEG source imaging. *Clin. Neurophysiol.* 115, 2195–2222. doi: 10.1016/j.clinph.2004.06.001

Musso, F., Brinkmeyer, J., Mobascher, A., Warbrick, T., and Winterer, G. (2010). Spontaneous brain activity and EEG microstates. A novel EEG/fMRI analysis approach to explore resting-state networks. *Neuroimage* 52, 1149–1161. doi: 10.1016/j.neuroimage.2010.01.093

Nichols, T. E., and Holmes, A. P. (2002). Nonparametric permutation tests for functional neuroimaging: a primer with examples. *Hum. Brain Mapp.* 15, 1–25. doi: 10.1002/hbm.1058

Nishida, K., Morishima, Y., Yoshimura, M., Isotani, T., Irisawa, S., Jann, K., et al. (2013). EEG microstates associated with salience and frontoparietal networks in frontotemporal dementia, schizophrenia and Alzheimer's disease. *Clin. Neurophysiol.* 124, 1106–1114. doi: 10.1016/j.clinph.2013.01.005

Pascual-Marqui, R. D., Michel, C. M., and Lehmann, D. (1995). Segmentation of brain electrical activity into microstates: model estimation and validation. *IEEE Trans. Biomed. Eng.* 42, 658–665. doi: 10.1109/10.391164

Picchioni, D., Fukunaga, M., Carr, W. S., Braun, A. R., Balkin, T. J., Duyn, J. H., et al. (2008). fMRI differences between early and late stage-1 sleep. *Neurosci. Lett.* 441, 81–85. doi: 10.1016/j.neulet.2008.06.010

Raichle, M. E., MacLeod, A. M., Snyder, A. Z., Powers, W. J., Gusnard, D. A., and Shulman, G. L. (2001). A default mode of brain function. *Proc. Natl. Acad. Sci. U S A* 98, 676–682. doi: 10.1073/pnas.98.2.676

Schlegel, F., Lehmann, D., Faber, P. L., Milz, P., and Gianotti, L. R. R. (2012). EEG microstates during resting represent personality differences. *Brain Topogr.* 25, 20–26. doi: 10.1007/s10548-011-0189-7

Smith, S. M. (2002). Fast robust automated brain extraction. *Hum. Brain Mapp.* 17, 143–155. doi: 10.1002/hbm.10062

Smith, S. M., Fox, P. T., Miller, K. L., Glahn, D. C., Fox, P. M., Mackay, C. E., et al. (2009). Correspondence of the brain's functional architecture during activation and rest. *Proc. Natl. Acad. Sci. U S A* 106, 13040–13045. doi: 10.1073/pnas.0905267106

Smith, S. M., Jenkinson, M., Woolrich, M. W., Beckmann, C. F., Behrens, T. E. J., Johansen-Berg, H., et al. (2004). Advances in functional and structural MR image analysis and implementation as FSL. *Neuroimage* 23, S208–S219. doi: 10.1016/j.neuroimage.2004.07.051

Smith, S. M., Miller, K. L., Moeller, S., Xu, J., Auerbach, E. J., Woolrich, M. W., et al. (2012). Temporally-independent functional modes of spontaneous brain activity. *Proc. Natl. Acad. Sci. U S A* 109, 3131–3136. doi: 10.1073/pnas.1121329109

Srinivasan, N., and Baijal, S. (2007). Concentrative meditation enhances preattentive processing: a mismatch negativity study. *Neuroreport* 18, 1709–1712. doi: 10.1097/wnr.0b013e3282f0d2d8

Takahashi, T., Murata, T., Hamada, T., Omori, M., Kosaka, H., Kikuchi, M., et al. (2005). Changes in EEG and autonomic nervous activity during meditation and their association with personality traits. *Int. J. Psychophysiol.* 55, 199–207. doi: 10.1016/j.ijpsycho.2004.07.004

Tei, S., Faber, P. L., Lehmann, D., Tsujiuchi, T., Kumano, H., Pascual-Marqui, R. D., et al. (2009). Meditators and non-meditators: EEG source imaging during resting. *Brain Topogr.* 22, 158–165. doi: 10.1007/s10548-009-0107-4

Vincent, J. L., Patel, G. H., Fox, M. D., Snyder, A. Z., Baker, J. T., Van Essen, D. C., et al. (2007). Intrinsic functional architecture in the anaesthetized monkey brain. *Nature* 447, 83–86. doi: 10.1038/nature05758

Wallace, B. A. (1999). The buddhist tradition of samatha: methods for refining and examining consciousness. *J. Conscious. Stud.* 6, 175–187.

Xu, J., Vik, A., Groote, I. R., Lagopoulos, J., Holen, A., Ellingsen, O., et al. (2014). Nondirective meditation activates default mode network and areas associated with memory retrieval and emotional processing. *Front. Hum. Neurosci.* 8:86. doi: 10.3389/fnhum.2014.00086

Yuan, H., Zotev, V., Phillips, R., Drevets, W. C., and Bodurka, J. (2012). Spatiotemporal dynamics of the brain at rest–exploring EEG microstates as electrophysiological signatures of BOLD resting state networks. *Neuroimage* 60, 2062–2072. doi: 10.1016/j.neuroimage.2012.02.031

Zalesky, A., Fornito, A., Cocchi, L., Gollo, L. L., and Breakspear, M. (2014). Time-resolved resting-state brain networks. *Proc. Natl. Acad. Sci. U S A* 111, 10341–10346. doi: 10.1073/pnas.1400181111

13

A 12-Week Cycling Training Regimen Improves Gait and Executive Functions Concomitantly in People with Parkinson's Disease

Alexandra Nadeau[1,2,3], Ovidiu Lungu[1,2,4,5], Catherine Duchesne[1,2,3], Marie-Ève Robillard[1,2], Arnaud Bore[1,2], Florian Bobeuf[1,6], Réjean Plamondon[7], Anne-Louise Lafontaine[1,2,8], Freja Gheysen[9], Louis Bherer[1,6,10,11] and Julien Doyon[1,2,3]**

[1] Research Center of the University Institute of Geriatrics of Montreal, Montreal, QC, Canada, [2] Functional Neuroimaging Unit, Montreal, QC, Canada, [3] Department of Psychology, University of Montreal, Montreal, QC, Canada, [4] Department of Psychiatry, University of Montreal, Montreal, QC, Canada, [5] Centre for Research in Aging, Donald Berman Maimonides Geriatric Centre, Montreal, QC, Canada, [6] PERFORM Centre, Concordia University, Montreal, QC, Canada, [7] Department of Electrical Engineering, Polytechnique Montreal, Montreal, QC, Canada, [8] McGill Movement Disorder Clinic, McGill University, Montreal, QC, Canada, [9] Department of Movement and Sport Sciences, Ghent University, Ghent, Belgium, [10] Department of Medicine, University of Montreal, Montreal, QC, Canada, [11] Montreal Heart Institute, Montreal, QC, Canada

Edited by:
Stephane Perrey,
University of Montpellier, France

Reviewed by:
Johanna Wagner,
University of California,
San Diego, USA
João Manuel R. S. Tavares,
University of Porto, Portugal
Wei Peng Teo,
Deakin University, Australia

***Correspondence:**
Alexandra Nadeau
alexandra.nadeau.3@umontreal.ca
Julien Doyon
julien.doyon@umontreal.ca

Background: There is increasing evidence that executive functions and attention are associated with gait and balance, and that this link is especially prominent in older individuals or those who are afflicted by neurodegenerative diseases that affect cognition and/or motor functions. People with Parkinson's disease (PD) often present gait disturbances, which can be reduced when PD patients engage in different types of physical exercise (PE), such as walking on a treadmill. Similarly, PE has also been found to improve executive functions in this population. Yet, no exercise intervention investigated simultaneously gait and non-motor symptoms (executive functions, motor learning) in PD patients.

Objective: To assess the impact of aerobic exercise training (AET) using a stationary bicycle on a set of gait parameters (walking speed, cadence, step length, step width, single and double support time, as well as variability of step length, step width and double support time) and executive functions (cognitive inhibition and flexibility) in sedentary PD patients and healthy controls.

Methods: Two groups, 19 PD patients (Hoehn and Yahr $\leq$2) and 20 healthy adults, matched on age and sedentary level, followed a 3-month stationary bicycle AET regimen.

Results: Aerobic capacity, as well as performance of motor learning and on cognitive inhibition, increased significantly in both groups after the training regimen, but only PD patients improved their walking speed and cadence (all $p < 0.05$; with no change in the step length). Moreover, in PD patients, training-related improvements in aerobic capacity correlated positively with improvements in walking speed ($r = 0.461$, $p < 0.05$).

Conclusion: AET using stationary bicycle can independently improve gait and cognitive inhibition in sedentary PD patients. Given that increases in walking speed were obtained through increases in cadence, with no change in step length, our findings suggest that gait improvements are specific to the type of motor activity practiced during exercise (i.e., pedaling). In contrast, the improvements seen in cognitive inhibition were, most likely, not specific to the type of training and they could be due to indirect action mechanisms (i.e., improvement of cardiovascular capacity). These results are also relevant for the development of targeted AET interventions to improve functional autonomy in PD patients.

Keywords: Parkinson's disease, exercise, gait, aerobic, stationary bicycle

INTRODUCTION

Parkinson's disease (PD) is a neurodegenerative pathology characterized by progressive motor symptoms, including gait modifications leading to balance instability (Bello et al., 2010). Patients can also develop several non-motor complications, such as depression, sleep disturbances and cognitive impairments like executive dysfunctions (Speelman et al., 2011) and deficits in procedural learning (Clark et al., 2014; Ruitenberg et al., 2015). Despite advances in pharmacological agents and surgical procedures that could be employed in PD patients to alleviate the primary motor signs of the disease, these treatment options often fail to improve the whole range of symptoms observed in PD and side effects are common (Bloem et al., 2004). Recently, exercise has been proposed as an adjuvant therapy that may help in alleviating multiple symptoms, but very little is know about the impact and the mechanisms of such alternatives.

Despite the fact that the link between gait and cognitive functions, especially executive functions, is well documented in aging research (Springer et al., 2006; Yogev-Seligmann et al., 2008; Liu-Ambrose et al., 2010; Martin et al., 2013), to date, only a few studies have investigated the same relationship in PD patients. In contrast, there is growing evidence documenting the association between standing balance and gait initiation with cognition in PD population, but in a dual-tasking context (Fernandes et al., 2015, 2016). The latter have shown that some cognitive processes, such as executive functions, processing speed and semantic fluency (Smulders et al., 2013; Stegemoller et al., 2014) are associated with some gait parameters and functional mobility in PD. In addition, several studies have shown independently that non-pharmacological treatment approaches, such as physical exercise (PE), do improve various gait parameters in PD (Mehrholz et al., 2010; Li et al., 2012; Shu et al., 2014; Arcolin et al., 2015), on the one hand, and executive functions, on the other hand (Tanaka et al., 2009). Yet, evidence that this type of intervention can simultaneously improve motor (such gait) and non-motor symptoms (executive functions, motor learning) in PD is non-existent and the mechanisms by which training produces changes in both of these components remain unknown.

We have recently reported that an aerobic exercise training (AET) regimen using a stationary bicycle is not only safe for PD patients in early stages of the disease, but that it has also improved aerobic capacity as well as cognitive inhibition and motor sequence learning (MSL; Duchesne et al., 2015). In the current study, our main objective was to assess the effects of an AET regimen using stationary bicycling on gait parameters in sedentary people with PD (not reported in the previous study). As a second objective, we set out to compare these effects to those observed in healthy adults (HA) in order to determine whether this type of intervention has a different impact depending on the participant's health status. In addition, as a third objective, we intended to evaluate the associations between exercise-related changes in gait (not reported in the previous study) with those seen in cardiovascular capacity, executive functions and motor sequence capacity (Duchesne et al., 2015). We hypothesized that: (1) bicycle training would improve gait parameters in all participants (especially speed and cadence based on the specificity of the bicycle training), but especially those diagnosed with PD, (2) such improvements in gait parameters would correlate with other AET-related improvements, such as cardiovascular capacity, cognitive inhibition and the capacity to learn a new sequence of movements, and that (3) these relations would be moderated by disease.

MATERIALS AND METHODS

Participants

In order to be eligible for the study, all participants (HA and those with PD) had to be right-handed, sedentary, and aged between 40 and 80 years old. They were screened for the presence of possible dementia score between 24 and 30 needed on the Mini Mental State Evaluation (Folstein et al., 1975) or on the Montreal Cognitive Assessment (Marinus et al., 2011) and appropriateness for testing in an MRI environment (e.g., no metallic implants that could interfere with testing, no claustrophobia). The Physical Activity Readiness Questionnaire (PAR-Q) was used to verify the participant's safety in participating in a physical program. Exclusion criteria included other neurological disorders, and comorbidities likely to affect gait, smoking or heart diseases. Importantly, HA were matched with PD patients with respect to sex distribution, age, education as well as cognitive and fitness levels. PD patients had to be classified as stage 1 or 2 according to Hoehn and Yahr's scale based upon evaluation of a certified neurologist (A-LL). Participants who were under medication continued their treatment all throughout the study (testing and training). This study was carried out in accordance with the recommendations of the research ethics committees' guidelines of the Research Center of the University Institute of

Geriatrics of Montreal, which approved the protocol. Written and informed consent was obtained from each participant in this study. Demographic characteristics of the samples are presented in **Table 1**.

Exercise Intervention Protocol

Prior to engaging in the training regimen, all participants were cleared by a physician, who analyzed the electrocardiogram (ECG) at rest in order to rule out any cardiac anomalies. The aerobic exercise intervention was designed to improve cardiorespiratory fitness with an exercise intensity prescription based on each participant's maximal aerobic power output achieved at maximum volume of oxygen (VO_2 peak) uptake assessed on the pre-test day (ACMS, 2006). Recumbent bicycles were used to train participants. Duration of the exercise program started at 20 min and 60% of intensity per session, and was then increased by steps of 5 min and 5% of intensity every week, until participants reached 40 min of training at 80% intensity. Bike speed was maintained at 60 revolutions per minute (RPM). As such, to achieve the desired bike resistance power and adjust intensity level (if needed), the work intensity was based on power output (Watt), controlling for participant's heart rate. In addition, rate of perceived exertion (Borg scale; Borg, 2012) was assessed during each training session. The program lasted 12 weeks, with three training sessions per week. A participation rate equivalent to 75% of the sessions was achieved by each participant included in the data analyzes. Trained kinesiologists supervised all sessions.

Assessments

Participants were evaluated on a variety of outcome measures before the intervention and immediately after completion of the 3-month exercise program.

Lower limb capacities were assessed with the GaitMat II (E.Q. Inc., Chalfont, PA, USA; Barker et al., 2006). The GaitMat II consists of a 7.8-m long walkway and its computer software, which controls the mat sensors and calculates different metrics of gait. The mat is also equipped with initial and final 1 m inactive sections that allow acceleration and deceleration of the participant locomotion. One trial consisted of participants walking the full length of the Mat at their self-selected walking speed. After a practice of two trials, participants completed four more trials for data collection and measurements (walking speed, cadence, step length, step width, single and double support time, as well as variability of step length, step width and double support time).

To evaluate the patient's mood, the Beck Depression Inventory (BDI; Beck et al., 1961) and the Beck Anxiety Inventory

TABLE 1 | Demographic data.

Characteristics	HA	PD	Group differences
Demographic information			
Age (years)	64 ± 8.19	59 ± 7.11	$p = 0.06$
Ratio men/women	8/12	10/0	$p = 0.07$
Education (years)	15.7 ± 2.36	15.05 ± 2.78	$p = 0.43$
Overall cognitive level			
Cognition (MMSE/MoCA)	29.18 ± 1.25	28.4 ± 1.34	$p = 0.28$
	29.56 ± 1.51	27.21 ± 1.85	$p = 0.08$
Psychological well-being			
Depression (BDI)	4.8 ± 4.5	10.5 ± 8.3	$p < 0.01$
Anxiety (BAI)	2.1 ± 2.7	8.6 ± 9.4	$p < 0.01$
Executive functions			
Inhibition (Stroop, in s)	115.4 ± 4.7	128.5 ± 6.7	$p = 0.12$
Flexibility (TMT, in s)	75.0 ± 6.4	85.5 ± 10.5	$p = 0.39$
Clinical variables			
UPDRS III	N/A	21.84 ± 6.16	N/A
Duration of disease (years)	N/A	8.1 ± 9.12	N/A
Hoehn and Yahr	N/A	2.1 ± 0.2	N/A
Gait parameters			
Walking speed (m/s)	1.14 ± 0.03	1.10 ± 0.04	0.386
Cadence (steps/min)	115.49 ± 2.00	110.05 ± 2.72	0.116
Step length (m)	0.593 ± 0.064	0.598 ± 0.080	0.833
Step width (m)	0.207 ± 0.032	0.215 ± 0.035	0.455
Single support time (s)	0.401 ± 0.006	0.417 ± 0.009	0.154
Double support time (s)	0.12 ± 0.01	0.13 ± 0.01	0.339
Step length variability	0.012 ± 0.009	0.011 ± 0.006	0.737
Step width variability	0.009 ± 0.007	0.011 ± 0.007	0.593
Double support time variability	0.009 ± 0.002	0.007 ± 0.001	0.905

Means ± SD. HA, healthy adults; PD, Parkinson's diseases individuals; N/A, non-applicable; s, seconds; m, meters; min, minute.

(BAI; Beck et al., 1988) were used. Also, executive functions were assessed, precisely cognitive inhibition and flexibility. Participants' inhibitory aptitude was assessed using a version of the Stroop test with three different conditions (naming, reading, and interference). Each condition contained 100 stimuli (i.e., words, colored rectangles, words in colors) printed on a 21.5 cm × 28 cm sheet of paper. In the reading condition, participants had to read the words (red, green, blue, and yellow) printed in black. In the naming condition, subjects had to name of the rectangles. In the third condition (interference), individuals needed to name the color of the ink in which the words were written. In the latter condition, the meaning of each word had to be ignored, as it was incongruent with the color to name (i.e., the word "blue" written in yellow). The trail Making Test (TMT) was used to assess subjects' flexibility functions. The first part of the test (TMT A) included numbers from 1 to 25, circled and written on a 21.5 cm × 28 cm sheet of paper. Participants were asked to connect with a pencil, as fast as possible, the numbers in numerical order. In contrast, the second part (TMT B) included numbers from 1 to 13 and letters from A to L. Subjects were asked to connect, as fast as possible, a number followed by a letter in numerical and alphabetic order, respectively (i.e., 1-A-2-B-etc.). The participants' capacity in MSL was evaluated during a functional magnetic resonance imaging session, where they had to perform an implicit serial reaction time task (Nissen and Bullemer, 1987). More details of the complete fitness, psychological, neuropsychological and motor learning evaluations can be found in our previous study by Duchesne et al. (2015).

Statistical Analysis

A repeated model ANOVA was used to test the effect of AET on primary and secondary outcomes in PD participants. In addition, a mixed model ANCOVA was carried out to assess group differences pre-post AET, as well as the effect of training within each group and group differences at baseline and after AET for all gait parameters. BDI scores and age were used as covariates for all analyses to account for group differences in sentiments of depression and age, two factors that may impact gait parameters such walking speed (Rochester et al., 2008). In order to account for the effect of multiple comparisons, the statistical significance was adjusted using the Bonferroni method. All results were expressed as means ± standard deviations for descriptive statistics. Pearson linear correlations between walking speed, cadence and step length with aerobic capacity, executive functions (inhibition and flexibility) and MSL (performance and learning scores) were tested to figure out if there is a link between gait and these factors among PD participants only. We then employed Hayes's (2009) free add-on SPSS macro to test whether the disease (present/absent) moderated the relationship between gait parameters and other variables of interest, i.e., if the relation between variables in PD is in the same direction than the group of reference. Training-related changes in cognitive scores, MSL, and aerobic capacity constituted the independent variables in the moderation model, while gait parameters that changed significantly as a result of training corresponded to the outcome variable. Analyses were conducted using SPSS 21.0 (IBM, Armonk, NY, USA). The level of statistical significance for all tests was set at $p < 0.05$.

RESULTS

Forty-four participants (21 PD patients and 23 HA) were deemed eligible to enroll in the study after the completion of the first evaluation. However, between the evaluation and the beginning of the exercise program, two HA decided to withdraw from the project for personal reasons. One PD participant and one HA were excluded after the beginning of the training regimen for health security reasons. Only one PD patient was excluded from analysis after AET regimen completion because of extreme results on several outcomes, even if this person respected all inclusion criteria. In the end, a total of 39 persons (19 PD patients and 20 HA) were analyzed. All demographic characteristics and initial values of the study participants are described in **Table 1**. There was no difference between groups for any of the gait parameters at baseline.

Following the 12-week AET, repeated measures ANOVA indicated that PD participants showed significant improvements for the walking speed ($F_{1,18} = 6.154$, $p < 0.05$), the step length ($F_{1,18} = 5.828$, $p < 0.05$) and the single support time ($F_{1,18} = 4.771$, $p < 0.05$), with a trend for cadence ($F_{1,18} = 4.211$, $p = 0.055$). When using the mixed ANCOVA model, the effect observed in PD for walking speed and single support time remained the same while the one obtained for step length disappeared (**Figure 1**). However, the trend observed for the cadence became significant when using covariates such the age and the BDI ($p < 0.05$). In addition, the groups did not differ significantly neither in pre- or post-comparisons, nor in regards to AET-related changes. All other gait parameters did not change significantly following the aerobic training ($ps > 0.05$) (**Table 2**).

Significant between-sessions differences were found in both groups for outcomes related to aerobic capacity (VO_2 peak), MSL capacity and cognitive inhibition (all $p < 0.05$), indicating that the training improved participants' fitness, procedural learning and cognitive inhibition, regardless of the health status. Given that these results were analyzed in detail and reported elsewhere (Duchesne et al., 2015), they are presented here only for reader's convenience in the Supplementary material (Supplementary Figure S1). However, these data were used to test the correlation with gait parameters among PD participants. We observed a significant association only between the walking speed at the post-test and the aerobic capacity after the AET ($r = 0.461$, $p < 0.05$, $N = 19$). No correlation was observed between other gait parameters and cognition or MSL.

A multiple regression model was then employed to investigate whether the association between pre-post change in walking speed and change in fitness depended upon the presence of disease (i.e., moderation). The relationship between change in fitness and change in walking speed was significantly moderated by the presence of the disease (R^2 increase due to the interaction: $F_{1,32} = 4.34$, $p < 0.05$; conditional effect of change in fitness on change in walking speed: HA $t = -1.08$, $p = 0.29$, PD $t = 1.79$, $p = 0.08$). Specifically, patients with PD who increased

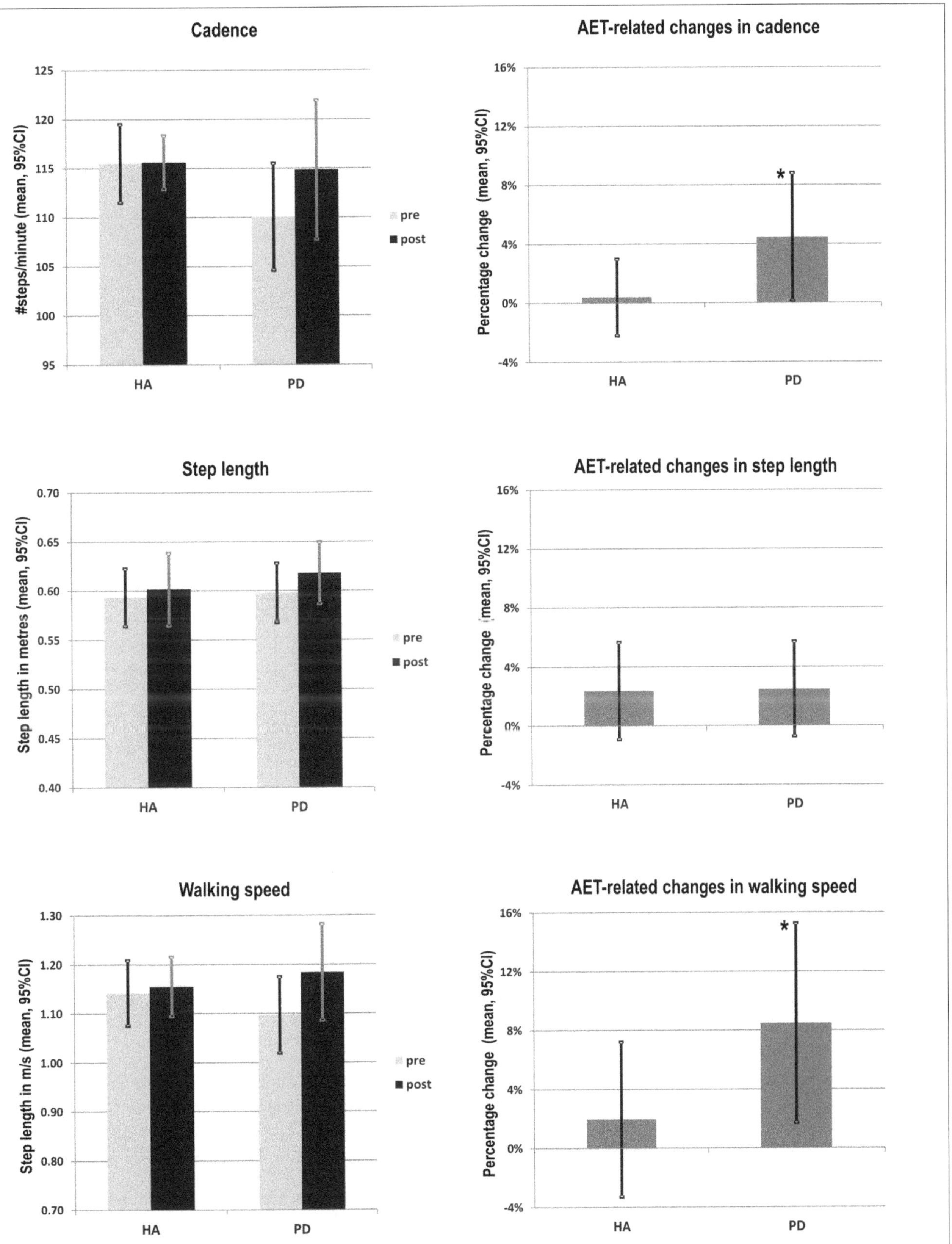

FIGURE 1 | AET-related changes in walking speed, cadence and step length in PD patients and healthy adults. *Indicate statistically significant differences pre- to post- training ($p < 0.05$). HA, healthy adults; PD, Parkinson's diseases patients.

TABLE 2 | Spatiotemporal gait parameters during self-selected speed condition.

Gait variables	HC		PD		Statistical significance for the independent variables		
	Pre-AET	Post-AET	Pre-AET	Post-AET	AET	Group	Interaction
Walking speed (m/s)	1.14 ± 0.03	1.16 ± 0.03	1.10 ± 0.04	1.18 ± 0.05†	$p = 0.28$	$p = 0.91$	$p = 0.27$
Cadence (steps/min)	115.49 ± 2.00	115.61 ± 1.37	110.05 ± 2.72	114.84 ± 3.53†	$p = 0.15$	$p = 0.70$	$p = 0.10$
Step length (m)	0.593 ± 0.064	0.602 ± 0.066	0.598 ± 0.08	0.618 ± 0.069	$p = 0.71$	$p = 0.73$	$p = 0.98$
Step width (m)	0.207 ± 0.032	0.213 ± 0.028	0.215 ± 0.035	0.222 ± 0.037	$p = 0.381$	$p = 0.727$	$p = 0.962$
Single support time (s)	0.401 ± 0.006	0.398 ± 0.004	0.417 ± 0.009	0.384 ± 0.015†	**$p < 0.05$***	$p = 0.83$	**$p < 0.05$***
Double support time (s)	0.120 ± 0.010	0.117 ± 0.004	0.130 ± 0.010	0.136 ± 0.013	$p = 0.25$	$p = 0.24$	$p = 0.21$
Step length variability	0.52 ± 0.01	0.52 ± 0.01	0.55 ± 0.01	0.53 ± 0.02	$p = 0.15$	$p = 0.41$	$p = 0.17$
Step width variability	0.010 ± 0.007	0.011 ± 0.008	0.011 ± 0.007	0.008 ± 0.010	$p = 0.166$	$p = 0.983$	$p = 0.509$
Double support time variability	0.009 ± 0.010	0.006 ± 0.003	0.007 ± 0.004	0.033 ± 0.077	$p = 0.417$	$p = 0.160$	$p = 0.087$

No significant differences between groups at baseline were found. Means ± SD. †A significant within-group difference from baseline. HA, Healthy adults; PD, Parkinson's disease patients; m, meters; s, second(s); min, minute; AET, aerobic exercise training. Bolded terms emphasize statistical differences.

their cardiorespiratory capacities the most also showed the best improvement in walking speed (**Figure 2**). By contrast, there was no significant relationship between these variables in HA (HA group: $\beta = -0.162$, $p = 0.505$; PD group: $\beta = 0.596$, $p = 0.027$). Also, no relationship between gait parameters and motor skill learning or executive functions was found alone or when investigating the moderation of these relationships by the presence of the disease.

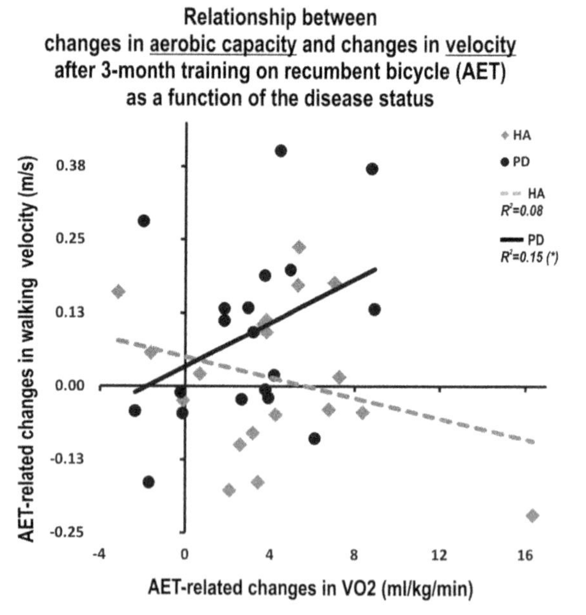

FIGURE 2 | Moderating effect of the disease on the relationship between AET-related changes in walking speed and aerobic capacity. *Indicate statistically significant differences pre- to post- training ($p < 0.05$). HA, healthy adults; PD, Parkinson's disease; AET, aerobic exercise training; m, meters, sec, second, ml: milliliters, kg, kilogram, min, minute.

DISCUSSION

In the current study, we investigated the effects of an AET regimen using stationary bicycling on gait parameters in sedentary HA and in PD patients. As reported previously by our group (Duchesne et al., 2015), such training regimen improved cardiovascular capacity, executive functions and motor learning capacities in both groups. Here, we report that AET also had a significant positive impact on cadence and walking speed in the PD group. Moreover, the presence of the disease mediated the relationship between aerobic capacity and walking speed, as the improvement in fitness correlated positively with that in walking speed of PD patients only. Contrary to our expectations, we did not find significant relationships between AET-related changes in gait parameters and cognition.

Importantly and as predicted, however, the present study yielded significant increases in walking speed and cadence in the PD group. The latter findings are consistent with previous studies indicating that 4–12 weeks of treadmill training improved walking speed, step length and step-to-step variability (Herman et al., 2009). This is also in accordance with other reports that resistance training, tai chi and physical therapy lead to improvements in walking speed and step length (Pellecchia et al., 2004; Li et al., 2012). Until now, studies on stationary bicycle training used forced exercise paradigm and observed improvements of dexterity, tremor and bradykinesia (Burini et al., 2006; Ridgel et al., 2009; Alberts et al., 2011). Finally, the fact that we did not find significant improvements in step length in PD patients, but observed significant increases in walking speed and cadence, may be due to the nature of our AET program. Indeed, the pedaling rhythm during exercising has a built-in cadence, and thus, it is expected that training-specific effect of bicycling would be more pronounced in terms of cadence, as compared to other gait parameters. This is similar to the mechanism by which treadmill training will impact more step length and walking speed, rather than other gait variables (Fisher et al., 2008; Herman et al., 2009).

Contrary to our expectations, there was no significant relationship between changes in PD participants' executive functions, MSL, cardiovascular capacity and gait parameters. We had hypothesized that we would find a positive and significant relation between executive functions and gait in the PD group, mostly because previous evidence suggested that some elements of cognition such as working memory and attention capacities, were associated with gait abnormalities in PD (Smulders et al., 2013). Our hypothesis was based on the fact that in a recent study, Sohmiya et al. (2012) found significant correlation between frontal assessment battery scores and changes in gait following physical therapy (Sohmiya et al., 2012). Yet it is important to note that in that study, PD patients with high, but not low, executive functioning scores improved walking speed, stride and step length after physical training. Furthermore, unlike in our sample, PD participants in these studies were in more advanced stages of the disease. Thus this suggests that the relationship between gait and executive functions may be more evident as the disease progresses, hence possibly explaining why we did not observe any relation between gait parameters and other cognitive and learning functions. The fact that AET improved certain gait parameters and cognitive functions, but that these changes did not correlate with each other suggest that independent action mechanisms underlie this therapeutic improvements, at least at this stage of the disease.

We used moderation analyses to investigate the extent to which age influenced the relationship between changes in participants' fitness levels as well as their executive functioning and motor learning capacities on the one hand, and gait parameters, on the other hand. Using such an approach, we found a significant moderation effect for the disease variable only, regarding the relationship between AET-related improvements in aerobic capacity and those in walking speed. It has previously been suggested that motor abilities in the PD population, such as gait, could be affected by various health conditions. For example, a decrease in cardiorespiratory capacity has been shown to affect walking speed (Skidmore, 2008). Therefore, our results, especially the positive correlation between improvements in VO_2 peak and those in walking speed in PD patients only, seem to support this hypothesis. In addition, they suggest that motor abilities may be improved in PD via non-pharmacological means, such as aerobic PE.

The main objective of our study was to assess of AET in PD patients. We used the HA group to explore the possibility that AET may have a differential impact as a function of disease. However, we found no significant differences between these two groups in regards to any of the primary and secondary outcomes, neither in pre-, post- or AET-related changes. This is in contrast with the few studies that compared gait parameters in these two populations (Frenkel-Toledo et al., 2005; Bello et al., 2008). Thus, although conjectural, the reason why we did not observe any group differences may be that we recruited PD patients that were in the early phase of the disease (i.e., Hoehn and Yahr stage 1 or 2), compared to previous reports which included patients in more advanced stages (Frenkel-Toledo et al., 2005; Bello et al., 2008).

Several mechanisms have been proposed to explain physical training-related improvements similar to those seen in the present study. Some of these include direct effects on the central nervous system based upon an optimisation of the medication intake by easing its absorption (Speelman et al., 2011) or through increased corticomotor excitability (Fisher et al., 2008) and dopaminergic neurotransmission (Petzinger et al., 2010). Other proposed mechanisms have been more indirect and include increased cortical vascularisation, synaptic plasticity and neurogenesis (Speelman et al., 2011). These processes, which could be mediated by neurotrophic factors, would lead to structural and functional brain changes. Although the present study does not allow identifying the mechanism(s) that could explain the effects of AET on gait measures reported here, one can nevertheless assume that some brain structural and functional changes could be at the origin of such clinical outcomes. For example, in rodents, regional gray matter volume in a region equivalent to supplementary motor area (SMA) in humans has shown to be correlated positively with the total distance run by the animal following 7 days of exercise (Sumiyoshi et al., 2014). Similar increases, in both white and gray matter, have been reported in a group of older sedentary human adults after participation in a 6-month aerobic training regimen (Colcombe et al., 2006). Furthermore, a recent study using resting state functional magnetic resonance imaging found significant changes in activity in sensorimotor areas in a group of young individuals after 20 min of aerobic exercise (Rajab et al., 2014), while a couple of studies demonstrated that functional brain activity in motor areas increased proportional to the movement rate on a pedaling task executed during scanning (Mehta et al., 2012). Finally, increased SMA activation was observed during motor imagery of locomotor-related tasks (Malouin et al., 2003) as well as during real locomotion as measured by electrophysiological studies showing SMA modulation during walking (Petersen et al., 2012; Wagner et al., 2012, 2014; Seeber et al., 2015). Thus despite the scarcity of studies assessing cerebral structural and functional changes in relation to gait parameters and aerobic training in humans, the above mentioned studies provide basic evidence that AET can have a direct impact on the brain. Given the lack of neuroimaging studies looking at the effect of PE in PD, further investigations are needed to directly assess these mechanisms in PD patients using neuroimaging techniques.

An issue that merits discussion would be the role of medication. There is evidence that medication itself may have a differential effect on movement rate and amplitude, as demonstrated by past research (Espay et al., 2009, 2010, 2011; Stegemöller et al., 2009; Teo et al., 2013, 2014). In the current study, we believed that medication did not play a major role influencing the outcomes for PD patients. The reason is that patients were always on their medication during both pre and post evaluations, their medication did not change and more importantly, assessments always took place at the same time of the day.

Although our findings help increasing our knowledge base about the effects of AET on gait, the current study has some limitations. A limitation of the present study was the lack of an additional training condition controlling for the type and intensity of exercise that PD patients performed over the 3-month period. However, despite this shortcoming, we believe that the results of the current study are theoretically and clinically relevant as they suggest that the use of AET using stationary bicycle can have a beneficial impact in persons suffering from PD. Another limitation is the fact that we only assessed two cognitive functions, inhibition and flexibility, which are the most commonly used in the PD literature. Therefore, one cannot exclude the possibility that other cognitive domains may show correlations with gait parameters following physical training.

From a clinical perspective, the use of high-intensity exercise is now a common rehabilitation method in PD. It is important to note that the AET effects in the current study were observed after a moderate to a high intensity exercise regimen (half of the program was performed at 80% of maximal intensity). Thus, with its stable and comfortable sitting posture, our results suggest that AET with a stationary bicycle is not only a viable, but also a safe training procedure for PD patients in stage 1 and 2 of the disease. Further studies are still needed in order to assess the safety and feasibility of a training regimen on stationary bicycle in patients in more advanced stages of the disease who are showing greater physical limitations such as balance impairments, as well as to evaluate the long-term benefits of this training method. Yet, despite such limitations, our study shows that stationary bicycle can be successfully used to improve gait functions in PD patients. The main contribution of the current study thus stems from the fact that our findings are showing AET-related improvements in a gait parameter (walking speed) is crucial for the daily functioning of sedentary patients who are in the initial stages of the disease. Therefore, we believe that this result is another step closer to developing a reliable strategy to stimulate an active lifestyle in patients with PD, taking into account safety issues and each patient's individual capacities.

ETHICS STATEMENT

RNQ- Research Ethics Mixed Committee. The protocol was approved by a research committee to ensure the full security of the participants. The consent form was read with participants before to obtain their agreement to participate.

AUTHOR CONTRIBUTIONS

Research project conception: CD, RP, FG, LB, and JD; Research project organization: CD, M-ÈR, AB, FB, and JD; Research project execution: AN, CD, M-ÈR, FB, and A-LL. Statistical analysis: AN and OL. Manuscript writing: AN, OL, and JD; Manuscript review and critique: AN, CD, OL, M-ÈR, AB, FB, RP, A-LL, FG, LB, and JD.

ACKNOWLEDGMENTS

The results of the present study do not constitute endorsement by ACSM. The authors wish to thank Dr. Juan Manuel Villalpando and Dr. Thien Tuong Minh Vu who kindly accepted to supervise physical assessment during testing.

REFERENCES

ACMS (2006). *American College of Sports Medicine's Guidelines for Exercise Testing and Prescription.* Philadelphia, PA: Lippincott Williams & Wilkins.

Alberts, J. L., Linder, S. M., Penko, A. L., Lowe, M. J., and Phillips, M. (2011). It is not about the bike, it is about the pedaling: forced exercise and parkinso's disease. *Exerc. Sport Sci. Rev.* 39, 177–186. doi: 10.1097/JES.0b013e31822cc71a

Arcolin, I., Pisano, F., Delconte, C., Godi, M., Schieppati, M., Mezzani, A., et al. (2015). Intensive cycle ergometer training improves gait speed and endurance in patients with Parkinson's disease: a comparison with treadmill training. *Restor. Neurol. Neurosci.* 34, 125–138. doi: 10.3233/RNN-150506

Barker, S., Craik, R., Freedman, W., Herrmann, N., and Hillstrom, H. (2006). Accuracy, reliability, and validity of a spatiotemporal gait analysis system. *Med. Eng. Phys.* 28, 460–467. doi: 10.1016/j.medengphy.2005.07.017

Beck, A. T., Epstein, N., Brown, G., and Steer, R. A. (1988). An inventory for measuring clinical anxiety: psychometric properties. *J. Consult. Clin. Psychol.* 56, 893–897. doi: 10.1037/0022-006X.56.6.893

Beck, A. T., Ward, C. H., Mendelson, M., Mock, J., and Erbaugh, J. (1961). An inventory for measuring depression. *Arch. Gen. Psychiatry* 4, 561–571. doi: 10.1001/archpsyc.1961.01710120031004

Bello, O., Marquez, G., Camblor, M., and Fernandez-Del-Olmo, M. (2010). Mechanisms involved in treadmill walking improvements in Parkinson's disease. *Gait Posture* 32, 118–123. doi: 10.1016/j.gaitpost.2010.04.015

Bello, O., Sanchez, J. A., and Fernandez-del-Olmo, M. (2008). Treadmill walking in Parkinson's disease patients: adaptation and generalization effect. *Mov. Disord.* 23, 1243–1249. doi: 10.1002/mds.22069

Bloem, B. R., Hausdorff, J. M., Visser, J. E., and Giladi, N. (2004). Falls and freezing of gait in Parkinson's disease: a review of two interconnected, episodic phenomena. *Mov. Disord.* 19, 871–884. doi: 10.1002/mds.20115

Borg, G. A. V. (2012). *"The Borg CR10 Scale Folder." A Method for Measuring Intensity of Experience.* Hasselby: Borg perception, 1–4.

Burini, D., Farabollini, B., Iacucci, S., Rimatori, C., Riccardi, G., Capecci, M., et al. (2006). A randomised controlled cross-over trial of aerobic training versus Qigong in advanced Parkinson's disease. *Eur. Medicophys.* 42, 231–238.

Clark, G. M., Lum, J. A. G., and Ullman, M. T. (2014). A meta-analysis and meta-regression of serial reaction time task performance in Parkinson's disease. *Neuropsychology* 28, 945–958. doi: 10.1037/neu0000121

Colcombe, S. J., Erickson, K. I., Scalf, P. E., Kim, J. S., Prakash, R., McAuley, E., et al. (2006). Aerobic exercise training increases brain volume in aging humans. *J. Gerontol. A Biol. Sci. Med. Sci.* 61, 1166–1170. doi: 10.1093/gerona/61.11.1166

Duchesne, C., Lungu, O., Nadeau, A., Robillard, M. E., Boré, A., Bobeuf, F., et al. (2015). Enhancing both motor and cognitive functioning in Parkinson's disease: aerobic exercise as a rehabilitative intervention. *Brain Cogn.* 99, 68–77. doi: 10.1016/j.bandc.2015.07.005

Espay, A. J., Beaton, D. E., Morgante, F., Gunraj, C. A., Lang, A. E., and Chen, R. (2009). Impairments of speed and amplitude of movement in Parkinson's disease: a pilot study. *Mov. Disord.* 24, 1001–1008. doi: 10.1002/mds.22480

Espay, A. J., Giuffrida, J. P., Chen, R., Payne, M., Mazzella, F., Dunn, E., et al. (2011). Differential response of speed, amplitude, and rhythm to dopaminergic medications in Parkinson's disease. *Mov. Disord.* 26, 2504–2508. doi: 10.1002/mds.23893

Espay, A. J., Lang, A. E., and Chen, R. (2010). "Effect of movement frequency on repetitive finger movements in patients with Parkinson's disease. *Mov. Disord.* 25, 252–252. doi: 10.1002/mds.22930

Fernandes, Â., Coelho, T., Vitória, A., Ferreira, A., Santos, R., Rocha, N., et al. (2015). Standing balance in individuals with Parkinson's disease during single and dual-task conditions. *Gait Posture* 42, 323–328. doi: 10.1016/j.gaitpost.2015.06.188

Fernandes, Â., Sousa, A. S. P., Rocha, N., and Tavares, J. M. (2016). Parkinson's disease and cognitive-motor dual-task: is motor prioritization possible in the early stages of the disease? *J. Mot. Behav.* 48, 377–383. doi: 10.1080/00222895.2015.1105194

Fisher, B. E., Wu, A. D., Salem, G. J., Song, J., Lin, C. H., Yip, J., et al. (2008). The effect of exercise training in improving motor performance and corticomotor excitability in people with early Parkinson's disease. *Arch. Phys. Med. Rehabil.* 89, 1221–1229. doi: 10.1016/j.apmr.2008.01.013

Folstein, M. F., Folstein, S. E., and McHugh, P. R. (1975). "Mini-Mental State". A practical method for grading the cognitive state of patients for the clinician. *J. Psychiatr. Res.* 12, 189–198. doi: 10.1016/0022-3956(75)90026-6

Frenkel-Toledo, S., Giladi, N., Peretz, C., Herman, T., Gruendlinger, L., Hausdorff, J. M., et al. (2005). Treadmill walking as an external pacemaker to improve gait rhythm and stability in Parkinson's disease. *Mov. Disord.* 20, 1109–1114. doi: 10.1002/mds.20507

Hayes, A. F. (2009). *Statistical Methods for Communication Science*. Mahwah, NJ: Lawrence Erlbaum Associates, Inc.

Herman, T., Giladi, N., and Hausdorff, J. M. (2009). Treadmill training for the treatment of gait disturbances in people with Parkinson's disease: a mini-review. *J. Neural Transm.* 116, 307–318. doi: 10.1007/s00702-008-0139-z

Li, F., Harmer, P., Fitzgerald, K., Eckstrom, E., Stock, R., Galver, J., et al. (2012). Tai chi and postural stability in patients with Parkinson's disease. *N. Engl. J. Med.* 366, 511–519. doi: 10.1056/NEJMoa1107911

Liu-Ambrose, T., Nagamatsu, L. S., Graf, P., Beattie, B. L., Ashe, M. C., and Handy, T. C. (2010). Resistance training and executive functions: a 12-month randomized controlled trial. *Arch. Intern. Med.* 170, 170–178. doi: 10.1001/archinternmed.2009.494

Malouin, F., Richards, C. L., Jackson, P. L., Dumas, F., and Doyon, J. (2003). Brain activations during motor imagery of locomotor-related tasks: a PET study. *Hum. Brain Mapp.* 19, 47–62. doi: 10.1002/hbm.10103

Marinus, J., Verbaan, D., van Hilten, J. J., Dalrymple-Alford, J. C., Nakas, C. T., Macaskill, M. R., et al. (2011). The MoCA: well-suited screen for cognitive impairment in Parkinson disease. *Neurology* 76, 1944–1945. doi: 10.1212/WNL.0b013e318219dc77

Martin, K. L., Blizzard, L., Wood, A. G., Srikanth, V., Thomson, R., Sanders, L. M., et al. (2013). Cognitive function, gait, and gait variability in older people: a population-based study. *J. Gerontol. A Biol. Sci. Med. Sci.* 68, 726–732. doi: 10.1093/gerona/gls224

Mehrholz, J., Friis, R., Storch, A., Pohl, M., Elsner, B., and Hirsch, K. (2010). Treadmill training for patients with Parkinson's disease. *Cochrane Database. Syst. Rev.* 8:CD007830. doi: 10.1002/14651858.CD007830

Mehta, J. P., Verber, M. D., Wieser, J. A., Schmit, B. D., and Schindler-Ivens, S. M. (2012). The effect of movement rate and complexity on functional magnetic resonance signal change during pedaling. *Motor Control* 16, 158–175. doi: 10.1123/mcj.16.2.158

Nissen, M. J., and Bullemer, P. (1987). Attentional requirements of learning: evidence from performance measures. *Cogn. Psychol.* 19, 1–32. doi: 10.1016/0010-0285(87)90002-8

Pellecchia, M. T., Grasso, A., Biancardi, L. G., Squillante, M., Bonavita, V., and Barone, P. (2004). Physical therapy in Parkinson's disease: an open long-term rehabilitation trial. *J. Neurol.* 251, 595–598. doi: 10.1007/s00415-004-0379-2

Petersen, T. H., Willerslev-Olsen, M., Conway, B. A., and Nielsen, J. B. (2012). The motor cortex drives the muscles during walking in human subjects. *J. Physiol.* 590, 2443–2452. doi: 10.1113/jphysiol.2012.227397

Petzinger, G. M., Fisher, B. E., Van Leeuwen, J. E., Vukovic, M., Akopian, G., Meshul, C. K., et al. (2010). Enhancing neuroplasticity in the basal ganglia: the role of exercise in Parkinson's disease. *Mov. Disord.* 25, S141–S145. doi: 10.1002/mds.22782

Rajab, A. S., Crane, D. E., Middleton, L. E., Robertson, A. D., Hampson, M., and MacIntosh, B. J. (2014). A single session of exercise increases connectivity in sensorimotor-related brain networks: a resting-state fMRI study in young healthy adults. *Front. Hum. Neurosci.* 8:625. doi: 10.3389/fnhum.2014.00625

Ridgel, A. L., Vitek, J. L., and Alberts, J. L. (2009). Forced, not voluntary, exercise improves motor function in Parkinson's disease patients. *Neurorehabil. Neural Repair* 23, 600–608. doi: 10.1177/1545968308328726

Rochester, L., Nieuwboer, A., Baker, K., Hetherington, V., Willems, A.-M., Kwakkel, G., et al. (2008). Walking speed during single and dual tasks in Parkinson's disease: Which characteristics are important? *Mov. Disord.* 23, 2312–2318. doi: 10.1002/mds.22219

Ruitenberg, M. F. L., Duthoo, W., Santens, P., Notebaert, W., and Abrahamse, E. L. (2015). Sequential movement skill in Parkinson's disease: a state-of-the-art. *Cortex* 65, 102–112. doi: 10.1016/j.cortex.2015.01.005

Seeber, M., Scherer, R., Wagner, J., Solis-Escalante, T., and Müller-Putz, G. R. (2015). High and low gamma EEG oscillations in central sensorimotor areas are conversely modulated during the human gait cycle. *Neuroimage* 112, 318–326. doi: 10.1016/j.neuroimage.2015.03.045

Shu, H.-F., Yang, T., Yu, S. X., Huang, H. D., Jiang, L. L., Gu, J. W., et al. (2014). Aerobic exercise for parkinson's disease: a systematic review and meta-analysis of randomized controlled trials. *PLoS ONE* 9:e100503. doi: 10.1371/journal.pone.0100503

Skidmore, F. M. (2008). Pilot safety and feasibility study of treadmill aerobic exercise in Parkinson disease with gait impairment. *J. Rehabil. Res. Dev.* 45, 117–124. doi: 10.1682/JRRD.2006.10.0130

Smulders, K., van Nimwegen, M., Munneke, M., Bloem, B. R., Kessels, R. P., and Esselink, R. A. (2013). Involvement of specific executive functions in mobility in Parkinson's disease. *Parkinsonism Relat. Disord.* 19, 126–128. doi: 10.1016/j.parkreldis.2012.06.010

Sohmiya, M., Wada, N., Tazawa, M., Okamoto, K., and Shirakura, K. (2012). Immediate effects of physical therapy on gait disturbance and frontal assessment battery in Parkinson's disease. *Geriatr. Gerontol. Int.* 13, 630–637. doi: 10.1111/j.1447-0594.2012.00953.x

Speelman, A. D., van de Warrenburg, B. P., van Nimwegen, M., Petzinger, G. M., Munneke, M., and Bloem, B. R. (2011). How might physical activity benefit patients with Parkinson disease? *Nat. Rev. Neurol.* 7, 528–534. doi: 10.1038/nrneurol.2011.107

Springer, S., Giladi, N., Peretz, C., Yogev, G., Simon, E. S., and Hausdorff, J. M. (2006). Dual-tasking effects on gait variability: the role of aging, falls, and executive function. *Mov. Disord.* 21, 950–957. doi: 10.1002/mds.20848

Stegemöller, E. L., Simuni, T., and MacKinnon, C. (2009). Effect of movement frequency on repetitive finger movements in patients with Parkinson's disease. *Mov. Disord.* 24, 1162–1169. doi: 10.1002/mds.22535

Stegemoller, E. L., Wilson, J. P., Hazamy, A., Shelley, M. C., Okun, M. S., Altmann, L. J., et al. (2014). Associations between cognitive and gait performance during single- and dual-task walking in people with Parkinson disease. *Phys. Ther.* 94, 757–766. doi: 10.2522/ptj.20130251

Sumiyoshi, A., Taki, Y., Nonaka, H., Takeuchi, H., and Kawashima, R. (2014). Regional gray matter volume increases following 7days of voluntary wheel running exercise: a longitudinal VBM study in rats. *Neuroimage* 98, 82–90. doi: 10.1016/j.neuroimage.2014.04.075

Tanaka, K., de Quadros, A. C. Jr., Santos, R. F., Stella, F., Gobbi, L. T., and Gobbi, S. (2009). Benefits of physical exercise on executive functions in older people with Parkinson's disease. *Brain Cogn.* 69, 435–441. doi: 10.1016/j.bandc.2008.09.008

Teo, W. P., Rodrigues, J. P., Mastaglia, F. L., and Thickbroom, G. W. (2013). Comparing kinematic changes between a finger-tapping task and unconstrained finger flexion–extension task in patients with Parkinson's disease. *Exp. Brain Res.* 227, 323–331. doi: 10.1007/s00221-013-3491-7

Teo, W.-P., Rodrigues, J. P., Mastaglia, F. L., and Thickbroom, G. W. (2014). Modulation of corticomotor excitability after maximal or sustainable-rate repetitive finger movement is impaired in Parkinson's disease and is reversed by levodopa. *Clin. Neurophysiol.* 125, 562–568. doi: 10.1016/j.clinph.2013.09.004

Wagner, J., Solis-Escalante, T., Grieshofer, P., Neuper, C., Müller-Putz, G., and Scherer, R. (2012). Level of participation in robotic-assisted treadmill walking modulates midline sensorimotor EEG rhythms in able-bodied subjects. *Neuroimage* 63, 1203–1211. doi: 10.1016/j.neuroimage.2012.08.019

Wagner, J., Solis-Escalante, T., Scherer, R., Neuper, C., and Müller-Putz, G. (2014). It's how you get there: walking down a virtual alley activates premotor and parietal areas. *Front. Hum. Neurosci.* 8:93. doi: 10.3389/fnhum.2014.00093

Yogev-Seligmann, G., Hausdorff, J. M., and Giladi, N. (2008). The role of executive function and attention in gait. *Mov. Disord.* 23, 329–342. doi: 10.1002/mds.21720

14

Cardiorespiratory Fitness is Associated with Selective Attention in Healthy Male High-School Students

*Eivind Wengaard[1], Morten Kristoffersen[1], Anette Harris[2] and Hilde Gundersen[1]**

[1]Department of Sport and Physical Education, Western Norway University of Applied Sciences, Bergen, Norway,
[2]Department of Psychosocial Science, Faculty of Psychology, Institute of Psychosocial Science, University of Bergen, Bergen, Norway

Edited by:
Claudia Voelcker-Rehage,
Technische Universität Chemnitz,
Germany

Reviewed by:
Keita Kamijo,
Waseda University, Japan
Daniel Sanabria,
University of Granada, Spain

***Correspondence:**
Hilde Gundersen
hsg@hvl.no

Background: Previous studies have shown associations of physical fitness and cognition in children and in younger and older adults. However, knowledge about associations in high-school adolescents and young adults is sparse. Thus, the aim of this study was to evaluate the association of physical fitness, measured as maximal oxygen uptake ($\dot{V}O_{2max}$), muscle mass, weekly training, and cognitive function in the executive domains of selective attention and inhibitory control, in healthy male high-school students.

Methods: Fifty-four males (17.9 ± 0.9 years, 72 ± 11 kg and 182 ± 7 cm) completed a $\dot{V}O_{2max}$ test, a body composition test and a visual cognitive task based on the Posner cue paradigm with three types of stimuli with different attentional demands (i.e., stimuli presentation following no cue, valid cue or invalid cue presentations). The task consisted of 336 target stimuli, where 56 (17%) of the target stimuli appeared without a cue (no cue), 224 (67%) appeared in the same rectangle as the cue (valid cue) and 56 (17%) appeared in the rectangle opposite to the cue (invalid cue). Mean reaction time (RT) and corresponding errors was calculated for each stimuli type. Total task duration was 9 min and 20 s In addition, relevant background information was obtained in a questionnaire.

Results: Linear mixed model analyses showed that higher $\dot{V}O_{2max}$ was associated with faster RT for stimuli following invalid cue (Estimate = −2.69, SE = 1.03, $p = 0.011$), and for stimuli following valid cue (Estimate = −2.08, SE = 1.03, $p = 0.048$). There was no association of muscle mass and stimuli ($F = 1.01$, $p = 0.397$) or of weekly training and stimuli ($F = 0.99$, $p = 0.405$).

Conclusion: The results suggest that cardiorespiratory fitness is associated with cognitive performance in healthy male high-school students in the executive domains of selective attention.

Keywords: aerobic fitness, VO_2max, cognitive function, cue-target paradigm, attention

INTRODUCTION

In recent years, researchers have become increasingly interested in investigating possible impacts of physical activity and physical fitness on cognitive functions, and several studies have suggested that higher physical fitness levels are associated with cognitive benefits (Guiney and Machado, 2013; Dupuy et al., 2015; Cox et al., 2016).

The vast majority of research has been conducted with older adults (above 50 years), and shows positive associations of physical activity and cognitive function (Colcombe and Kramer, 2003), as well as a reduced risk of age-related cognitive decline (Paillard et al., 2015). Recently, a growing number of studies have shown positive associations between physical fitness and cognitive function in developing children and young adolescents (Hillman et al., 2009; Chaddock et al., 2011; Fedewa and Ahn, 2011; Esteban-Cornejo et al., 2015). Positive associations are also reported in young adults (Themanson and Hillman, 2006; Kamijo and Takeda, 2009), however with inconsistent findings (Scisco et al., 2008; Hayes et al., 2014). Knowledge about the associations in high-school adolescents and young adults are still sparse (Cox et al., 2016).

Given that executive functions develop throughout the childhood and decline with age (Friedman et al., 2009), the effects of physical fitness may be elusive in high-school students and in young adults where cognition is developmentally peaking (Hayes et al., 2014). As a result, specific and sensitive methods of measurement are required. In general, a large number of different methods of measurement have been employed in research in this field, as well as different definitions of cognitive function (Biddle and Asare, 2011). Dupuy et al. (2015) have stressed that a major weakness in many studies is the fact that fitness is often measured by subjective self-reports or through submaximal tests. An objective measure of cardiorespiratory fitness, $\dot{V}O_{2max}$, was therefore chosen in the present study, in addition to self-reported weekly physical activity and objectively measured muscle mass.

In general, previous research indicates that the association of physical fitness and cognitive function is stronger for tasks requiring higher level of executive functioning (Colcombe and Kramer, 2003; Hillman et al., 2009; Pontifex et al., 2011; Guiney and Machado, 2013), particularly those tasks related to different aspects of attentional ability such as inhibition and task switching (Themanson et al., 2008; Guiney and Machado, 2013; Buckley et al., 2014). A cognitive task with different attentional load was therefore chosen in the present study to investigate the association of physical fitness and cognitive load.

In terms of age, the high-students in our study came close to what could be categorized as young adulthood, thus the study adds to previous work done on subjects in late adolescence or young adulthood. Our study further contributes to previous work exploring associations between physical fitness and selective attention performed on this age group.

Thus, the aim of this study was to investigate if physical fitness was associated with cognitive function in healthy male high-school students. To do this, participants completed a $\dot{V}O_{2max}$ test, answered questions regarding weekly physical activity, underwent a body composition test and performed a pc-based visuospatial attention task to determine performance in the executive domains of selective attention and inhibitory control. The Posner cue target paradigm (Posner, 1980) was chosen to study the association of cardiorespiratory fitness and attention capacity to stimuli with different attentional load. Responding to stimuli presented after an invalid cue is particularly demanding, compared to stimuli following valid cue and no cue presentations, as it involves an interaction between goal-directed actions and inhibition of reflexive bottom-up processing of attention initiated by the distracting cue. To have a homogeneous population, only males were included. The main hypothesis was that higher physical fitness is associated with faster reaction time (RT) for all stimuli categories, due to better selective attention and inhibitory control. Moreover, we expected to find the fastest RT for stimuli following valid cue, followed by invalid cue and no cue.

MATERIALS AND METHODS

Participants

Out of the 85 young male students attending two different high schools in Norway, 66 (77.7%) were recruited, with 54 (63.5%) participants (17.9 ± 0.9 years, 72 ± 11 kg and 182 ± 7 cm) completing both the physical test and cognitive task.

Procedures

Information regarding the study was sent via e-mail to the principals of two different high schools in Norway, and they replied quickly, expressing their willingness to participate in the study. An information meeting was then arranged at which the students who were interested in participating in the study, signed informed consent forms. When recruiting participants, it was made clear that both trained/active and untrained/sedentary participants were needed.

Data was collected in the course of 6 weeks, from September–November 2015. The tests were conducted in two independent test-runs for all participants, one for the physical tests (Day A) and one for the cognitive task (Day B; **Figure 1**). The cognitive task was performed between 10:15 and 15:22. On average, there was 12 ± 10 days between tests. All physical tests were conducted in the physiological test lab at Bergen University College, and the cognitive task was mainly completed at the students' respective schools. Five to ten minutes before the participants started with the cognitive performance task, they completed a web-based electronic questionnaire.

All participants were told to dress appropriately for the physical tests, wearing shorts or pants, a t-shirt and running shoes. Participants were asked if they had felt ill during the last week before the test, especially with symptoms of fever and/or

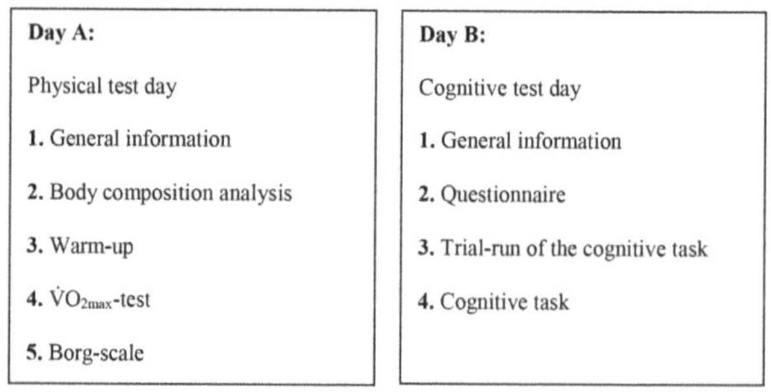

FIGURE 1 | Test-sequence of day A and day B.

impaired general condition. Participants were excluded if they had been diagnosed with heart disease, asthma or any type of disease that could potentially affect their cardiorespiratory system in a strenuous exercise test. Before testing, all participants were informed orally of the test procedures and were given the opportunity to ask questions regarding the tests. In addition, they were asked not to engage in any strenuous physical exercise the day before the physical test as this could affect the results.

Body Composition

A direct segmental multi-frequency bioelectrical impedance analysis (DSM-BIA) for determining body composition (body weight (kg), muscle mass (%)) was performed using the In-Body720 (Biospace Co. Ltd, Seoul, Korea) body composition analyzer (Lim et al., 2009; Tompuri et al., 2015). Standard procedures were followed for all participants.

Cardiorespiratory Fitness Test

The test started with a 10-min warm-up with a gradient of 1.7% on a motorized treadmill (Woodway PPS 55, USA) where the velocity was gradually increased until the participant maintained a heart rate (HR) in the area of 73%–82% of age-predicted maximum HR (HR_{max}). Following a short rest period (<3 min), an incremental test protocol was followed with a treadmill-gradient of 5.3% and a start velocity of 8 km $\cdot$ t^{-1}. The manual test protocol was controlled by the test leader, whom increased the speed by 1 km $\cdot$ t^{-1} each minute until volitional exhaustion. Notifications of the amount of time left to complete each speed and the amount of time left until the apparatus would attain a new sample registration were given throughout. When each participant was nearing possible exhaustion (respiratory exchange ratio >1), the test leader asked if a speed increase would be tolerable; the participant then had the opportunity, through the use of different hand signals, to agree to a velocity increase of 1 km $\cdot$ t^{-1} or 0.5 km $\cdot$ t^{-1}, or to maintain the same speed.

Oxygen uptake was measured using a computer that was connected to a metabolic system with a 4.2-Liter (L) mixing chamber, containing baffles (Oxycon Pro, Erich Jaeger GmbH, Hoechberg, Germany). A full system calibration was performed before the testing of each group of participants, and a volume calibration using a 3 L calibration syringe with an accuracy of 1/2 ± of 1% (Hans Rudolph Inc., Shawnee, KS, USA) was regularly performed between and during the testing of each group. Gas calibration was performed using a container that held 300 L of a gas mixture (Riessner-Gase GmbH, Carefusion, Germany) with a mixture ratio of carbon dioxide (5.84 vol. %), oxygen (15.00 vol. %), nitrogen (79.16 vol. %). Measurements of oxygen uptake were continuously recorded and saved at 30-s intervals. HR was monitored every fifth seconds using the RS400 (Polar, Kempele, Finland).

The average value of the two highest consecutive $\dot{V}O_2$ values (30-s intervals) for each participant, in any interval registration, was recorded as their individual $\dot{V}O_{2max}$. $\dot{V}O_{2max}$ was defined when two of three criteria were satisfied (Dupuy et al., 2015): (1) attaining a $\dot{V}O_2$-plateau; (2) attaining a HR >90% or equivalent to their age-predicted maximum (i.e., 220 minus age); and (3) attaining a respiratory exchange ratio >1.1.

Cognitive Performance Task

A visual cognitive task based on the Posner cue paradigm was used to assess response time (RT), accuracy and inhibition (Posner, 1980; Posner and Cohen, 1984; Gundersen et al., 2007; Irgens-Hansen et al., 2015; **Figure 2**). The task was performed on a 13.3″ laptop, and was programmed with E-prime 2.0, standard version (Psychology Software Tools, Inc.).

The participants were instructed to fixate on the crosshair in the middle of the screen (**Figure 2A**), and to respond as fast as they could by pressing "l" on the keyboard when the target stimulus (an asterisk) appeared in the right rectangle and "d" when the target stimulus appeared in the left rectangle. Sometimes during the task, the frame on one of the rectangles became broader (a cue) before the target stimulus appeared. Participants were told to ignore the cue stimulus and only press the key when the target stimulus appeared.

All participants were instructed orally and performed a small practice run before the actual task to make sure they had understood the procedure. The task duration was 9 min and 20 s, and it was carried out in a quiet location without distractions (usually a small classroom), wearing hearing protectors to exclude distracting noise.

Three different stimuli categories appeared in the task: "no cue", "valid cue" and "invalid cue". If the target stimuli appeared in one of the rectangles without a cue, this was called a no cue presentation (**Figure 2B**). If the target stimulus appeared within the rectangle with a broader frame, it was called a valid cue presentation (**Figure 2C**). The third category applied when the target stimulus appeared in the opposite rectangle to the cue location, and was called an invalid cue presentation (**Figure 2D**).

The task consisted of 336 target stimuli, with each stimulus being presented for 500 ms with an interstimuli-interval (time between stimulus) of between 600 ms and 1400 ms. The inter-

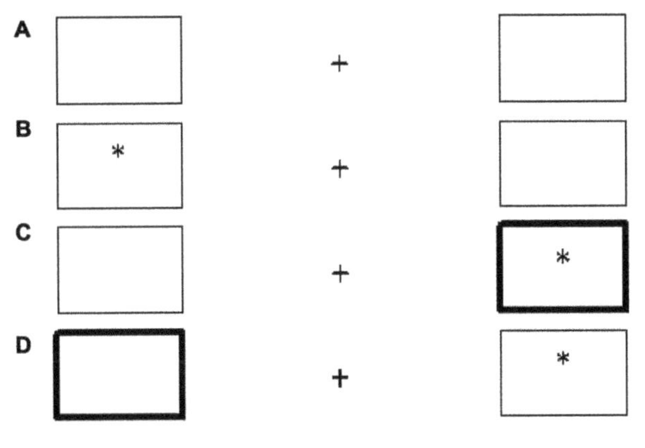

FIGURE 2 | Cognitive performance task. **(A)** Standard output screen display with a crosshair and two horizontal rectangles. **(B)** Target stimulus appears without cue (no cue). **(C)** Target stimulus appears following a cue (valid cue). **(D)** Target stimulus appears opposite to cue rectangle (invalid cue).

stimuli interval was selected from a set of fixed values (600, 700, 900, 1000 and 1200 ms). The order of the inter-stimuli interval, stimuli and cues was fixed for all participants, with mean interstimuli-interval of 825 ± 253 ms for no cue stimuli, 1108 ± 112 ms for valid stimuli and 1164 ± 236 for invalid stimuli presentations. The cue appeared in 50% of the cases 200 ms before the target stimuli, and in 50% of the cases 400 ms before the target stimulus would appear. Fifty-six (17%) of the target stimuli would appear without a cue (no cue), 224 (67%) would appear in the same rectangle as the cue (valid cue), and 56 (17%) would appear in the rectangle opposite to the cue (invalid cue).

RT (i.e., processing speed) and response accuracy were recorded and stored on the laptop for each trial. Mean RT for stimuli following no cue, valid cue and invalid cue were calculated for each participant. Error rate for the different stimuli categories were presented in percentage. Registration of responses before the target stimulus appeared, and responses during the first 149 ms. after target stimuli presentation were defined as erroneous responses (Amano et al., 2006). If an erroneous response was corrected by pressing a second time before the next stimulus was presented, it was still considered an erroneous response.

Questionnaire

The questionnaire included questions about weekly physical activity (1 = less than once a week, 2 = 1–2 time a week, 3 = 3–4 times a week, 4 = 5–6 times a week, 5 = 7–8 times a week, 6 = 9–10 times a week), and variables that previously have been associated with cognitive performance in visuospatial tests, like ADHD diagnosis (yes/no; McDonald et al., 1999), dyslexia (yes/no; Franceschini et al., 2012), daily nicotine use (yes/no; Heishman et al., 2010) and daily video-game playing (minutes; Green and Bavelier, 2003). In order to calculate the potential covariate effects of alertness on the association of cardiorespiratory fitness and cognitive performance, the participants were also asked to rate their present alertness level on a 5-point Likert scale, ranging from 1 (not alert at all) to 5 (highly alert).

Ethics

The study was conducted in accordance with the Helsinki declaration. All participants were informed about the study and signed an informed consent form before participating. Participants could withdraw from the study at any point, and results were treated anonymously. Norwegian Social Science Data Services (NSD) approved the study (reference number: 44551).

Data Analysis

The descriptive data is shown as range, mean ± standard deviation (SD). The data was checked for outliers and the preliminary analysis ensured no violation of the assumptions of normality.

To investigate if physical fitness affected RT differently for stimuli following no cue, valid cue and invalid cue, a linear mixed model was applied. Stimuli (no cue, valid cue and invalid cue) were used as repeated measure and subject as random intercept. Main effect of RT for the different stimuli categories, and interactions between RT for the different stimuli and $\dot{V}O_{2max}$, muscle mass and weekly training were included in the model. Furthermore, the model was adjusted for daily video-game playing, time-point of cognitive testing and alertness. *Post hoc* test with Bonferroni correction was performed to evaluate differences in RT between the different stimuli. A model with a first autoregressive (AR1) covariance structure and maximum likelihood of 10,000 iterations was applied showing an acceptable model fit (AIC = 1454).

Because no participants reported being diagnosed with ADHD, only three participants reported dyslexia and seven reported daily nicotine use, those variables were not included in the regression analyses. For all statistical analyses, *p*-values of <0.05 were considered statistically significant. SPSS® version 23.0 (IBM Corporation, Armonk, NY, USA) for Windows® was used for all the statistical analyses.

RESULTS

A significant main effect of stimuli (F = 6.01, p = 0.003) was found. Faster RT was seen on stimuli following valid cue (Estimate = −146.89, SE = 43.42, p = 0.001), but not on stimuli following no cue (Estimate = −65.62, SE = 32.96, p = 0.051) when invalid cue was the reference. However, *post hoc* analyses with Bonferroni correction showed significant differences between all stimuli categories. RT to stimuli following invalid cues were slower compared to valid cue (Mean differences = 59.94, SE = 2.81, p < 0.001) and faster compared to stimuli following no cue (Mean differences = −23.16, SE = 2.13, p < 0.001). RT to valid cue was faster compared to no cue (Mean differences = −83.10, SE = 2.8, p < 0.001). For mean values, see **Table 1**.

TABLE 1 | An overview of scores from the physical, cognitive and questionnaire assessments of the participants (n = 54).

	Mean ± SD	Range
RT (ms)		
Stimuli after no cues	376 ± 31	313–451
Stimuli after valid cues	293 ± 28	239–364
Stimuli after invalid cues	353 ± 35	278–429
Errors (%)		
Stimuli after no cues	3.3 ± 3.0	0–14.3
Stimuli after valid cues	5.9 ± 5.0	0.5–20.5
Stimuli after invalid cues	10.0 ± 7.6	0–32.1
$\dot{V}O_2$ max (ml/min/kg)	54.2 ± 4.9	41.9–66.7
Muscle mass (%)	49.8 ± 3.3	40.4–54.5
Weekly training sessions:		
Less than once a week	9%	
1–2	24%	
3–4	33%	
5–6	19%	
7–8	13%	
9–10	2%	
Daily video game playing (min)	73 ± 67	0–360
Time-point of cognitive testing	11:50 ± 1.0	10:15–15:22
Alertness	3.5 ± 0.8	1–5

Data is presented as mean ± standard deviation (SD) and range (min-max).

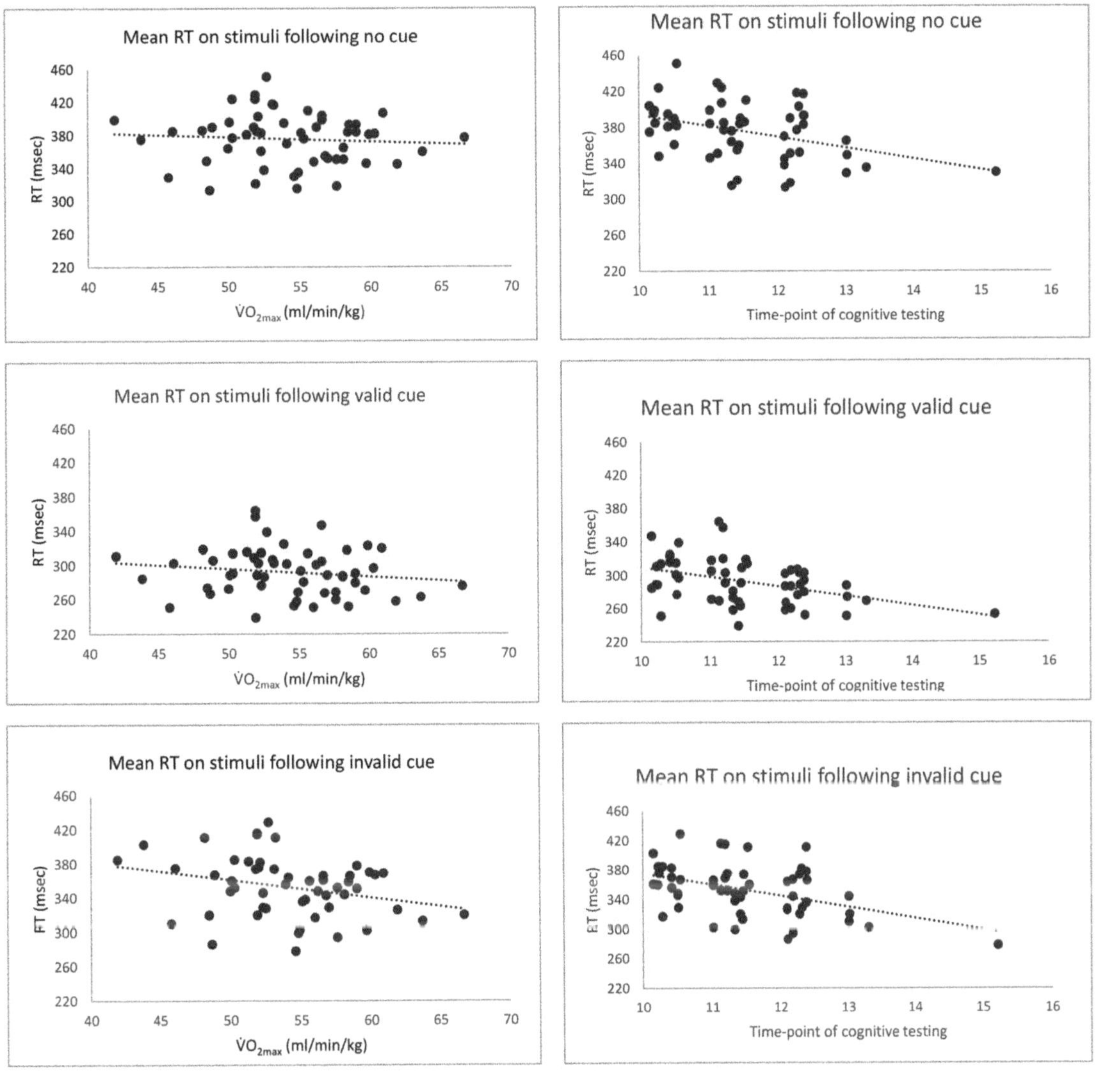

FIGURE 3 | An overview of correlations between $\dot{V}O_{2max}$ (ml/min/kg) and time-point of cognitive testing, and mean reaction time (RT; ms) to stimuli following no cue, valid cue and invalid cue for each participant. The dotted lines represent the linear trend.

Moreover, there was a significant interaction of $\dot{V}O_{2max}$ and stimuli ($F = 3.67$, $p = 0.017$). Higher $\dot{V}O_{2max}$ was associated with faster RT for stimuli following invalid cue (Estimate = −2.69, SE = 1.03, $p = 0.011$), and for stimuli following valid cue (Estimate = −2.08, SE = 1.03, $p = 0.048$), but not for stimuli following no cue (Estimate = −1.16, SE = 1.03, $p = 0.266$). There was no interaction of muscle mass and stimuli ($F = 1.01$, $p = 0.397$) or of weekly training and stimuli ($F = 0.99$, $p = 0.405$). Time-point of cognitive testing was the only covariate that contributed significantly to the model ($F = 14.14$, $p < 0.001$) with significantly slower RT in the morning (Estimate = −12.32, SE = 3.28, $p < 0.001$). See **Figure 3** for an overview of correlations between RTs of the different stimuli and $\dot{V}O_{2max}$ and for the RTs of the different stimuli and the time-point of cognitive testing.

DISCUSSION

Our results showed a significant interaction of $\dot{V}O_{2max}$ and RTs for the different stimuli categories. The interaction was significant for stimuli following valid and invalid cues, with an association between higher $\dot{V}O_{2max}$ and faster RT. There was also a significant association between time-point of cognitive testing and RT, with slower RT in the morning.

The findings of the present study show an association between higher $\dot{V}O_{2max}$ and faster RT for stimuli following both valid and invalid cues. Both stimuli conditions initiate a reflexive bottom-up attraction of attention due to the appearing peripheral cue, but differ in their demand as the most often appearing valid cue (67%) does not demand inhibition. The invalid condition (17%) will therefore demand more of a volitional top-down control when having to inhibit the most probable response.

Higher $\dot{V}O_{2max}$ seems to be beneficial in conditions initiated by cues through a faster processing speed of information, indicating a relationship between cardiorespiratory fitness and selective attention and inhibitory control in conditions where facilitation occurs.

Our findings are in agreement with a previous study by Themanson et al. (2008) showing that higher fit individuals exhibited a better top-down control of attention, and a better modulation of responses to tasks measuring selective attention. In addition, our results support previous studies showing that physical fitness yield favorable effects on executive functions (Gomez-Pinilla and Hillman, 2013; Erickson et al., 2014; Dupuy et al., 2015; Guiney et al., 2015; Szuhany et al., 2015; Luque-Casado et al., 2016). No interaction between $\dot{V}O_{2max}$ and RT on stimuli following no cue in the present study may be due to a lower attentional demand, or to the lack of priming in that stimuli category.

Our results showed fastest RT for stimuli following valid cue, followed by invalid cue and no cue. As our results show, cueing was consistently associated with faster RT, possibly reflecting a higher internal activation and increased responsiveness to upcoming target stimulus caused by the priming effect (Mangun and Hillyard, 1991; Gabay and Henik, 2008; Hayward and Ristic, 2013). Lack of priming may explain the slowest RT for stimuli following no cue. Slowest RT for no cue could also be related to the shorter interstimuli-interval. Time-point for cognitive testing were associated with RT with highest RT in the morning, supporting common knowledge of the circadian variation in alertness and performance (Van Dongen and Dinges, 2010).

$\dot{V}O_{2max}$ was the only significant physical fitness-predictor of cognitive performance in the present study. Our finding is in accordance with previous studies showing that cardiorespiratory fitness is regarded as one of the components of physical fitness mostly associated with cognitive performance (Ruiz-Ariza et al., 2017).

It is worth noting that there are recent studies failing to demonstrate the fitness-executive function hypothesis (Verburgh et al., 2014; Ballester et al., 2015). Moreover, Belsky et al. (2015) found that children with higher IQ scores grew up to be adults who were less sedentary and less obese, and in turn, had better cardiorespiratory fitness. They suggest that socioeconomic status, household and neuroselection must be considered when investigating the fitness-executive function hypothesis. Thus, more studies including other explanatory factors is needed.

Participants in the present study demonstrated an above average cardiorespiratory fitness ($\dot{V}O_{2max}$ score of 54.2 ± 4.9 mL $\cdot$ kg^{-1} $\cdot$ min^{-1}) compared to the age-relative norm of the population (46–50 mL $\cdot$ kg^{-1} $\cdot$ min^{-1}; Shvartz and Reibold, 1990). Thus, we cannot exclude a greater association of $\dot{V}O_{2max}$ and cognitive function in participants whose mean score is closer to the population average, given normally distributed $\dot{V}O_{2max}$ scores.

Limitations and Strengths

Due to the general limitations of a cross-sectional design, it is impossible to establish cause and effect in this study. In addition, the above average fitness of the participants has some implications for generalizability. The fact that the study exclusively recruited males and that the sample size is relatively small contributes to this generalization problem. Moreover, the spatial visual attention task used in the present study may not be appropriate to identify whether the cueing effects are due to endogenous spatial orienting driven by probability manipulation, attentional capture (peripheral cues), stimulus-response compatibility, or a mixture of all of them. The strengths of the study are the use of direct measures of $\dot{V}O_{2max}$ and a pc-based cognitive performance task with different attentional loads and the homogeneous group regarding age and gender.

CONCLUSION

The findings of this study show that cardiorespiratory fitness is associated with cognitive performance in healthy male high-school students. Our results suggest that cardiorespiratory fitness may be associated with better modulation of bottom-up and top-down processes in tasks involving selective attention. More research is needed to increase the knowledge about factors affecting cognitive function.

Implications for Future Research

This study contributes to the limited number of studies investigating the influence of physical fitness on the components of selective attention and inhibition in male high-school students. More studies are needed to further assess the association of physical fitness and attentional tasks demanding inhibitory control, and how this relates to the ability to maintain attention.

AUTHOR CONTRIBUTIONS

All authors participated in planning the experiment. EW, MK and HG participated in data collection. All authors have participated in conception of this manuscript, and have assisted in revising the manuscript for important content. EW and HG wrote the first draft of the manuscript, and all authors have provided final approval of the enclosed manuscript.

ACKNOWLEDGMENTS

Thanks to all the participants who volunteered to take part in this study; their participation is greatly appreciated. Thanks also to the principals and teachers at the schools for their cooperation, and to Esben Martinsen, Cecilie Hannevig and Henrik Hysing-Dahl for their assistance in parts of the physiological testing.

REFERENCES

Amano, K., Goda, N., Nishida, S., Ejima, Y., Takeda, T., and Ohtani, Y.

(2006). Estimation of the timing of human visual perception from magnetoencephalography. *J. Neurosci.* 26, 3981–3991. doi: 10.1523/jneurosci.4343-05.2006

Ballester, R., Huertas, F., Yuste, F. J., Llorens, F., and Sanabria, D. (2015). The relationship between regular sports participation and vigilance in male and female adolescents. *PLoS One* 10:e0123898. doi: 10.1371/journal.pone.0123898

Belsky, D. W., Caspi, A., Israel, S., Blumenthal, J. A., Poulton, R., and Moffitt, T. E. (2015). Cardiorespiratory fitness and cognitive function in midlife: neuroprotection or neuroselection? *Ann. Neurol.* 77, 607–617. doi: 10.1002/ana.24356

Biddle, S. J., and Asare, M. (2011). Physical activity and mental health in children and adolescents: a review of reviews. *Br. J. Sports Med.* 45, 886–895. doi: 10.1136/bjsports-2011-090185

Buckley, J., Cohen, J., Kramer, A. F., McAuley, E., and Mullen, S. P. (2014). Cognitive control in the self-regulation of physical activity and sedentary behavior. *Front. Hum. Neurosci.* 8:747. doi: 10.3389/fnhum.2014.00747

Chaddock, L., Pontifex, M. B., Hillman, C. H., and Kramer, A. F. (2011). A review of the relation of aerobic fitness and physical activity to brain structure and function in children. *J. Int. Neuropsychol. Soc.* 17, 975–985. doi: 10.1017/s1355617711000567

Colcombe, S., and Kramer, A. F. (2003). Fitness effects on the cognitive function of older adults a meta-analytic study. *Psychol. Sci.* 14, 125–130. doi: 10.1111/1467-9280.t01-1-01430

Cox, E. P., O'Dwyer, N., Cook, R., Vetter, M., Cheng, H. L., Rooney, K., et al. (2016). Relationship between physical activity and cognitive function in apparently healthy young to middle-aged adults: a systematic review. *J. Sci. Med. Sport* 19, 616–628. doi: 10.1016/j.jsams.2015.09.003

Dupuy, O., Gauthier, C. J., Fraser, S. A., Desjardins-Crèpeau, L., Desjardins, M., Mekary, S., et al. (2015). Higher levels of cardiovascular fitness are associated with better executive function and prefrontal oxygenation in younger and older women. *Front. Hum. Neurosci.* 9:66. doi: 10.3389/fnhum.2015.00066

Erickson, K. I., Leckie, R. L., and Weinstein, A. M. (2014). Physical activity, fitness, and gray matter volume. *Neurobiol. Aging* 35, S20–S28. doi: 10.1016/j.neurobiolaging.2014.03.034

Esteban-Cornejo, I., Tejero-Gonzalez, C. M., Sallis, J. F., and Veiga, O. L. (2015). Physical activity and cognition in adolescents: a systematic review. *J. Sci. Med. Sport* 18, 534–539. doi: 10.1016/j.jsams.2014.07.007

Fedewa, A. L., and Ahn, S. (2011). The effects of physical activity and physical fitness on children's achievement and cognitive outcomes: a meta-analysis. *Res. Q. Exerc. Sport* 82, 521–535. doi: 10.1080/02701367.2011.10599785

Franceschini, S., Gori, S., Ruffino, M., Pedrolli, K., and Facoetti, A. (2012). A causal link between visual spatial attention and reading acquisition. *Curr. Biol.* 22, 814–819. doi: 10.1016/j.cub.2012.03.013

Friedman, D., Nessler, D., Cycowicz, Y. M., and Horton, C. (2009). Development of and change in cognitive control: a comparison of children, young adults, and older adults. *Cogn. Affect. Behav. Neurosci.* 9, 91–102. doi: 10.3758/cabn.9.1.91

Gabay, S., and Henik, A. (2008). The effects of expectancy on inhibition of return. *Cognition* 106, 1478–1486. doi: 10.1016/j.cognition.2007.05.007

Gomez-Pinilla, F., and Hillman, C. (2013). The influence of exercise on cognitive abilities. *Compr. Physiol.* 3, 403–428. doi: 10.1002/cphy.c110063

Green, C., and Bavelier, D. (2003). Action video game modifies visual selective attention. *Nature* 423, 534–537. doi: 10.1038/nature01647

Guiney, H., Lucas, S. J., Cotter, J. D., and Machado, L. (2015). Evidence cerebral blood-flow regulation mediates exercise-cognition links in healthy young adults. *Neuropsychology* 29, 1–9. doi: 10.1037/neu0000124

Guiney, H., and Machado, L. (2013). Benefits of regular aerobic exercise for executive functioning in healthy populations. *Psychon. Bull. Rev.* 20, 73–86. doi: 10.3758/s13423-012-0345-4

Gundersen, H., Helland, C. A., Raeder, M. B., Hugdahl, K., and Wester, K. (2007). Visual attention in patients with intracranial arachnoid cysts. *J. Neurol.* 254, 60–66. doi: 10.1007/s00415-006-0280-2

Hayes, S. M., Forman, D. E., and Verfaellie, M. (2014). Cardiorespiratory fitness is associated with cognitive performance in older but not younger adults. *J. Gerontol. B. Psychol. Sci. Soc. Sci.* 71, 474–482. doi: 10.1093/geronb/gbu167

Hayward, D. A., and Ristic, J. (2013). Measuring attention using the Posner cuing paradigm: the role of across and within trial target probabilities. *Front. Hum. Neurosci.* 7:205. doi: 10.3389/fnhum.2013.00205

Heishman, S. J., Kleykamp, B. A., and Singleton, E. G. (2010). Meta-analysis of the acute effects of nicotine and smoking on human performance. *Psychopharmacology* 210, 453–469. doi: 10.1007/s00213-010-1848-1

Hillman, C. H., Buck, S. M., Themanson, J. R., Pontifex, M. B., and Castelli, D. M. (2009). Aerobic fitness and cognitive development: event-related brain potential and task performance indices of executive control in preadolescent children. *Dev. Psychol.* 45:114. doi: 10.1037/a0014437

Irgens-Hansen, K., Gundersen, H., Sunde, E., Baste, V., Harris, A., Bråtveit, M., et al. (2015). Noise exposure and cognitive performance: a study on personnel on board Royal Norwegian Navy vessels. *Noise Health* 17, 320–327. doi: 10.4103/1463-1741.165057

Kamijo, K., and Takeda, Y. (2009). General physical activity levels influence positive and negative priming effects in young adults. *Clin. Neurophysiol.* 120, 511–519. doi: 10.1016/j.clinph.2008.11.022

Lim, J. S., Hwang, J. S., Lee, J. A., Kim, D. H., Park, K. D., Jeong, J. S., et al. (2009). Cross-calibration of multi-frequency bioelectrical impedance analysis with eight-point tactile electrodes and dual-energy X-ray absorptiometry for assessment of body composition in healthy children aged 6–18 years. *Pediatr. Int.* 51, 263–268. doi: 10.1111/j.1442-200X.2008.02698.x

Luque-Casado, A., Perakakis, P., Hillman, C. H., Kao, S. C., Llorens, F., Guerra, P., et al. (2016). Differences in sustained attention capacity as a function of aerobic fitness. *Med. Sci. Sports Exerc.* 48, 887–895. doi: 10.1249/mss.0000000000000857

Mangun, G. R., and Hillyard, S. A. (1991). Modulations of sensory-evoked brain potentials indicate changes in perceptual processing during visual-spatial priming. *J. Exp. Psychol. Hum. Percept. Perform.* 17, 1057–1074. doi: 10.1037/0096-1523.17.4.1057

McDonald, S., Bennett, K. M. B., Chambers, H., and Castiello, U. (1999). Covert orienting and focusing of attention in children with attention deficit hyperactivity disorder. *Neuropsychologia* 37, 345–356. doi: 10.1016/s0028-3932(98)00078-5

Paillard, T., Rolland, Y., and de Souto Barreto, P. (2015). Protective effects of physical exercise in Alzheimer's disease and Parkinson's disease: a narrative review. *J. Clin. Neurol.* 11, 212–219. doi: 10.3988/jcn.2015.11.3.212

Pontifex, M. B., Raine, L. B., Johnson, C. R., Chaddock, L., Voss, M. W., Cohen, N. J., et al. (2011). Cardiorespiratory fitness and the flexible modulation of cognitive control in preadolescent children. *J. Cogn. Neurosci.* 23, 1332–1345. doi: 10.1162/jocn.2010.21528

Posner, M. I. (1980). Orienting of attention. *Q. J. Exp. Psychol.* 32, 3–25.

Posner, M. I., and Cohen, Y. (1984). "Components of visual orienting," in *Attention and Performance X: Control of Language Processes* (Vol 32), eds H. Bouma and D. G. Bouwhuis (Hillsdale: Erlbaum), 531–556.

Ruiz-Ariza, A., Grao-Cruces, A., de Loureiro, N. E. M., and Martínez-López, E. J. (2017). Influence of physical fitness on cognitive and academic performance in adolescents: a systematic review from 2005–2015. *Int. Rev. Sport Exerc. Psychol.* 10, 108–133. doi: 10.1080/1750984x.2016.1184699

Scisco, J. L., Leynes, P. A., and Kang, J. (2008). Cardiovascular fitness and executive control during task-switching: an ERP study. *Int. J. Psychophysiol.* 69, 52–60. doi: 10.1016/j.ijpsycho.2008.02.009

Shvartz, E., and Reibold, R. C. (1990). Aerobic fitness norms for males and females aged 6 to 75 years: a review. *Aviat. Space Environ. Med.* 61, 3–11.

Szuhany, K. L., Bugatti, M., and Otto, M. W. (2015). A meta-analytic review of the effects of exercise on brain-derived neurotrophic factor. *J. Psychiatr. Res.* 60, 56–64. doi: 10.1016/j.jpsychires.2014.10.003

Themanson, J. R., and Hillman, C. H. (2006). Cardiorespiratory fitness and acute aerobic exercise effects on neuroelectric and behavioral measures of action monitoring. *Neuroscience* 141, 757–767. doi: 10.1016/j.neuroscience.2006.04.004

Themanson, J. R., Pontifex, M. B., and Hillman, C. H. (2008). Fitness and action monitoring: evidence for improved cognitive flexibility in young adults. *Neuroscience* 157, 319–328. doi: 10.1016/j.neuroscience.2008.09.014

Tompuri, T. T., Lakka, T. A., Hakulinen, M., Lindi, V., Laaksonen, D. E., Kilpeläinen, T. O., et al. (2015). Assessment of body composition by dual-energy X-ray absorptiometry, bioimpedance analysis and anthropometrics in children: the Physical Activity and Nutrition in Children study. *Clin. Physiol. Funct. Imaging* 35, 21–33. doi: 10.1111/cpf.12118

Van Dongen, H. P. A., and Dinges, D. F. (2010). "Circadian rhythms in fatigue, alertness and performance," in *Principles and Practice of Sleep Medicine*, 3rd Edn. eds M. H. Kryger, T. Roth and W. C. Dement (Philadelphia, PA: Elsevier Saunders), 391–399.

Verburgh, L., Konigs, M., Scherder, E. J., and Oosterlaan, J. (2014). Physical exercise and executive functions in preadolescent children, adolescents and young adults: a meta-analysis. *Br. J. Sports Med.* 48, 973–979. doi: 10.1136/bjsports-2012-091441

15

Computer Enabled Neuroplasticity Treatment: A Clinical Trial of a Novel Design for Neurofeedback Therapy in Adult ADHD

Benjamin Cowley[1,2]*, *Édua Holmström*[3], *Kristiina Juurmaa*[2], *Levas Kovarskis*[3] *and Christina M. Krause*[2]

[1] BrainWork Research Centre, Finnish Institute of Occupational Health, Helsinki, Finland, [2] Cognitive Brain Research Unit, Cognitive Science, Institute of Behavioural Sciences, University of Helsinki, Helsinki, Finland, [3] Formally affiliated with Faculty of Behavioural Sciences, University of Helsinki, Helsinki, Finland

Edited by:
Soledad Ballesteros,
Universidad Nacional de Educación a Distancia, Spain

Reviewed by:
Lutz Jäncke,
University of Zurich, Switzerland
Juliana Yordanova,
Bulgarian Academy of Sciences, Bulgaria

***Correspondence:**
Benjamin Cowley
benjamin.cowley@ttl.fi

Background: We report a randomized controlled clinical trial of neurofeedback therapy intervention for ADHD/ADD in adults. We focus on internal mechanics of neurofeedback learning, to elucidate the primary role of cortical self-regulation in neurofeedback. We report initial results; more extensive analysis will follow.

Methods: Trial has two phases: intervention and follow-up. The intervention consisted of neurofeedback treatment, including intake and outtake measurements, using a waiting-list control group. Treatment involved ~40 h-long sessions 2–5 times per week. Training involved either theta/beta or sensorimotor-rhythm regimes, adapted by adding a novel "inverse-training" condition to promote self-regulation. Follow-up (ongoing) will consist of self report and executive function tests.

Setting: Intake and outtake measurements were conducted at University of Helsinki. Treatment was administered at partner clinic Mental Capital Care, Helsinki.

Randomization: We randomly allocated half the sample then adaptively allocated the remainder to minimize baseline differences in prognostic variables.

Blinding: Waiting-list control design meant trial was not blinded.

Participants: Fifty-four adult Finnish participants (mean age 36 years; 29 females) were recruited after screening by psychiatric review. Forty-four had ADHD diagnoses, 10 had ADD.

Measurements: Symptoms were assessed by computerized attention test (T.O.V.A.) and self-report scales, at intake and outtake. Performance during neurofeedback trials was recorded.

Results: Participants were recruited and completed intake measurements during summer 2012, before assignment to treatment and control, September 2012. Outtake measurements ran April-August 2013. After dropouts, 23 treatment and 21 waiting-list participants remained for analysis.
Initial analysis showed that, compared to waiting-list control, neurofeedback promoted improvement of self-reported ADHD symptoms, but did not show transfer of learning to T.O.V.A. Comprehensive analysis will be reported elsewhere.

Trial Registration: "Computer Enabled Neuroplasticity Treatment (CENT)," ISRCTN13915109.

Keywords: neurofeedback, attention deficit/hyperactivity disorder, attention deficit disorder, adult, randomized controlled trial, waiting list control, learning curves, learning transfer

1. INTRODUCTION

Attention Deficit/Hyperactivity Disorder (ADHD) is a neurobiological condition which can strongly affect several areas of life: lower socio-economic status, less satisfaction with employment and marriage, as well as common co-occurrence of conditions like addiction and depression. Epidemiology research has estimated the prevalence of ADHD among adults to be 4.4%. Subtypes of ADHD have been identified including Inattentive (ADHD-I), Hyperactive (ADHD-H) and combined (ADHD-C). However, the nature of the disease and most effective method of treatment are still not well understood.

This open-label clinical trial is a test of neurofeedback (NFB) as a treatment intervention for ADHD or ADD-diagnosed adults[1]. The intervention is based on the NFB training regimes "theta-beta" (TB) and "sensorimotor rhythm" (SMR). These regimes train self-regulation of power in specific bands of the EEG frequency spectrum, through the principle of operant conditioning. The trial also includes the novel addition of a third type of training, "inverse training," designed to help investigate the relationship between NFB learning performance (the requirement to self-regulate) and the specific effects of each training regime. This follows recent calls for increased focus on the internal mechanics of the NFB process by Gevensleben et al. (2014) and Zuberer et al. (2015), in order to attempt more than just another simple test of efficacy.

We test intervention efficacy in a between-subjects manner using a waiting-list control (WLC) group. The trial thus relies on three different levels of measurements: neurophysiological, cognitive, and behavioral; and examines their relationship across multiple time-points. Transfer of learning is measured by: questionnaires tapping ADHD/ADD symptoms that participants filled out at four time-points during the intervention; and by performance on a continuous performance test. More importantly, given our focus on mechanics, we also test specific effects of the NFB training regimes by analysing within-subjects learning curves (LCs) of the treatment group, which represent how they learn to self-regulate their EEG-band activity.

At the time of writing this is an ongoing two phase trial, where phase 1 included intake measurements, NFB intervention, and outtake (all complete), and phase 2 will include follow-up measurements and WLC treatment opportunity (pending). In addition to the protocol structure, we report an initial group-comparison result from the first phase, showing mixed outcomes for efficacy. This result is primarily included to illustrate the importance of the planned within-subjects analysis for obtaining clear insights from the data gathered.

1.1. Attention Deficit/Hyperactive Disorder

Models seeking to explain the cognitive neuropsychological problems associated with ADHD include disturbance of attention, cortical arousal, and executive functions (for review see e.g., Sergeant et al., 2003; Seidman, 2006). However, a meta-analysis by Huang-Pollock and Nigg (2003) discarded the explanatory value of attention, at least in individuals diagnosed with the combined subtype of ADHD. Increasingly, ADHD is not seen as a disorder of attention at all but as a disorder in key aspects of self-regulation and executive functions (Nigg, 2005). One caveat is the growing consensus that the executive function "single deficit" model cannot sufficiently explain ADHD (Nigg, 2005; Pennington, 2005; Sonuga-Barke, 2005). Studies indicate that not all persons with ADHD have executive function deficits — at least as measured by laboratory tests.

Cortical arousal models in ADHD are closely related to the attentional concept of alerting as proposed by Posner and Petersen (1990), reflecting right-lateralized vigilance network with noradrenergic involvement. These models emphasize deficiencies in the early stages of information processing as a result of under-arousal in cortical systems (Sergeant et al., 1999). EEG and ERP findings tend to support this model in that they reveal excess slow-wave activity in adults with ADHD (Bresnahan et al., 1999). Support also comes from consistent findings of deficit in the continuous performance test (CPT) d-prime parameter, which can be considered a consensus index of arousal (Losier et al., 1996). Epstein et al. (2003) found that the d-prime demonstrated very robust relationships to the 18 DSMV-IV ADHD symptoms.

EEG studies suggest that ADHD might stem either from a maturational lag or a developmental deviation (Barry et al., 2003). Maturational lag models require that EEG measures from an individual with ADHD would be considered normal in a younger person, and implies that ADHD adults grow out of their immature EEG activity with increasing age (Mann et al., 1992). Whereas in the developmental deviation model, ADHD is conceptualized as resulting from an abnormality in the functioning of the central nervous system, unlikely to change without targeted intervention.

Abbreviations: ADHD, Attention Deficit/Hyperactivity Disorder; ADD, Attention Deficit Disorder; BCIA, Biofeedback Certification International Alliance; CENT, Computer Enabled Neuroplasticity Treatment; CNV, Contingent Negative Variation; IBS, Institute of Behavioral Science; MCC, Mental Capital Care (clinic); NFB, neurofeedback; RCT, randomized controlled trial; SCP, Slow Cortical Potentials (neurofeedback training regime); SMR, SensoriMotor Rhythm (neurofeedback training regime); TB, Theta/Beta (neurofeedback training regime); T.O.V.A., Test Of Variables of Attention; UoH, University of Helsinki; WLC, waiting list control.

[1]The ICD-10 diagnosis classification system is in use in Finland where the study was conducted. Both ADD and ADHD are used as diagnoses, the former referring to the predominantly inattentive type, as opposed to predominantly hyperactive or combined types.

Longitudinal studies, reviewed by Bresnahan et al. (1999), that followed participants up till adulthood revealed that although there is a significant reduction of slow wave activity in both the ADHD and the control group with increasing age, absolute and relative theta activity remained elevated through adolescence into adulthood (Bresnahan and Barry, 2002). Interestingly, with increasing age, the level of beta activity produced by adults with ADHD was normalized in the frontocentral regions. The most consistent finding from EEG studies of ADHD in adults is increased absolute power in theta, clearly visible in frontocentral areas (Bresnahan et al., 1999; Lazzaro et al., 1999; Clarke et al., 2001). Such findings contradict the maturational lag model, as the difference in slow activity does not disappear with increasing age.

By contrast, the hypo-arousal developmental deviation model originally proposed by Satterfield et al. (1974) has been supported by cerebral blood flow and positron emission tomography studies (Lou et al., 1989; Zametkin et al., 1990). This model proposes that ADHD results from cortical under-arousal, and the observed atypical slow wave activity confirms the existence of altered brain activity among adults with ADHD. Hypo-arousal is thought to correlate with both beta and SMR (sensory motor rhythm, also called low beta), because in normal functioning, increased beta is associated with mental activity, and decreased SMR with physical activity.

Much of the existing research has identified maturational lag or hypo-arousal as the underlying cause of ADHD. Although these models have initiated extensive research, they have failed to clarify the aetiology of the disorder (Bresnahan et al., 1999). Thus, the literature suggests that, at least in adult ADHD, aetiological specificity is lacking; with the consequence that traditional treatments targeted at ADHD as a single disorder are unlikely to be reliable. In contrast, personalized medicine emphasizes heterogeneity within a given disorder, relying on biomarkers or endophenotypes to guide different treatments.

1.2. Neurofeedback

NFB, also called EEG biofeedback, is operant conditioning of specific temporal, spatial and frequency features extracted from scalp-recorded electrical potentials (Lubar and Shouse, 1976). Feedback is presented to the treated individual in the form of positive and negative reinforcers (in this study: visual reinforcers) whenever their ongoing EEG features meet or fail to meet a predefined criterion. The aim of NFB is to learn to gain control of those EEG features over time.

Literature supports the efficacy of NFB for children with ADHD (Arns et al., 2009, 2014b; Micoulaud-Franchi et al., 2014). Part of its value is that NFB can be personalized to suit the specific clinical presentation, provided that there is requisite theoretical and observational data to guide the personalization.

NFB has been described as a mechanism that can stimulate cortical arousal and/or regulate cortical oscillations, which in turn may influence such cognitive activity as attention (Vernon et al., 2003). The specific effect has been described variously as following one of two models, termed by Gevensleben et al. (2014) as "conditioning- and-repairing model" vs. "skill-acquisition model." This implies that the effect of NFB may be to repair a presumed cause of disorder to normalize behavior, or instead may be a tool to enhance cognitive performance (see Gevensleben et al., 2014 for a thorough discussion).

It has been suggested that, besides the neurophysiological aspects of NFB, treatment outcome depends greatly on the subjective involvement of the patient. Calderon and Thompson (2004) have conceptualized biofeedback as a three-step process that consists of

- becoming aware of a physiological response,
- learning to control the response, and
- transferring control of the response to everyday life.

The first two steps of the model — becoming aware and learning to control the electrical activity of the brain — constitute NFB learning. The third step refers to *transfer* of the NFB learning, measured here by performance on a neurocognitive test as well as self-reported ADHD related symptoms.

This study employs two kinds of separate NFB training regimes: theta/beta and sensimotor-rhythm. Additionally, we included a novel "inverse mode" of training, which is a modification of each of these two regimes. Finally, transfer trials during which the patient is given no visual feedback were included toward the end of the trial.

Theta/beta (TB) training regime assumes a theta power that is elevated above normal, and therefore uses an inhibition target for theta power and a reinforcement target for beta power. EEG recording is often at a frontal site. The rationale behind TB training has been described in at least two different ways: as the rectification of cortical hypoarousal (Barry et al., 2003), and as the reinforcement of working memory (Vernon et al., 2003).

Sensimotor-rhythm (SMR) training regime reinforces beta power, usually low or mid beta, often with an inhibition target for theta. The site is above the sensorimotor strip, often lateral, such that the beta oscillations correspond to the sensorimotor rhythm. The rationale for SMR training has been proposed as either facilitating attention (Vernon et al., 2003), or the improvement of sleep through an increase in beta spindles, with concomitant effects on cognitive function (Arns et al., 2014a).

It is important to note, that NFB learning is anchored in two scientific theories, but occurrence of NFB learning as such tests only one of these. On the one hand, NFB learning relies on the cortical arousal model of ADHD that emphasizes under-arousal in the cortical systems with excess slow wave activity affecting information processing (Sergeant et al., 1999; Barry et al., 2003). Based on this model, the NFB training aims at increasing fast-wave activity (in this study: SMR and beta bands) and decreasing slow-wave activity (in this study: theta) (Barry et al., 2003). However, NFB learning as such does not test whether the underlying problem of ADHD is under-arousal; what it does test is the operant conditioning of EEG activity. NFB learning is conceptualized in terms of changes in the amount of time a patient manages to move his/her EEG features in the required direction during training sessions as a result of learning to self-regulate cortical oscillations. Zuberer et al. (2015) argue that NFB outcomes should be tested by examination of the learning curves.

Thus, it is clear that, although aetiological and thus clinical specificity for ADHD is lacking, all NFB treatment regimes share a common goal of promoting self-regulation. On the other hand, some more modern NFB regimes have a more explicit approach to self-regulation than their older cousins. For example, Slow Cortical Potentials (SCP) training uses two opposed cortical regulation targets (Mayer et al., 2013), to be trained in random consecutive order. The two most common NFB training regimes TB and SMR do not include such an explicit set of counter-poised targets to induce self-regulation, relying instead on a single target of reinforcement/inhibition, which is trained repeatedly.

The target of SCP training is the Contingent Negative Variation (CNV) Event Related Potential, which Mayer et al. defined as a slow negative shift over central sites that develops following the presentation of warning stimulus while expecting an imperative stimulus that requires a response (Mayer et al., 2015). Thus, while SCP directly addresses self-regulation, it does so only for a single correlate of attention. Other cortical correlates of attention processes are addressed by other NFB training regimes, e.g., cortical hypo-arousal in TB, or spontaneous motor activation in SMR. However, these training regimes have no specific component designed to promote self-regulation.

Therefore, to the standard TB and SMR training regimes we have introduced a mode of "inverse training" (denoted iTB and iSMR), in order to explore the effect of adding an SCP-like approach to these unidirectional training regimes. This takes the form of an extra target in each regime, where the reinforcer/inhibitor is the exact opposite of the norm (see Methods).

TB and SMR training regimes are based on sub-second frequency-band features, so they are not directly comparable with SCP which feeds back the time domain DC component. However, from our point of view, there are at least three motivating reasons to test the "inverse training" self-regulatory modes of TB and SMR.

First, the neurological effect of TB and SMR remains unclear, due to the competing explanatory models. This study will not lay all questions to rest, but it does pursue a novel line of inquiry. Second, "inverse training" should aid the subjective experience of self-regulation, as it does in SCP; after all from the clinical point of view, NFB training in any training regime relies on the patient's own "mental strategy," reinforced by feedback-free transfer trials. Third, combining the above two issues, the participants have the opportunity to learn the experiential correlate of the inverse neural state, and thus learn to be able to activate OR deactivate cortical resources at will. If we accept, for example, that TB trains the activation of cortical arousal, then the experiential correlate of inverse TB (iTB) might be more appropriate when the individual needs to enter a state of calm reflection. Similarly, SMR implies activation of the sensorimotor strip, which in turn implies quietude of bodily motor-neuron activity; however inverse SMR (iSMR) might be more appropriate when particular task activity calls for so-called kinaesthetic intelligence. This conceptualization of the process would follow the "skill-acquisition" model of Gevensleben et al. (2014). That is, the patient would gain a tool to enhance cognitive performance, as opposed (or in addition) to repairing a presumed cause of disorder.

Although earlier work (Lubar and Shouse, 1976; Monastra et al., 2005), including meta-analysis by Snyder and Hall (2006), has shown support for a single-trait model of ADHD (an elevated theta-beta ratio), others have argued that research results and clinical application should be interpreted with more regard for variability of individuals (Arns et al., 2008). Hammond (2010) goes into this issue in detail, illustrating the heterogeneity in quantitative EEG (qEEG) patterns associated with symptoms and discussing the requirements and need for qEEG analysis guided by normative databases. Johnstone et al. (2005) provided a review of such databases, along with a review of qEEG profiles, which are manifestations seen between genome and behavioral that they term "intermediate" EEG endophenotypes. They called for QEEG endophenotype-guided NFB treatments to provide non-pharmacological interventions to help the subgroup of non-responders to traditional treatments, or complement traditional treatments in certain cases.

Especially in adults, who are subject to maturation effects across a broad age range, ADHD is a heterogeneous disorder with an uncertain treatment situation. In other words, some might have executive function deficits and might possibly benefit from TB over the prefrontal cortex; while some might benefit more from the characteristic behavioral correlate of SMR, that is, immobility as well as reduction of muscular tension (Chase and Harper, 1971; Howe and Sterman, 1972), thus facilitating the self-regulation of attention through mechanisms similar to mindfulness meditation (Zylowska et al., 2008). For this reason, in this study TB and SMR training regimes are assigned in a personalized fashion based on EEG spectral profiles (see Methods).

1.2.1. Outline

In the rest of this paper, following the CONSORT guidelines, we first document the Methods and design of the trial, including participant criteria, intervention details, objectives, outcome measures, sample size calculation, randomization procedure and other allocation details, plus statistical analysis. Next, we provide existing results from the trial as it stands, primarily regarding how the treatment stage was run, along with preliminary analyses of group comparison outcomes. Finally we discuss issues arising from the trial design and implementation, as well as the implications of the preliminary analyses and future work.

2. METHODS/DESIGN

2.1. Participants

Inclusion criteria were scores on Adult ADHD Self Report Scale (ASRS) (Kessler et al., 2005), and Brown -ADHD scale (BADDS) (Brown, 1996) indicating presence of ADHD, as well as:

- pre-existing diagnosis of ADHD or ADD,
- nonexistence of neurological diagnoses,
- age 18–60 years,
- IQ score >80 measured by a qualified psychologist using WAIS IV (Wechsler, 2008)

Exclusion criteria included extreme outlier scores in the scales of

- Generalized Anxiety Disorder (Spitzer et al., 2006),

- Beck Depression Inventory (Beck et al., 1996),
- Alcohol Use Disorders Identification Test (Saunders et al., 1993),
- the Mood Disorder Questionnaire (Hirschfeld et al., 2000),
- test of prodromal symptoms of psychosis (Heinimaa et al., 2003), and
- the Dissociative experiences scale (Liebowitz, 1992) for dissociative symptoms.

Thresholds for exclusion were not fixed but at the discretion of the consulting psychiatrist. Use of medication for ADHD was not an exclusion criterion but participants were asked not to make changes in medication during the time of the training. Informed consent was obtained from each subject in accordance with the Declaration of Helsinki.

Self-report tests were distributed and submitted by mail. Psychiatric consultations were performed at the private practice of the psychiatrist; IQ testing was performed at the testing room of the University of Helsinki (UoH) Institute of Behavioral Sciences (IBS); both in central Helsinki.

2.1.1. Ethical Approval

Written informed consent for participation was obtained from all participants before entering the study. The protocol followed the Declaration of Helsinki for the rights of the participants and the procedures of the study. An ethical approval of the present research protocol for all participants was obtained from The Ethical Committee of the Hospital District of Helsinki and Uusimaa, 28/03/2012, 621/1999, 24 §. Participants were not remunerated.

2.1.2. Clinic of Treatment

The clinic for intervention sessions was required to be centrally located in Helsinki, to be staffed by licensed psychiatrist in case of emergencies, and to have recognition by the Association for Finnish Work. Technicians were required to have a primary degree in a discipline related to human psychology; they were also required to take a 3-month training course provided at the UoH based on principles of the Biofeedback Certification International Alliance (BCIA).

2.2. Intervention

The experimental treatment was a novel neurofeedback (NFB) intervention, based on the well-known operant conditioning NFB training regimes "theta-beta" (TB) and "sensorimotor rhythm" (SMR); with the novel addition of a self-regulatory component designed to address the heterogeneity and aetiological uncertainty of ADHD in the adult population. The comparator was a WLC group. The WLC design places a randomly assigned control group on hiatus, while the active treatment is applied to the randomly assigned treatment group. The WLC group should receive treatment after the follow-up assessment at 24 months post-treatment, without experimental oversight.

Participants who volunteered in response to advertisements were recruited at time T0. Contact with the psychiatrist and psychologist for screening followed at time T1.

Successfully screened participants were taken to the intake measurement at time T2, where they performed the T.O.V.A. test along with eyes-open and closed baselines, while scalp EEG was recorded. The individual alpha peak frequency (IAPF) of each participant was estimated from band power analysis of eye-opened and eye-closed baseline conditions (Lansbergen et al., 2011). The boundaries of each EEG frequency band for each participant are defined with respect to IAPF, e.g., theta is IAPF$\times$0.4 to IAPF$\times$0.6.

After randomization between treatment and WLC groups at time T3, we assigned participants in the NFB treatment group to either TB or SMR training based on their IAPF-adjusted theta/beta ratio. Those with theta/beta ratio >1 ($n = 9$) received reinforcement for simultaneous increase in beta and decrease in theta (over power estimated from per-session baseline) at electrode Fz. The rest ($n = 16$) got reinforcement for increase in SMR and decrease in theta at electrode C4. Band powers within the NFB training regimes are adjusted by IAPF.

Treatment was administered using the following hardware and software set up. The EEG amplifier was the Enobio ambulatory device (Neuroelectrics SL, Barcelona)[2], with streaming Bluetooth connection to standard Windows 8 desktop computers. The software was developed within the project, as described in Cowley et al. (forthcoming). Briefly, the system is based on OpenViBE signal acquisition framework[3], with a Qt frontend, and is available open source[4].

NFB interventions were standardized by scheduling of the training sessions: session duration was fixed; and training blocks per session, sessions per week, timing of the break from training, and total duration of training were all constrained to equalize the intervention. At time T4, treatment group participants began their treatment by being briefed about all aspects of the NFB training regimes, e.g., length, frequency, purpose. Finally for the first phase, outcome measures were taken at time T5, when all participants in the treatment group had completed 40 sessions NFB.

In the first phase the care providers were monitored by both the lead researcher and responsible psychiatrist on separate occasions, with interviews to ascertain their self-assessment of performance. Both care providers and patients were given self-assessment questionnaires to describe their working relationships.

The second phase of the trial is ongoing at time of writing. Beginning with re-recruitment at T6, phase two consists of a follow-up measurement for all, and treatment option for WLC participants. Follow-up measurements include the ASRS and BADDS self-reports. Treatment for the WLC group will not be NFB, but will consist of a game-like computerized attention training intervention, without concurrent recording of EEG.

2.3. Objectives

Our RCT research questions (RQs) follow Calderon and Thompson (2004), since we first examine NFB learning "within subjects," and second examine the transfer of NFB learning

[2] http://www.neuroelectrics.com/.
[3] http://openvibe.inria.fr/.
[4] https://github.com/CBRUhelsinki/CENTplatform.

comparing the treatment group to a WLC group. Within this paper, we report only first-stage analysis, namely the comparison between groups addressed by H2a and H3c below (see Results).

2.3.1. Learning in NFB

The NFB learning metric reflects the proportion of time during training when EEG signals are in the target state; the "learning curve" is thus characterized by a signal evolving over blocks and sessions of training. The shapes or slopes of participants LCs are rarely reported in the NFB literature: analysis tends to focus on transfer outcomes compared to a control group. However, clinical observations commonly indicate that learning occurs. Also, NFB learning in this study was manipulated with the addition of the "inverse-training" mode. The LCs resulting from normal, inverse and transfer training blocks should each be slope-positive, because they each require a similar act of concentration which the participants are practicing throughout training. Finally, the profile of the LCs over sessions which combine all training types should be slope-positive, because training with counter-poised targets increases the need to self-regulate. Thus, we propose the following hypotheses:

- H1a: "normal" NFB training results in positive-slope LCs.
- H1b: "inverse" NFB training results in positive-slope LCs.
- H1c: "transfer" NFB training results in positive-slope LCs.

2.3.2. Transfer: Attention Test and Self-Reported Symptoms

Due to meta-analyses that find that NFB is efficacious for reduction of inattention (Arns et al., 2009), transfer of learning is expected to result in more improvement-over-baseline of the treatment group, compared with a control group, at the continuous performance test (CPT) Test Of Variables of Attention (T.O.V.A.) applied before and after training. Furthermore, those participants who perform better in baseline T.O.V.A. (lower scores), are expected to learn quicker during the NFB training.

- H2a: the treatment group will achieve better T.O.V.A. performance, and improve more after training, than the WLC.
- H2b: a better baseline T.O.V.A. score will predict better baseline NFB performance and better NFB learning.

Severity of subjective symptoms of ADHD/ADD should be reduced by the transfer of NFB learning to the ability to self-regulate. We also expect this effect to be dose-dependent, such that participants with better NFB performance (steeper positive slope) should present a higher rate of change in reported symptoms (steeper negative slope). Finally, the treatment group is expected to report fewer symptoms than the control group in the outcome measurement.

- H3a: NFB training will result in a negative linear trend in reported ADHD/ADD symptoms.
- H3b: the NFB LC profile will correlate with reported ADHD/ADD symptoms.
- H3c: the treatment group will report greater improvements in ADHD/ADD symptoms than the WLC.

2.4. Outcomes

Primary outcome measures include learning curve assessment, T.O.V.A., ASRS, and Digit span. These measures fall into two categories: (1) between-group comparison of NFB and WLC groups; and (2) within-subjects tests for treatment group. Primary measures are all comparative, truly experimental, and hypothesis-driven.

Secondary outcome measures include pre- and post-treatment vigilance measurement with an EEG protocol (Olbrich et al., 2012); also per-session self-report of circadian patterns, mood, excitement, effort and frustration; and the Pittsburgh Sleep Quality Index (PSQI) administered pre-, post- and at two intermediate points during treatment. These measures were taken to explore the additional research question of the relationship between sleep quality and NFB performance.

Additional methods taken to assess the quality of measurements include

- placebo expectation reports (Borkovec and Sibrava, 2005) asked before and at halfway through the treatment,
- the novel participant-technician interaction questionnaire, designed to assess the participants' experience of their interaction with the technician. Based on the guidelines of the "Framework for Measuring Impact"[5], we created what they term "specifically developed questions." This option was especially appropriate given the requirement to translate any existing measure, which would limit validity. The questionnaire was a set of ten simple questions such as "has my trainer supported me during my neurofeedback training?" Responses were made on a six-point Likert-scale from "0-not at all" to "5-enough," for a scoring range of 0–50.

2.5. Sample Size

The power calculation of $N = 60$ was based on an estimated effect size for neurofeedback of 0.9, alpha at 0.05 and Power at 0.95 (for an independent samples t-test, estimate based on studies including Egner and Gruzelier, 2004; Rossiter, 2004a,b; Arns et al., 2009). Recent work has shown an effect size of 0.73 for a purely adult population (Mayer et al., 2012), but we can still maintain $N = 60$ by assuming power $= 0.85$, since this is equivalent to an phase 1 trial where the motivation is greater to minimize Type I error than Type II. This also contributes to our motivation to use a WLC along with the principle that NFB is closer in nature to a behavioral intervention than a drug trial, and thus double-blinding is unwarranted and unethical.

2.6. Randomization Procedure

We assign patients to test or control groups using a procedure that controls for selection bias, and known and unknown sources of external variance due to prognostic variables; the procedure is based on combined randomization and adaptive allocation.

Simple randomization prevents biased selection and meets the assumptions of uniform assignment probability made in standard inferential procedures. However, it does not guarantee equal group sizes and can lead to baseline imbalance in prognostic variables such as age, gender or disease severity. Equal group sizes

[5]http://www.measuringimpact.org/home.

can be obtained using blocking, while baseline imbalance can be helped by using blocking stratified over prognostic variables, although the number of variables which can be used is small. This limitation is surmounted by adaptive allocation, exemplified by minimization methods: these are not strictly random but allow tight control of balance of multiple prognostic variables (see e.g., Roberts and Torgerson, 1998 on methodological issues).

In their review of recommendations of assignment method, (Scott et al., 2002, p. 671) found a general support for minimization with a random element in smaller trials. Our approach follows: X% random blocking followed by 100-X% minimization (0<X<100). The algorithm is:

1. Simple blocked random allocation of X% patients (of those currently recruited).
2. For the next 100−X% of patients, reassign patients based on minimization.
3. Using a distance measure, make the assignment that results in the smaller inter-group distance.
4. For every new assignment decrement the number of possible new assignments to that group, to maintain equal group sizes.

Assignment was balanced over age, sex, education, IQ, diagnosis (ADHD vs. ADD), comorbities from diagnosis, comorbities from administered scales, and ASRS subtype score, and tested between groups to show no statistically significant differences (see **Table 1** below). The same tests returned null when run after any change in relative group composition, due to e.g., drop-outs. Thus, groups did not differ in terms of symptom severity, diagnosis, IQ or demographic features at assignment.

Given that the initial allocation of patients is random, further non-random selections will also be random at the population level. Even if the minimization assignments cannot be considered random, the overall assignment retains a proportional amount of randomness equivalent to X, similar to more complex biased-coin approaches. In this trial X was set equal to 50.

The most important caveat of the approach is that variables used in minimization must be included as covariates during analysis, to avoid potentially misleading results.

Technicians must be assigned to treatment and control group by recruitment on-demand, as the group treatment phases were separated in time.

TABLE 1 | Demographic and clinical characteristics for NFB and WLC groups.

		Treatment	Control	Statistical testing		
		N = 25	*N* = 29	*t*	*df*	*p*
Age	Mean	35.72	36.45	−0.259	52	0.797
	Std. Dev.	9.66	10.86			
WAIS-IV: VCI	Mean	113.68	113.59	0.035	52	0.972
	Std. Dev.	10.33	9.37			
WAIS-IV: POI	Mean	113.44	112.69	0.194	52	0.847
	Std. Dev.	11.87	15.87			
				χ^2	*df*	*p*
Gender	Female	14 (56%)	15 (52%)	0.99	1	0.753
	Male	11 (44%)	14 (48%)			
Education	Primary	6 (24%)	5 (17%)	0.470	2	0.791
	Secondary	15 (60%)	18 (62%			
	Tertiary	4 (16%)	6 (21%)			
ADHD/ADD	ADHD	21 (84%)	23 (79%)	0.196	1	0.658
	ADD	4 (16%)	6 (21%)			

2.6.1. Allocation Concealment

Participants were randomly assigned by use of computerized algorithm detailed above, at one time, directly after all intake measurements and before the start of NFB treatment.

2.6.2. Implementation

The allocation algorithm was designed and implemented by the lead researcher; the direct contact with participants for enrolment and assignment was handled by a technician working for the MCC clinic.

2.6.3. Blinding

Due to the fact that the trial used waiting list for the control group, assessment was not blinded. Thus, after assignment, all participants and researchers/technicians had access to the assignment information. As mentioned above, since NFB is closer in nature to a behavioral intervention than a drug trial, double-blinding would be unwarranted and unethical.

2.7. Statistical Methods

Independent variables for group comparison include NFB training regime (TB vs. SMR), participant age and gender, and assigned group (treatment vs. WLC group). Dependent variables (DVs) for group comparison include the T.O.V.A. and the ASRS self-report.

T.O.V.A. variables, based on response times (RT) and error rates, include RT variability (RTV) indicating consistency; mean RT; Omission errors (OM) indicating inattention; Commission errors (COM) indicating impulsivity; as well as the D-prime score. D-prime is described as a measure of "perceptual sensitivity" and has been suggested as an index of arousal (Losier et al., 1996). T.O.V.A. variables are standardized in the analysis.

To evaluate the effect of NFB on T.O.V.A., we created five new variables by subtracting the baseline scores from the outcome measurement scores: RTV-change, mean RT-change, OM-change, COM-change, and D-prime-change. These T.O.V.A. change scores are subsequently compared for the treatment group and the WLC, using independent samples *t*-test. The Levene's test showed that the variances for the two groups were similar. Consequently, the independent samples *t*-test was run with equal variances assumed.

MANOVA was subsequently used to evaluate the effect of NFB training, compared to the WLC, in the outcome measures on the five dependent variables of T.O.V.A.

ASRS consists of 18 items tapping the frequency of recent DSM-IV criterion symptoms of adult ADHD, including a scale for Inattention (IA, max 36 points) and a scale for Hyperactivity-Impulsivity (HI, max 36 points). We calculated differences of scores between baseline and outcome measurements to create IA-change and HI-change scores. These difference scores are subsequently compared for the NFB and the control group, using independent samples t-test.

The Levene's test showed that the variances in IA-change were statistically significantly different in the two groups ($F = 4.36$, $p < 0.05$). As a result, the independent samples t-test for IA-change was run with equal variances not assumed. The opposite was the case for the variable HI-change.

In all our random coefficient models the intercept and slope are separately estimated for each participant. That is, the coefficients are estimated for each participant for the linear regression equation as follows: Score = Intercept + B (Session).

All participants were treated with NFB at a single center. All technicians were equivalently trained and capable; therefore clustering of participants per technician was based simply on scheduling logistics.

3. RESULTS

Results primarily describe the specific details of the intervention implementation. Also, as stated, a preliminary between-subjects comparison was performed after phase one to assess intervention efficacy under a conventional analysis model. Thus, we report the two straightforward pre- to post-treatment outcome measures which are comparable between-groups: T.O.V.A. and ASRS. The ambiguous results of this conventional approach, especially in an unblinded context, supports the motivation to extend the analysis with LC modeling. We therefore include these results in the protocol report because they constitute an informative part of the trial design going into the second phase.

3.1. Participant Flow

Eighty-two adults were recruited through cooperating clinics Mental Capital Care, Neuromental and YTHS; also by newspaper advertisement and posting to online forums for the Helsinki-based ADHD society of Finland. Of this, 19 dropped out of the trial before completing the screening process, due to various issues.

Sixty-three participants were screened by a psychiatrist and a psychologist prior to the training, resulting in nine participants screened out of the trial due to one or more failures to meet the criteria. The remainder ($n = 54$) consisted of 29 females, 25 males, mean age 36 std.dev. 10 years, with 44 ADHD and 10 ADD diagnoses.

Participants were split equally between treatment ($n = 27$) and control groups ($n = 27$); however two switched from treatment group (final $n = 25$) to control group (final $n = 29$) for personal reasons. From these assignments, eight dropped out from the WLC group (including one participant whose pre-test measurement data was then deleted by request), and two from the treatment group. Thus, 23 treatment group, and 21 WLC group cases (total $n = 44$) were available for analysis. The trial progression is shown in detail in **Figure 1**.

Out of those who completed NFB, five participants did not complete treatment on the pre-defined schedule, of which three exceeded by more than a week. Delays were due to personal reasons, causing a number of cancelations of scheduled sessions, which is a regularly observed phenomenon in this diagnostic group.

3.1.1. Implementation of Intervention

In practice, NFB training consisted of ~40 sessions (range: 38–41) during 2–4 months. There was a mid-training pause of nominally 2 weeks. Patients came to the sessions 2–5 times a week. One session lasted ~1 h, subdivided into self-report of mood, excitement, hours slept and hours awake; electrode attachment; baseline measurement; 5–7 units of 5 min NFB trials; and debrief including self-report of effort and frustration. During each session, patients played different NFB "game" trials during which they got immediate visual reinforcement for classifier-matching states in their EEG. The scores per game trial are baseline-adjusted and averaged per session to form characteristic LCs. The content and purpose of the training sessions followed a phased timeline:

1. Tutorial stage, for becoming accustomed to NFB, two practice sessions: participants were given normal NFB trials with baseline thresholds adjusted by a constant factor to make the training easier;
2. Beginner stage, for NFB training, 18 sessions up to halfway break: normal NFB with non-adjusted baseline thresholds;
3. Intermediate stage, for learning to self-regulate, ten sessions from half-way to session 30: normal training blocks were gradually reduced in number to half per session, and inverse training blocks introduced in their place;
4. Expert stage, for transfer training, ten sessions until session 40: as Intermediate stage, but also with one to two "transfer" trials with no feedback stimuli.

3.1.2. Recruitment

As shown in **Figure 1**, participants were recruited in May/June 2012, with intake measurements during July/August 2012. Randomization took place in early September; treatment began September 17, 2012. Outtake measurements ran from April until August 2013.

Follow-up measurements are planned for start of 2016.

3.2. Baseline Data

The participants who began the trial ($n = 54$, 29 females) had mean age 36 years (std.dev. 10 years), with 44 ADHD and 10 ADD diagnoses. The characteristics per group are shown below in **Table 1**.

All intervention sessions were performed at the Mental Capital Care (MCC) clinic premises in Helsinki, which met all requirements described above. Technicians were recruited to administer the NFB from IBS and MCC; they were trained at UOH over a 3 month period; four of the team also attended the Biofeedback Certification International Alliance (BCIA)-accredited introductory course at the Brainclinics education and treatment center, Netherlands.

3.2.1. Numbers Analyzed

The analysis included 23 participants in the treatment group, and 21 participants in the WLC group. Given that dropouts were not analyzed, this analysis was not by intention-to-treat.

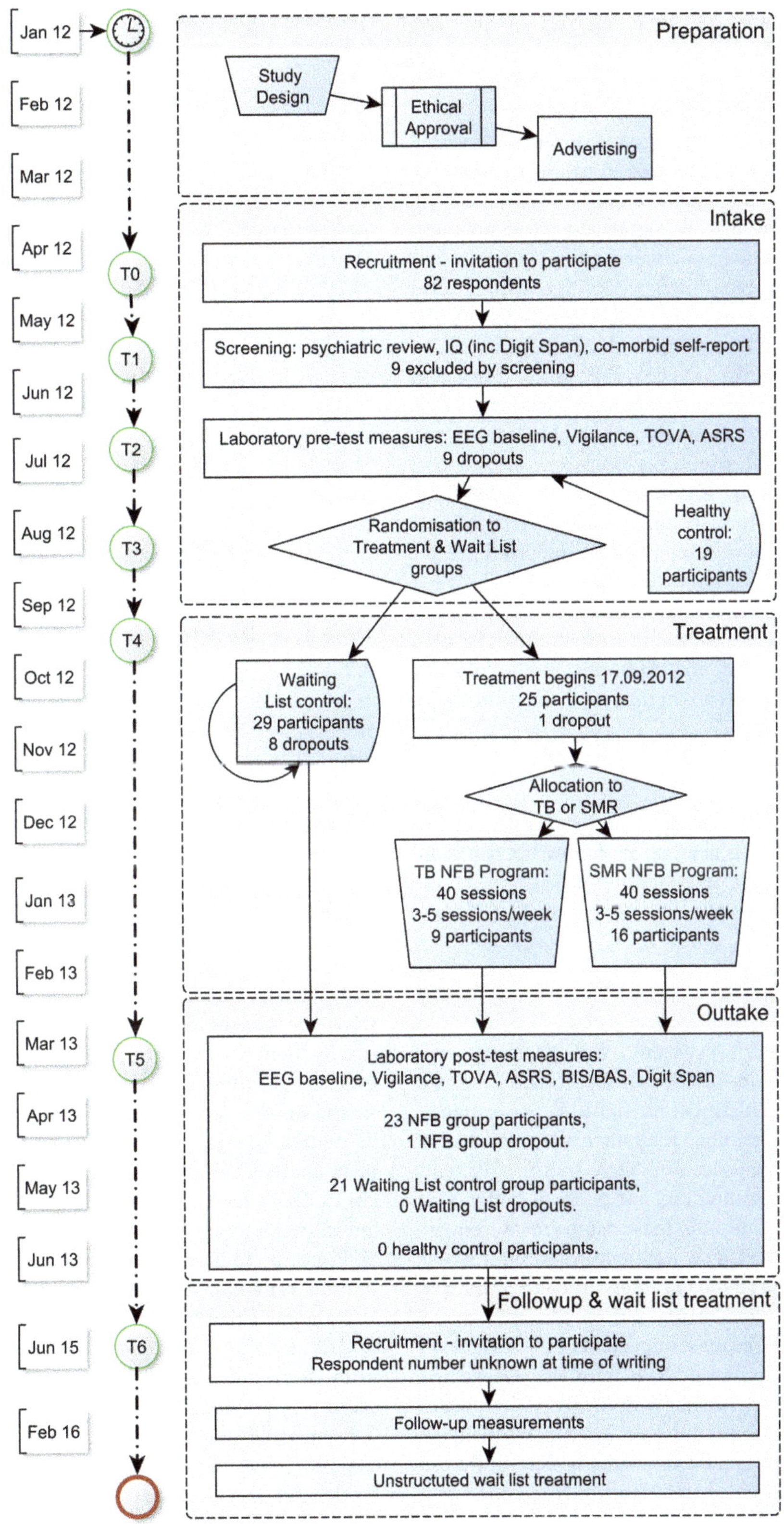

FIGURE 1 | Flow chart of assessments and treatments in the CENT trial.

3.3. Outcomes and Estimation

For H2a we find no support after analysis of the five T.O.V.A. indexes; **Table 2** shows their mean differences between baseline and post-training. Changes in these variables were not significantly different for the NFB group than for the WLC. Results of the MANOVA at the outcome measurement revealed that on the Wilks' Lambda the difference in means between the NFB and WLC did not reach significance [$F_{(5, 38)} = 0.45$, $p > 0.05$]. Thus, NFB training had no significant effect on the 5 indexes of T.O.V.A. at the end of the intervention.

Table 3 presents the mean difference of the two indexes between baseline and post-training and the results of the independent sample t-tests comparing IA-change and HI-change between NFB group and WLC. The NFB group presented a higher reduction of inattention symptoms than the WLC $t_{(36.03)} = -2.14$, $p < 0.05$. Similarly, while the NFB group presented a reduction of HI symptoms from baseline to post-training, the WLC presented an increase in HI symptoms $t_{(44)} = -2.42$, $p < 0.05$. Thus, we find statistically significant support for H3c. That is, the treatment group reported greater improvements in ADHD/ADD symptoms than the WLC.

A more detailed analysis concerning the rest of the hypotheses will follow in a separate paper. As treating the hypotheses H1a-b, H2b, and H3a-b requires substantial additional methodological reporting, addressing them does not fit the scope of a clinical trial report.

3.3.1. Adverse Effects

No adverse effects were observed in the treatment group. Further investigation of this question is planned for follow-up, using the state-oriented self-report items described above.

TABLE 2 | Groups statistics for RTV-change, mean RT-change, OM-change, COM-change and D-prime-change scores from baseline to outcome.

	N	Mean	Std.	*t*	*df*	*p*
RTV-change				0.343	42	0.739
NFB group	23	−5.56	40.13			
WLC	21	−9.44	34.15			
Mean RT-change				0.132	42	0.896
NFB group	23	−3.37	16.23			
WLC	21	−3.94	11.85			
OM-change				1.19	39	0.240
NFB group	23	10.10	72.73			
WLC	21	−46.25	198.84			
COM-change				0.517	42	0.608
NFB group	23	6.19	27.49			
WLC	21	1.81	28.67			
D-prime-change				−0.016	42	0.987
NFB group	23	1.50	45.30			
WLC	21	1.72	44.73			

TABLE 3 | Groups statistics for IA-change and HI-change scores.

	N	Mean	Std	*t*	*df*	*p*
IA-change				−2.14	36.03	0.039
NFB group	25	−1.2	2.17			
WLC	21	−0.14	1.06			
HI-change				−2.42	44	0.020
NFB group	25	−1.08	2.31			
WLC	21	0.38	1.65			

4. DISCUSSION

4.1. Interpretation

Regarding the relationship between NFB learning and performance in the continuous performance test, H2a proposed that the NFB group will achieve better T.O.V.A. performance, and improve more after training, than the WLC. Results of this study did not find evidence for such transfer. Patients participating in the NFB training did not perform better than WLC on the 5 indexes of T.O.V.A. in the outcome measurement. This result can be interpreted in at least two ways. On the one hand, it can be a sign of the all too common problem of transfer of training (Green and Bavelier, 2012).

Lack of transfer is one of the most important of the several key obstacles pertaining to the effect of NFB trainings (Gazzaniga, 2009, p. 94). Because brain plasticity is highly task specific, training in a specific task shows little or no improvement on related tasks. On the other hand, the results of this study can mean that NF learning bears no relationship to performance on any indexes of the T.O.V.A. test. This would contradict the findings of Losier et al. (1996) who considered the D-prime index of T.O.V.A. a consensus index of arousal, which is, in turn, assumed to be a manifestation of excessive slow wave brain waves in ADHD patients (Barry et al., 2003).

H3c suggested that the NFB group will report greater improvements in ADHD symptoms than the WLC. Results show the change of IA was significant. Patients did perceive a reduction of inattention symptoms over the course of the training. Furthermore, this perceived reduction of inattention symptoms differed significantly from the perceived reduction of inattention symptoms of the control group. This supports the meta-analysis by Arns et al. (2009) concluding that NFB has large effect sizes on inattention. In the index of HI, no negative linear trend was found. Interestingly however, patients in the NFB group did perceive a significantly larger reduction of these symptoms over the course of the training than the control group.

It might be that the training indeed resulted in some reduction of IA and HI symptoms. This interpretation gets support from theories claiming that ADHD is, in effect, pathology of executive functions that cannot be tapped by neurocognitive tests, but can instead be measured by self-reported questionnaires (Rabbitt, 1997; Brown, 2009, pp. 81–116). Alternatively, the results can also be interpreted as an example of the so called Hawthorne effect (Green and Bavelier, 2012). Establishing the presence of experience-dependent learning effects is not always straightforward. It is well documented, that individuals who take an active interest in their performance tend to improve more, or evaluate their improvement more positively. The Hawthorne effect can lead to powerful subjective improvements that have little to do with the specific cognitive training regimen being studied reflecting motivational factors instead.

If the training caused the decreased symptoms, a higher rate of learning should have a relationship to the rate of ADHD symptom decrease under the training. Therefore further analyses of this trial will examine the relationship between NFB LCs and the trend of self-reported ADHD symptoms.

Also, the different learning performance levels across the group should reflect different long term effects, to be measured during the second phase in a within-subjects analysis. This contrasts with the effect from the interaction-derived placebo which is relatively constant for all participants (per group), and presumably "fades away" quickly after the phase one intervention. Thus, second phase measurements will be analyzed with respect to NFB LCs.

Though this is a relatively small study, we believe the analysis of learning curve questions is a novel and useful contribution. As noted by Arns (personal communication, 2012):

> "In any Neurofeedback study it is very important to track and have an indication of 'learning.' If neurofeedback fails to demonstrate a clinical effect and there is no indication that learning actually took place, one can't draw any conclusions about neurofeedback. In an analogy, if one employs operant conditioning to [teach] a rat to press a lever, and the rat does not learn to press the lever, then it is incorrect to conclude that 'operant conditioning' does not work. This means that maybe the operant conditioning procedure was not implemented effectively. The same applies to neurofeedback, and this is further illustrated by the study from Roger DeBeuss. His study employed sub-optimal parameters e.g., auto-thresholding, 'game' feedback and an 'unconventional' training regime (engagement index) making it likely harder to learn. On the group level they found no effects of neurofeedback in ADHD, however, when separating learners from non-learners based on session data they did find an effect."

Questions of efficacy on the other hand are still a matter of controversy in the literature. WLC controls are not accepted as sufficient evidence by some. Double blind control through sham NFB was not chosen for this study because of the discussed lack of general understanding of ADHD. This lack, combined with the extremely contingent nature of NFB which depends heavily on non-specific aspects of treatment, implies that even if a double blind RCT showed large effect for NFB the causal mechanisms would still not be clear. A true resolution to this issue is probably only possible by running the kind of large sham NFB RCT called for by others; we choose instead to side-step this debate and focus on questions of internal comparisons within the method.

There is no blinding in this open-label WLC study, except at random assignment to groups. Other control paradigms may be preferred in pharmacological interventions; however there are a number of arguments in support of WLC, in the context of NFB. The WLC is a minimum viable control for non-specific effects of history, maturation, repeated testing, instrument drift, statistical regression, selection bias, and population inhomogeneity effects (Mohr et al., 2009). There is no control for non-specific or placebo effects; however this is still a valid experimental control design. Among other things, WLC controls for expectation and attention (Hawthorne) effects, whereby the notion that at some future point treatment will be provided (and life will improve) is by itself able to produce improvement. Additionally, longitudinal (rather than parallel) designs control for maturation, regression to the mean, instrument drift and practice effects; also time threats to validity (the same effect occurring 2 years in a row in different samples rules out external non-seasonal temporal causes for the effect. Seasonal causes with a WLC group should be ruled out by staggered application i.e., 2nd treatment starting in spring).

Technicians can be considered equally skilled and expert. All began as neurofeedback novices before the trial. Qualification history was varied. Due to availability, only some began their training with attendance at the Biofeedback Certification International Alliance (BCIA)-accredited introductory course at the Brainclinics education and treatment center, Netherlands. However, all five then shared 3 months training at UoH premises, including extensive peer review work, which helped to disseminate and pool the knowledge across the group.

4.2. Generalizability

External validity asks the question of "generalizability": to what populations, settings, treatment variables and measurement variables can this effect be generalized? While the question of external validity is never completely answerable, it is of particular interest for intervention research (Campbell et al., 1966, pp. 171–246). Campbell et al. (1966) note that there is a recurrent reluctance among researchers to accept Hume's truism that induction or generalization is never fully justified logically. While the problems of internal validity are solvable within the limits of the logic of probability statistics, the problems of external validity are not logically solvable in any neat, conclusive way (Campbell et al., 1966, p. 17). Generalization always involves extrapolation into a realm not represented in one's sample. Here, the issue of sample bias is of importance. If an experimental study is conducted with voluntary patients from a given district, they might have characteristics that cause the experimental treatment to be more effective than it would be in other populations. However, for ethical reasons, intervention studies are impossible to conduct without the informed consent of the research subjects. It is obvious, that a "true" experimental design is in practice impossible with a fully representative sample of a given country, let alone all ADHD patients in the world. It must be emphasized that the results of an experiment "probe" but do not "prove" a theory. An adequate hypothesis is one that has repeatedly survived such probing, but it may always be displaced by a new probe. Many findings in experimental psychology gain generalizability not through the nature of the setting in which they occurred, but through their ability to establish a theory of basic mental processes that are implicated in many tasks.

4.3. Overall Evidence

After preliminary analysis, the trial did not find evidence for a transfer of learning that was the intended benefit of the intervention. Since the intervention's goal is symptomatic improvement outside the laboratory, the results underline how the transfer-problem limits the potential benefits. Patients did perceive a reduction of Inattention symptoms over the course of training, yet this change was not reflected in better performance in the continuous performance test (T.O.V.A.).

We propose that in the absence of any other evidence, one should consider these self-report results as due to placebo by default. The improvement in self-reported symptoms might not be specifically due to NFB, but due to employment of goal-oriented attention in general. At present, we can not rule out the possibility that the individuals would also report improvement if all other factors were held equal but NFB was swapped for some other exercise that requires concentration. That is, our preliminary results did not support the effectiveness of NFB in alleviating the symptoms of AHDH/ADD.

Nevertheless, keeping in mind the core aim of studying mechanisms and models of NFB, the CENT trial is on track to provide the necessary evidence. As Seidman (2006) suggest, an adequate neuropsychological model of ADHD should utilize measures from multiple domains to be able to encompass subtypes and multiple deficits. Combining neuropsychological, neurophysiological and behavioral measures, we aim toward an evaluation of structure-function relationships in NFB treatment for adult ADHD.

AUTHOR CONTRIBUTIONS

BC designed and implemented the study and wrote the draft text; EH conducted the statistical analyses and contributed to the draft; KJ and LK contributed to the study design and implementation, and the draft; CK contributed to the study design and the draft.

ACKNOWLEDGMENTS

The authors wish to thank Svetlana Kirjanen, Mona Moisala, Marko Repo, Hanna Björkstrand, Tanja Hyttinen, Jari Torniainen, Teemu Itkonen, Markus Kivikangas for their part in running the trial; also Laura Hokkanen and Jari Lipsanen for assistance with the work of EH. Partly funded by Finnish science agency TEKES, project #440078.

REFERENCES

Arns, M., Feddema, I., and Kenemans, J. L. (2014a). Differential effects of theta/beta and SMR neurofeedback in ADHD on sleep onset latency. *Front. Hum. Neurosci.* 8:1019. doi: 10.3389/fnhum.2014.01019

Arns, M., Gunkelman, J., Breteler, M., and Spronk, D. (2008). EEG phenotypes predict treatment outcome to stimulants in children with ADHD. *J. Integr. Neurosci.* 7, 421–438. doi: 10.1142/S0219635208001897

Arns, M., Heinrich, H., and Strehl, U. (2014b). Evaluation of neurofeedback in ADHD: the long and winding road. *Biol. Psychol.* 95, 108–115. doi: 10.1016/j.biopsycho.2013.11.013

Arns, M., Ridder, S. D., Strehl, U., Breteler, M., and Coenen, A. (2009). Efficacy of neurofeedback treatment in ADHD: the effects on inattention, impulsivity and hyperactivity: a meta-analyis. *Clin. Eeg. Neurosci.* 40, 180–189. doi: 10.1177/155005940904000311

Barry, R. J., Clarke, A. R., and Johnstone, S. J. (2003). A review of electrophysiology in attention-deficit/hyperactivity disorder: I. Qualitative and quantitative electroencephalography. *Clin. Neurophysiol.* 114, 171–183. doi: 10.1016/S1388-2457(02)00362-0

Beck, A., Steer, R., and Brown, G. (1996). *BDI-II, Beck Depression Inventory: Manual, 2 Edn.* Boston, MA: Harcourt Brace.

Borkovec, T. D., and Sibrava, N. J. (2005). Problems with the use of placebo conditions in psychotherapy research, suggested alternatives, and some strategies for the pursuit of the placebo phenomenon. *J. Clin. Psychol.* 61, 805–818. doi: 10.1002/jclp.20127

Bresnahan, S. M., Anderson, J. W., and Barry, R. J. (1999). Age-related changes in quantitative EEG in attention- deficit/hyperactivity disorder. *Biol. Psychiatry* 46, 1690–1697.

Bresnahan, S. M., and Barry, R. J. (2002). Specificity of quantitative EEG analysis in adults with attention deficit hyperactivity disorder. *Psychiatry Res.* 112, 133–144. doi: 10.1016/S0165-1781(02)00190-7

Brown, T. E. (1996). *Brown Attention-Deficit Disorder Scales, Manual.* San Antonio: Harcourt Brace.

Brown, T. E. (2009). *ADHD Comorbidities : Handbook for ADHD Complications in Children and Adults.* Washington, DC: American Psychiatric Pub.

Calderon, K. S., and Thompson, W. W. (2004). Biofeedback relaxation training: a rediscovered mind-body tool in public health. *Am. J. Health Studies* 19, 185–194.

Campbell, D. T., Stanley, J. C., and Gage, N. L. (1966). *Experimental and Quasi-Experimental Designs for Research.* Chicago, Il: R. McNally.

Chase, M., and Harper, R. (1971). Somatomotor and visceromotor correlates of operantly conditioned 1214 c/sec sensorimotor cortical activity. *Electroencephalogr. Clin. Neurophysiol.* 31, 85–92.

Clarke, A. R., Barry, R. J., McCarthy, R., and Selikowitz, M. (2001). Excess beta activity in children with attention-deficit/hyperactivity disorder: an atypical electrophysiological group. *Psychiatry Res.* 103, 205–218. doi: 10.1016/S0165-1781(01)00277-3

Cowley, B., Torniainen, J., Itkonen, T., and Rabenel, R. (forthcoming). Computer enabled neuroplasticity treatment: a modular, extensible platform for neurofeedback with lightweight wearable EEG devices. *PeerJ Comput. Sci.*

Egner, T., and Gruzelier, J. (2004). EEG biofeedback of low beta band components: frequency-specific effects on variables of attention and event-related brain potentials. *Clin. Neurophysiol.* 115, 131–139. doi: 10.1016/S1388-2457(03)00353-5

Epstein, J. N., Erkanli, A., Conners, C. K., Klaric, J., Costello, J. E., and Angold, A. (2003). Relations between Continuous Performance Test performance measures and ADHD behaviors. *J. Abnormal Child Psychol.* 31, 543–554. doi: 10.1023/A:1025405216339

Gazzaniga, M. S. (2009). *The Cognitive Neurosciences, 4 Edn.* Cambridge, MA: MIT Press .

Gevensleben, H., Moll, G. H., Rothenberger, A., and Heinrich, H. (2014). Neurofeedback in attention-deficit/hyperactivity disorder - different models, different ways of application. *Front. Hum. Neurosci.* 8:846. doi: 10.3389/fnhum.2014.00846

Green, C. S., and Bavelier, D. (2012). Learning, attentional control and action video games. *Curr. Biol.* 22, R197–R206. doi: 10.1016/j.cub.2012.02.012

Hammond, D. C. (2010). The need for individualization in neurofeedback: heterogeneity in QEEG patterns associated with diagnoses and symptoms. *Appl. Psychophysiol. Biofeedback* 35, 31–36. doi: 10.1007/s10484-009-9106-1

Heinimaa, M., Salokangas, R. K. R., Ristkari, T., Plathin, M., Huttunen, J., Ilonen, T., et al. (2003). PROD-screen–a screen for prodromal symptoms of psychosis. *Intern. J. Methods Psychiatric Res.* 12, 92–104. doi: 10.1002/mpr.146

Hirschfeld, R. M., Williams, J. B., Spitzer, R. L., Calabrese, J. R., Flynn, L., Keck, P. E. Jr., et al. (2000). Development and validation of a screening instrument for bipolar spectrum disorder: the Mood Disorder Questionnaire. *Am. J. Psychiatry* 157, 1873–1875. doi: 10.1176/appi.ajp.157.11.1873

Howe, R. C., and Sterman, M. B. (1972). Cortical-subcortical EEG correlates of suppressed motor behavior during sleep and waking in the cat. *Electroencephalogr. Clin. Neurophysiol.* 32, 681–695.

Huang-Pollock, C. L., and Nigg, J. T. (2003). Searching for the attention deficit in attention deficit hyperactivity disorder: the case of visuospatial orienting. *Clin. Psychol. Rev.* 23, 801–830. doi: 10.1016/S0272-7358(03)00073-4

Johnstone, J., Gunkelman, J., and Lunt, J. (2005). Clinical database development: characterization of EEG phenotypes. *Clin. EEG Neurosci.* 36, 99–107. doi: 10.1177/155005940503600209

Kessler, R. C., Adler, L., Ames, M., Demler, O., Faraone, S., Hiripi, E., et al. (2005). The World Health Organization Adult ADHD Self-Report Scale (ASRS): a short screening scale for use in the general population. *Psychol. Med.* 35, 245–256. doi: 10.1017/S0033291704002892

Lansbergen, M. M., Arns, M., van Dongen-Boomsma, M., Spronk, D., and Buitelaar, J. K. (2011). The increase in theta/beta ratio on resting-state EEG in boys with attention-deficit/hyperactivity disorder is mediated by slow alpha peak frequency. *Progr. Neuro Psychopharmacol. Biol. Psychiatry* 35, 47–52. doi: 10.1016/j.pnpbp.2010.08.004

Lazzaro, I., Gordon, E., Li, W., Lim, C. L., Plahn, M., Whitmont, S., et al. (1999). Simultaneous EEG and EDA measures in adolescent attention deficit hyperactivity disorder. *Intern. J. Psychophysiol.* 34, 123–134.

Liebowitz, M. R. (1992). Dissociative experiences scale. *Am. J. Psychiatry* 149, 719.

Losier, B. J., McGrath, P. J., and Klein, R. M. (1996). Error patterns on the continuous performance test in non-medicated and medicated samples of children with and without ADHD: a meta-analytic review. *J. Child Psychol. Psychiatry All. Discipl.* 37, 971–987.

Lou, H. C., Henriksen, L., Bruhn, P., Bø rner, H., and Nielsen, J. B. (1989). Striatal dysfunction in attention deficit and hyperkinetic disorder. *Archiv. Neurol.* 46, 48–52.

Lubar, J. F., and Shouse, M. N. (1976). EEG and behavioral changes in a hyperkinetic child concurrent with training of the sensorimotor rhythm (SMR): a preliminary report. *Biofeedback Self Regul.* 1, 293–306.

Mann, C. A., Lubar, J. F., Zimmerman, A. W., Miller, C. A., and Muenchen, R. A. (1992). Quantitative analysis of EEG in boys with attention-deficit-hyperactivity disorder: controlled study with clinical implications. *Pediatric Neurol.* 8 30–36.

Mayer, K., Wyckoff, S. N., Schulz, U., and Strehl, U. (2012). Neurofeedback for adult attention-deficit/hyperactivity disorder: investigation Of slow cortical potential neurofeedback preliminary results. *J. Neurother.* 16, 37–45. doi: 10.1080/10874208.2012.650113

Mayer, K., Wyckoff, S. N., and Strehl, U. (2013). One size fits all? Slow cortical potentials neurofeedback: a review. *J. Attent. Disorders* 17, 393–409. doi: 10.1177/1087054712468053

Mayer, K., Wyckoff, S. N., and Strehl, U. (2015). Underarousal in Adult ADHD: how are peripheral and cortical arousal related? *Clin. EEG Neurosci.* doi: 10.1177/1550059415577544. [Epub ahead of print].

Micoulaud-Franchi, J.-A., Geoffroy, P. A., Fond, G., Lopez, R., Bioulac, S., and Philip, P. (2014). EEG neurofeedback treatments in children with ADHD: an updated meta-analysis of randomized controlled trials. *Front. Hum. Neurosci.* 8:906. doi: 10.3389/fnhum.2014.00906

Mohr, D. C., Spring, B., Freedland, K. E., Beckner, V., Arean, P., Hollon, S. D., et al. (2009). The selection and design of control conditions for randomized controlled trials of psychological interventions. *Psychother. Psychosomat.* 78, 275–284. doi: 10.1159/000228248

Monastra, V. J., Lynn, S., Linden, M., Lubar, J. F., Gruzelier, J., and LaVaque, T. J. (2005). Electroencephalographic biofeedback in the treatment of attention-deficit/hyperactivity disorder. *Appl. Psychophysiol. Biofeedback* 30, 95–114. doi: 10.1007/s10484-005-4305-x

Nigg, J. T. (2005). Neuropsychologic theory and findings in attention-deficit/hyperactivity disorder: the state of the field and salient challenges for the coming decade. *Biol. Psychiatry* 57, 1424–1435. doi: 10.1016/j.biopsych.2004.11.011

Olbrich, S., Sander, C., Minkwitz, J., Chittka, T., Mergl, R., Hegerl, U., et al. (2012). EEG vigilance regulation patterns and their discriminative power to separate patients with major depression from healthy controls. *Neuropsychobiology* 65, 188–194. doi: 10.1159/000337000

Pennington, B. F. (2005). Toward a new neuropsychological model of attention-deficit/hyperactivity disorder: subtypes and multiple deficits. *Biol. Psychiatry* 57, 1221–1223. doi: 10.1016/j.biopsych.2005.03.010

Posner, M. I., and Petersen, S. E. (1990). The attention system of the human brain. *Ann. Rev. Neurosci.* 13, 25–42.

Rabbitt, P. (1997). *Methodology of Frontal and Executive Function.* Hove, UK: Psychology Press.

Roberts, C., and Torgerson, D. (1998). Understanding controlled trials: randomisation methods in controlled trials. *BMJ* 317, 1301–1310.

Rossiter, T. (2004a). The effectiveness of neurofeedback and stimulant drugs in treating AD/HD: Part I. Review of methodological issues. *Appl. Psychophysiol. Biofeedback* 29, 95–112. doi: 10.1023/B:APBI.0000026636.13180.b6

Rossiter, T. (2004b). The effectiveness of neurofeedback and stimulant drugs in treating AD/HD: Part II. Replication. *Appl. Psychophysiol. Biofeedback* 29, 233–243. doi: 10.1007/s10484-004-0383-4

Satterfield, J. H., Cantwell, D. P., and Satterfield, B. T. (1974). Pathophysiology of the hyperactive child syndrome. *Arch. Gen. Psychiatry* 31, 839–844.

Saunders, J. B., Aasland, O. G., Babor, T. F., de la Fuente, J. R., and Grant, M. (1993). Development of the alcohol use disorders identification test (AUDIT): WHO collaborative project on early detection of persons with harmful alcohol consumption–II. *Addiction (Abingdon, England)* 88, 791–804.

Scott, N. W., McPherson, G. C., Ramsay, C. R., and Campbell, M. K. (2002). The method of minimization for allocation to clinical trials. *Controll. Clin. Trials* 23, 662–674. doi: 10.1016/S0197-2456(02)00242-8

Seidman, L. J. (2006). Neuropsychological functioning in people with ADHD across the lifespan. *Clin. Psychol. Rev.* 26, 466–485. doi: 10.1016/j.cpr.2006.01.004

Sergeant, J., Oosterlaan, J., and van der Meere, J. (1999). "Information processing and energetic factors in attention-deficit/hyperactivity disorder," in *Handbook of Disruptive Behavior Disorders SE - 4*, eds H. Quay and A. Hogan (New York, NY: Kluwer Academic/Plenum Publishers), 75–104.

Sergeant, J. A., Geurts, H., Huijbregts, S., Scheres, A., and Oosterlaan, J. (2003). The top and the bottom of ADHD: a neuropsychological perspective. *Neurosci. Biobehav. Rev.* 27, 583–592. doi: 10.1016/j.neubiorev.2003.08.004

Snyder, S. M., and Hall, J. R. (2006). A meta-analysis of quantitative EEG power associated with attention-deficit hyperactivity disorder. *J. Clin. Neurophysiol.* 23, 440–455. doi: 10.1097/01.wnp.0000221363.12503.78

Sonuga-Barke, E. J. S. (2005). Causal models of attention-deficit/hyperactivity disorder: from common simple deficits to multiple developmental pathways. *Biol. Psychiatry* 57, 1231–1238. doi: 10.1016/j.biopsych.2004.09.008

Spitzer, R. L., Kroenke, K., Williams, J. B. W., and Löwe, B. (2006). A brief measure for assessing generalized anxiety disorder: the GAD-7. *Archiv. Int. Med.* 166, 1092–1097. doi: 10.1001/archinte.166.10.1092

Vernon, D., Egner, T., Cooper, N., Compton, T., Neilands, C., Sheri, A., et al. (2003). The effect of training distinct neurofeedback protocols on aspects of cognitive performance. *Inter. J. Psychophysiol.* 47, 75–85. doi: 10.1016/S0167-8760(02)00091-0

Wechsler, D. (2008). *Wechsler Adult Intelligence Scale: Technical and Interpretive Manual, 4th Edn.* San Antonio, TX: Pearson.

Zametkin, A. J., Nordahl, T. E., Gross, M., King, A. C., Semple, W. E., Rumsey, J., et al. (1990). Cerebral glucose metabolism in adults with hyperactivity of childhood onset. *New England J. Med.* 323, 1361–1366.

Zuberer, A., Brandeis, D., and Drechsler, R. (2015). Are treatment effects of neurofeedback training in children with ADHD related to the successful regulation of brain activity? A review on the learning of regulation of brain activity and a contribution to the discussion on specificity. *Front. Hum. Neurosci.* 9:135. doi: 10.3389/fnhum.2015.00135

Zylowska, L., Ackerman, D. L., Yang, M. H., Futrell, J. L., Horton, N. L., Hale, T. S., et al. (2008). Mindfulness meditation training in adults and adolescents with ADHD: a feasibility study. *J. Att. Disorders* 11, 737–746. doi: 10.1177/1087054707308502

16

The Posterior Parietal Cortex Subserves Precise Motor Timing in Professional Drummers

Bettina Pollok[1], *Katharina Stephan*[2], *Ariane Keitel*[1], *Vanessa Krause*[1]* *and Nora K. Schaal*[2]

[1]*Medical Faculty, Institute of Clinical Neuroscience and Medical Psychology, Heinrich-Heine University Duesseldorf, Duesseldorf, Germany,* [2]*Department of Experimental Psychology, Heinrich-Heine University Duesseldorf, Duesseldorf, Germany*

Edited by:
Louis Bherer, Université de Montréal, Canada

Reviewed by:
Takako Fujioka, Stanford University, USA
Filippo Brighina, University of Palermo, Italy
Simone Dalla Bella, University of Montpellier 1, France

***Correspondence:**
Vanessa Krause
vanessa.krause@uni-duesseldorf.de

The synchronization task is a well-established paradigm for the investigation of motor timing with respect to an external pacing signal. It requires subjects to synchronize their finger taps in synchrony with a regular metronome. A specific significance of the posterior parietal cortex (PPC) for superior synchronization in professional drummers has been suggested. In non-musicians, modulation of the excitability of the left PPC by means of transcranial direct current stimulation (tDCS) modulates synchronization performance of the right hand. In order to determine the significance of the left PPC for superior synchronization in drummers, we here investigate the effects of cathodal and anodal tDCS in 20 professional drummers on auditory-motor synchronization of the right hand. A continuation and a reaction time task served as control conditions. Moreover, the interaction between baseline performance and tDCS polarity was estimated in precise as compared to less precise synchronizers according to median split. Previously published data from 16 non-musicians were re-analyzed accordingly in order to highlight possible differences of tDCS effects in drummers and non-musicians. TDCS was applied for 10 min with an intensity of 0.25 mA over the left PPC. Behavioral measures were determined prior to and immediately after tDCS. In drummers the overall analysis of synchronization performance revealed significantly larger tap-to-tone asynchronies following anodal tDCS with the tap preceding the tone replicating findings in non-musicians. No significant effects were found on control tasks. The analysis for participants with large as compared to small baseline asynchronies revealed that only in drummers with small asynchronies tDCS interfered with synchronization performance. The re-analysis of the data from non-musicians indicated the reversed pattern. The data support the hypothesis that the PPC is involved in auditory-motor synchronization and extend previous findings by showing that its functional significance varies with musical expertise.

Keywords: anticipation, brain plasticity, musicians, synchronization, transcranial direct current stimulation (tDCS)

INTRODUCTION

Timing abilities are essential for precise movement execution, in particular when movements have to be executed with respect to external events. The ability to predict such events increases movement accuracy and reduces attentional demands. A well-established paradigm to investigate motor timing with respect to an external signal is the so-called synchronization task, which requires subjects to synchronize their own finger taps with respect to a regular metronome (reviewed in Repp and Su, 2013). Despite the simplicity of this task, non-musicians typically show the so-called negative asynchrony, which is characterized by the tap preceding the tone by several tens of milliseconds (for a review, see Repp and Su, 2013). Motor timing relies on a cerebello-thalamo-cortical network (Pollok et al., 2005; Pecenka et al., 2013; for reviews, see Coull and Nobre, 2008; Chen et al., 2009). Core timing functions have been related to the basal ganglia (Malapani et al., 1998) and the cerebellum, which has been particularly linked to the stabilization of movements with respect to external events (Ivry et al., 2002; Spencer et al., 2005; for a review, see Molinari et al., 2003) as well as to the anticipation of sensory events (Tesche and Karhu, 2000). On a cortical level precise motor timing engages parietal as well as primary motor and premotor areas (Karabanov et al., 2009; Pecenka et al., 2013; for a review see Coull and Nobre, 2008). A specific relevance of the dorsal premotor cortex (dPMC) for precise movement timing with respect to auditory stimuli has been found suggesting that the dPMC integrates auditory information with motor actions (Chen et al., 2006, 2008, 2009; for a review, see Zatorre et al., 2007).

Drummers (Krause et al., 2010a,b) and percussionists (Manning and Schutz, 2016) show superior synchronization performance as compared to non-musicians and even as compared to professional pianists (Krause et al., 2010a,b). This behavioral advantage has been related to a stronger functional interaction between the thalamus and the posterior parietal cortex (PPC), suggesting a specific significance of the PPC for synchronization accuracy (Krause et al., 2010b). The term synchronization accuracy refers to the mean temporal distance between the onsets of the auditory pacing signal and the finger-tap as well as its variability. Noteworthy, although the data by Krause et al. (2010b) reveal evidence for a stronger involvement of the dPMC in professional musicians as compared to non-musicians, the dPMC cannot account for superior synchronization in drummers, since no significant differences between drummers and pianists were found. The PPC has been related to sensorimotor integration possibly acting as sensorimotor interface (Andersen, 1997; Andersen and Buneo, 2003) as well as to anticipatory motor control, which suggests that movements can be planned and executed not only with respect to actual but also to anticipated sensory events (Beudel et al., 2009; reviewed in Blakemore and Sirigu, 2003). Due to the regularity of the pacing signal, the synchronization task allows the investigation of anticipatory motor control. In line with this hypothesis, faster reaction times with respect to temporally predictable visual cues have been particularly related to increased activation of the inferior PPC (Coull et al., 2016).

Although neuroimaging studies reveal important insights into brain areas involved in a certain task, the results do not necessarily allow a conclusion regarding their functional significance for task execution. In order to estimate the functional relevance of different brain areas within a network, non-invasive brain stimulation methods like transcranial direct current or magnetic stimulation (tDCS/TMS) can be applied. These methods allow the modulation of cortical excitability. Evidence exists that tDCS changes the resting membrane potential in a polarity specific manner. While anodal tDCS increases the likelihood of neural firing by depolarization of neurons, cathodal tDCS yields hyperpolarization of cell bodies (Lang et al., 2005; reviewed in Stagg and Nitsche, 2011; Shin et al., 2015). Stimulation after-effects are assumed to rely on changes of inhibitory and excitatory synapses (reviewed in Stagg and Nitsche, 2011).

Previous studies showed that modulation of the PPC excitability by 1 Hz repetitive TMS (rTMS; Krause et al., 2012) or tDCS (Krause et al., 2014) changes synchronization accuracy in non-musicians as indicated by larger tap-to-tone asynchronies following anodal tDCS (Krause et al., 2014) and smaller asynchronies following inhibitory 1 Hz rTMS (Krause et al., 2012). Since in non-musicians no significant effects were found in the continuation and reaction tasks, we hypothesized that the PPC is particularly involved in anticipatory motor control. The present study aims at investigating whether this area is causally involved in superior synchronization in professional drummers. To this end, anodal and cathodal tDCS was applied to the left PPC and effects on synchronization as well as continuation accuracy and reaction times of the right hand were determined. Assuming a specific significance of the PPC for anticipatory motor control, we expected effects of tDCS: (*i*) on synchronization accuracy only; and (*ii*) being evident particularly in precise drummers.

MATERIALS AND METHODS

Participants

Twenty professional drummers (19 male) aged between 19 years and 63 years (34.3 $\pm$ 2.6 years; mean $\pm$ standard error of the mean; SEM) were included in the present study. Sample size was determined with respect to our previous study (Krause et al., 2014) revealing relatively large effect sizes. The mean lateralization ratio according to the Edinburgh Handedness Inventory (Oldfield, 1971) was 96.3 $\pm$ 0.7 indicating that all participants were right-handed. They were either students of a music college or worked as professional musicians in an orchestra or as music teachers. Nineteen participants were formally educated on the instrument for 13.7 $\pm$ 1.2 years on average (range 5–24 years). One participant learned the instrument by self-education without any formal training. Mean age at the beginning of formal training was 9.9 $\pm$ 1.3 years (range 3–21 years). Mean duration of regular practice was 17.2 $\pm$ 2.6 years.

In addition, data from 16 healthy non-musicians (6 male) with a mean age of 23.7 $\pm$ 1.0 years were re-analyzed (Krause et al., 2014) in order to determine a possible interaction between baseline performance and musical expertise on tDCS effects. Right-handedness was indicated by a mean lateralization ratio of 85.0 $\pm$ 4.3. This group was labeled non-musicians since they never had regularly practiced an instrument.

Subjects with personal or family history of epileptic seizures or other neurological or psychiatric disorders, cardiac pacemaker or intracranial metal implants or intake of central nervous system-effective medication were not included in the study.

Ethics

The study was carried out in accordance with the standards set by the latest revision of the Declaration of Helsinki. Experimental procedures were approved by the local ethics committee (Heinrich-Heine University Duesseldorf; study number 3347). Participants gave their written informed consent prior to participation.

Experimental Paradigm

Participants were naïve with respect to the exact hypotheses of the study. None of them had received electrical brain stimulation before. Participants and the main investigator were blinded with respect to the type of tDCS until the end of the experiment. To this end, a second investigator ran the DC stimulator which was covered by a paperboard in order to hide the exact stimulation type. The order of tDCS conditions was counterbalanced across subjects. Timing abilities were measured by means of the: (*i*) synchronization paradigm which was always followed by; a (*ii*) continuation task; and a (*iii*) simple reaction time task. The order of tasks (synchronization-continuation vs. reaction time tasks) was counterbalanced across participants and tDCS sessions. During synchronization the subjects were instructed to tap with their right index finger in synchrony with an auditory pacing signal presented with a regular stimulus onset asynchrony (SOA) of 900 ms. Length of the pacing signal was 100 ms. After 30 taps the pacing signal stopped and subjects continued with the same rhythm for another 30 taps (continuation task). Reaction times were measured with respect to the same auditory signal being presented at varying SOAs of 1.000, 1.500 and 2.000 ms. In total 60 reactions were recorded for each individual. Behavioral data prior to and immediately after tDCS were measured by a photoelectric barrier mounted on a pad. For stimulus presentation and recording of behavioral data E-Prime® 2.0 software was applied (Psychology Software Tools, Sharpsburg, MD, USA). Prior to data acquisition a short practice run was implemented in order to familiarize the subjects with the tasks. No specific training was conducted. During each experimental session, subjects were comfortably seated in a reclining chair. They were instructed to relax and to keep their eyes open during the entire experiment.

Transcranial Direct Current Stimulation

tDCS was applied using a battery driven DC stimulator (NeuroConn GmbH, Ilmenau, Germany) with a pair of rubber electrodes (3×3 cm^2) nestling between saline-soaked sponges. According to our previous study (Krause et al., 2014) the stimulation electrode was fixed above the left PPC and the reference electrode was placed over the contralateral orbit (Nitsche and Paulus, 2000; Moliadze et al., 2010). Self-adhesive bandages (Coban^{TM}, 3M Deutschland GmbH, Neuss, Germany) were used for the fixation of the electrodes. Anodal as well as cathodal tDCS was applied during rest for 10 min, respectively, with an intensity of 0.25 mA, resulting in a current density of 27.77 μA/cm^2 below electrodes. In line with our previous study (Krause et al., 2014) the relatively weak stimulation intensity was chosen in order to adjust the current density for the electrode size. A previous study has shown that smaller stimulation electrodes in combination with lower intensities result in higher tDCS focality (Nitsche et al., 2007). We tried to reduce the probability of primary motor cortex (M1) co-stimulation by the application of 3×3 cm^2 stimulation electrodes along with lower stimulation intensities. The current was ramped up and down over additional 10 s at the beginning and the end of stimulation, respectively. Impedance was kept below 10 kΩ. Mean impedance was 8.2 ± 0.4 kΩ. An interval of at least 1 week was interspersed between anodal and cathodal tDCS sessions in order to avoid carryover effects. Stimulation was in accordance with established safety protocols (Nitsche et al., 2003; Iyer et al., 2005). In order to monitor the quality of blinding, subjects were asked to estimate the respective stimulation condition by a questionnaire. To this end, at the end of each session they were asked to decide whether they had received either anodal or cathodal tDCS.

The PPC was localized by means of a neuronavigation system (LOCALITE, Sankt Augustin, Germany) using a standard brain. The stimulation target was set to the Talairach coordinates (*x*, *y*, *z*) −25, −46, 62 corresponding to Brodmann area (BA) 7 (**Figure 1**).

In order to ensure that the stimulated area does not overlap with the M1, M1 was localized by means of single pulse TMS using a standard figure of eight coil with an outer winding diameter of 80 mm (MC-B 70) being connected to a MagPro stimulator (Mag Venture, Hückelhoven, Germany). The coil was placed tangentially to the scalp with the handle pointing backwards and laterally at about 45° away from the midline inducing an initial posterior-anterior current flow in the brain. The magnetic stimulus had a biphasic waveform with a pulse width of about 300 μs. In a first step, the optimal cortical representation of the first dorsal interosseous (FDI) muscle was determined by eliciting motor evoked potentials (MEPs; for an overview see Kobayashi and Pascual-Leone, 2003). Then, the point which evoked the largest motor response of the FDI muscle was determined as motor hot spot by moving the coil in 0.5 cm steps anterior, posterior, medial and lateral to this area. The mean distance between the left M1 hot spot and the stimulated area corresponding to the left PPC was 4.6 ± 0.2 cm.

Data Analysis

Synchronization performance and reaction times were determined as the temporal distance between tap and tone onsets. Continuation performance was determined as the mean inter-tap interval (ITI) and calculated by the temporal distance between two subsequent tap onsets. In addition, the inter-tap variability was calculated for the continuation task as determined by the mean standard deviation of the ITI. Accordingly, the tap-to-tone variability was determined for the synchronization task as indicated by the mean standard deviation of the temporal distance between tap and tone onsets. The first three taps of each run were excluded from the analysis. Data which were two standard deviations below

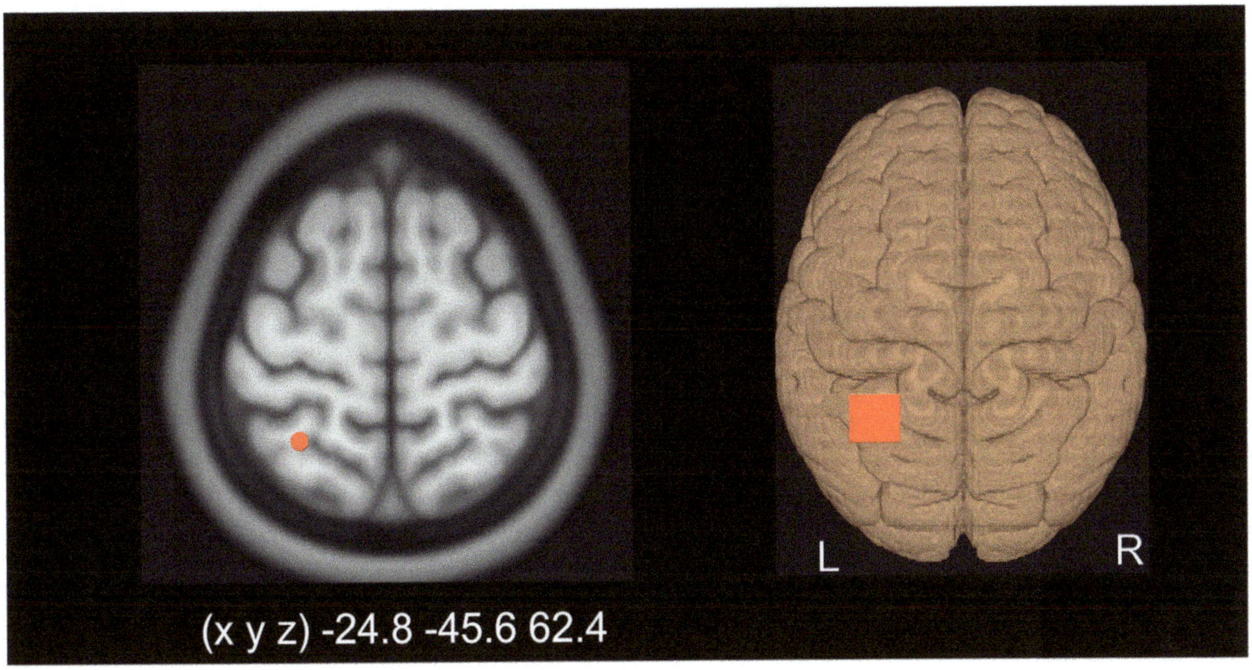

FIGURE 1 | Application of transcranial direct current stimulation (tDCS). The target area was set to Talairach coordinates *(x, y, z)* −25, −46, 62 corresponding to Brodmann area (BA) 7 (left). The right part of the figure schematically illustrates the electrode montage over the left posterior parietal cortex (PPC). Please note that the reference electrode was placed over the contralateral orbit.

or above individual and group means were identified as outliers and discarded. Less than 5% of individual data per condition were removed prior to the final analysis. The number of outliers did not significantly differ between stimulation conditions ($p > 0.14$). Due to this procedure synchronization and continuation data from one subject and reaction times from two other subjects were excluded. Analysis of variance (ANOVA) with factors *stimulation* (anodal vs. cathodal) and *time* (pre vs. post) were calculated for each task (synchronization, continuation, reaction), respectively. *T*-tests were applied for *post hoc* analysis.

In order to determine whether tDCS effects vary depending on baseline performance, the data were additionally split with respect to baseline median of the tap-to-tone asynchrony (synchronization task) and ITI (continuation task), respectively and were analyzed separately for subjects with performance levels above (large asynchronies) and below (small asynchronies) group median. A comparable procedure has been recently used for the investigation of tDCS effects on spatial attention depending on age (Learmonth et al., 2015). Median was calculated for each baseline measurement, respectively. In addition, data from our previous study investigating the effects of tDCS over the left PPC on motor timing in non-musicians (Krause et al., 2014) were re-analyzed with respect to baseline performance in the same way. This analysis aimed at investigating whether and to what extent effects of tDCS might vary with musical expertise and baseline performance.

RESULTS

Blinding

In the first measurement 6 and in the second measurement 5 out of 20 participants correctly indicated the tDCS type, suggesting that blinding was successful.

Synchronization Task

The analysis of the tap-to-tone asynchrony revealed a significant *stimulation* × *time* interaction ($F_{(1,18)} = 6.71$, $p = 0.02$; **Figure 2**). This interaction was due to larger tap-to-tone asynchronies following anodal stimulation as compared to baseline ($t_{(18)} = 2.31$, $p = 0.03$), while no significant effect following cathodal stimulation was found ($t_{(18)} = -1.58$, $p = 0.13$). Comparison of baseline performance between tDCS conditions revealed a trend towards significance ($t_{(18)} = 1.97$, $p = 0.06$). Neither a significant main effect of *stimulation* ($F_{(1,18)} = 0.06$, $p = 0.45$) nor *time* ($F_{(1,18)} = 0.49$, $p = 0.49$) was evident.

Effect of Age and Amount of Musical Training

Since the age at the beginning of formal musical training was quite variable across subjects, we compared subjects with early (i.e., starting the formal training below the age of 8 years) and late onset of musical practice (i.e., > 8 years) according to median split. The analysis did not reveal a significant main effect of *age* ($F_{(1,15)} = 10.79$; $p = 0.23$) or a significant interaction with this factor ($p > 0.34$). Moreover, no significant correlation:

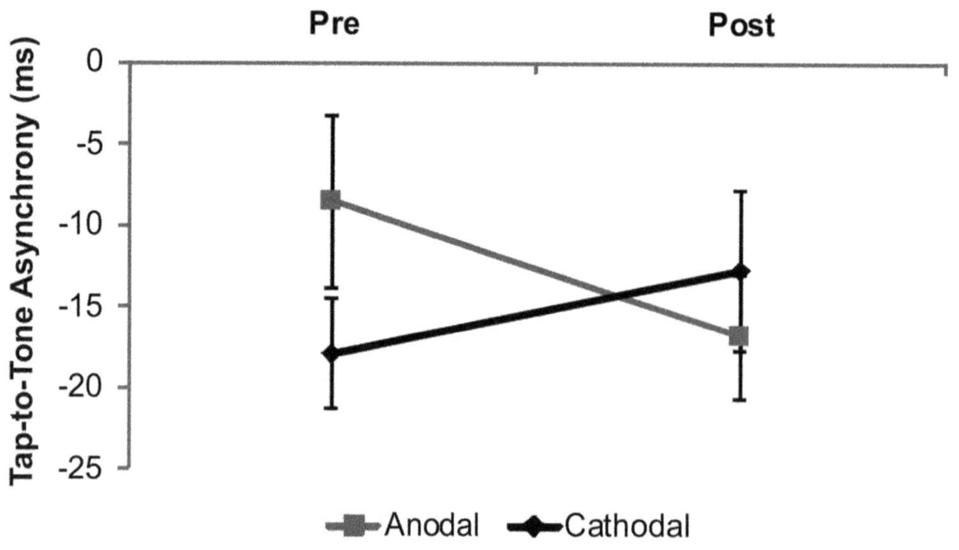

FIGURE 2 | Results from the overall analysis in drummers. The analysis revealed a significant increase of the tap-to-tone asynchrony following anodal tDCS while no significant effects occurred following cathodal tDCS. Error bars indicate the standard error of the mean (SEM).

(*i*) between years of musical education; or (*ii*) duration of daily practice on the instrument with the amount of the tap-to-tone asynchrony was observed ($p > 0.5$).

Effects of Baseline Performance

Analysis for drummers with large baseline asynchronies according to median split revealed neither significant main effects (*stimulation*: $F_{(1,9)} = 0.09$, $p = 0.78$; *time*: $F_{(1,9)} = 1.48$, $p = 0.26$) nor a significant *stimulation* × *time* interaction ($F_{(1,9)} = 0.83$, $p = 0.39$). In drummers with small baseline asynchronies—however—the interaction turned out to be significant ($F_{(1,9)} = 12.85$, $p = 0.01$). *Post hoc* analyses revealed a significant shift from a mean positive to a mean negative asynchrony following anodal tDCS as compared to baseline ($t_{(8)} = 3.94$, $p = 0.003$) while no significant effect was found following cathodal tDCS ($t_{(8)} = -1.09$, $p = 0.31$). Mean asynchronies were significantly different during baseline ($t_{(8)} = 4.14$, $p = 0.003$), but not after tDCS ($t_{(8)} = -1.24$, $p = 0.252$). No significant main effect of factor *stimulation* was found ($F_{(1,9)} = 0.22$, $p = 0.65$) while factor *time* showed a trend towards significance ($F_{(1,9)} = 4.82$, $p = 0.06$). Data are summarized in **Figure 3**.

The observed baseline differences raised the question whether behavioral tDCS effects indeed occur due to tDCS or may arise simply due to such baseline differences. In order to estimate the effect of baseline performance on post-tDCS synchronization, we additionally calculated regression analyses with post-tDCS synchronization as the dependent and baseline performance as the predictor variable. The analysis revealed significant effects in drummers with large baseline asynchronies (anodal tDCS: $F_{(1,7)} = 13.40$, $p = 0.001$, $R^2 = 0.66$, $\beta = 0.81$; cathodal tDCS: $F_{(1,7)} = 6.13$, $p = 0.04$, $R^2 = 0.47$, $\beta = 0.68$). In drummers with small baseline asynchronies post-tDCS synchronization was not significantly associated with baseline performance in the anodal condition ($F_{(1,8)} = 1.09$, $p = 0.328$, $R^2 = 0.120$, $\beta = 0.346$) while in the cathodal condition a trend emerged ($F_{(1,7)} = 5.03$, $p = 0.060$, $R^2 = 0.418$, $\beta = 0.647$).

The analysis of synchronization variability as indicated by the standard deviation of the tap-to-tone asynchrony did not reveal significant main effects or interactions neither for the entire group nor for the sub-group analysis ($p > 0.09$).

Continuation Task

The analysis of ITI and inter-tap variability across the entire group did not reveal significant main effects or an interaction ($p > 0.13$). In subjects with large ITIs, a significant main effect of *time* was found ($F_{(1,8)} = 11.38$, $p = 0.01$) which was due to smaller ITIs post tDCS (904.41 ± 4.09 ms) as compared to pre-tDCS ITIs (916.74 ± 2.95 ms). A trend emerged for *stimulation* ($F_{(1,8)} = 3.57$, $p = 0.09$) which was characterized by smaller ITIs in the cathodal (903.19 ± 4.09 ms) as compared to anodal tDCS (916.74 ± 5.23 ms). The *stimulation* × *time* interaction ($F_{(1,8)} = 0.27$, $p = 0.62$) was not significant. The analysis of the data from subjects with small ITIs revealed a trend for *time* ($F_{(1,8)} = 4.90$, $p = 0.06$) and a non-significant effect of *stimulation* ($F_{(1,8)} = 0.009$, $p = 0.92$). The *time* × *stimulation* interaction was again not significant ($F_{(1,8)} = 0.30$, $p = 0.60$). The trend of factor *time* can be explained by smaller ITIs prior to (882.91 ± 3.00 ms) as compared to post tDCS performance (897.18 ± 5.63 ms).

Reaction Times

The analysis revealed neither significant main effects of factors *stimulation* ($F_{(1,17)} = 0.08$, $p = 0.78$) and *time* ($F_{(1,17)} = 0.41$, $p = 0.53$) nor a significant interaction ($F_{(1,17)} = 1.29$, $p = 0.27$).

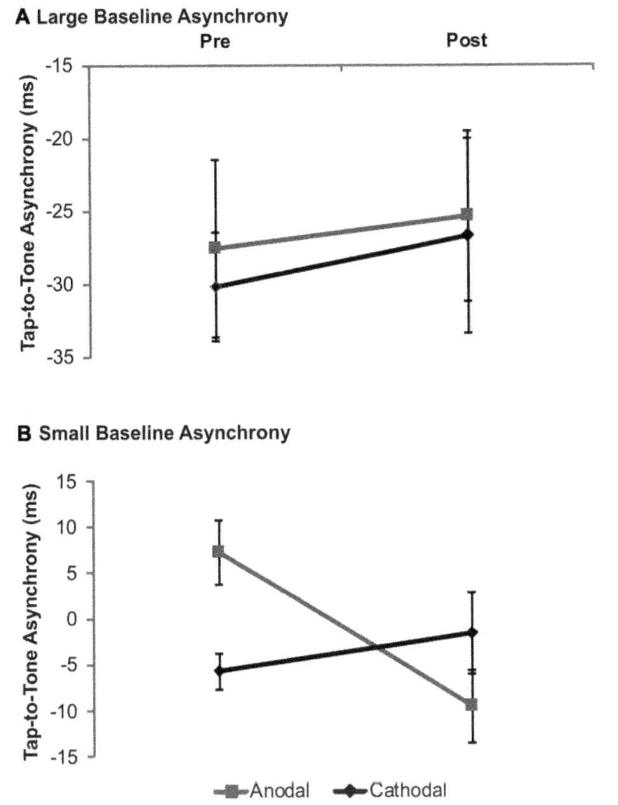

FIGURE 3 | Analysis of tDCS effects on synchronization accuracy depending on baseline performance in drummers. Data were split according to group median of the tap-to-tone asynchrony during baseline. In drummers with large tap-to-tone asynchronies **(A)** no significant effects depending on tDCS polarity were observed while in participants with small asynchronies **(B)** anodal tDCS significantly modulated the tap-to-tone asynchrony. Error bars indicate the SEM.

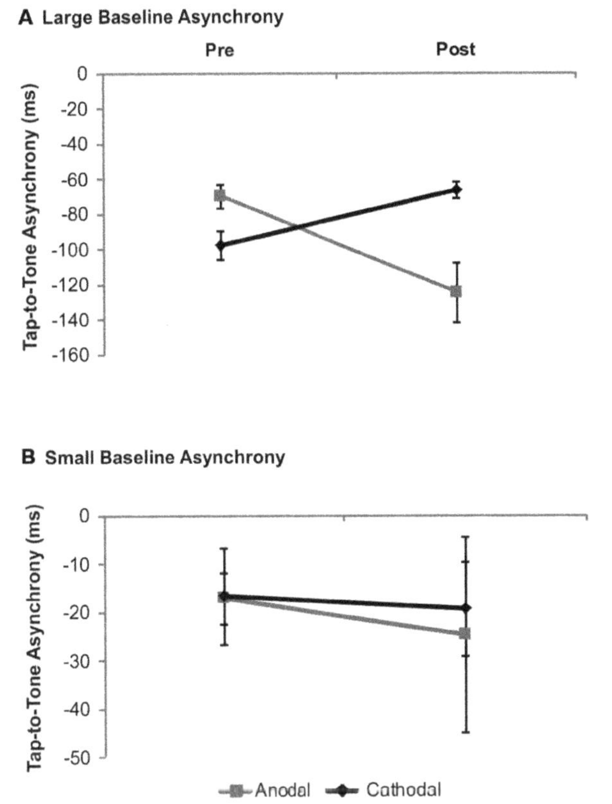

FIGURE 4 | Analysis of tDCS effects on synchronization accuracy depending on baseline performance in non-musicians. Data were split according to group median of the tap-to-tone asynchrony during baseline. In non-musicians with large tap-to-tone asynchronies **(A)** anodal tDCS resulted in significantly larger asynchronies, while in subjects with small baseline asynchronies **(B)** no significant tDCS effects were found. Error bars indicate the SEM.

Synchronization in Non-Musicians

In order to test whether in non-musicians tDCS effects vary with baseline performance as shown in drummers, we re-analyzed the data published previously (Krause et al., 2014). In participants with small baseline asynchronies neither significant main effects of *stimulation* ($F_{(1,6)} = 0.03$, $p = 0.86$) and *time* ($F_{(1,7)} = 0.28$, $p = 0.61$) nor a significant *stimulation* × *time* interaction ($F_{(1,6)} = 0.04$, $p = 0.85$) emerged. In contrast to this, in participants with large baseline asynchronies a significant *stimulation* × *time* interaction ($F_{(1,6)} = 14.21$, $p = 0.01$) was evident suggesting larger tap-to-tone asynchronies following anodal tDCS ($t_{(6)} = 2.80$; $p = 0.03$) while following cathodal tDCS a trend towards smaller asynchronies was found ($t(6) = -2.33$; $p = 0.06$). Neither significant main effects of *stimulation* ($F_{(1,6)} = 1.71$, $p = 0.24$) nor *time* ($F_{(1,6)} = 0.92$, $p = 0.37$) were found. While the comparison of baseline asynchronies revealed a trend towards significance ($t_{(6)} = 2.23$, $p = 0.07$) significant differences emerged following tDCS ($t(6) = -3.01$, $p = 0.024$). Results are summarized in **Figure 4**.

Again, we calculated regression analyses with post-tDCS synchronization as dependent and baseline performance as predictor variable. In participants with small baseline asynchronies no significant effect in the anodal ($F_{(1,5)} = 1.80$, $p = 0.24$, $R^2 = 0.26$, $\beta = 0.51$), but in the cathodal condition emerged ($F_{(1,5)} = 9.55$, $p = 0.03$, $R^2 = 0.66$, $\beta = 0.81$). In participants with large baseline asynchronies no significant effect was found (anodal: $F_{(1,5)} = 0.46$, $p = 0.53$, $R^2 = 0.08$, $\beta = 0.29$; cathodal: $F_{(1,5)} = -1.64$, $p = 0.16$, $R^2 = 0.35$, $\beta = -0.59$).

Finally, we analyzed whether effects of tDCS on the size of the negative asynchrony is modulated by continuation performance. To this end analysis of covariance (ANCOVA) was calculated with pre-tDCS ITIs in the continuation task as co-variate. In drummers this analysis resulted in a non-significant effect of *time* in the anodal condition ($F_{(1,16)} = 0.02$, $p = 0.89$) while in non-musicians the significant effect of *time* remained unaffected ($F_{(1,11)} = 5.11$, $p = 0.05$). No modulation following cathodal tDCS was found for either group.

DISCUSSION

The analysis across the entire group suggests that anodal tDCS over the left PPC in professional drummers yields an increase of the tap-to-tone asynchrony of the right hand while no significant effect on reaction times was found. The data are in line with the hypothesis that the PPC is involved in precise auditory-motor synchronization, but not in motor control per se. The overall-effects in drummers resembled the effects observed in non-musicians (Krause et al., 2014). The sub-group analysis with respect to baseline performance suggests that tDCS influenced synchronization in drummers with small asynchronies only. In contrast to this, in non-musicians tDCS was found to modulate the tap-to-tone asynchrony in participants with large asynchronies. The data support the functional significance of the left PPC for auditory-motor synchronization of the right hand (Krause et al., 2012, 2014) and extend these findings by showing that behavioral tDCS effects vary depending on baseline performance and musical expertise. While in professional drummers the PPC seems to be relevant for exactly keeping the rhythm, in non-musicians, this area might be rather related to prevent the participants from deviating from a given pace within a broader range.

Motor Timing in Musicians

Structural as well as functional reorganization in the musician's brain is well-established (e.g., Schlaug, 2001; Münte et al., 2002; Gaser and Schlaug, 2003; Herholz and Zatorre, 2012). Early musical practice drives gray matter plasticity in the ventral premotor cortex (vPMC; Bailey et al., 2014) and white matter volume in the cerebellum (Baer et al., 2015). These changes were correlated with accuracy in an auditory rhythmic synchronization task, which requires subjects to synchronize their finger taps with respect to rhythms varying in their metrical complexity. The vPMC has been particularly related to visuo-motor integration (for a review, see Chen et al., 2009). Interestingly enough, activation changes in this area are not sensitive to the metrical structure of a rhythm as supported by a brain imaging study (reviewed in Chen et al., 2009), suggesting that it is less involved in higher-order aspects of movement control. In contrast to this, it has been suggested that the dPMC plays a crucial role for auditory-motor integration in a synchronization task (Pollok et al., 2008; for a review, see Chen et al., 2009). Findings by Chen et al. (2009) furthermore showed that activity within auditory cortices and the dPMC varies with metrical salience as determined by functional magnetic resonance imaging (fMRI).

A possible contribution of the dorsal PPC (BA 7) for motor timing in musicians has less attracted the literature so far. A recently published study suggests its involvement in the processing of rhythmic deviations in musicians after a short-term sensorimotor training (Lappe et al., 2016). This finding is in line with the hypothesis that processing of temporal and spatial stimuli relies on auditory as well as parietal and prefrontal brain areas (Di Pietro et al., 2004; Koch et al., 2009). The present results extend the current knowledge by providing evidence for the hypotheses that: (*i*) this area is indeed involved in anticipatory motor control; and (*ii*) that its functional involvement varies with the size of the baseline asynchrony as well as with musical expertise.

In contrast to the observed tDCS effects on synchronization performance, tDCS did not affect continuation performance as well as simple reaction times in a polarity-specific manner.

Nevertheless, the sub-group analysis of drummers with large baseline ITIs revealed a main effect of *time* as well as a trend towards significance of factor *stimulation*. The main effect of *time* was characterized by larger ITIs prior to as compared to post-tDCS performance. In contrast to this, in drummers with small ITIs a trend of this factor was due to larger ITIs post-tDCS as compared to pre-stimulation performance. Since we did not find a polarity-specific effect, we cannot exclude the possibility that this result reflects training or unspecific tDCS effects. Interestingly enough, results from the ANCOVA suggest that in drummers post-tDCS synchronization performance is modulated by pre-stimulation continuation efficiency. This finding suggests interdependency between both tasks in this group revealing evidence for the hypothesis that in drummers the PPC might be crucial for precise motor timing independent of a pacing signal. All in all this analysis may suggest that motor timing is differentially controlled in drummers as compared to non-musicians.

PPC and Motor Timing

Precise motor timing is associated with a cerebello-thalamo-cortical network (Karabanov et al., 2009; Pecenka et al., 2013; for a review, see Coull and Nobre, 2008; Chen et al., 2009). Besides primary and premotor areas, the PPC has been suggested to be of particular importance for superior synchronization in professional drummers using magnetoencephalography (MEG; Krause et al., 2010b). Results from that study revealed evidence for a significantly stronger functional interaction between the thalamus and the PPC in professional drummers. Those data provide additional evidence for a stronger functional interaction between the thalamus and the dPMC, but this was found in professional pianists as well and thus this interaction less likely accounts for superior synchronization observed in drummers.

A recent study investigating patients with brain lesions following stroke suggests that lesions of the left but not the right PPC impair accuracy in the double-step task requiring the modification of an ongoing arm movement (Mutha et al., 2014). Accordingly, inhibitory TMS over the left PPC disturbed this ability (Desmurget et al., 1999) and increased parietal activation was shown when an ongoing action had to be modified (Mars et al., 2007). These data suggest a critical role of the left PPC for action modification in particular when movements were guided by actual and predicted sensory information. Furthermore, the present findings are in line with studies suggesting the involvement of parietal and premotor areas in motor timing (Coull et al., 2013; for a review, see Coull and Nobre, 2008). However, it should be stressed that those data reveal evidence for a specific relevance of the inferior PPC for precise timing while the present data reveal evidence for the contribution of its superior part. Given a stronger involvement of the inferior PPC in visuo-motor integration (for a review, see Chen et al., 2009), this apparent discrepancy can be explained by different modalities of sensory cues used in the studies: in the present study auditory pacing signals were applied while in the studies by Coull et al. (2013) visual stimuli were used.

The present data are in contrast with those from Vicario et al. (2013) showing overestimation of reproduced time intervals following cathodal tDCS over the right PPC and reduced variability following left PPC cathodal stimulation. It should be stressed that reproduction of temporal intervals in the supra-second range was investigated in that study, possibly requiring visuo-spatial attention. Thus, it is likely that the behavioral effects observed by Vicario et al. (2013) are mediated by attentional changes following right PPC tDCS. Combining those data with data from the present study, one may conclude that the PPC may differentially contribute to auditory-motor synchronization in the sub- and supra-second range. But, we realize that this interpretation remains speculative at the moment.

We argue in favor of a specific relevance of the PPC for auditory-motor synchronization, although tDCS may have affected somatosensory processing or auditory-somatosensory integration rather than motor control. Indeed previous studies suggest that tDCS applied to the PPC modulates multisensory integration of one's own body (for a review, see Azañón and Haggard, 2009). Thus, it remains open whether the effect observed in the present study is indeed due to changes of auditory-motor synchronization or due to a modulation of the necessary somatosensory input.

A Possible Contribution of the Primary Motor Cortex

Previous studies suggest that TMS (Koch et al., 2007; Karabanov et al., 2013) as well as tDCS over the PPC (Rivera-Urbina et al., 2015) yield changes of M1 excitability likely due to a modulation of functional connectivity between both areas (Rivera-Urbina et al., 2015). Since effects occurred at relatively long intervals of 10 and 15 ms, they are likely due to a modulation of polysynaptic pathways possibly involving the basal ganglia and/or the thalamus (Rivera-Urbina et al., 2015). The feasibility to affect cortical-subcortical connectivity by tDCS has been previously proven by combining neuroimaging studies with tDCS applied to M1 (Polania et al., 2012). Results from other studies reveal further evidence for monosynaptic connections between M1 and PPC (Koch et al., 2007; Koch and Rothwell, 2009; Karabanov et al., 2013), which were particularly found in the inferior parietal sulcus, an area that has been related to visuo-motor interaction (Cohen and Andersen, 2002; Grefkes and Fink, 2005). Regarding the dorsal PPC it was found that the strength of functional M1-PPC connectivity varies during learning being stronger at the beginning and returning back to baseline after training (Karabanov et al., 2012). Due to the simplicity of the synchronization paradigm and due to the fact that the subjects were not trained on the task, the effects observed here are less likely due to learning induced changes of M1 excitability. In addition, previous results from our group do not support this hypothesis since in non-musicians tDCS applied to M1 did not result in changes of the tap-to-tone asynchrony (Krause et al., 2014). Those data suggest that M1 seems to be involved more strongly in motor implementation rather than in motor timing. The assumption that M1 and PPC differentially contribute to motor control has been supported by a study investigating the effects of tDCS over both areas on skilled motor function (Convento et al., 2014). Finally, if the present results were indeed due to changes of M1 excitability, we would expect a general effect on movement execution independent of movement type. We would not exclude the possibility that PPC tDCS affected M1 excitability, but the observed behavioral effects appear to be less likely due to such changes.

Why Does Anodal tDCS Increase the Asynchrony?

The primary mechanisms underlying tDCS effects are most likely alterations of the resting membrane state (for reviews, see Stagg and Nitsche, 2011; Shin et al., 2015). Based on stimulation effects on cortico-spinal excitability as determined by MEP changes, it has been suggested that anodal tDCS yields enhanced motor-cortical excitability while cathodal stimulation results in the reversed effect (for reviews, see Stagg and Nitsche, 2011; Shin et al., 2015). However, improved performance following cathodal tDCS has been found in attentional (Weiss and Lavidor, 2012) and complex perceptional tasks (Antal et al., 2004) as well as planning abilities (Dockery et al., 2009).

In a previous study we applied inhibitory rTMS over the left and right PPC, respectively and found smaller tap-to-tone asynchronies as compared to baseline following left PPC rTMS (Krause et al., 2012). Assuming that PPC is relevant for the comparison between predicted and actual sensory feedback (Blakemore and Sirigu, 2003), we brought forward the hypothesis that this potentially time-consuming mechanism is important for complex motor tasks, but detrimental to the relatively easy synchronization task (Krause et al., 2012).

We would like to stress that in precise drummers the asynchrony changed from a mean positive prior to tDCS to a mean negative asynchrony after stimulation, but the size of the asynchrony was comparable. Thus, for this group the assumption of larger tap-to-tone asynchronies following anodal tDCS does not sustain. Nevertheless, although the asynchrony was not found to be larger in terms of absolute values after anodal stimulation, the data suggest that tDCS interferes with synchronization accuracy, but the effect varies depending on baseline performance.

The present results support previous findings by Krause et al. (2014) and reveal further evidence for the involvement of the PPC in anticipatory motor control over motor control in general.

Limitations

A main limitation of the present study is the lack of a sham condition. Thus, tDCS effects can be estimated by comparison with baseline performance only. Unexpectedly, the tap-to-tone asynchrony at baseline differed between tDCS conditions. This raises the question whether post-tDCS effects were driven by baseline differences. In order to clarify this issue, regression analyses were calculated. Assuming that post-tDCS synchronization performance was mainly driven by baseline differences, one would expect a significant regression in drummers with small and in non-musicians with large baseline asynchronies. However, this result was not provided by the analyses weakening the hypothesis that effects on synchronization accuracy occurred due to baseline differences. We would therefore argue that the modulation of synchronization performance indeed reflects a "real" tDCS effect, rather than an effect of pre-tDCS performance.

Another limitation of the analysis might be seen in the sub-group analysis with respect to the median split of baseline performance. This analysis: (*i*) does not consider the continuous nature of the outcome measures (i.e., synchronization and continuation); and (*ii*) does not allow the investigation of the most precise as compared to the most imprecise performance. Nevertheless, we would like to stress that the investigation of such extreme groups was not the aim of the present study. The data should be seen as a piece of evidence for the hypothesis that the functional significance of the PPC might vary depending on the interaction between baseline performance and musical expertise.

In addition, we acknowledge that drummers and non-musicians were not matched with respect to age and gender. For that reason we did not directly compare both groups. However, despite smaller tap-to-tone asynchronies in drummers, the overall effect of tDCS on synchronization performance was comparable in both groups. Thus, we would argue that the results of the sub-group analysis are less likely due to such group differences.

Finally, we realize that although the tap-to-tone asynchrony is usually negative in non-musicians, it can be even positive, particularly in musicians. Thus, the comparison of the tap-to-tone asynchrony between different conditions and groups might result in misleading findings (i.e., individuals always tapping close to the pacing signal will show a mean asynchrony comparable to other individuals producing larger but positive and negative asynchronies). Thus, mean values need to be interpreted cautiously, and a proper interpretation of synchronization data requires the consideration of the variability across subjects.

CONCLUSION

The present results suggest that the functional relevance of the PPC for precise auditory-motor synchronization might differ depending on musical expertise. While in drummers the PPC might be relevant for keeping exactly the pace, in non-musicians the PPC might be rather related to prevent the participants from deviating from a given pace within a broader range.

AUTHOR CONTRIBUTIONS

BP: conception and design of the experiment, data collection and analyses, interpretation of the data, drafting the article; KS: data collection and analyses; AK: data collection, interpretation of the data, critical revision of the article; VK: conception and design of the experiment, data collection, interpretation of the data, critical revision of the article; NKS: conception and design of the experiment, interpretation of the data, critical revision of the article.

ACKNOWLEDGMENTS

We would like to thank Dr. Markus Butz for his valuable comments on the manuscript.

REFERENCES

Andersen, R. A. (1997). Multimodal integration for the representation of space in the posterior parietal cortex. *Philos. Trans. R. Soc. Lond. B Biol. Sci.* 352, 1421–1428. doi: 10.1098/rstb.1997.0128

Andersen, R. A., and Buneo, C. A. (2003). Sensorimotor integration in posterior parietal cortex. *Adv. Neurol.* 93, 159–177.

Antal, A., Nitsche, M. A., Kruse, W., Kincses, T. Z., Hoffmann, K. P., and Paulus, W. (2004). Direct current stimulation over V5 enhances visuomotor coordination by improving motion perception in humans. *J. Cogn. Neurosci.* 16, 521–527. doi: 10.1162/089892904323057263

Azañón, E., and Haggard, P. (2009). Somatosensory processing and body representation. *Cortex* 45, 1078–1084. doi: 10.1016/j.cortex.2009.01.006

Baer, L. H., Park, M. T., Bailey, J. A., Chakravarty, M. M., Li, K. Z., and Penhune, V. B. (2015). Regional cerebellar volumes are related to early musical training and finger tapping performance. *Neuroimage* 109, 130–139. doi: 10.1016/j.neuroimage.2014.12.076

Bailey, J. A., Zatorre, R. J., and Penhune, V. B. (2014). Early musical training is linked to gray matter structure in the ventral premotor cortex and auditory-motor rhythm synchronization performance. *J. Cogn. Neurosci.* 26, 755–767. doi: 10.1162/jocn_a_00527

Beudel, M., Renken, R., Leenders, K. L., and de Jong, B. M. (2009). Cerebral representations of space and time. *Neuroimage* 44, 1032–1040. doi: 10.1016/j.neuroimage.2008.09.028

Blakemore, S. J., and Sirigu, A. (2003). Action prediction in the cerebellum and in the parietal lobe. *Exp. Brain Res.* 153, 239–245. doi: 10.1007/s00221-003-1597-z

Chen, J. L., Penhune, V. B., and Zatorre, R. J. (2008). Moving on time: brain network for auditory-motor synchronization is modulated by rhythm complexity and musical training. *J. Cogn. Neurosci.* 20, 226–239. doi: 10.1162/jocn.2008.20.2.226

Chen, J. L., Penhune, V. B., and Zatorre, R. J. (2009). The role of auditory and premotor cortex in sensorimotor transformations. *Ann. N Y Acad. Sci.* 1169, 15–34. doi: 10.1111/j.1749-6632.2009.04556.x

Chen, J. L., Zatorre, R. J., and Penhune, V. B. (2006). Interactions between auditory and dorsal premotor cortex during synchronization to musical rhythms. *Neuroimage* 32, 1771–1781. doi: 10.1016/j.neuroimage.2006.04.207

Cohen, Y. E., and Andersen, R. A. (2002). A common reference frame for movement plans in the posterior parietal cortex. *Nat. Rev. Neurosci.* 3, 553–562. doi: 10.1038/nrn873

Convento, S., Bolognini, N., Fusaro, M., Lollo, F., and Vallar, G. (2014). Neuromodulation of parietal and motor activity affects motor planning and execution. *Cortex* 57, 51–59. doi: 10.1016/j.cortex.2014.03.006

Coull, J. T., Cotti, J., and Vidal, F. (2016). Differential roles for parietal and frontal cortices in fixed versus evolving temporal expectations: dissociating prior from posterior temporal probabilities with fMRI. *Neuroimage* 141, 40–51. doi: 10.1016/j.neuroimage.2016.07.036

Coull, J. T., Davranche, K., Nazarian, B., and Vidal, F. (2013). Functional anatomy of timing differs for production versus prediction of time intervals. *Neuropsychologia* 51, 309–319. doi: 10.1016/j.neuropsychologia.2012.08.017

Coull, J. T., and Nobre, A. C. (2008). Dissociating explicit timing from temporal expectation with fMRI. *Curr. Opin. Neurobiol.* 18, 137–144. doi: 10.1016/j.conb.2008.07.011

Desmurget, M., Epstein, C. M., Turner, R. S., Prablanc, C., Alexander, G. E., and Grafton, S. T. (1999). Role of the posterior parietal cortex in updating reaching movements to a visual target. *Nat. Neurosci.* 2, 563–567. doi: 10.1038/9219

Di Pietro, M., Laganaro, M., Leemann, B., and Schnider, A. (2004). Receptive amusia: temporal auditory processing deficit in a professional musician following a left temporo-parietal lesion. *Neuropsychologia* 42, 868–877. doi: 10.1016/j.neuropsychologia.2003.12.004

Dockery, C. A., Hueckel-Weng, R., Birbaumer, N., and Plewnia, C. (2009). Enhancement of planning ability by transcranial direct current stimulation. *J. Neurosci.* 29, 7271–7277. doi: 10.1523/JNEUROSCI.0065-09.2009

Gaser, C., and Schlaug, G. (2003). Brain structures differ between musicians and non-musicians. *J. Neurosci.* 23, 9240–9245.

Grefkes, C., and Fink, G. R. (2005). The functional organization of the intraparietal sulcus in humans and monkeys. *J. Anat.* 207, 3–17. doi: 10.1111/j.1469-7580.2005.00426.x

Herholz, S. C., and Zatorre, R. J. (2012). Musical training as a framework for brain plasticity: behavior, function, and structure. *Neuron* 76, 486–502. doi: 10.1016/j.neuron.2012.10.011

Iyer, M. B., Mattu, U., Grafman, J., Lomarev, M., Sato, S., and Wassermann, E. M. (2005). Safety and cognitive effect of frontal DC brain polarization in healthy individuals. *Neurology* 64, 872–875. doi: 10.1212/01.WNL.0000152986.07469.e9

Ivry, R. B., Spencer, R. M., Zelaznik, H. N., and Diedrichsen, J. (2002). The cerebellum and event timing. *Ann. N Y Acad. Sci.* 978, 302–317. doi: 10.1111/j.1749-6632.2002.tb07576.x

Karabanov, A. N., Blom, O., Forsman, L., and Ullén, F. (2009). The dorsal auditory pathway is involved in performance of both visual and auditory rhythms. *Neuroimage* 44, 480–488. doi: 10.1016/j.neuroimage.2008.08.047

Karabanov, A. N., Chao, C. C., Paine, R., and Hallett, M. (2013). Mapping different intra-hemispheric parietal-motor networks using twin coil TMS. *Brain Stimul.* 6, 384–389. doi: 10.1016/j.brs.2012.08.002

Karabanov, A. N., Jin, S. H., Joutsen, A., Poston, B., Aizen, J., Ellenstein, A., et al. (2012). Timing-dependent modulation of the posterior parietal cortex-primary motor cortex pathway by sensorimotor training. *J. Neurophysiol.* 107, 3190–3199. doi: 10.1152/jn.01049.2011

Kobayashi, M., and Pascual-Leone, A. (2003). Transcranial magnetic stimulation in neurology. *Lancet Neurol.* 2, 145–156. doi: 10.1016/S1474-4422(03)00321-1

Koch, G., Fernandez Del Olmo, M., Cheeran, B., Ruge, D., Schippling, S., Caltagirone, C., et al. (2007). Focal stimulation of the posterior parietal cortex increases the excitability of the ipsilateral motor cortex. *J. Neurosci.* 27, 6815–6822. doi: 10.1523/JNEUROSCI.0598-07.2007

Koch, G., Oliveri, M., and Caltagirone, C. (2009). Neural networks engaged in milliseconds and seconds time processing: evidence from transcranial magnetic stimulation and patients with cortical or subcortical dysfunction. *Philos. Trans. R. Soc. Lond. B Biol. Sci.* 364, 1907–1918. doi: 10.1098/rstb.2009.0018

Koch, G., and Rothwell, J. C. (2009). TMS investigations into the task-dependent functional interplay between human posterior parietal and motor cortex. *Behav. Brain Res.* 202, 147–152. doi: 10.1016/j.bbr.2009.03.023

Krause, V., Bashir, S., Pollok, B., Caipa, A., Schnitzler, A., and Pascual-Leone, A. (2012). 1 Hz rTMS of the left posterior parietal cortex (PPC) modifies sensorimotor timing. *Neuropsychologia* 50, 3729–3735. doi: 10.1016/j.neuropsychologia.2012.10.020

Krause, V., Pollok, B., and Schnitzler, A. (2010a). Perception in action: the impact of sensory information on sensorimotor synchronization in musicians and non-musicians. *Acta Psychol.* 133, 28–37. doi: 10.1016/j.actpsy.2009.08.003

Krause, V., Schnitzler, A., and Pollok, B. (2010b). Functional network interactions during sensorimotor synchronization in musicians and non-musicians. *Neuroimage* 52, 245–251. doi: 10.1016/j.neuroimage.2010.03.081

Krause, V., Weber, J., and Pollok, B. (2014). The posterior parietal cortex (PPC) mediates anticipatory motor control. *Brain Stimul.* 7, 800–806. doi: 10.1016/j.brs.2014.08.003

Lang, N., Siebner, H. R., Ward, N. S., Lee, L., Nitsche, M. A., Paulus, W., et al. (2005). How does transcranial DC stimulation of the primary motor cortex alter regional neuronal activity in the human brain? *Eur. J. Neurosci.* 22, 495–504. doi: 10.1111/j.1460-9568.2005.04233.x

Lappe, C., Lappe, M., and Pantev, C. (2016). Differential processing of melodic, rhythmic and simple tone deviations in musicians—an MEG study. *Neuroimage* 124, 898–905. doi: 10.1016/j.neuroimage.2015.09.059

Learmonth, G., Thut, G., Benwell, C. S., and Harvey, M. (2015). The implications of state-dependent tDCS effects in aging: behavioural response is determined by baseline performance. *Neuropsychologia* 74, 108–119. doi: 10.1016/j.neuropsychologia.2015.01.037

Malapani, C., Rakitin, B., Levy, R., Meck, W. H., Deweer, B., Dubois, B., et al. (1998). Coupled temporal memories in Parkinson's disease: a dopamine-related dysfunction. *J. Cogn. Neurosci.* 10, 316–331. doi: 10.1162/089892998562762

Manning, F. C., and Schutz, M. (2016). Trained to keep a beat: movement-related enhancements to timing perception in percussionists and non-percussionists. *Psychol. Res.* 80, 532–542. doi: 10.1007/s00426-015-0678-5

Mars, R. B., Piekema, C., Coles, M. G., Hulstijn, W., and Toni, I. (2007). On the programming and reprogramming of actions. *Cereb. Cortex* 17, 2972–2979. doi: 10.1093/cercor/bhm022

Moliadze, V., Antal, A., and Paulus, W. (2010). Boosting brain excitability by transcranial high frequency stimulation in the ripple range. *J. Physiol.* 588, 4891–4904. doi: 10.1113/jphysiol.2010.196998

Molinari, M., Leggio, M. G., De Martin, M., Cerasa, A., and Thaut, M. (2003). Neurobiology of rhythmic motor entrainment. *Ann. N Y Acad. Sci.* 999, 313–321. doi: 10.1196/annals.1284.042

Münte, T. F., Altenmuller, E., and Jäncke, L. (2002). The musician's brain as a model of neuroplasticity. *Nat. Rev. Neurosci.* 3, 473–478. doi: 10.1038/nrn843

Mutha, P. K., Stapp, L. H., Sainburg, R. L., and Haaland, K. Y. (2014). Frontal and parietal cortex contributions to action modification. *Cortex* 57, 38–50. doi: 10.1016/j.cortex.2014.03.005

Nitsche, M. A., Doemkes, S., Karaköse, T., Antal, A., Liebetanz, D., Lang, N., et al. (2007). Shaping the effects of transcranial direct current stimulation of the human motor cortex. *J. Neurophysiol.* 97, 3109–3117. doi: 10.1152/jn.01312.2006

Nitsche, M. A., Liebetanz, D., Lang, N., Antal, A., Tergau, F., and Paulus, W. (2003). Safety criteria for transcranial direct current stimulation (tDCS) in humans. *Clin. Neurophysiol.* 114, 2220–2222; author reply 2222–2223. doi: 10.1016/s1388-2457(03)00235-9

Nitsche, M. A., and Paulus, W. (2000). Excitability changes induced in the human motor cortex by weak transcranial direct current stimulation. *J. Physiol.* 527, 633–639. doi: 10.1111/j.1469-7793.2000.t01-1-00633.x

Oldfield, R. C. (1971). The assessment and analysis of handedness: the Edinburgh inventory. *Neuropsychologia* 9, 97–113. doi: 10.1016/0028-3932(71)90067-4

Pecenka, N., Engel, A., and Keller, P. E. (2013). Neural correlates of auditory temporal predictions during sensorimotor synchronization. *Front. Hum. Neurosci.* 7:380. doi: 10.3389/fnhum.2013.00380

Polania, R., Paulus, W., and Nitsche, M. A. (2012). Modulating cortico-striatal and thalamo-cortical functional connectivity with transcranial direct current stimulation. *Hum. Brain Mapp.* 33, 2499–2508. doi: 10.1002/hbm.21380

Pollok, B., Gross, J., Müller, K., Aschersleben, G., and Schnitzler, A. (2005). The cerebral oscillatory network associated with auditorily paced finger movements. *Neuroimage* 24, 646–655. doi: 10.1016/j.neuroimage.2004.10.009

Pollok, B., Rothkegel, H., Schnitzler, A., Paulus, W., and Lang, N. (2008). The effect of rTMS over left and right dorsolateral premotor cortex on movement timing of either hand. *Eur. J. Neurosci.* 27, 757–764. doi: 10.1111/j.1460-9568.2008.06044.x

Repp, B. H., and Su, Y. H.(2013). Sensorimotor synchronization: a review of recent research (2006–2012). *Psychon. Bull. Rev.* 20, 403–452. doi: 10.3758/s13423-012-0371-2

Rivera-Urbina, G. N., Batsikadze, G., Molero-Chamizo, A., Paulus, W., Kuo, M. F., and Nitsche, M. A. (2015). Parietal transcranial direct current stimulation modulates primary motor cortex excitability. *Eur. J. Neurosci.* 41, 845–855. doi: 10.1111/ejn.12840

Schlaug, G. (2001). The brain of musicians. A model for functional and structural adaptation. *Ann. N Y Acad. Sci.* 930, 281–299. doi: 10.1111/j.1749-6632.2001.tb05739.x

Shin, Y. I., Foerster, A., and Nitsche, M. A. (2015). Transcranial direct current stimulation (tDCS)—application in neuropsychology. *Neuropsychologia* 69, 154–175. doi: 10.1016/j.neuropsychologia.2015.02.002

Spencer, R. M., Ivry, R. B., and Zelaznik, H. N. (2005). Role of the cerebellum in movements: control of timing or movement transitions? *Exp. Brain Res.* 161, 383–396. doi: 10.1007/s00221-004-2088-6

Stagg, C. J., and Nitsche, M. A. (2011). Physiological basis of transcranial direct current stimulation. *Neuroscientist* 17, 37–53. doi: 10.1177/1073858410386614

Tesche, C. D., and Karhu, J. J. (2000). Anticipatory cerebellar responses during somatosensory omission in man. *Hum. Brain Mapp.* 9, 119–142. doi: 10.1002/(SICI)1097-0193(200003)9:3<119::AID-HBM2>3.3.CO;2-I

Vicario, C. M., Martino, D., and Koch, G. (2013). Temporal accuracy and variability in the left and right posterior parietal cortex. *Neuroscience* 245, 121–128. doi: 10.1016/j.neuroscience.2013.04.041

Weiss, M., and Lavidor, M. (2012). When less is more: evidence for a facilitative cathodal tDCS effect in attentional abilities. *J. Cogn. Neurosci.* 24, 1826–1833. doi: 10.1162/jocn_a_00248

Zatorre, R. J., Chen, J. L., and Penhune, V. B. (2007). When the brain plays music: auditory-motor interactions in music perception and production. *Nat. Rev. Neurosci.* 8, 547–558. doi: 10.1038/nrn2152

Steps to Health in Cognitive Aging: Effects of Physical Activity on Spatial Attention and Executive Control in the Elderly

*Giancarlo Condello[1], Roberta Forte[2], Simone Falbo[2], John B. Shea[3], Angela Di Baldassarre[4], Laura Capranica[1] and Caterina Pesce[2]**

[1] Sport Performance Laboratory, Department of Movement, Human and Health Sciences, Italian University of Sport and Movement "Foro Italico", Rome, Italy, [2] Exercise and Cognition Laboratory, Department of Movement, Human and Health Sciences, Italian University of Sport and Movement "Foro Italico", Rome, Italy, [3] Ergonomics Laboratory, School of Public Health, Indiana University Bloomington, Bloomington, IN, USA, [4] Department of Medicine and Aging Sciences, School of Medicine and Health Sciences, "G. d'Annunzio" University of Chieti-Pescara, Chieti, Italy

Edited by:
Claudia Voelcker-Rehage, Chemnitz University of Technology, Germany

Reviewed by:
Florentino Huertas Olmedo, Universidad Católica de Valencia San Vicente Mártir, Spain
Terry McMorris, University of Chichester, UK

***Correspondence:**
Caterina Pesce
caterina.pesce@uniroma4.it

The purpose of this study was to investigate whether physical activity (PA) habits may positively impact performance of the orienting and executive control networks in community-dwelling aging individuals and diabetics, who are at risk of cognitive dysfunction. To this aim, we tested cross-sectionally whether age, ranging from late middle-age to old adulthood, and PA level independently or interactively predict different facets of the attentional performance. Hundred and thirty female and male individuals and 22 adults with type 2 diabetes aged 55–84 years were recruited and their daily PA (steps) was objectively measured by means of armband monitors. Participants performed a multifunctional attentional go/no-go reaction time (RT) task in which spatial attention was cued by means of informative direct cues of different sizes followed by compound stimuli with local and global target features. The performance efficiency of the orienting networks was estimated by computing RT differences between validly and invalidly cued trials, that of the executive control networks by computing local switch costs that are RT differences between switch and non-switch trials in mixed blocks of global and local target trials. In regression analyses performed on the data of non-diabetic elderlies, overall RTs and orienting effects resulted jointly predicted by age and steps. Age predicted overall RTs in low-active individuals, but orienting effects and response errors in high-active individuals. Switch costs were predicted by age only, with larger costs at older age. In the analysis conducted with the 22 diabetics and 22 matched non-diabetic elderlies, diabetic status and daily steps predicted longer and shorter RTs, respectively. Results suggest that high PA levels exert beneficial, but differentiated effects on processing speed and attentional networks performance in aging individuals that partially counteract the detrimental effects of advancing age and diabetic status. In conclusion, adequate levels of overall PA may positively impinge on brain efficiency and attentional control and should be therefore promoted by actions that support lifelong PA participation and impact the built environment to render it more conducive to PA.

Keywords: attentional networks, reaction time, active lifestyle, late middle-aged, old, diabetes

INTRODUCTION

The rectangularization of the life expectancy curve and the increasing proportion of 'graying' population (Spirduso et al., 2005) urges societies toward a more comprehensive understanding of how to ensure health and quality of life of aging people. Awareness is increasing that physical activity (PA) is one of the major lifestyle-related health determinants with benefits that go beyond physical health also in advanced age (Netz et al., 2005; World Health Organization, 2007; Ballesteros et al., 2015). Over the past decades, there has been a rise and fall of interest for the different facets of PA-elicited health outcomes due to reasons ranging from epidemiological trends to methodological advancements. The worldwide overweight and insulin resistance epidemic has led to advocate for PA in aging with the aim to ensure health-appropriate levels of PA and caloric expenditure (Ryan, 2010). On the other hand, methodological advancements in cognitive and especially neuroscientific research have allowed to accumulate evidence on the beneficial impact of PA on several aspects of brain health and cognitive efficiency in the aging population with or without chronic diseases (Bherer et al., 2013; Prakash et al., 2015; Young et al., 2015; Gajewski and Falkenstein, 2016).

Age-related chronic diseases are frequently associated with cognitive impairment. Population aging appears to be the most important demographic change to the prevalence of diabetes, one of the four main types of non-communicable diseases across the world (World Health Organization, 2015) projected to double from 2000 to 2030 (Wild et al., 2004) and demonstrated to be a risk factor for cognitive decline and dysfunction as early as middle-age (Kodl and Seaquist, 2008; Nooyens et al., 2010; Luchsinger, 2012; Umegaki, 2014). Thus in recent years, the focus of PA interventions has been extended from sole physical to brain health effects. Designed, structured PA interventions (Espeland et al., 2016), as well as physically active habits as simply walking (Yaffe et al., 2001; Abbott et al., 2004) seem beneficial to counteract cognitive aging of older adults with and without diabetes, even though health-related covariates may limit effect size (Devore et al., 2009).

Echoing the title of a European framework to promote PA for health ("Steps to health," World Health Organization, 2007), we extend the notion of the health-enhancing effects of PA to an aspect of cognitive health in aging people – the efficiency of attentional control – that has still received scarce consideration in research on the influence of PA on cognition. Particularly, the present study investigates the relation of PA habits of aging individuals with and without diabetes, as objectively assessed in terms of daily steps, to the efficiency of the attentional systems responsible for the orienting of attention and the executive control, which seem to undergo different trajectories of age-related deterioration from middle-age to older adulthood (Zhou et al., 2011).

Recent advancements in neurosciences suggest that these attentional systems rely on two interactive, but anatomically distinct networks each (Dosenbach et al., 2008; Petersen and Posner, 2012; Vossel et al., 2014). The orienting of attention is handled by both a more dorsal and a ventral network that act cooperatively to enable individuals to flexibly control attention in relation to top-down goals and bottom-up sensory stimulation (Corbetta and Shulman, 2002; Vossel et al., 2014). The dorsal network, including parietal regions, as the intraparietal sulcus, but also a small set of frontal locations, particularly in the frontal eye fields, allows for strategic control over attention according to the information delivered by environmental cues. The ventral network, including the ventral frontal cortex and the temporoparietal junction, comes into play when the focus of attention is erroneously engaged by misleading cues and must be therefore disengaged and shifted in a task-relevant direction (Petersen and Posner, 2012).

Executive control is guaranteed by the interplay of two distinct networks too: the fronto-parietal and the cingulo-opercular components. The first seems responsible for the adaptability, the second for the stability of top-down task control (Dosenbach et al., 2008). Particularly, the fronto-parietal network, including lateral frontal and parietal regions and particularly the dorsolateral prefrontal cortex, is supposed to initiate executive control and handle its ongoing adjustment for conflict resolution on a trial-by-trial basis. The cingulo-opercular network, including the anterior cingulate cortex, the anterior insula and frontal regions as the frontal operculum, appears to ensure a stable 'set maintenance' over trials by monitoring the preparatory allocation of attention especially in presence of competing attentional sets (Luks et al., 2002; Petersen and Posner, 2012).

After the seminal meta-analysis by Colcombe and Kramer (2003), showing that executive functions of older adults are more improved by PA than lower-level functions, researchers have confirmed such larger or selective effects and devoted noticeable efforts to further differentiate PA effects on specific aspects of executive vs. non-executive function (Gajewski and Falkenstein, 2016). Executive function is responsible for crucial aspects of cognition as planning of goal-oriented actions, monitoring of cognitive operations and behavioral adaptability (Diamond, 2013). Thus, this special focus on PA effects on executive function is well justified, but has led, with specific regard to the PA-attention relationship, to a disproportional interest for the attentional networks responsible for executive control and to a relative neglect of the other attentional networks the executive control network is strictly intertwined with. The study of PA effects on attentional orienting is mainly limited to the effects of acute bouts of exercise in young active adults (Pesce et al., 2007b; Huertas et al., 2011; Sanabria et al., 2011; Luque-Casado et al., 2013; Chang et al., 2015; Llorens et al., 2015). The only two attentional orienting studies performed with older adults have tested the moderation of acute exercise effects by chronic PA participation (Pesce et al., 2007a, 2011).

The lack of aging studies that examine the separate and joint effects of chronic PA on the orienting and executive control networks is surprising, because such networks contribute in an intertwined manner to the ability to allocate attention in response to expectations and environmental stimuli (Petersen and Posner, 2012) that is relevant to functioning and safety of older adults in everyday life (Bédard et al., 2006). Several situations, as in house hold or road traffic, require the ability to decide where and what to pay attention in advance, as a traffic light for pedestrians, coupling go/no-go actions, but also to re-orient attention rapidly to changes in the environment, as a car unexpectedly approaching, or selecting from the set of possible locomotor actions the most adequate to key features of the situation, avoiding distraction from other irrelevant sources.

Thus, the primary aim of the present study was to investigate whether active PA habits have a similar or differentiated impact – if any – on the performance of the orienting and executive control networks in aging. Of the large body of cognitive research that has investigated the interplay between age and PA (Young et al., 2015; Gajewski and Falkenstein, 2016), most studies have used age and PA levels as categorical variables. When, rarely, direct/indirect measures of PA were used as continuous predictors (e.g., Bixby et al., 2007), age was accounted for as a covariate, thus neglecting the potential interaction between PA and age. Also as regards age, mostly younger and older age classes were compared, whereas the interesting transition phase of late middle-age, characterized by a unique interplay between covert neural and overt behavioral changes (Berchicci et al., 2012) remains relatively underinvestigated. Since specific aspects of the attentional orienting (Pesce et al., 2007a) and executive control networks (Hillman et al., 2006; Themanson et al., 2006) seem benefited by PA at old age, we hypothesized that aging and PA level may have interactive effects on the different facets of the attentional performance across a wide range of ages from late middle-age to old adulthood.

The second aim, related to the first one, was to investigate whether aging diabetics, who are at risk of poor cognition (Luchsinger, 2012), may profit from the expected attentional benefits of being physically active. Although PA and exercise training is considered a major therapeutic modality for type 2 diabetes, persons affected by this pathology usually exhibit lower levels of PA and related lower levels of cardiovascular fitness (Albright et al., 2000). This may prevent diabetics from successful cognitive aging, which is linked to physically active habits (Young et al., 2015) through different mechanisms and above all the enhancement and maintenance of cardiovascular fitness (Stillman et al., 2016). Recent evidence suggests that the mechanisms through which PA affects cognitive function may differ for aging persons by diabetes status, since beneficial cognitive outcomes of PA were found in diabetic elderlies, but not in co-aged individuals without diabetes (Espeland et al., 2016). Thus, we hypothesized to find more pronounced benefits in diabetics than in non-diabetics. Espeland et al.'s (2016) study addressed global cognition and memory. Nevertheless, of particular concern is evidence showing that among the broad range of cognitive functions impaired by type 2 diabetes, there is executive function (Qiu et al., 2006; Okereke et al., 2008). Given the critical role that executive control plays in functional abilities relevant for everyday life of aging people (Rucker et al., 2012; Forte et al., 2013, 2015), we deemed relevant to examine if a physically active lifestyle counteracts the deterioration of the ability to exert executive control over attention in this special population.

MATERIALS AND METHODS

This study was carried out in accordance with the recommendations of "Umberto I" hospital of the First Rome University with written informed consent from all subjects. All subjects gave written informed consent in accordance with the Declaration of Helsinki. The protocol was approved by the Ethics Committee of the "Umberto I" hospital of the First Rome University.

Participants

Hundred and thirty participants (68 females and 62 males) were recruited according to the following eligibility criteria: (i) age between 55 and 84 years; (ii) not self-reported diagnosis of psychiatric or somatic illnesses, (iii) normal or corrected-to-normal vision. Also, they were stratified sampled for age class (Spirduso et al., 2005): late middle-aged (55–64 years = 48), young-old (65–74 years = 44), and old adults (75–84 years = 38). Within each age class, they were further stratified sampled for their declared PA level to ensure a balanced presence of sedentary and physically active individuals and master athletes (runners and swimmers) engaged in regular structured physical PA/training for ≥ 3 ($n = 42$), ≥ 2 ($n = 46$), or < 2 ($n = 42$) sessions/week, respectively.

To address the secondary aim of this study, also a sample of 22 late middle-aged, young-old, and old adults with type 2 diabetes (55–64 = 5; 65–74 = 12; 75–84 = 5) was recruited. Accordingly to literature (Hu et al., 1999), a case of diabetes was considered confirmed if at least one of the following criteria was reported: (1) one or more classic symptoms (excessive thirst, polyuria, weight loss, hunger) and fasting plasma glucose levels of at least 140 mg/dL (7.8 mmol/L), or random plasma glucose levels of at least 200 mg/dL (11.1 mmol/L); (2) at least two elevated plasma glucose concentrations on different occasions [fasting levels of at least 140 mg/dL (7.8 mmol/L), random plasma glucose levels of at least 200 mg/dL (11.1 mmol/L), and/or concentrations of at least 200 mg/dL after 2 h or more shown by oral glucose tolerance testing] in the absence of symptoms; (3) treatment with hypoglycemic medication (insulin or oral hypoglycemic agent).

Health, Physical Activity, and Anthropometric Assessment

Participants answered the AAHPERD (American Alliance for Health, Physical Education, Recreation and Dance) exercise/medical history questionnaire (Osness et al., 1996) ascertaining their activity level, educational background, dietary habits, tobacco smoking and alcohol consumption, medication use and history of PA.

Daily PA was measured under free-living conditions using the SenseWear Pro3 armband (BodyMedia, Pittsburgh, PA, USA). The use of SenseWear Pro armband has been already validated in older adults (Mackey et al., 2011). The armband is a monitor that integrates the information gathered by the two axis accelerometers and sensors (i.e., skin and near body temperature, heat flux, and galvanic skin response) with sex, age, height, weight, smoking status, and handedness of the user. It provides proprietary algorithms to give quantitative information (e.g., number of daily steps, locomotor activity intensity, and energy expenditure; Di Blasio et al., 2016) about an individual's habitual PA involving any form of locomotion as activities at workplace, sports, conditioning, house holding. The descriptive characteristics of the participants were entered into the software program (SenseWear Professional 8; BodyMedia) before the monitoring was initialized. The participants wore the armband on the right arm over the triceps muscle at the midpoint between the acromion and olecranon processes. According to reliability criteria reported in the literature, participants wore the armband for seven entire and consecutive days, 24 h a day except during water-based activities (Scheers et al., 2012), with a wear time of at least 540 min/day on weekdays and 480 min/day on weekend days (Di Blasio et al., 2016). From the default information given by the software, the mean value of steps of 7 days was used for the statistical analysis.

Standing height to the nearest 0.1 cm and body mass to the nearest 0.1 kg, were measured using a portable stadiometer (Seca 220, GmbH & Co., Hamburg, Germany) and a balance scale (Seca 761, GmbH & Co., Hamburg, Germany), respectively. Body mass index (BMI, kg*m^{-2}) was computed. Background information on the participants, as main health, lifestyle and anthropometric characteristics are reported in **Table 1** separately for non-diabetic and diabetic individuals and for the three age classes (late middle-aged, young-old, old).

Attentional Assessment

The attentional test, developed by Pesce et al. (2003) by means of the Experimental Run Time System (ERTS, BeriSoft Cooperation), has been applied in aging research to investigate the effects of acute bouts of exercise and those of chronic PA participation on performance of the attentional networks responsible for orienting (Pesce et al., 2007a, 2011) and executive control (Pesce and Audiffren, 2011). The testing took place either in the morning or in the afternoon, according to participants' availability, avoiding the time before 9 am, between 1 and 3 pm, and after 7 pm to minimize undesired reaction time (RT) variability due to circadian vigilance fluctuation.

Apparatus and Stimuli

Participants were seated in a dimly lit room at a distance of 60 cm from a PC-driven video screen. Four visual displays were used: the instruction, presented on the screen only one time at the beginning of the experimental session, and three types of stimuli, sequentially presented on the screen at each trial. They were a central fixation point, a spatial cue of variable size, and a compound stimulus. The fixation point was a tilted "T" of 0.4° × 0.4° and the spatial cue was an empty box of 1° × 1° or 5° × 5°. The compound stimulus was a large letter (4.6° × 4.6°) made of 13–17 small letters (0.6° × 0.6°) spaced 0.4° in a 5 × 5 matrix. The large letter and its small elements represented the global and local level of the compound stimulus, respectively. The large letter could be an A, E, F, or H; the small elements were the remaining letters. The fixation point, the large box and the following compound stimulus were centered on the screen; the small box could randomly appear at one of the locations of the elements composing the compound stimulus.

The Attentional Task

Each trial consisted of the sequence of events represented in **Figure 1**. In five sixths of the trials (go trials), the compound stimulus contained a target letter (e.g., "H," **Figures 1**, **2**) either at the global or at the local level. Participants had to react as soon as possible to the target letter by pressing a RT-key with the right index finger while gazing at the fixation point. In the remaining trials (no-go trials), the compound stimulus did not contain the target letter and participants had to refrain from responding. Responses to no-go trials or responses with RTs shorter than 200 ms or longer than 2,500 ms were considered errors (anticipations and delayed responses, respectively) and were discarded. The response caused the offset of the compound stimulus for the next trial to begin after an inter-trial interval of 1,000 ms.

In 80% of the go trials, the size of the cue and that of the upcoming target were matched: a large cue was followed by a global target and a small cue by a local target at the same location (validly cued trials, **Figure 2** left). In the remaining 20% of trials, cue and target size were mismatched (invalidly cued trials, **Figure 2** right). Before the experiment, participants were instructed to focus their attention on the area of the visual field delimited by the spatial cue, without shifting their gaze, in order to react as soon as possible to a predefined target letter that would probably match cue size. Further instructions were aimed at forcing participants, in the case of cue-target mismatching, to directly switch from the global to the local level (attentional zooming in) or from the local to the global level (zooming out), avoiding visual search strategies. It was explained that when a large cue was not followed by a global target letter, the target was the local letter at the center of the screen; when a small cue was not followed by a local target letter at the cued location, the target was the global letter (**Figure 2**, right).

There were two blocks of 76 trials, one with short (150 ms) time interval between the onset of the cue and the onset of the target stimulus that follows (cue-target Stimulus-Onset-Asynchrony, SOA) and one with long (500 ms) SOA, lasting 3–4 min depending on SOA and reaction speed of the participant. Each block included four warm-up trials, 60 go trials and 12 no-go trials. Short and long SOAs were blocked and not randomized within blocks to avoid a bias in target expectancy. If SOAs were randomized within blocks, the probability (and therefore expectancy) of the target would increase after the short SOA was passed without target occurrence.

Testing was preceded by one block of practice trials to ensure that set acquisition reached a learning asymptote in both younger and older individuals. The minimum amount of practice (40 trials) could be automatically prolonged until a criterion frequency of 80% correct responses was reached. The order of the two blocks of trials with short and long SOA within each task, as well as the use of two of four possible target letters were counterbalanced across participants. Also, to reduce potential threats to internal validity deriving from the use of four different letters, all possible combinations with the remaining non-target

TABLE 1 | Background characteristics of the participants: gender, anthropometric data, steps, education, number of medications and diseases, retirement, smoking, and alcohol habits.

	Non-diabetics (*n* = 130)			Diabetics (*n* = 22)		
	Late middle-aged (55–64 years)	**Young-old (65–74 years)**	**Old (75–84 years)**	**Late middle-aged (55–64 years)**	**Young-old (65–74 years)**	**Old (75–84 years)**
Gender						
Female (*n*)	25	21	16	1	4	1
Male (*n*)	23	23	22	4	8	4
Height (m)	1.68 ± 0.09	1.64 ± 0.09	1.62 ± 0.09	1.66 ± 0.03	1.64 ± 0.08	1.69 ± 0.03
Body mass (kg)	75.2 ± 14.4	72.2 ± 12.4	68.3 ± 9.6	88.2 ± 13.0	78.6 ± 13.6	78.9 ± 8.5
BMI (kg/m^2)	26.4 ± 3.8	26.9 ± 3.4	26.1 ± 3.4	32.0 ± 6.0	29.1 ± 4.0	27.5 ± 2.9
Step (mean)	11488 ± 3473	11285 ± 3847	9146 ± 3401	9354 ± 3878	9402 ± 3823	6801 ± 1286
Educational level						
<High school (*n*)	6	12	14	4	7	1
High school (*n*)	25	24	15	1	4	1
College (*n*)	17	8	9	0	1	3
Drugs (*n*)	2.0 ± 1.9	3.0 ± 2.6	3.8 ± 3.4	3.8 ± 3.0	4.4 ± 2.4	5.2 ± 1.9
Diseases (*n*)	1.0 ± 1.4	2.5 ± 2.1	3.4 ± 2.5	6.6 ± 3.9	4.6 ± 2.5	5.6 ± 2.6
Retirement						
Yes (*n*)	21	41	34	2	10	5
No (*n*)	27	3	4	3	2	0
Smoking						
No (*n*)	20	25	20	1	5	3
In the past (*n*)	19	16	13	2	6	2
Yes (*n*)	9	3	5	2	1	0
Alcohol						
No (*n*)	22	12	14	2	3	3
Occasionally (*n*)	26	32	24	3	9	2

letters at the global and local level of the compound stimuli were balanced and randomized within blocks. Cue sizes and target levels were balanced and randomized within blocks. Particularly, the 50% frequency of global or local target occurrence allowed to balance the priming effects between consecutive global- or local-target trials (Robertson, 1996) that were estimated as a measure of switch costs (see "Switch Costs").

PRELIMINARY COMPUTATIONS AND ANALYSES

Trials with response errors (responses with RTs shorter than 200 ms or longer than 2,500 ms) were discarded and median RTs were computed for correct trials separately for each type of trial. Median instead of mean RTs were used because of the disproportional contribution of outliers on mean RTs and the appropriateness of median values for positively skewed distributions, as RTs usually are, as long as RT differences, not absolute RTs, are relevant (Pesce et al., 2003). Thus, computations of RT differences of interest were performed on median RT data of correct trials to isolate the performance of the (i) orienting and (ii) executive control networks from the performance of the processing systems that, handling incoming stimuli and producing outputs, contribute to general information processing speed. Specifically, we computed (i) RT differences that reflect the efficiency of the exogenous (automatic) and endogenous (intentional) control of attentional orienting (Lauwereyns, 1998) and (ii) switch costs that reflect how an individual is able to cope with the cognitive flexibility requirements of the attentional task (Rogers and Monsell, 1995).

Attentional Orienting Effects

As common in spatial cueing paradigms (Chica et al., 2014), attentional orienting effects were generated by manipulating the validity of the spatial cue: cue and target size where most probably matching and only rarely mismatching (80 and 20% probability, respectively). Consequently, participants were expected to react faster on validly cued trials with targets matching in size the antecedent cue (**Figure 2**, left) and slower on invalidly cued trials with cue-target mismatching (**Figure 2**, right). To estimate the time needed to refocus attention when a misleading cue leads to focus attention at the wrong spatial scale, RT differences between invalidly and validly cued trials were computed as follows (**Figure 2**):

1. $RT_{(\text{small cue} - \text{global target})} - RT_{(\text{small cue} - \text{local target})}$ = zooming out effect
2. $RT_{(\text{large cue} - \text{local target})} - RT_{(\text{large cue} - \text{global target})}$ = zooming in effect

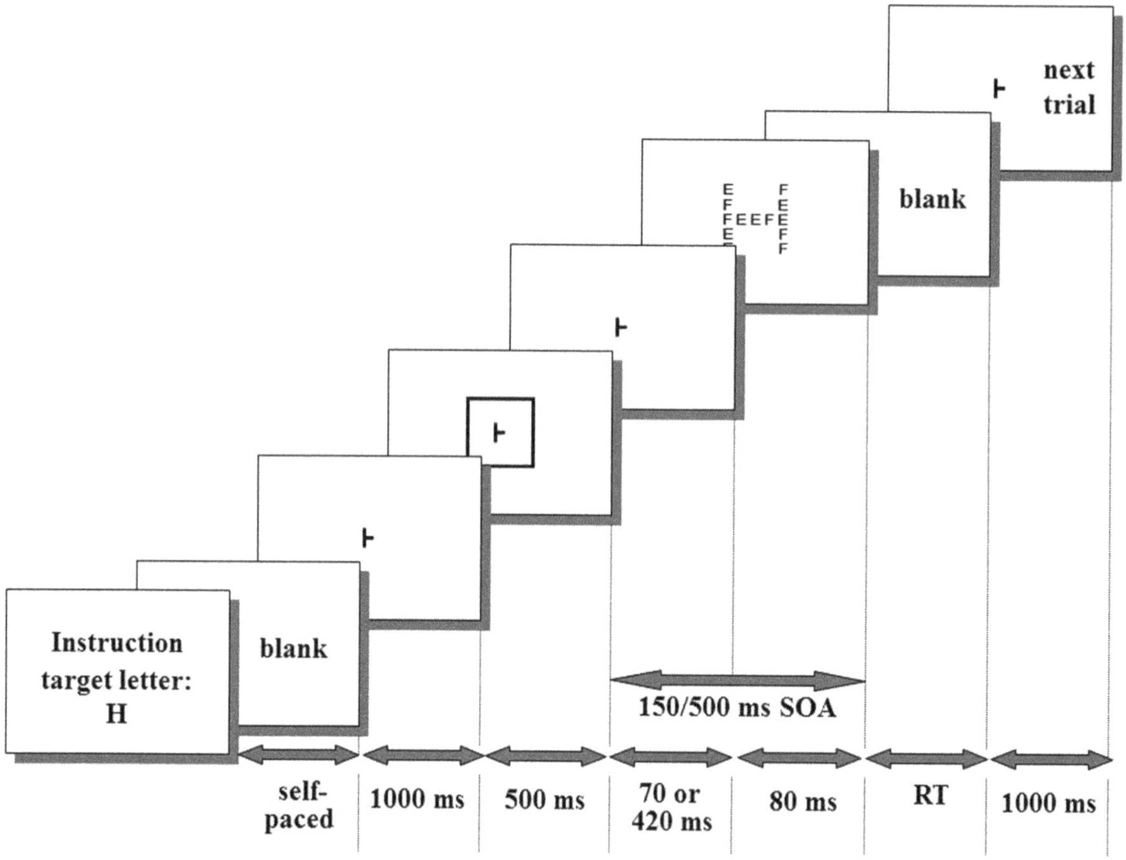

FIGURE 1 | Timing of the event sequence within a trial. As an example, the cue is large and the target letter ("H") matches in size with the cue.

The attentional task was originally designed to tap the exogenous and endogenous control of attentional orienting jointly within the same task (Pesce et al., 2003). The abrupt onset of the direct cue was expected to elicit an automatic, short-lasting orienting of attention toward the cued area affecting performance at short SOA (Stoffer, 1993; Lamb et al., 2000). The informative value of the direct cues as to where the upcoming target should occur was expected to generate a lower-rising spatial expectancy affecting performance especially at longer SOA. Traditional views attributed the exogenous, stimulus-driven and the endogenous, intentional control of attention allocation to the ventral and dorsal networks, respectively. In recent years, this dichotomy has been replaced by a more interactive view attributing to the dorsal and ventral networks a joint role in both exogenous and endogenous control of attentional orienting to locations and features (Macaluso and Doricchi, 2013; Vossel et al., 2014). Thus, to have an overall estimate of the joint activity of the two networks responsible for attentional orienting, the above RT differences were computed merging short- and long-SOA trials. Means and standard deviations of median RTs calculated for the four types of trials used for the calculation of attentional orienting effects and the RT differences that reflect zooming in/out effects are presented in **Table 2**.

Switch Costs

The structure of the present attentional task allowed assessing executive function by computing a classical index of cognitive flexibility and executive control of cognitive processes, labeled specific (or local) switch cost (Rogers and Monsell, 1995; Kiesel et al., 2010). Since the attentional task was composed of equally frequent trials with global or local target stimulus dimensions, presented in a random order within heterogeneous blocks, participants had to switch between global and local attending. In general terms, in tasks involving the switching between two tasks A and B within heterogeneous trial blocks, trial n + 1 may be a repetition of task A or B (A–A or B–B) or an alternation of tasks A and B (A–B or B–A). Specific switch costs are computed as the difference between the RT for repetition trials and the RT for switch trials. Especially when task switching is explicitly cued, switch costs are proven to index the duration of a true executive control process of task set reconfiguration that must suppress the proactive interference from the previous, no longer appropriate stimulus-response mapping and activate a new relevant task set (Jost et al., 2008).

In the present experiment, switches between global and local target features of complex visual stimuli were explicitly cued by the preceding spatial cue. To isolate the switch costs from differential attention orienting effects of validly vs. invalidly

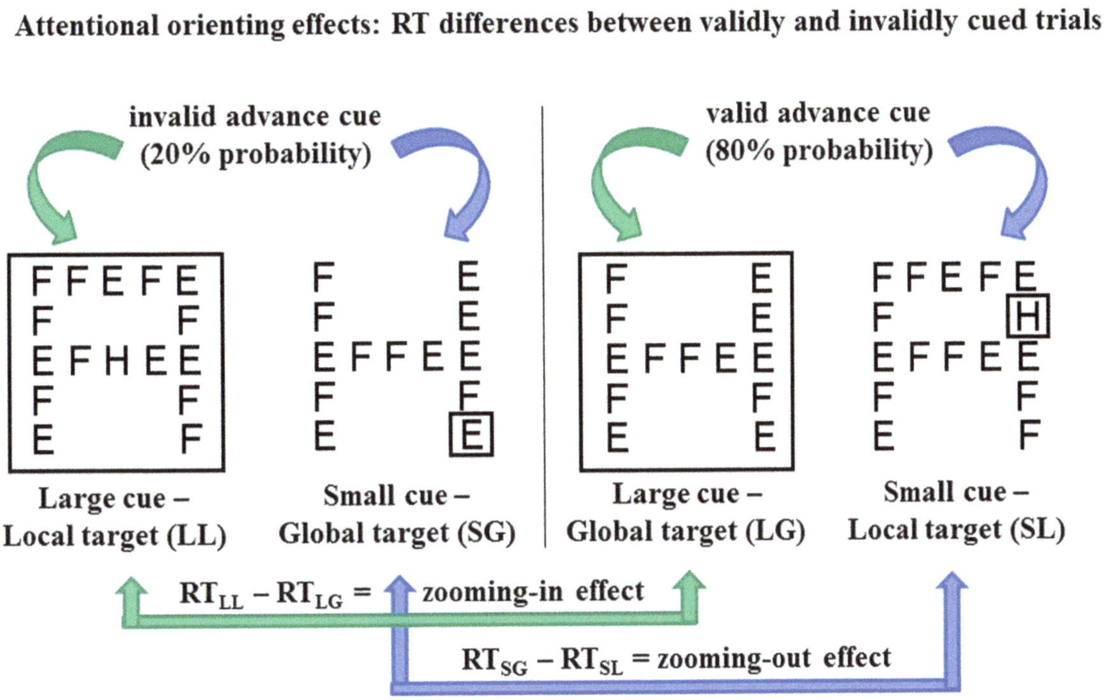

FIGURE 2 | Schematic representation of four types of trials (with "H" as target letter for example). Left: invalidly cued trials with cue-target mismatching, right: validly cued trials with cue-target matching. Bottom: computation of RT differences between invalidly and validly cued trials as estimates of attentional zooming in (right) and zooming out (left) effects.

cued targets, only trials with cue-target matching (80% of trials, comprising equally frequent large cue global target and small cue-local target trials) were used for switch costs computation. Each trial was coded as "switch trial" or "non-switch trial" according to whether it was preceded by a trial with a target at the different or the same object level, respectively. Thus, four types of trials were identified (**Figure 3**):

(1) switch to global (STG, i.e., a global target trial preceded by a local target trial);
(2) non-switch global (NSG, i.e., a global target trial preceded by a global target trial);
(3) switch to local (STL, i.e., a local target trial preceded by a global target trial);
(4) non-switch local (NSL, i.e., a local target trial preceded by a local target trial).

Median RTs were computed separately for each type of trial. Means and standard deviations of median RTs calculated for the four types of trials are presented in **Table 3**. Switch costs were calculated as RT differences between switch trials and non-switch trials, representing an estimate of the time required to switch from attending to the global level of a visual object on trial n to attending to the local level on trial n + 1, or vice versa:

1. local-to-global switch cost = $RT_{STG} - RT_{NSG}$ (**Figure 3**, top).
2. global-to-local switch cost = $RT_{STL} - RT_{NSL}$ (**Figure 3**, bottom).

TABLE 2 | Means ± SD of median Reaction Times (ms) of community-dwelling non-diabetic elderlies (*n* = 130) and co-aged diabetics (*n* = 22, within brackets) calculated for the four types of validly/invalidly cued trials and reaction time (RT) differences computed to estimate spatial cueing (zooming) effects.

Type of trial	RT ± SD	RT difference
Invalidly cued SG trials	800 ± 209 (754 ± 153)	Zooming out effect: 10 ± 288 (−111 ± 227)
Validly cued SL trials	790 ± 189 (865 ± 181)	
Invalidly cued LL trials	789 ± 277 (779 ± 127)	Zooming in effect: 119 ± 298 (43 ± 174)
Validly cued LG trials	669 ± 122 (736 ± 166)	
All go trials	762 ± 134 (784 ± 109)	

SG, small cue-global target; LL, large cue-local target; SL, small cue-local target; LG, large cue-global target. Data are collapsed across short and long Stimulus-Onset Asynchronies (SOAs).

Error Rates

Three types of error rates were calculated: real response errors (responses to no-go trials), anticipated responses (RTs shorter than 200 ms), and delayed responses (RTs longer than 2,500 ms). They were computed both as overall error rates and separately for the different types of experimental conditions used to obtain attentional orienting effects and switch costs (**Table 4**). Since anticipated

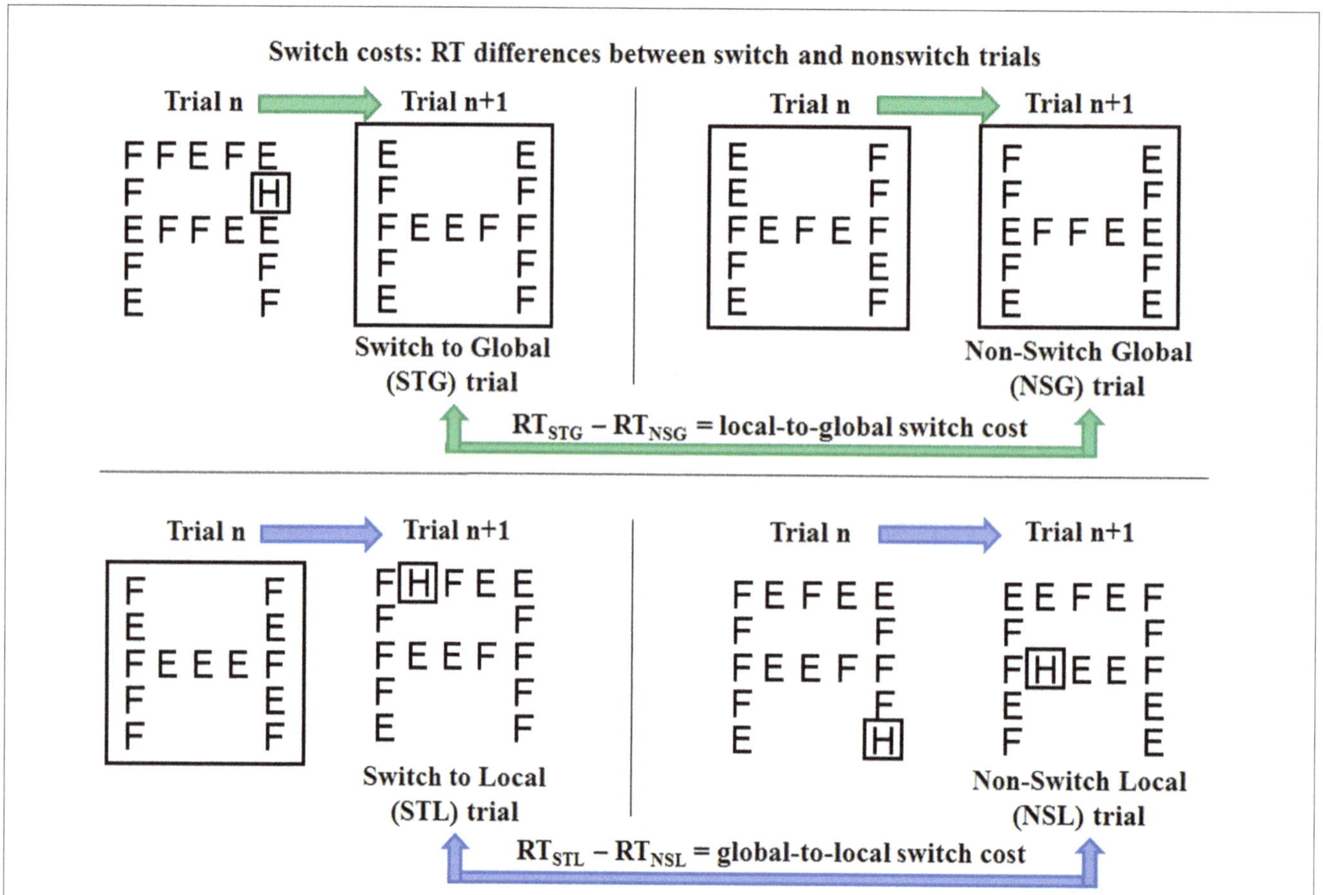

FIGURE 3 | Schematic representation of the four types of switch and non-switch trials with global and local targets ("H" in the example) and computation of RT differences between switch and non-switch trials as estimates of local to global (top) and global to local (bottom) switch costs.

responses were overall very low (2%), they were not analyzed further.

RESULTS

Effects of Age and Physical Activity in Aging Individuals

The first question regarded whether the efficiency of the attentional networks responsible for attentional orienting and executive control are differentially affected by transitions from late middle-aged to young-old and old adulthood and whether physically active habits may counteract the hypothesized age-related deterioration. To address this question, RT differences of community-dwelling aging individuals, computed to estimate attentional orienting effects and switch costs, were regressed on age with daily steps as moderator and gender and BMI as covariates. The rationale for including BMI as a covariate was that we aimed at disentangling the role played by habitual PA from weight status, whose independent or joint influence on cognition across the lifespan and in aging is still an issue of debate (Memel et al., 2016; Chang et al., 2017), but goes beyond the aim of the present study.

TABLE 3 | Means ± SD of median Reaction Times (ms) of community-dwelling non-diabetic elderlies (n = 130) and co-aged diabetics (n = 22, within brackets) calculated for the four types of switch and non-switch trials used to compute RT differences as estimates of switch costs.

Type of trial	RT ± SD	RT difference
Switch to global (STG)	697 ± 187 (811 ± 210)	Switch to global: 87 ± 158 (155 ± 172)
Non-switch global (NSG)	610 ± 142 (656 ± 185)	
Switch to local (STL)	754 ± 233 (837 ± 231)	Switch to local: −6 ± 156 (5 ± 165)
Non-switch local (NSL)	760 ± 223 (832 ± 235)	

Data are collapsed across SOAs.

This moderated regression model entailed the following steps: (1) computing the interaction variable by multiplying age and daily steps (after centering them); (2) performing a hierarchical multiple regression analysis for the prediction of RT by age, daily steps, and their interaction term. Gender and BMI were statistically controlled for by entering them in a first block, while the individual predictors (age and daily steps) were entered

TABLE 4 | Average percentage errors of community-dwelling non-diabetic elderlies (n = 130) and co-aged diabetics (n = 22, within brackets) calculated for the four types of validly/invalidly cued go trials and the two types of no-go trials.

Type of trial	Anticipated responses (%)	Delayed responses (%)	Response errors (%)
Small-cue trials:			21% (20%)
Invalidly cued SG trial	1% (0%)	33% (25%)	
Validly cued SL trial	3% (0%)	25% (26%)	
Large-cue trials:			20% (17%)
Invalidly cued LL trial	1% (0%)	25% (20%)	
Validly cued LG trial	2% (0%)	13% (14%)	
All go trials	2% (0%)	21% (20%)	
All no-go trials			21% (18%)

SG, small cue-global target; LL, large cue-local target; SL, small cue-local target; LG, large cue-global target.

in a second block and their interaction term in a third block. (3) In case, the interaction term significantly predicted RT, *post hoc* analysis through simple slope test was performed (Aiken and West, 1991). The statistical significance was set at $p < 0.05$.

Also overall reaction speed (absolute RTs), as well as accuracy (response errors and delayed responses) data were submitted to the same regression analysis models. This allowed ensuring that larger RT differences of interest would not be merely due to longer RTs in absolute terms, or that smaller RT differences would merely reflect a shift in speed-accuracy trade-off setpoint. For instance, if older adults would show, as expected, longer RTs, this might lead to proportionally larger zooming effects and switch costs, which are RT differences. If such longer RTs and correspondently larger RT differences would be paralleled by lower rates of responses to no-go trials, it might be just due to the fact that older individuals traded speed for accuracy.

Since no reference data for *a priori* power analysis for multiple regression were available from aging studies with the employed attentional variables, *post hoc* achieved power (1−β) was computed with the G*Power program (Faul et al., 2009).

Reaction Speed

The results of the analysis performed on overall RT are presented in **Table 5**, left. There was a gender difference in RT in favor of females (744 ± 126 vs. 782 ± 141 ms) and a direct relationship between age and RT, indicating that RT slows down with increasing age. However, there was a further small, but significant percentage of variance explained by the interaction between age and daily steps, suggesting that the effect of age on RT was moderated by the activity level. Simple slope testing (**Figure 4**) showed a buffering effect of the moderator on the predictor. While in low-active adults, older age predicted longer RT, this negative effect of age on RT was not present in high-active adults along the entire age range from late middle-age to old adulthood. *Post hoc* observed power (1−β) was 0.99.

Attentional Orienting Effects

The results of the analysis performed on attentional orienting effects are presented in **Table 5**, middle, separately for the two directions of the attentional zooming. This distinction was deemed necessary because the size of the two effects differed greatly, with zooming out effects being averagely almost absent with a huge interindividual variability (**Table 2**). Regardless of zooming direction, there was a significant prediction by age. Additionally for zooming out, there was a further small, but significant percentage of variance explained by the interaction between age and daily steps. In contrast to what observed in the case of overall RT, simple slope testing showed an inverse relationship between age and the size of the attentional zooming effect and an amplifying effect of the moderator (**Figure 5A**). While low-active adults showed an averagely almost absent zooming out effect regardless of age, high-active adults showed such effect, but with an age-related decrement from late middle-aged to old adulthood. Visual inspection of single slopes showed a similar, but non-significant pattern of results for zooming in effects (**Figure 5B**). *Post hoc* observed power (1−β) from the analysis of zooming out and zooming in effects was 0.98 and 0.88, respectively.

Switch Costs

The results of the analysis performed on switch costs are presented in **Table 5**, right, separately for the two directions of local-to-global and global-to-local switches. Similar to what explained for the zooming effects, this distinction was deemed necessary also for switches of attention between global and local features of visual objects. Also in this case, the effect in one switch direction was averagely not detectable (i.e., small negative value, **Table 3**). Results of the regression analysis evidenced only a small, but significant prediction by age of local-to-global switch costs, with increasing switch costs at older age. This direct relationship was not moderated by PA level (**Figure 6**). *Post hoc* observed power (1−β) from the analysis of local-to-global and global-to-local switch costs was 0.82 and 0.54, respectively.

Error Rates

The same model of regression analysis performed on delayed responses yielded a large percentage of variance explained by age (R^2 = 0.24, std β = 0.49, t = 5.86, p < 0.001). The older the person, the larger the amount of delayed responses (**Figure 7A**). This age effect was not moderated by PA level, whereas an interactive prediction by age and PA level emerged from the analysis of response errors (R^2 = 0.10, std β = 0.23, t = 2.62, p = 0.010). Simple slope testing (**Figure 7B**) showed that high-active adults, as compared to their low-active counterparts, had lower rates of responses to no-go trials at late middle-age, but higher rates at old adulthood, due to the presence of an incremental trend as a function of age in high-active participants only. *Post hoc* observed power (1−β) from the analysis of delayed responses and response errors was 1.0 and 0.97, respectively.

TABLE 5 | Hierarchical regression models testing moderated prediction of overall RT, attentional orienting (zooming) effects, and switch costs in community-dwelling elderlies (n = 130).

	Overall RT			Zooming effects			Switch costs		
	Beta (Std.)	***t***	***p***	**Beta (Std.)**	***t***	***p***	**Beta (Std.)**	***t***	***p***
Factors in block 1									
Gender	0.69	−2.24	0.027	n.s.	n.s.	n.s. (out)	n.s.	n.s.	n.s. (LtG)
				n.s.	n.s.	n.s. (in)	n.s.	n.s.	n.s. (GtL)
Body Mass Index	n.s.	n.s.	n.s.	n.s.	n.s.	n.s. (out)	n.s.	n.s.	n.s. (LtG)
				n.s.	n.s.	n.s. (in)	n.s.	n.s.	n.s. (GtL)
R^2			0.05			0.02 (out)			0.01 (LtG)
						<0.01 (in)			0.01 (GtL)
Factors in block 2									
Age	0.17	1.96	0.053	−0.35	−3.88	<0.001 (out)	0.23	2.41	0.018 (LtG)
				−0.26	−2.78	=0.006 (in)	n.s.	n.s.	n.s. (GtL)
Daily steps	n.s.	n.s.	n.s.	n.s.	n.s.	n.s.	n.s.	n.s.	n.s. (LtG)
							n.s.	n.s.	n.s. (GtL)
R^2 change			0.05			0.09 (out)			0.05 (LtG)
						0.06 (in)			0.02 (GtL)
Factor in block 3									
Age × Daily steps	−0.27	−3.14	0.002	−0.20	−2.35	0.020 (out)	n.s.	n.s.	n.s. (LtG)
				n.s.	n.s.	n.s. (in)	n.s.	n.s.	n.s. (GtL)
R^2 change			0.05			0.04 (out)			<0.01 (LtG)
						<0.01 (in)			<0.01 (LtG)
			Total R^2 = 0.17			Total R^2 = 0.14 (out)			Total R^2 = 0.06 (LtG)
						=0.07 (in)			=0.03 (GtL)

Total R^2 explained and standardized β coefficients with t-values and significance level are reported. out, in = spatial attentional zooming out or zooming in effects; LtG, GtL = local-to-global or global-to-local switch costs.

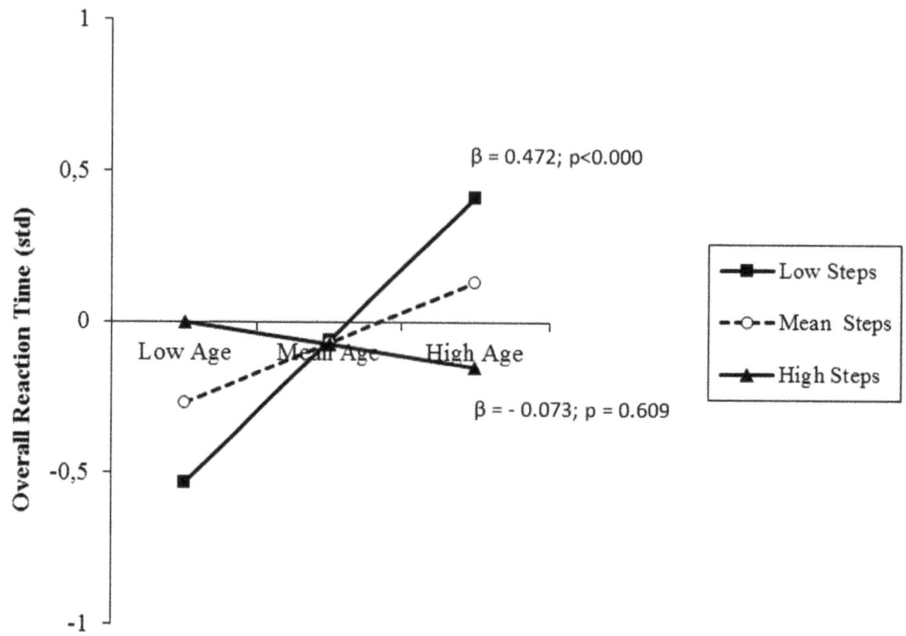

FIGURE 4 | prediction of overall reaction time (RT) accrued by age and moderated by physical activity (PA) level (daily steps). Solid lines: change in the slope of the predictor for high vs. low PA levels (1 SD change); β values and their significance are also reported.

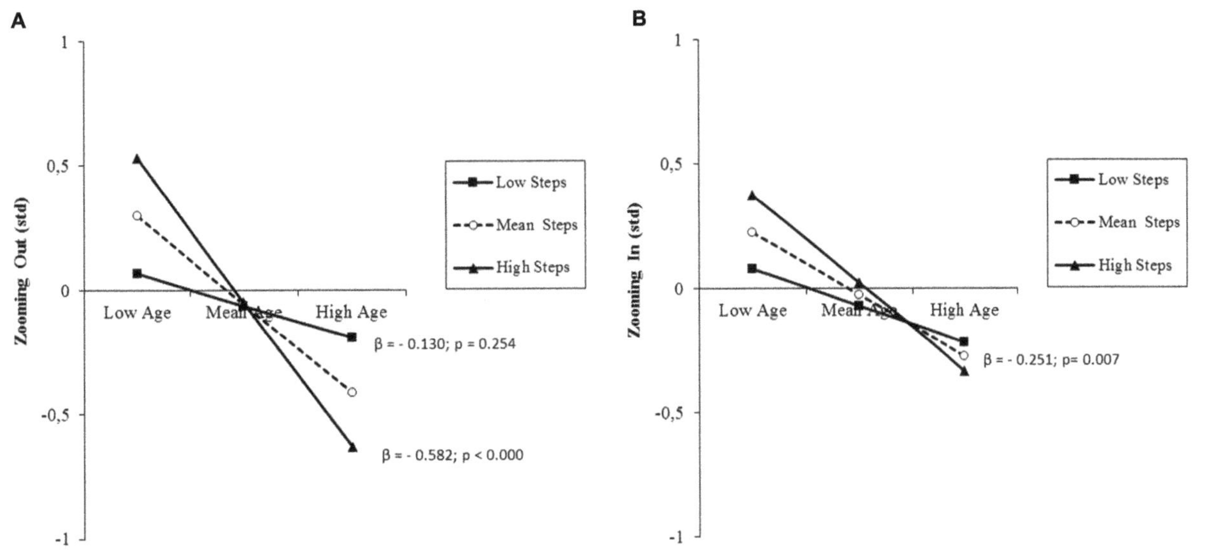

FIGURE 5 | (A) Prediction of attentional zooming out effects accrued by age and moderated by PA level (daily steps); **(B)** prediction of attentional zooming in effects accrued by age without any significant moderation by PA level. Solid lines: change in the slope of the predictor for high vs. low PA levels (1 *SD* change); β values and their significance are reported for each single slope of the moderated prediction **(A)**, or for the main slope (dotted line) of the non-moderated prediction **(B)**.

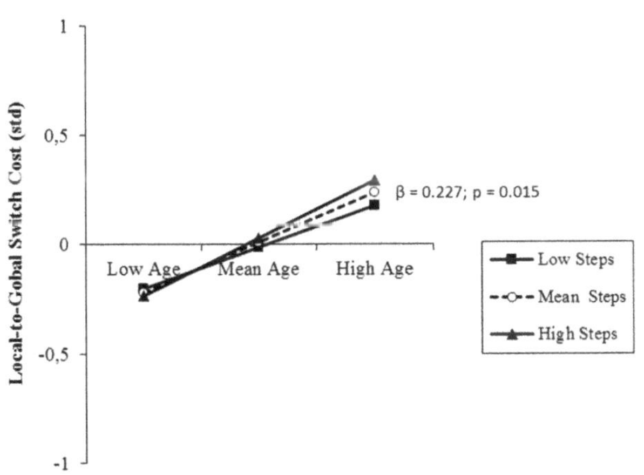

FIGURE 6 | Prediction of local-to-global switch costs accrued by age without any significant moderation by PA level (daily steps). Solid lines: non-significant change in the slope of the predictor for high vs. low PA levels (1 *SD* change); β value and its significance are reported for the main slope (dotted line) of the non-moderated prediction.

Effects of Diabetic Status and Physical Activity in Aging Individuals

The second question of the present study regarded whether the diabetic status affects the cognitive functions of interest and PA level may buffer diabetes-related cognitive impairments. To address this question, further regression analyses were performed on the same dependent variables, but contrasting the data of the 22 late middle-aged, young-old, and old adults with type 2 diabetes recruited for this study with those of a subsample of 22 non-diabetic individuals selected from the main sample. Matching criteria for selection were: gender, age (± 1 year), and mean number of daily steps closest to that of the diabetic and non-diabetic participants (correlation between daily steps of age- and gender-matched pairs of diabetic participants: $r = 0.96$, $p < 0.001$). By matching diabetics and non-diabetics for daily steps, we aimed at isolating the hypothesized attentional differences due to the diabetic status from those expectedly due to lower PA levels and related lower fitness in diabetics (Albright et al., 2000), according to the cardiovascular fitness hypothesis of chronic PA effects on cognition (Stillman et al., 2016). In a moderated regression model, BMI was statistically controlled for by entering it in a first block, while the individual predictors (diabetic/non-diabetic status and daily steps) were entered in a second block and their interaction term in a third block.

Reaction Speed

The results of the analysis performed on overall RT showed that diabetic status, and daily steps inversely predicted reaction speed ($R^2 = 0.16$; diabetic status: std $\beta = 0.29$, $t = 2.15$, $p = 0.038$; daily steps: std $\beta = -0.27$, $t = -2.09$, $p = 0.043$), after accounting for the significant prediction accrued by BMI ($R^2 = 0.16$, std $\beta = 0.30$, $t = 2.21$, $p = 0.033$). Diabetics showed longer RTs than their non-diabetic counterparts (**Figure 8A**), but a similar, inverse relationship between higher PA level and shorter RT (**Figure 8B**). The relationship between BMI and RT was direct, with a higher weight predicting longer RT in both diabetics and their non-diabetic counterparts, who marginally ($p = 0.06$) differed in BMI (diabetics: 29.4 ± 4.4; non-diabetics: 27.3 ± 4.43). *Post hoc* observed power (1−β) was 0.99. Moreover, to estimate if the absence of interaction between diabetic status and daily steps reflected truly independent effects, or a lack of power (Stone-Romero et al., 1994), a further *post hoc* power analysis for differences between slopes in moderated regression

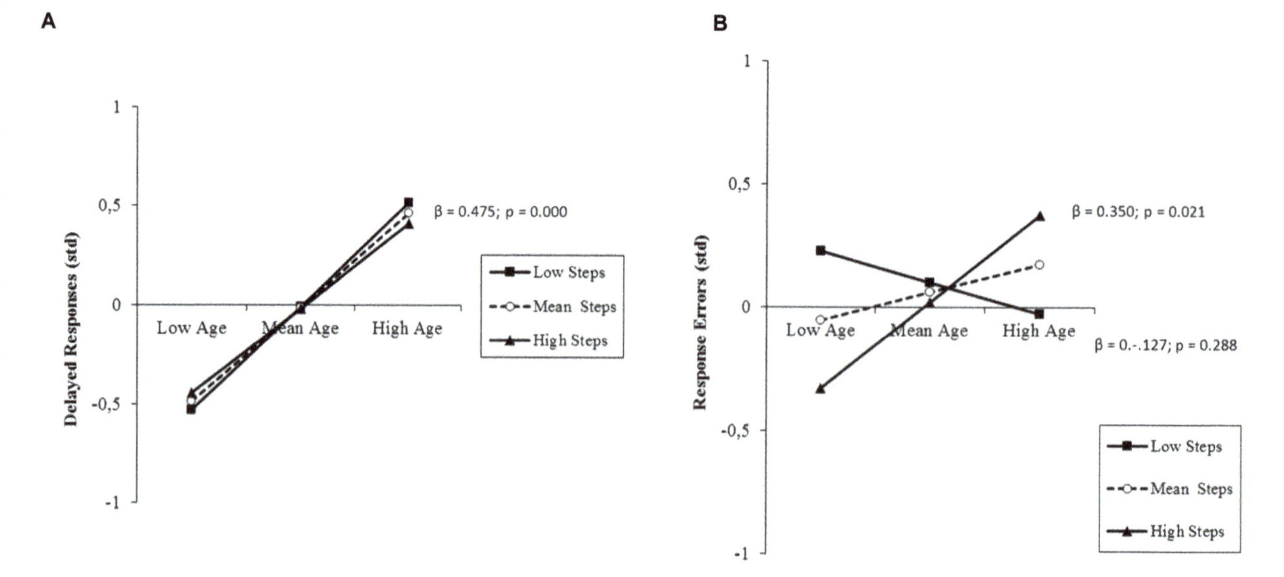

FIGURE 7 | (A) Prediction of delayed responses to go trials accrued by age without any significant moderation by PA level (daily steps); **(B)** prediction of response errors (responses to no-go trials) accrued by age and moderated by PA level. Solid lines: change in the slope of the predictor for high vs. low PA levels (1 *SD* change); β values and their significance are reported for the main slope (dotted line) of the non-moderated prediction **(A)**, or for each single slope of the moderated prediction **(B)**.

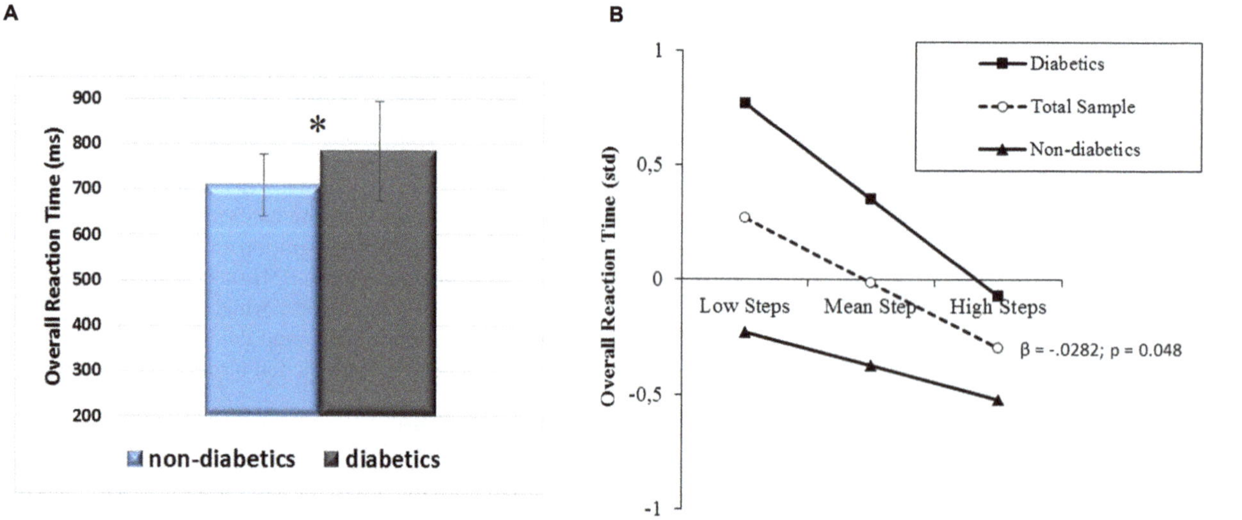

FIGURE 8 | (A) Overall RT differences between diabetic and non-diabetic aging individuals (mean ± SD) and **(B)** prediction of overall RT accrued by PA level (daily steps) independently of diabetic/non-diabetic status. Solid lines: change in the slope of the predictor for diabetic vs. non-diabetic aging individuals; β values and their significance are reported for the main slope (dotted line) of the non-moderated prediction. $^{*}p < 0.05$.

with diabetic/non-diabetic status as a dichotomous moderator was computed. Its low value (0.26) indicated lack of power.

Attentional Orienting Effects, Switch Costs, and Error Rates

Although descriptive statistics show noticeable differences in zooming out effects and local-to-global switch costs, regression analyses did not reveal any significant prediction of RT difference and accuracy variables accrued by health status and/or PA level. *Post hoc* observed power (1−β) from the analysis of zooming out and zooming in effects, local-to-global and global-to-local switch costs was 0.46, 0.49, 0.61, and 0.42, respectively.

DISCUSSION

The present study aimed to investigate the independent and interactive effects of aging and objectively measured PA levels on performance of the orienting and executive control networks in community-dwelling aging individuals and diabetics. In sum, the results show a pattern of effects suggesting that there is a generalized detrimental impact of aging on information processing speed, attentional effects, and performance accuracy. However, being physically active seems to partially dampen this age-related deterioration, exerting a protective effect on processing speed and on the ability to orient attention toward locations and objects in the visual field, as well as avoiding an age-related shift toward accurate, but slowed performance on the speed-accuracy trade-off. Instead, different from the general claim that PA is especially beneficial to executive function (Colcombe and Kramer, 2003; Gajewski and Falkenstein, 2016), physically active habits appear to neither outweigh, nor attenuate the detrimental effect of aging on the executive control processes involved in task set reconfiguration. Furthermore, diabetic status and PA level resulted to affect processing speed in opposite directions, whereas they did not affect the performance of the orienting and executive control networks as reflected in orienting effects and switch costs.

To our knowledge, this was the first study of PA effects on cognition in aging people to investigate the performance of the orienting and executive control networks in combination in one task. Previous research combining the investigation of different attentional networks have been performed only in the area of acute exercise research by adopting Posner and Petersen's (1990) attention network test that combines in one task warning signals prior to targets (alerting), cues that direct attention toward potential target locations (orienting) and target stimuli surrounded by congruent or incongruent flankers (executive control; Huertas et al., 2011; Chang et al., 2015). Differently, the attentional test developed by Pesce et al. (2003) and used for the present study merges typical features of the spatial orienting paradigm (Chica et al., 2014) with hierarchically built visual objects that contain global or local target features (Navon, 1977). The use of direct and informative cues with different cue-target SOAs and a low percentage of misleading cues allows tapping the initially exogenous and then strategic control over attention according to the informative value of the cue and the attentional re-orienting following miscued targets, led by the dorsal and ventral networks, respectively (Corbetta and Shulman, 2002; Petersen and Posner, 2012). The initial blocked task instruction, followed by the random presentation of global and local targets allows tapping true executive processes of stable set maintenance and adjustment of executive control on a trial-by-trial basis to switch attention between global and local attending led by the cingulo-opercular and fronto-parietal networks, respectively.

First, older age predicted lengthened RT, but only in the case of low-active individuals (**Figure 4**). This is in line with evidence of generalized slowing of information processing speed at old age (Birren and Fisher, 1995) and results of previous aging studies performed with the present attentional paradigm, which showed faster reaction speed in older athletes than in sedentary co-aged individuals (Pesce et al., 2005, 2007a, 2011). However, results also suggest that from late middle-age to old adulthood there is a differential shift in speed-accuracy trade-off setpoint between low-active and high-active individuals. In fact, high-active late middle-aged individuals showed averagely longer RTs (**Figure 4**), but lower rates of responses to no-go trials (**Figure 7B**). The pattern of results was reversed at older age, since high-active individuals were faster in responding than their low-active counterparts, but made more response errors. It seems that with increasing age, low-active older adults trade speed for maintaining accuracy as a compensatory strategy (Spirduso et al., 2005), whereas high-active individuals trade accuracy for maintaining speed of performance.

High PA levels seem also to dampen the age-related decline of efficiency of the orienting system. It must be pointed out that the size of the RT differences computed to estimate orienting effects and switch costs has an opposite meaning. As regards the orienting (zooming) effect, it represents the difference in RT between validly and invalidly cued trials. A large RT difference means that the individual was able to strategically orient attention toward the cued area, thus shortening the RT to validly cued target and had to pay a RT cost in the rare cases of miscued targets. This ability seems relatively scarce in low-active individuals already at late middle-age, when high-active individuals instead show a preservation of orienting ability reflected in a higher orienting effect (**Figure 5A**). Nevertheless, the active lifestyle no longer seems to buffer the age-related deterioration in old adulthood. The negligible size of the zooming out effect is attributable to the fact older adults show a typical local attending deficit (Pesce et al., 2005) that lengthens RT particularly when local targets and the preceding cue are not presented foveally, as it is the case for RT on valid local cue-local target trials that was used as subtrahend for the computation of the zooming out effect (**Figure 2**). The huge interindividual variability in zooming out effect is therefore an indicator that some individuals succeeded in overcoming the typical age-related local attending deficit, thus showing a positive zooming out effect, but other did not. A similar, but non-significant trend emerged for the zooming in effect (**Figure 5B**).

The graphical representation suggests that those, who succeeded were high-active late middle-aged individuals. Since orienting effects are RT differences, the larger effect in high-active late middle-aged individuals would be meaningless if it would be paralleled by a corresponding increment in absolute RT. This was not the case, as they showed lowest RTs. This strengthens the interpretation that being physically active helps overcoming age-related attending deficits. Intriguing neuroimaging evidence, while confirming the hypothesis that gains in cardiovascular fitness lead to enhanced neural efficiency, also shows a unique relationship between coordination training at old age and increased activation in the visuo-spatial orienting network (Voelcker-Rehage et al., 2011). The counteracting effect of overall PA on the age-related decline of attention orienting performance found in the present study might be therefore attributable, at least in part, to the coordinative demands of being physically active, since our objective measure of overall PA tapped a variety of possible activities at workplace, sports, house holding.

However, in studies of aging effects on the attentional networks, the most pronounced deterioration has been reported for the executive control network (Mahoney et al., 2010), which is also reported to be the primary locus of the beneficial effects of PA and exercise (Etnier and Chang, 2009), particularly at old age (Colcombe and Kramer, 2003; Gajewski and Falkenstein, 2016). In the present study, we focused on cognitive flexibility, a core executive function needed to switch attention between tasks that we measured by means of local switch costs. In contrast to the orienting effect, whose size reflected the ability to exert top-down control over attention to adhere to task requirements, local switch costs represented the inability to adjust executive control flexibly according to the unpredictable need to switch between global and local attending. Thus, the higher the switch cost, the lower the efficiency of the executive control. This type of costs is indeed thought to reflect the executive processes needed to deactivate a previous task set in favor of the actually relevant one. Differently from many other aspects of executive function that are benefited by PA, this type of cost was not positively affected by the PA level of the participants, but only negatively by age (**Figure 6**). This age-related decline was observed only for local-to-global switch costs, because global-to-local switch costs were biased by interacting spatial orienting effects. The strong automatic capture of attention by small cues interfered with the allocation of attention to visual objects (Goldsmith and Yeari, 2003), overweighing the persistence of attention on the last attended object that should facilitate RT in the case of consecutive local target trials used as subtrahend for the computation of the global-to-local switch cost (**Figure 3**; Pesce and Audiffren, 2011).

In sum, our findings parallel and extend to overall PA the notion that regular participation in exercise training, regardless of exercise mode, facilitates reaction speed, but is uninfluential on local switch costs (Dai et al., 2013). In their study across the lifespan, Pesce and Audiffren (2011) found that age and sport expertise independently predicted lower switch costs, whereas we could not find any effect by PA level. Taken together, the result suggests that not PA *per se*, but the cognitive demands inherent in many sports may be the mediator of PA effects on the executive control networks and particularly the fronto-parietal network (Pesce, 2012). This hypothesis refers to the "cognitive component skills approach" (Voss et al., 2010), suggesting that sport-related cognitive expertise may transfer to sport-unspecific tasks requiring fundamental cognitive abilities. The interpretation of the absence of PA effects on switch costs in the present study is in accordance with the finding that not PA, but cognitive training interventions in aging seem to have the potential to positively impinge on the plasticity of those specific processes and underlying neural substrate responsible for task switching ability (Gajewski and Falkenstein, 2012).

The second aim of the study was to investigate whether in aging diabetics, who are at risk of poor cognition and especially executive dysfunction (Qiu et al., 2006; Okereke et al., 2008; Luchsinger, 2012), a physically active lifestyle counteracts the deterioration of the ability to exert executive control over attention, which is particularly relevant for this special population. The outcomes of this study do not show impairments of specific aspects of the attentional networks performance as compared to non-diabetic co-aged participants, but only a worse information processing speed (**Figure 8A**). A physically active lifestyle seems beneficial to their processing speed to the same extent as it benefits performance of non-diabetic aging individuals. This means that the vascular pathologies that characterize the diabetic status and may be responsible for cerebrovascular disease and cognitive dysfunction (Luchsinger, 2012; Umegaki, 2014) can be counteracted – at least in terms of efficiency of the processes responsible for perceiving and responding – by physically active habits. Instead, the question if an active lifestyle counteracts the deterioration of the attention networks performance in diabetics needs further exploration, since this study resulted underpowered for that type of variables.

The study has further limitations that must be addressed. Merging the spatial orienting paradigm with the task switching between global and local stimulus features has the advantage to tap different attention networks with one task, but also led to some biases. One reason for the absence of PA effects on switch costs might be the relatively small size of such costs probably due to the presence of a spatial cue to switch. This anticipated information, typical of cueing paradigms, generally results in smaller switch costs (Wasylyshyn et al., 2011). This reflects an influence of the orienting network on the executive network, with the latter taking advantage from the information provided by the first to revolve a conflict and switch sooner (Callejas et al., 2005). Furthermore, the spatial cueing with small cues narrowed and captured attention, overweighing the global-to-local switch effect (Goldsmith and Yeari, 2003; Pesce and Audiffren, 2011). It is therefore possible that in our study, due to the influence of the advance cues on local switch costs, benefits by PA level could be detected only for attention orienting.

Thus, an outlook for future research is to use an interactionist approach to the study of PA effects on the attentional networks in aging (Callejas et al., 2005). The present study assessed local switch costs in heterogeneous blocks of spatially cued trials, but did not consider global switch costs in homogeneous trial blocks. Instead, beneficial PA effects in aging could be found for both local and global switch costs in uncued task switching (Hillman et al., 2006; Themanson et al., 2006). An interactionist approach with/without spatial cueing in both heterogeneous and homogeneous blocks of trials might further our understanding of whether the orienting of attention, preserved by an active lifestyle at least in late middle-age, is able to raise the efficiency of the executive control networks responsible for the adaptability of top-down control on a trial-by-trial basis and the stability of top-down control for set maintenance, respectively (Dosenbach et al., 2008).

A reason that may have prevented to detect a buffering effect of PA on the attentional performance of diabetics, as instead found for the orienting performance of non-diabetics, is the relatively small sample size and the intrinsically low power of moderated multiple regression analysis, particularly when the moderator is a dichotomous variable (Stone-Romero and Anderson, 1994; Stone-Romero et al., 1994). Extending the sample of diabetic elderlies can help distinguish true absence of PA effects on the attentional networks from power and generalizability issues of this convenience sample.

CONCLUSION

Adequate levels of PA may positively influence the brain processes and systems responsible for information processing speed and the strategic control of the orienting of attention, but seem uninfluential on the ability to exert executive control for switching attention, which, instead, seems positively influenced by participation in cognitively demanding sports (Pesce and Audiffren, 2011). The differential association of physically and/or cognitively challenging activities to different attentional functions may provide the basis to design interventions for successful attentional aging tailored to exploit the multifaceted nature of the concept of an enriched environment, including PA and challenging cognitive tasks (Hertzog et al., 2009; Kraft, 2012). Given the broad range of unstructured, daily-life activities and structured exercise or grassroots/competitive sports composing overall PA levels measured in this study, our results add to the evidence that both daily-life PA as walking (Yaffe et al., 2001; Abbott et al., 2004) and sports participation (Pesce et al., 2007a; Zhao et al., 2016) may act as protective factors against cognitive decline in elderlies. These two main components of an active lifestyle (Condello et al., 2016) should be promoted by actions that impact the built environment to render it more conducive to PA (Saelens and Handy, 2008) and support physically active habits and sport participation until old age (Baker et al., 2010).

AUTHOR CONTRIBUTIONS

GC: Data acquisition with relevant role in data acquisition coordination, analysis and interpretation and drafting of the work, final approval of the version to be published and agreement to be accountable for all aspects of the work. RF: Data interpretation, drafting and critical revision of the work for important intellectual content with specific contribution as regards aging issues, final approval of the version to be published and agreement to be accountable for all aspects of the work. SF: Data acquisition and analysis, contribution to drafting the work, final approval of the version to be published and agreement to be accountable for all aspects of the work. JS: Interpretation of data and critical revision of the work for important intellectual content, final approval of the version to be published and agreement to be accountable for all aspects of the work. ADB: Interpretation of data and critical revision of the work for important intellectual content, final approval of the version to be published and agreement to be accountable for all aspects of the work. LC: Contribution to conception of the work with relevant role in project coordination, critical revision of the work, final approval of the version to be published and agreement to be accountable for all aspects of the work. CP: Main role in the conception and design of the work, creation of the attentional test, data analysis and interpretation, drafting of the work with specific contribution as regards the physical activity-attention relationship, final approval of the version to be published and agreement to be accountable for all aspects of the work.

ACKNOWLEDGMENTS

We thank all the participants who took part in the study and the master students who cooperated to this research project. We also thank the National Pensioners' Federation of the Italian National Confederation of the Labor Unions (CISL), the national secretary of the Department of Social and Health Policies, Attilio Rimoldi and Brigida Modesti for their indispensable contribution to recruitment. Moreover, we thank both reviewers and particularly FHO for very detailed and precious suggestions.

REFERENCES

Abbott, R. D., White, L. R., Ross, G. W., Masaki, K. H., Curb, J. D., and Petrovitch, H. (2004). Walking and dementia in physically capable elderly men. *JAMA* 292, 1447–1453. doi: 10.1001/jama.292.12.1447

Aiken, L. S., and West, S. G. (1991). *Multiple Regression: Testing and Interpreting Interactions*. Newbury Park, CA: Sage.

Albright, A., Franz, M., Hornsby, G., Kriska, A., Marrero, D., Ullrich, I., et al. (2000). American college of sports medicine position stand. Exercise and type 2 diabetes. *Med. Sci. Sports Exerc.* 32, 1345–1360. doi: 10.1097/00005768-200007000-00024

Baker, J., Fraser-Thomas, J., Dionigi, R. A., and Horton, S. (2010). Sport participation and positive development in older persons. *Eur. Rev. Aging Phys. Act.* 7, 3–12. doi: 10.1007/s11556-009-0054-9

Ballesteros, S., Kraft, E., Santana, S., and Tziraki, C. (2015). Maintaining older brain functionality: a targeted review. *Neurosci. Biobehav. Rev.* 55, 453–477. doi: 10.1016/j.neubiorev.2015.06.008

Bédard, M., Leonard, E., McAuliffe, J., Weaver, B., Gibbons, C., and Dubois, S. (2006). Visual attention and older drivers: the contribution of inhibition of return to safe driving. *Exp. Aging Res.* 32, 119–135. doi: 10.1080/03610730500511918

Berchicci, M., Lucci, G., Pesce, C., Spinelli, D., and Di Russo, F. (2012). Prefrontal hyperactivity in older people during motor planning. *Neuroimage* 62, 1750–1760. doi: 10.1016/j.neuroimage.2012.06.031

Bherer, L., Erickson, K. I., and Liu-Ambrose, T. (2013). A review of the effects of physical activity and exercise on cognitive and brain functions in older adults. *J. Aging Res.* 2013:657508. doi: 10.1155/2013/657508

Birren, J. E., and Fisher, L. M. (1995). Aging and speed of behavior: possible consequences for psychological functioning. *Annu. Rev. Psychol.* 46, 329–353. doi: 10.1146/annurev.ps.46.020195.001553

Bixby, W. R., Spalding, T. W., Haufler, A. J., Deeny, S. P., Mahlow, P. T., Zimmerman, J. B., et al. (2007). The unique relation of physical activity to executive function in older men and women. *Med. Sci. Sports Exerc.* 39, 1408–1416. doi: 10.1249/mss.0b013e31806ad708

Callejas, A., Lupiàñez, J., Funes, M. J., and Tudela, P. (2005). Modulations among the alerting, orienting and executive control networks. *Exp. Brain Res.* 167, 27–37. doi: 10.1007/s00221-005-2365-z

Chang, Y. K., Chu, C. H., Chen, F. T., Hung, T. M., and Etnier, J. L. (2017). Combined effects of physical activity and obesity on cognitive function: independent, overlapping, moderator, and mediator models. *Sports Med.* 47, 449–468. doi: 10.1007/s40279-016-0589-7

Chang, Y. K., Pesce, C., Chiang, Y. T., Kuo, C. Y., and Fong, D. Y. (2015). Antecedent acute cycling exercise affects attention control: an ERP study using attention network test. *Front. Hum. Neurosci.* 9:156. doi: 10.3389/fnhum.2015.00156

Chica, A. B., Martín-Arévalo, E., Botta, F., and Lupiánez, J. (2014). The spatial orienting paradigm: how to design and interpret spatial attention experiments. *Neurosci. Biobehav. Rev.* 40, 35–51. doi: 10.1016/j.neubiorev.2014.01.002

Colcombe, S., and Kramer, A. F. (2003). Fitness effects on the cognitive function of older adults: a meta-analytic study. *Psychol. Sci.* 14, 125–130. doi: 10.1111/1467-9280.t01-1-01430

Condello, G., Man Ling, F. C., Bianco, A., Chastin, S., Cardon, G., Ciarapica, D., et al. (2016). Using concept mapping in the development of the EU-PAD framework (European-physical activity determinants across the life course): a DEDIPAC-study (2016). *BMC Public Health* 16:1145. doi: 10.1186/s12889-016-3800-8

Corbetta, M., and Shulman, G. L. (2002). Control of goal-directed and stimulus-driven attention in the brain. *Nat. Rev. Neurosci.* 3, 201–215. doi: 10.1038/nrn755

Dai, C. T., Chang, Y. K., Huang, C. J., and Hung, T. M. (2013). Exercise mode and executive function in older adults: an ERP study of task-switching. *Brain Cogn.* 83, 153–162. doi: 10.1016/j.bandc.2013.07.007

Devore, E. E., Hee Kang, J., Okereke, O., and Grodstein, F. (2009). Physical activity levels and cognition in women with type 2 diabetes. *Am. J. Epidemiol.* 170, 1040–1047. doi: 10.1093/aje/kwp224

Di Blasio, A., Napolitano, G., Di Donato, F., Izzicupo, P., Di Baldassarre, A., Modestini, E., et al. (2016). Analysis of female physical activity characteristics according to age and ponderal status in a free-living context: a study from a central Italy sample. *Sport Sci. Health* 12, 453–462. doi: 10.1007/s11332-016-0315-8

Diamond, A. (2013). Executive Functions. *Annu. Rev. Psychol.* 64, 135–168. doi: 10.1146/annurev-psych-113011-143750

Dosenbach, N. U., Fair, D. A., Cohen, A. L., Schlaggar, B. L., and Petersen, S. E. (2008). A dual-networks architecture of top-down control. *Trends Cogn. Sci.* 12, 99–105. doi: 10.1016/j.tics.2008.01.001

Espeland, M. A., Lipska, K., Miller, M. E., Rushing, J., Cohen, R. A., Verghese, J., et al. (2016). Effects of physical activity intervention on physical and cognitive function in sedentary adults with and without diabetes. *J. Gerontol. A Biol. Sci. Med. Sci.* doi: 10.1093/gerona/glw179 [Epub ahead of print].

Etnier, J. L., and Chang, Y. K. (2009). The effect of physical activity on executive function: a brief commentary on definitions, measurement issues, and the current state of the literature. *J. Sport Exerc. Psychol.* 31, 469–483. doi: 10.1123/jsep.31.4.469

Faul, F., Erdfelder, E., Buchner, A., and Lang, A. G. (2009). Statistical power analyses using G*Power 3.1: tests for correlation and regression analyses. *Behav. Res. Methods* 41, 1149–1160. doi: 10.3758/BRM.41.4.1149

Forte, R., Boreham, C. A. G., De Vito, G., Ditroilo, M., and Pesce, C. (2015). Health -related quality of life, executive function and dual task performance in healthy older individuals. *Int. J. Environ. Res. Publ. Health.* 12, 11328–11344. doi: 10.3390/ijerph120911328

Forte, R., Pesce, C., Costa Leite, J., De Vito, G., Gibney, E., Tomporowski, P. D., et al. (2013). Executive function moderates the role of physical fitness in determining functional ability of older individuals. *Aging Clin. Exp. Res.* 25, 291–298. doi: 10.1007/s40520-013-0044-7

Gajewski, P. D., and Falkenstein, M. (2012). Training-induced improvement of response selection and error detection in aging assessed by task switching: effects of cognitive, physical, and relaxation training. *Front. Hum. Neurosci.* 6:130. doi: 10.3389/fnhum.2012.00130

Gajewski, P. D., and Falkenstein, M. (2016). Physical activity and neurocognitive functioning in aging - a condensed updated review. *Eur. Rev. Aging Phys. Act.* 13:1. doi: 10.1186/s11556-016-0161-3

Goldsmith, M., and Yeari, M. (2003). Modulation of object-based attention by spatial focus under endogenous and exogenous orienting. *J. Exp. Psychol. Hum. Percept. Perform.* 29, 897–918. doi: 10.1037/0096-1523.29.5.897

Hertzog, C., Kramer, A. F., Wilson, R. S., and Lindenberger, U. (2009). Enrichment effects on adult cognitive development: can the functional capacity of older adults be preserved and enhanced? *Psychol. Sci. Public Interest* 9, 1–65. doi: 10.1111/j.1475-6811.2011.01373.x

Hillman, C. H., Kramer, A. F., Belopolsky, A. V., and Smith, D. P. (2006). A cross-sectional examination of age and physical activity on performance and event-related brain potentials in a task switching paradigm. *Int. J. Psychophysiol.* 59, 30–39. doi: 10.1016/j.ijpsycho.2005.04.009

Hu, F. B., Sigal, R. J., Rich-Edwards, J. W., Colditz, G. A., Solomon, C. G., Willett, W. C., et al. (1999). Walking compared with vigorous physical activity and risk of type 2 diabetes in women a prospective study. *JAMA* 282, 1433–1439. doi: 10.1001/jama.282.15.1433

Huertas, F., Zahonero, J., Sanabria, D., and Lupianez, J. (2011). Functioning of the attentional networks at rest vs. during acute bouts of aerobic exercise. *J. Sport Exerc. Psychol.* 33, 649–665. doi: 10.1123/jsep.33.5.649

Jost, K., Mayr, U., and Rösler, F. (2008). Is task switching nothing but cue priming? Evidence from ERPs. *Cogn. Affect. Behav. Neurosci.* 8, 74–84. doi: 10.3758/CABN.8.1.74

Kiesel, A., Steinhauser, M., Wendt, M., Falkenstein, M., Jost, K., Phillip, A., et al. (2010). Control and interference in task switching – a review. *Psychol. Bull.* 136, 849–874. doi: 10.1037/a0019842

Kodl, C. T., and Seaquist, E. R. (2008). Cognitive dysfunction and diabetes mellitus. *Endocr. Rev.* 29, 494–511. doi: 10.1210/er.2007-0034

Kraft, E. (2012). Cognitive function, physical activity, and aging: possible biological links and implications for multimodal interventions. *Neuropsychol. Dev. Cogn. B Aging Neuropsychol. Cogn.* 19, 248–263. doi: 10.1080/13825585.2011.645010

Lamb, R. L., Pond, H. M., and Zahir, G. (2000). Contributions of automatic and controlled processes to the analysis of hierarchical structures. *J. Exp. Psychol. Hum. Percept. Perform.* 26, 234–245. doi: 10.1037/0096-1523.26.1.234

Lauwereyns, J. (1998). Exogenous/endogenous control of space-based/object-based attention: four types of visual selection? *Eur. J. Cogn. Psychol.* 10, 41–74. doi: 10.1080/713752264

Llorens, F., Sanabria, D., and Huertas, F. (2015). The influence of acute intense exercise on exogenous spatial attention depends on physical fitness level. *Exp. Psychol.* 62, 20–29. doi: 10.1027/1618-3169/a000270

Luchsinger, J. A. (2012). Type 2 diabetes and cognitive impairment: linking mechanisms. *J. Alzheimers Dis.* 30(Suppl. 2), S185–S198. doi: 10.3233/JAD-2012-111433

Luks, T. L., Simpson, G. V., Feiwell, R. J., and Miller, W. L. (2002). Evidence for anterior cingulate cortex involvement in monitoring preparatory attentional set. *Neuroimage* 17, 792–802. doi: 10.1006/nimg.2002.1210

Luque-Casado, A., Zabala, M., Morales, E., Mateo-March, M., and Sanabria, D. (2013). Cognitive performance and heart rate variability: the influence of fitness level. *PLoS ONE* 8:e56935. doi: 10.1371/journal.pone.0056935

Macaluso, E., and Doricchi, F. (2013). Attention and predictions: control of spatial attention beyond the endogenous-exogenous dichotomy. *Front. Hum. Neurosci.* 7:685. doi: 10.3389/fnhum.2013.00685

Mackey, D. C., Manini, T. M., Schoeller, D. A., Koster, A., Glynn, N. W., Goodpaster, B. H., et al. (2011). Validation of an armband to measure daily energy expenditure in older adults. *J. Gerontol. A Biol. Sci. Med. Sci.* 66, 1108–1113. doi: 10.1093/gerona/glr101

Mahoney, J. R., Verghese, J., Goldin, Y., Lipton, R., and Holtzer, R. (2010). Alerting, orienting, and executive attention in older adults. *J. Int. Neuropsychol. Soc.* 16, 877–889. doi: 10.1017/S1355617710000767

Memel, M., Bourassa, K., Woolverton, C., and Sbarra, D. A. (2016). Body mass and physical activity uniquely predict change in cognition for aging adults. *Ann. Behav. Med.* 50, 397–408. doi: 10.1007/s12160-015-9768-2

Navon, D. (1977). Forest before trees: the precedence of global features in visual perception. *Cogn. Psychol.* 9, 353–383. doi: 10.1016/0010-0285(77)90012-3

Netz, Y., Wu, M. J., Becker, B. J., and Tenenbaum, G. (2005). Physical activity and psychological well-being in advanced age: a meta-analysis of intervention studies. *Psychol. Aging* 20, 272–284. doi: 10.1037/0882-7974.20.2.272

Nooyens, A. C., Baan, C. A., Spijkerman, A. M., and Verschuren, W. M. (2010). Type 2 diabetes and cognitive decline in middle-aged men and women. *Diabetes Care* 33, 1964–1969. doi: 10.2337/dc09-2038

Okereke, O. I., Kang, J. H., Cook, N. R., Gaziano, J. M., Manson, J. E., Buring, J. E., et al. (2008). Type 2 diabetes mellitus and cognitive decline in two large cohorts of community-dwelling older adults. *J. Am. Geriatr. Soc.* 56, 1028–1036. doi: 10.1111/j.1532-5415.2008.01686.x

Osness, W. H., Adrian, M., and Clak, B. (1996). *Functional Fitness Assessment for Adults Over 60 Years*, 2nd Edn. Dubuque, IA: Kendall/Hunt.

Pesce, C. (2012). Shifting the focus from quantitative to qualitative exercise characteristics in exercise and cognition research. *J. Sport Exerc. Psychol.* 34, 766–786. doi: 10.1123/jsep.34.6.766

Pesce, C., and Audiffren, M. (2011). Does physical activity switch-off switch costs? A study with younger and older athletes. *J. Sport Exerc. Psychol.* 33, 609–626. doi: 10.1123/jsep.33.5.609

Pesce, C., Capranica, L., Tessitore, A., and Figura, F. (2003). Focusing of visual attention under submaximal physical load. *Int. J. Sport Exerc. Psychol.* 1, 275–292. doi: 10.1080/1612197X.2003.9671719

Pesce, C., Cereatti, L., Casella, R., Baldari, C., and Capranica, L. (2007a). Preservation of visual attention in older expert orienteers at rest and under physical effort. *J. Sport Exerc. Psychol.* 29, 78–99.

Pesce, C., Cereatti, L., Forte, R., Crova, C., and Casella, R. (2011). Acute and chronic exercise effects on attentional control in older road cyclists. *Gerontology* 57, 121–128. doi: 10.1159/000314685

Pesce, C., Guidetti, L., Baldari, C., Tessitore, A., and Capranica, L. (2005). Visual attentional focusing in older individuals. *Gerontology* 51, 266–276. doi: 10.1159/000085123

Pesce, C., Tessitore, A., Casella, R., Pirritano, M., and Capranica, L. (2007b). Focusing of visual attention at rest and during physical exercise in soccer players. *J. Sports Sci.* 25, 1259–1270. doi: 10.1080/02640410601040085

Petersen, S. E., and Posner, M. I. (2012). The attention system of the human brain: 20 years after. *Annu. Rev. Neurosci.* 35, 73–89. doi: 10.1146/annurev-neuro-062111-150525

Posner, M. I., and Petersen, S. E. (1990). The attention system of the human brain. *Annu. Rev. Neurosci.* 13, 25–42. doi: 10.1146/annurev-neuro-062111-150525

Prakash, R. S., Voss, M. V., Erickson, K. I., and Kramer, A. F. (2015). Physical activity and cognitive vitality. *Annu. Rev. Psychol.* 66, 769–797. doi: 10.1146/annurev-psych-010814-015249

Qiu, W. Q., Price, L. L., Hibberd, P., Buell, J., Collins, L., Leins, D., et al. (2006). Executive dysfunction in homebound older people with diabetes mellitus. *J. Am. Geriatr. Soc.* 54, 496–501. doi: 10.1111/j.1532-5415.2005.00632.x

Robertson, L. C. (1996). Attentional persistence for features of hierarchical patterns. *J. Exp. Psychol. Gen.* 125, 227–249. doi: 10.1037/0096-3445.125.3.227

Rogers, R. D., and Monsell, S. (1995). Costs of a predictable switch between single cognitive tasks. *J. Exp. Psychol.* 124, 207–231. doi: 10.1037/0096-3445.124.2.207

Rucker, J. L., McDowd, J. M., and Kluding, P. M. (2012). Executive function and type 2 diabetes: putting the pieces together. *Phys. Ther.* 92, 454–462. doi: 10.2522/ptj.20100397

Ryan, A. S. (2010). Exercise in aging: its important role in mortality, obesity and insulin resistance. *Aging Health* 6, 551–563. doi: 10.2217/ahe.10.46

Saelens, B. E., and Handy, S. L. (2008). Built environment correlates of walking: a review. *Med. Sci. Sports Exerc.* 40(7 Suppl.), S550–S566. doi: 10.1249/MSS.0b013e31817c67a4

Sanabria, D., Morales, E., Luque, A., Gálvez, G., Huertas, F., and Lupiañez, J. (2011). Effects of acute aerobic exercise on exogenous spatial attention. *Psychol. Sport Exerc.* 12, 570–574. doi: 10.1016/j.psychsport.2011.04.002

Scheers, T., Philippaerts, R., and Lefevre, J. (2012). Variability in physical activity patterns as measured by the SenseWear Armband: how many days are needed? *Eur. J. Appl. Physiol.* 112, 1653–1162. doi: 10.1007/s00421-011-2131-9

Spirduso, W. W., Francis, K. L., and MacRae, P. G. (2005). "Health-related quality of life," in *Physical Dimensions of Aging*, 2nd Edn, eds W. W. Spirduso, K. L. Francis, and P. G. MacRae (Champaign, IL: Human Kinetics), 233–257.

Stillman, C. M., Cohen, J., Lehman, M. E., and Erickson, K. I. (2016). Mediators of physical activity on neurocognitive function: a review at multiple levels of analysis. *Front. Hum. Neurosci.* 10:626. doi: 10.3389/fnhum.2016.00626

Stoffer, T. H. (1993). The time course of the attentional zooming: a comparison of voluntary and involuntary allocation of attention to the levels of compound stimuli. *Psychol. Res.* 56, 189–196. doi: 10.1007/BF00572129

Stone-Romero, E. F., Alliger, G. M., and Aguinis, H. (1994). Type II error problems in the use of moderated multiple regression for the detection of moderating effects of dichotomous variables. *J. Manag.* 20, 167–178. doi: 10.1177/014920639402000109

Stone-Romero, E. F., and Anderson, L. E. (1994). Relative power of moderated multiple regression and the comparison of subgroup correlation coefficients for detecting moderating effects. *J. Appl. Psychol.* 79, 354–359. doi: 10.1037/0021-9010.79.3.354

Themanson, J. R., Hillman, C. H., and Curtin, J. J. (2006). Age and physical activity influences on action monitoring during task switching. *Neurobiol. Aging* 27, 1335–1345. doi: 10.1016/j.neurobiolaging.2005.07.002

Umegaki, H. (2014). Type 2 diabetes as a risk factor for cognitive impairment: current insights. *Clin. Interv. Aging* 9, 1011–1019. doi: 10.2147/CIA.S48926

Voelcker-Rehage, C., Godde, B., and Staudinger, U. M. (2011). Cardiovascular and coordination training differentially improve cognitive performance and neural processing in older adults. *Front. Hum. Neurosci.* 5:26. doi: 10.3389/fnhum.2011.00026

Voss, M. W., Kramer, A. F., Basak, C., Prakash, R. S., and Roberts, B. (2010). Are expert athletes 'expert' in the cognitive laboratory? A meta-analytic review of cognition and sport expertise. *Appl. Cogn. Psychol.* 24, 812–826. doi: 10.1002/acp.1588

Vossel, S., Geng, J. J., and Fink, G. R. (2014). Dorsal and ventral attention systems: distinct neural circuits but collaborative roles. *Neuroscientist* 20, 150–159. doi: 10.1177/1073858413494269

Wasylyshyn, C., Verhaeghen, P., and Sliwinski, M. J. (2011). Aging and task switching: a meta-analysis. *Psychol. Aging* 26, 15–20. doi: 10.1037/a0020912

Wild, S., Roglic, G., Green, A., Sicree, R., and King, H. (2004). Global prevalence of diabetes estimates for the year 2000 and projections for 2030. *Diabetes Care* 27, 1047–1053. doi: 10.2337/diacare.27.5.1047

World Health Organization (2007). *Steps to Health - A European Framework to Promote Physical Activity for Health.* Copenhagen: WHO Regional Office Europe.

World Health Organization (2015). *Noncommunicable Diseases.* Available at: http://www.who.int/mediacentre/factsheets/fs355/en/

Yaffe, K., Barnes, D., Nevitt, M., Lui, L. Y., and Covinsky, K. (2001). A prospective study of physical activity and cognitive decline in elderly women: women who walk. *Arch. Intern. Med.* 161, 1703–1708. doi: 10.1001/archinte.161.14.1703

Young, J., Angevaren, M., Rusted, J., and Tabet, N. (2015). Aerobic exercise to improve cognitive function in older people without known cognitive impairment. *Cochrane Database Syst. Rev.* 4:CD005381. doi: 10.1002/14651858.CD005381.pub4

Zhao, E., Tranovich, M. J., DeAngelo, R., Kontos, A. P., and Wright, V. J. (2016). Chronic exercise preserves brain function in master athletes when compared to sedentary counterparts. *Phys. Sportsmed.* 44, 8–13. doi: 10.1080/00913847.2016.1103641

Zhou, S. S., Fan, J., Lee, T. M., Wang, C. Q., and Wang, K. (2011). Age-related differences in attentional networks of alerting and executive control in young, middle-aged, and older Chinese adults. *Brain Cogn.* 75, 205–210. doi: 10.1016/j.bandc.2010.12.003

18

No Evidence that Short-Term Cognitive or Physical Training Programs or Lifestyles are Related to Changes in White Matter Integrity in Older Adults at Risk of Dementia

Patrick Fissler[1,2], Hans-Peter Müller[2], Olivia C. Küster[1,2], Daria Laptinskaya[1], Franka Thurm[3], Alexander Woll[4], Thomas Elbert[5], Jan Kassubek[2], Christine A. F. von Arnim[2] and Iris-Tatjana Kolassa[1]*

[1] Clinical and Biological Psychology, Institute of Psychology and Education, Ulm University, Ulm, Germany, [2] Department of Neurology, University Hospital Ulm, Ulm, Germany, [3] Department of Psychology, Technische Universität Dresden, Dresden, Germany, [4] Institute of Sports and Sports Science, Karlsruhe Institute of Technology, Karlsruhe, Germany, [5] Department of Psychology, University of Konstanz, Konstanz, Germany

Edited by:
Soledad Ballesteros,
National University of Distance Education, Spain

Reviewed by:
Betty M. Tijms,
VU University Medical Center, Netherlands
Joaquin Alberto Anguera,
University of California, San Francisco, USA

***Correspondence:**
Patrick Fissler
patrick.fissler@uni-ulm.de

Cognitive and physical activities can benefit cognition. However, knowledge about the neurobiological mechanisms underlying these activity-induced cognitive benefits is still limited, especially with regard to the role of white matter integrity (WMI), which is affected in cognitive aging and Alzheimer's disease. To address this knowledge gap, we investigated the immediate and long-term effects of cognitive or physical training on WMI, as well as the association between cognitive and physical lifestyles and changes in WMI over a 6-month period. Additionally, we explored whether changes in WMI underlie activity-related cognitive changes, and estimated the potential of both trainings to improve WMI by correlating training outcomes with WMI. In an observational and interventional pretest, posttest, 3-month follow-up design, we assigned 47 community-dwelling older adults at risk of dementia to 50 sessions of auditory processing and working memory training ($n = 13$), 50 sessions of cardiovascular, strength, coordination, balance and flexibility exercises ($n = 14$), or a control group ($n = 20$). We measured lifestyles trough self-reports, cognitive training skills through training performance, functional physical fitness through the Senior Fitness Test, and global cognition through a cognitive test battery. WMI was assessed via a composite score of diffusion tensor imaging-based fractional anisotropy (FA) of three regions of interest shown to be affected in aging and Alzheimer's disease: the genu of corpus callosum, the fornix, and the hippocampal cingulum. Effects for training interventions on FA outcomes, as well as associations between lifestyles and changes in FA outcomes were not significant. Additional analyses did show associations between cognitive lifestyle and global cognitive changes at the posttest and the 3-month follow-up ($\beta \geq 0.40, p \leq 0.02$) and accounting for changes in WMI did not affect these relationships. The targeted training outcomes were related to FA scores at baseline (cognitive training skills and FA composite score, $r_S = 0.68$, $p = 0.05$; functional physical fitness and fornix FA,

$r = 0.35, p = 0.03$). Overall, we found no evidence of a link between short-term physical or cognitive activities and WMI changes, despite activity-related cognitive changes in older adults at risk of dementia. However, we found positive associations between the two targeted training outcomes and WMI, hinting at a potential of long-term activities to affect WMI.

Keywords: white matter integrity, cognitive training, physical training, cognitive lifestyle, physical lifestyle, older adults, memory complaints, dementia

INTRODUCTION

An active cognitive and physical lifestyle can reduce the risk of cognitive decline (Valenzuela and Sachdev, 2006; Sofi et al., 2011; Ngandu et al., 2015) and dementia (Valenzuela and Sachdev, 2006; Hamer and Chida, 2009; Barnes and Yaffe, 2011). Cognitive training programs and video games showed cognitive benefits (Karbach and Verhaeghen, 2014; Lampit et al., 2014; Toril et al., 2014; Ballesteros et al., 2015), and first evidence indicated that cognitive training reduces the incidence of dementia over a 10-year period (Edwards et al., 2016). Similarly, physical activity has yielded promising results with regard to cognitive benefits (Smith et al., 2010; Nagamatsu et al., 2012; Kattenstroth et al., 2013).

Revealing the neurobiological mechanisms of the activity-induced prevention of cognitive decline and dementia could pave the way for an endogenous (Sale et al., 2014), personalized treatment approach (Cuthbert and Insel, 2013). By understanding the mechanisms of intervention effects, the identified neuropathological processes in a given patient can be targeted in an individualized fashion (Cuthbert and Insel, 2013). For example, cognitively impaired patients with deteriorated white matter integrity (WMI) may benefit more from an intervention that targets this microstructural impairment than a patient with the same behavioral syndrome but normal WMI.

However, our knowledge of the neurobiological mechanisms underlying the beneficial cognitive effects of an active lifestyle and training interventions is still in its infancy. Although there is initial evidence of functional and structural brain changes through cognitive and physical activity (Valenzuela et al., 2008, 2011; Erickson et al., 2011; Buschkuehl et al., 2012; Voss et al., 2012; Bennett D.A. et al., 2014; von Bastian and Oberauer, 2014; Constantinidis and Klingberg, 2016), the role of WMI in activity-related cognitive changes is largely unclear.

Cognitive and physical activity may increase WMI through activity-related myelination (Fields, 2015) that could lead to cognitive benefits. However, current evidence is inconsistent. While some studies support this mechanism for cognitive (Lövdén et al., 2010; Takeuchi et al., 2010; Engvig et al., 2011; Sagi et al., 2012; Steele et al., 2013; Salminen et al., 2016) and physical activities (Chaddock-Heyman et al., 2014; Svatkova et al., 2015), others do not (Voss et al., 2012; Chapman et al., 2013; Strenziok et al., 2014; Lampit et al., 2015). For example, Lampit et al. (2015) did not find cognitive training-induced changes in WMI, despite positive effects on global cognition, and Voss et al. (2012) did not observe positive effects on WMI following an extensive exercise program of three weekly 40-min sessions over the period of 1 year in a sample of 70 participants.

Moreover, there are four knowledge gaps in our understanding of physical and cognitive activity-related WMI changes. These comprise, first, training-induced WMI changes in tracts shown to be affected in cognitive aging and Alzheimer's disease (Head et al., 2004; Ringman et al., 2007; Madden et al., 2012; Wang et al., 2012; Kantarci, 2014; Salat, 2014), second, training-induced WMI changes in a population of older adults at risk of dementia, third, maintenance of training-induced WMI changes, and fourth, lifestyle-related WMI changes.

To address the inconsistent findings and the knowledge gaps, this study had two primary aims: First, to assess the immediate and long-term effects of cognitive and physical training programs on the integrity of tracts shown to be affected in cognitive aging and Alzheimer's disease (the genu of the corpus callosum, the fornix, and the hippocampal cingulum) in older adults at risk of dementia, and second, to investigate the relationship between cognitive and physical lifestyles and changes in WMI over the 6-month study period.

As additional analyses, we assessed the association at baseline between the two targeted training outcomes (cognitive training skills, functional physical fitness) and WMI in order to reveal the potential of training programs to affect WMI. Finally, we investigated whether changes in WMI could account for activity-related cognitive changes to understand whether changes in WMI underlie these cognitive changes.

For the cognitive training program, we used a computer-based training program targeting auditory processing and working memory that has been shown to have robust cognitive benefits (Smith et al., 2009; Zelinski et al., 2011, 2014; Bamidis et al., 2015; Shah et al., 2017). For the physical training program, we used a multimodal training regime based on a program that has previously been shown to have cognitive benefits (Thurm et al., 2011). The use of a multimodal exercise program is consistent with findings of larger cognitive benefits through combined aerobic and strength training versus aerobic exercise only (Colcombe et al., 2006; Smith et al., 2010).

With regard to our primary objectives, we hypothesized that the cognitive and physical training groups, in contrast to a passive control group, would exhibit an increase in the fractional anisotropy (FA) composite score at posttest and at the 3-month follow-up. We expected that self-reported active cognitive and physical lifestyles at baseline would be positively associated with changes in the FA composite score at both follow-ups.

MATERIALS AND METHODS

Study Design

This 10-week interventional, two-center, controlled clinical trial (Ulm and Konstanz, Germany) entailed a three-arm assessor-blinded study evaluating training- and lifestyle-related changes in WMI. This diffusion tensor imaging (DTI) study comprises a subsample of participants of the main study whose results on the cognitive outcomes have previously been reported (Küster et al., 2016). We found that the associations of an active lifestyle with cognitive changes over time were stronger than the effects of specifically designed cognitive or physical training interventions in the same period.

Participants

For inclusion in the study, participants had to be 55 or older, suffer from subjective memory complaints and either objective [Munich Verbal Learning Test (Ilmberger, 1988): average of the learning and free long-delayed recall trials below −1 *SD* of the age norm] or clinically apparent memory impairment (e.g., increased difficulty locating objects, keeping appointments, remembering conversations or events), have vision and hearing adjusted to normal, and be fluent in German. Exclusion criteria were a moderate or severe stage of dementia [Mini Mental State Examination (MMSE) < 20], changes in antidementive or antidepressive medication within 3 months prior to study initiation, a history of severe psychiatric or neurologic disorders, or physical impairment that would prevent participation in the physical training program. Participants without contraindications for magnet resonance imaging (MRI) were offered the opportunity to participate in the MRI subsample.

Subjects were recruited via newspaper articles, flyers, informative meetings at community centers, and personal contacts in the memory clinics of the University Hospital Ulm and the Reichenau Psychiatry Center in Konstanz. The study was approved by the Ethics Committees of the University of Konstanz and Ulm University, Germany. Participants gave written informed consent at screening visits before enrollment in the study.

Of the 122 individuals we screened, 65 were enrolled in the intervention study (Küster et al., 2016); of these, 47 participated in the MRI subsample and were assigned to a 10-week cognitive training group (five sessions/week, $n = 13$), a physical training group (five sessions/week, $n = 14$), or a passive control group ($n = 20$, see **Figure 1**).

The analysis included 39 participants (83% of all enrolled participants). Apart from the FA of the hippocampal cingulum, the three groups did not significantly differ in terms of demographics, FA outcomes, cognitive outcomes, lifestyles, or study-related data, even without adjusting for multiple comparisons (see **Table 1**).

Procedure

Outcome variables were assessed within 4 weeks before the 10-week intervention, within 4 weeks after the intervention, and another 3 months later to measure training and lifestyle-related changes in WMI. Due to logistic issues (e.g., limited available facilities, a highly selected study sample with more than 60% exclusions at screening, the required time commitment of participants, the limited time period between pretest and the start of the intervention, and the time slots of the physical training program), it was not possible to achieve the necessary number of included participants that allowed both randomized allocation and a sufficient number of participants to start a new group-based physical training program. To avoid any selection bias, the groups were matched in terms of age, education, gender, and MMSE. When a new physical training program started, all successfully screened participants were allocated to this group until the required number of participants was reached. During the other time periods, a minimization approach was implemented for the allocation of participants to the cognitive training and control groups in order to minimize group differences in age, gender, education, and MMSE. Neuropsychological outcome assessors were blind to the group allocation of participants. In rare cases, participants disclosed their group assignment during the neuropsychological assessment. The blinding of participants was not feasible due to the nature of the behavioral interventions.

Outcomes

MRI Analysis

Data recording

The MRI analysis was performed on 1.5 Tesla scanners at the two study centers, Ulm University (center 1, Magnetom Symphony, Siemens Medical) and the University of Konstanz (center 2, Intera, Philips Medical Systems). The DTI study protocol consisted of 2×30 gradient directions with $b = 1000$ s/mm^2 and two $b = 0$ gradient directions. At both centers, slice thickness was 2.5 mm and in-plane pixel size was 1.875 mm × 1.875 mm; 55 slices (128 pixels × 128 pixels) and 62 slices (128 pixels × 128 pixels) were recorded at center 1 and center 2, respectively. The echo time and repetition time were 28 and 3080 ms at center 1 and 70 ms and 8035 ms at center 2.

Data processing

DTI analysis was performed using the software package *Tensor Imaging and Fiber Tracking* (TIFT, Müller et al., 2007; Müller and Kassubek, 2013). For longitudinal data analysis, affine halfway linear registration (Menke et al., 2014) was employed. Pretest and posttest images were halfway-transformed, whereas follow-up images were affine transformed to the transformed pretest images. FA maps were calculated and smoothed with a Gaussian filter of 2 voxels full-width at the half maximum (FWHM, Madhyastha et al., 2014). Individualized FA templates were calculated by using FA maps of all available measurements of each individual. Based on these individualized FA templates, regions of interest (ROIs) were set. Because this processing procedure was implemented, Montreal Neurological Institute transformation was not necessary.

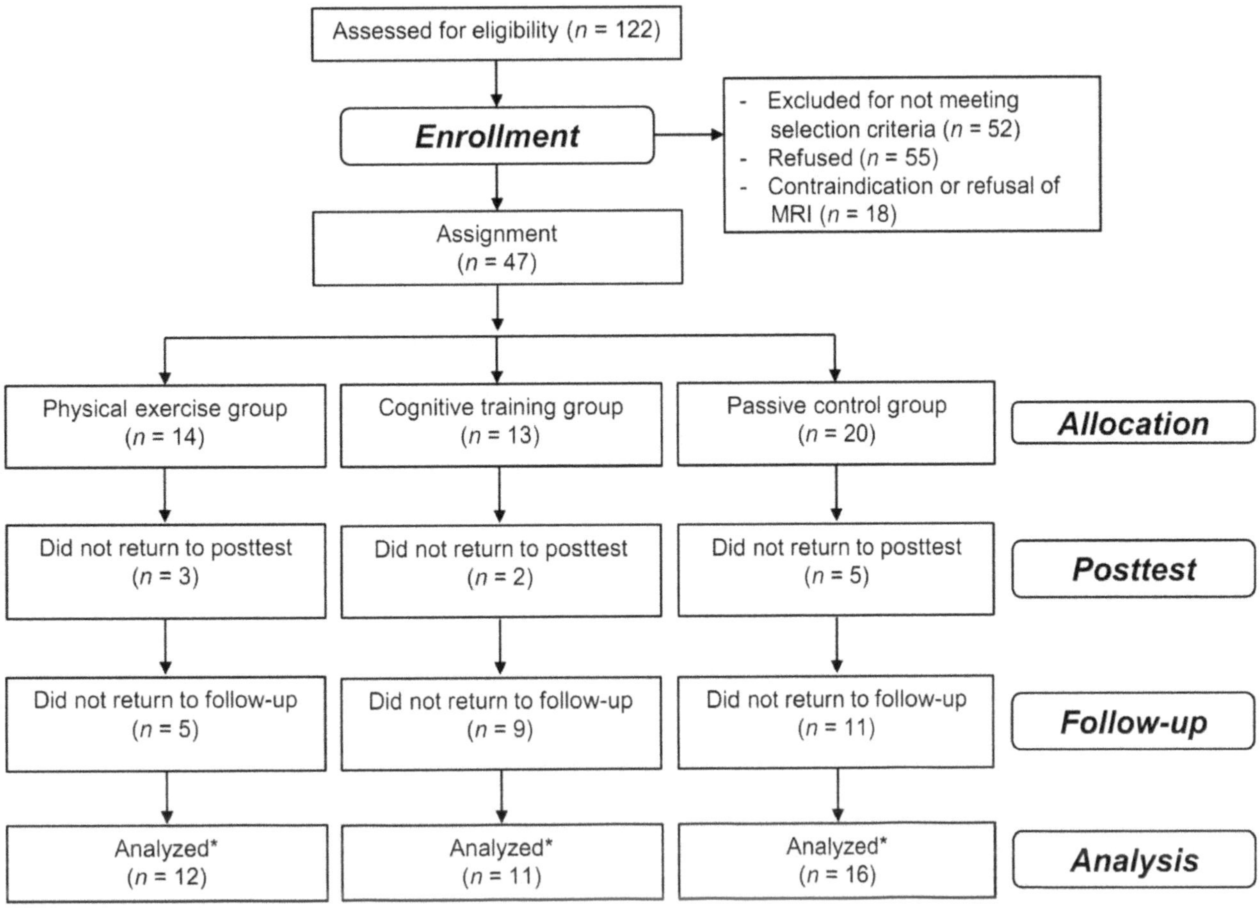

FIGURE 1 | Flow of participants. Flow of participants within the physical training, cognitive training, and passive control groups. *all participants that were assessed at least once at the posttest or at the 3-month follow up were included in the analysis using mixed-effects models that includes all time points in a single analysis without excluding participants with missing values at one time point.

Regions of Interest

Regions of interests were defined in an attempt to focus on white matter correlates of cognitive aging and Alzheimer's disease (Head et al., 2004; Ringman et al., 2007; Madden et al., 2012; Wang et al., 2012; Kantarci, 2014; Salat, 2014). To this end, the WM integrity of hippocampus-related limbic tracts and prefrontal cortex tracts were examined: the genu of the corpus callosum, the fornix and the hippocampal cingulum (see **Figure 2**). The tracts in the genu of the corpus callosum connect the two prefrontal cortices (Hofer and Frahm, 2006), and their white mater integrity has been shown to correlate with executive function (Madden et al., 2009). The fornix and the hippocampal cingulum interconnect the hippocampus with distributed brain areas; their WMI correlates with episodic memory (Bennett I.J. et al., 2014; Bennett and Stark, 2015; Ezzati et al., 2015).

Within the three ROIs (the genu of the corpus callosum, the fornix, and the hippocampal cingulum), two non-overlapping subregions were set and averaged in order to increase reliability. In the genu of the corpus callosum, the two 515-voxel subregions were set in the center of the genu of the midsagittal slice and six voxels to the right lateral direction in the center of the tract. In the fornix, the two 33-voxel subregions were set halfway between the anterior and posterior ends of the fornix in the center of the tract of the midsagittal slice and four voxels apart in the anterior-ventral direction in the center of the tract. In the hippocampal cingulum, the two 33-voxel subregions were set on the same coronal slice in the center of the tract in both hemispheres. The coronal slice was selected as the most anterior and dorsal area of the pyramidal tract. This slice - located anterior to the posterior commissure - generally cuts through the anterior pons and the midsection of the hippocampal cingulum.

The lower threshold for FA values was set to 0.2 to increase the probability that only white matter voxels would be included in the measurements (Kunimatsu et al., 2004). If fewer than 75% of all possible voxels in each subregion were above the threshold, it was lowered accordingly. Only in one participant did the threshold have to be lowered to 0.17 to include more than 75% of the fornix voxels.

TABLE 1 | Baseline characteristics of study groups.

Measure	Control group (n = 16)	Cognitive training (n = 11)	Physical training (n = 12)	p-value[a]
Demographic data				
Age, mean years ± *SD*	70.5 ± 5.0	71.4 ± 5.6	74.0 ± 5.2	0.22
Female, *n* (%)	8 (50%)	6 (55%)	9 (75%)	0.39
Education, mean years ± *SD*	15.1 ± 4.1	13.0 ± 4.2	13.9 ± 4.4	0.37
Fractional anisotropy data				
Composite score, mean FA ± *SD*	0.43 ± 0.04	0.44 ± 0.05	0.42 ± 0.04	0.40
gCC, mean FA ± *SD*	0.59 ± 0.05	0.58 ± 0.06	0.59 ± 0.06	0.85
Fornix, mean FA ± *SD*	0.37 ± 0.08	0.37 ± 0.06	0.33 ± 0.06	0.26
HC, mean FA ± *SD*	0.34 ± 0.05	0.38 ± 0.04	0.34 ± 0.04	0.05
Cognitive data				
MMSE, mean ± *SD*	28.3 ± 2.2	28.0 ± 1.7	27.8 ± 1.7	0.79
Global cognition, mean ± *SD*	−0.1 ± 1.2	0.2 ± 0.9	−0.1 ± 0.9	0.71
Executive function, mean ± *SD*	0.0 ± 1.0	0.3 ± 0.9	−0.2 ± 1.1	0.40
Episodic memory, mean ± *SD*	−0.1 ± 1.2	0.1 ± 1.0	0.1 ± 0.9	0.81
Lifestyle data				
Physical lifestyle, mean % ± *SD*	20.2 ± 8.8	20.3 ± 13.2	20.1 ± 9.2	>0.99
Cognitive lifestyle, mean % ± *SD*	43.3 ± 12.1	35.7 ± 15.9	36.3 ± 9.8	0.23
Study-related data				
Included in analysis, n/n_{group} (%)	16/20 (80%)	11/13 (85%)	12/14 (86%)	0.89

[a] *p-values of group comparisons refer to one-way ANOVA for continuous variables and to χ^2 tests for categorical variables. gCC, genu of the corpus callosum; HC, hippocampal cingulum; MMSE, Mini Mental State Examination; n, number of participants.*

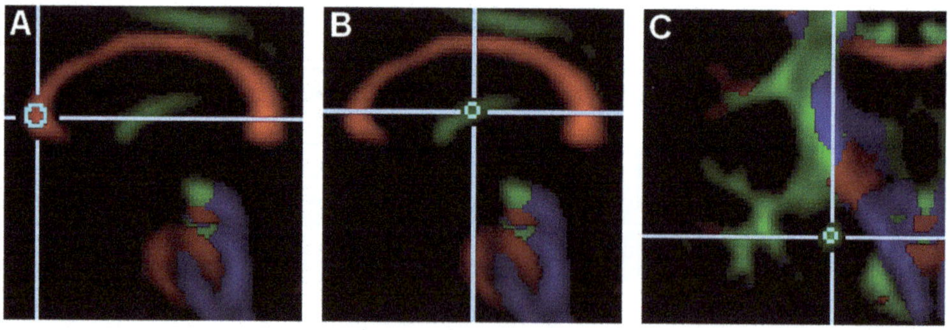

FIGURE 2 | Regions of interest. These examples depict a 515-voxel region of interest (ROI) in the genu of the corpus callosum (**A**, midsagittal slice), a 33-voxel ROI in the fornix (**B**, midsagittal slice), and a 33-voxel ROI in the left hippocampal cingulum (**C**, coronal slice).

Composite Score of WMI

A composite score of the three ROIs was constructed in order to increase statistical power by avoiding multiple comparison problems and by improving the reliability of the outcome. The composite score was calculated by averaging the FA values of the fornix, the hippocampal cingulum, and the genu of the corpus callosum.

Cognitive Outcomes

Global cognition, episodic memory, and executive functions were assessed through an extensive cognitive test battery. Principal component analysis served to construct the three composite scores (see Küster et al., 2016). The two composite scores for episodic memory and executive function represent the weighted average of the z-standardized cognitive test scores with loadings of at least $a_{ij} = 0.4$ on the respective components. The global cognition score represents the average of the two component scores.

The test battery consisted of the phonemic and semantic fluency tasks, the Trail Making Test (A and B) from the CERAD neuropsychological battery (Welsh et al., 1994), the forward and backward digit span, the digit symbol coding subtest from the Wechsler Adult Intelligence Scale-III (WAIS-III, Von Aster et al., 2006), the working-memory subtest from the Everyday Cognition Battery (Allaire and Marsiske, 1999), the free recall trial from the Alzheimer's Disease Assessment Scale – cognitive subscale (ADAS-cog, Ihl and Weyer, 1993), and the learning and free long-delayed recall trials from an adapted version of the California Verbal Learning Test (Munich Verbal Memory Test, Ilmberger, 1988).

Interventions

Cognitive Training

Participants were asked to complete a total of 50 h of computerized, home-based cognitive training within a period of 10 weeks, with five 1-h sessions per week. The training consisted of six different tasks targeting auditory processing and working memory (for details see Mahncke et al., 2006a,b; Küster et al., 2016). In each session, four different 15-min training tasks were completed. The order of the tasks varied in each session; moreover, the difficulty was adapted according to the participant's performance, and correct answers were positively reinforced. This training program was originally developed by Posit Science (San Francisco, CA, USA) and has been adapted and translated into German in a collaboration between Posit Science and the University of Konstanz. In the German version, a sound frequency discrimination task replaces the original auditory working memory task "listen and do" (see Mahncke et al., 2006b; Küster et al., 2016 for detailed training descriptions).

Physical Training

Participants were asked to attend a total of 20 sessions of a multimodal physical training program at the respective trial sites within a period of 10 weeks, with two 1-h sessions per week. The training was carried out in groups of 5–10 participants. In addition, a total of 30 sessions of a 20-min home-based physical training program was to be performed three times per week. These training sessions were documented by participants and monitored by the trainers. The multimodal training program involved aerobic, strength, coordination, balance, and flexibility elements and was designed in the form of an imaginary journey. The difficulty was adapted individually by the trainers to match the needs of participants. The structure of this training regime was based on a program that induced positive effects on cognition in a previous study on frail nursing-home residents (Thurm et al., 2011).

Passive Control Group

Wait-list control participants (controls) were asked to continue their daily life as usual and were given the opportunity to participate in one of the training programs after their follow-up assessment.

Assessment of Lifestyle

The cognitive and physical lifestyles of participants were assessed through the Community Healthy Activities Model Program for Seniors Physical Activity Questionnaire for Older Adults (CHAMPS, Stewart et al., 2001). This questionnaire describes 40 possible activities in the participants' daily life, categorized into physical activities (such as running, swimming, or bicycling) and cognitively challenging activities (such as playing card or board games, performing voluntary work, or playing a musical instrument; see Küster et al., 2016). Participants were asked to report the activities in which they had engaged in the previous four weeks. The number of completed activities was divided by the potential number of activities in each domain. These scores reflect the variety in the participants' cognitive and physical lifestyles, respectively.

Cognitive Training Skills

Cognitive training skills were measured by averaging the standardized training performance in the most frequently used cognitive training tasks: "high or low," "tell us apart," "sound replay," and "match it." Changes in cognitive training skills were measured in terms of the difference between the third and the last training session (the first two training sessions were guided by trainers). Unfortunately, the cognitive training data from two individuals were not properly stored and could not be included in the analysis.

Functional Physical Fitness

Functional physical fitness was assessed with four tasks from the Senior Fitness Test (Rikli and Jones, 2001): "chair stand," "chair sit-and-reach," "2-min step," and "8-feet up-and-go" which measure strength, flexibility, endurance, and agility, respectively. *Z*-standardized scores were averaged to create the functional physical fitness composite score.

Statistical Analyses

Statistical analyses were conducted using *R* version 3.2.1 for Windows (R Development Core Team, 2015). To assess baseline differences between the three groups, χ^2-tests and one-way analyses of variance were used for categorical variables and continuous variables, respectively.

Training- and Lifestyle-Related FA and Cognitive Changes

The effects of training interventions on WMI as well as lifestyle-related changes in WMI were assessed with linear mixed-effects models with maximum likelihood estimation (nlme package, Pinheiro et al., 2000). Group (with contrasts cognitive training vs. controls and physical training vs. controls), physical lifestyle, cognitive lifestyle, and time (with contrasts pre vs. post and pre vs. follow-up) were defined as fixed effects, and subject as the random intercept. Hypothesis-relevant effects were indicated by Group × Time, Physical Lifestyle × Time, and Cognitive Lifestyle × Time interactions. Hedges' *g* was based on the pretest standard deviation; this was calculated by the difference in change scores between (1) the physical training group vs. the control group and (2) the cognitive training group vs. the control group divided by the pooled baseline standard deviation corrected for bias in small samples (Lakens, 2013). Positive values indicate beneficial effects of the intervention. Standardized regression coefficients of cognitive and physical lifestyles predicting changes in outcomes were used as effect size measure for lifestyle-related outcome changes.

The Potential of the Two Training Programs to Affect White Matter Integrity

To assess the potential of the cognitive and physical training programs to improve hippocampus-related and prefrontal WMI, we performed two analyses: (1) at pretest, we assessed the cross-sectional correlations of cognitive training skills and functional physical fitness with FA and cognitive outcomes, and (2) we investigated the improvement in cognitive training skills and functional physical fitness within the respective training groups. For the analyses of cognitive training skills, we used non-parametric procedures (Spearman's rank correlation and Wilcoxon signed rank test for paired differences) due to the small sample size ($n = 9$).

Reliability of FA Scores

Retest-reliability was assessed through correlations between pretest and posttest scores within the total study sample including all three groups.

RESULTS

Effects of Cognitive and Physical Training on WMI and Cognition

We did not find a significant influence of the cognitive or physical training program on WMI compared to the control group, neither at the posttest (all *ps* $\geq$ 0.18 before adjustment of multiple comparisons; Hedges' *gs* $\leq$ 0.25) nor at the 3-month follow-up (all *ps* $\geq$ 0.16; Hedges' *gs* $\leq$ 0.31). Hedges' *gs* of the FA composite score were −0.09, 95% CI [−0.43, 0.22] at posttest and −0.14, 95% CI [−0.90, 0.57] at the 3-month follow-up for the cognitive training, and 0.03, 95% CI [−0.41, 0.47] at posttest and −0.18, 95% CI [−0.79, 0.40] at the 3-month follow-up for the physical training (see **Table 2**).

Likewise, we did not find a significant impact of both training programs on global cognition compared to the control group, neither at the posttest (all *ps* $\geq$ 0.09; Hedges' *gs* $\leq$ −0.16) nor at the 3-month follow-up (all *ps* $\geq$ 0.12; Hedges' *gs* $\leq$ −0.12; see **Table 2**).

Cognitive and Physical Lifestyle-Related Changes in WMI and Cognition

We did not find significant associations between self-reported cognitive and physical lifestyles at baseline and changes in WMI, neither at the posttest (all *ps* $\geq$ 0.08 before adjustment of multiple comparisons; all βs $\leq$ 0.34) nor at the 3-month follow-up (all *ps* $\geq$ 0.31 before adjustment of multiple comparisons; all βs $\leq$ 0.20). Effect sizes for the FA composite score were $\beta = 0.20$, 95% CI [−0.16, 0.56] at the posttest and $\beta = -0.04$, 95% CI [−0.54, 0.45] at the 3-month follow-up with respect to cognitive lifestyle, and $\beta = -0.04$, 95% CI [−0.40, 0.32] at the posttest and $\beta = 0.15$, 95% CI [−0.34, 0.64] at the 3-month follow-up with respect to physical lifestyle (see **Table 3**).

Despite the lack of significant lifestyle-related FA changes, we found an association between cognitive lifestyle and changes in both global cognition and episodic memory from the pretest to the posttest and to the 3-month follow-up (all *ps* $\leq$ 0.02, all βs $\geq$ 0.40; see **Figure 3** and **Table 3**).

Additional Analyses

The Potential of the Two Training Programs to Affect White Matter Integrity

Additional analyses showed that cognitive training skills at the start of the program were correlated with the FA composite score, $r_s = 0.68$, $p = 0.05$, indicating the potential of the cognitive training program to affect WMI and the fact that engagement in cognitive training taps the neural connections of interest (see **Figure 4**). Associations between the various ROIs and the cognitive training skills were similar, with medium to large effect sizes: fornix, $r_s = 0.50$, $p = 0.18$; hippocampal cingulum, $r_s = 0.33$, $p = 0.39$; genu of the corpus callosum, $r_s = 0.60$; $p = 0.01$.

In the cognitive training group, we found a significant increase in cognitive training skills over the training period, with a very large effect size, $g = 1.68$, $p = 0.008$. Performance changes in all four training tasks revealed medium to very large effect sizes: "match it," $g = 1.47$, $p = 0.02$; "sound replay," $g = 0.52$, $p = 0.20$; "high or low," $g = 0.89$, $p = 0.008$; "tell us apart," $g = 0.95$, $p = 0.10$.

Functional physical fitness was marginally significantly associated with the FA composite score, $r = 0.28$, $p = 0.08$, and significantly related to the fornix FA, $r = 0.35$, $p = 0.03$ (see **Figure 5**) indicating that interventions that target physical fitness have the potential to affect WMI.

In the physical training group, we found a significant increase in functional physical fitness over the study period, $p = 0.02$. This increase was marginally significant at the posttest, $\beta = 0.51$, $p = 0.07$, and significant at the 3-month follow-up, $\beta = 0.88$, $p = 0.007$.

Associations between Changes in Targeted Training Outcomes and FA Changes

Changes in cognitive training skills were not associated with changes in the FA composite score, $r_s = -0.27$, $p = 0.49$, or in global cognition, $r_s = 0.20$, $p = 0.61$. Likewise, changes in functional physical fitness did not correlate with changes in the FA composite score at posttest, $r = -0.19$, $p = 0.28$, or at follow-up, $r = 0.01$, $p = 0.96$, nor in global cognition at posttest, $r = -0.10$, $p = 0.58$, or at follow-up, $r = -0.14$, $p = 0.54$.

Reliability of FA Measures

Retest-reliability between pretest and posttest was high for the composite FA score, $r = 0.91$, and ranged from $r = 0.92$ for the genu of the corpus callosum to $r = 0.91$ for the fornix and $r = 0.80$ for the hippocampal cingulum.

DISCUSSION

We found no evidence of an effect of short-term cognitive or physical training programs on WMI in regions that have previously been shown to be affected in cognitive aging and Alzheimer's disease (the genu of the corpus callosum, the fornix, and the hippocampal cingulum) in a sample of older adults at risk of dementia (Head et al., 2004; Ringman et al., 2007; Madden et al., 2012; Wang et al., 2012; Kantarci, 2014; Salat,

TABLE 2 | Effects of training interventions.

Measure	Control group ($n = 16$)	Cognitive training ($n = 11$)			Physical training ($n = 12$)		
Time point	**Change (95% CI)**	**Change (95% CI)**	p^a	g^b	**Change (95% CI)**	p^a	g^b
Composite scores							
FA composite							
Posttest	0.0004 (−0.010 to 0.011)	−0.004 (−0.012 to 0.004)	0.57	−0.09	0.001 (−0.013 to 0.016)	0.85	0.03
3-month FU	0.0001 (−0.018 to 0.018)	−0.006 (−0.039 to 0.026)	0.41	−0.14	−0.007 (−0.023 to 0.008)	0.49	−0.18
Global cognition							
Posttest	0.53 (0.34 to 0.72)	0.35 (0.06 to 0.65)	0.32	−0.16	0.23 (−0.07 to 0.53)	0.09	−0.27
3-month FU	1.28 (1.00 to 1.56)	0.91 (0.00 to 1.81)	0.12	−0.33	1.14 (0.63 to 1.65)	0.61	−0.12
Specific scores							
gCC							
Posttest	0.013 (0.001 to 0.025)	−0.001 (−0.011 to 0.009)	0.18	−0.25	0.002 (−0.019 to 0.024)	0.45	−0.19
3-month FU	0.000 (−0.016 to 0.016)	0.013 (−0.001 to 0.027)	0.50	0.22	−0.017 (−0.043 to 0.009)	0.16	−0.29
Fornix							
Posttest	−0.018 (−0.034 to −0.002)	−0.003 (−0.022 to 0.016)	0.23	0.21	0.001 (−0.018 to 0.019)	0.18	0.25
3-month FU	−0.008 (−0.042 to 0.027)	−0.030 (−0.073 to 0.013)	0.17	−0.29	0.016 (−0.017 to 0.049)	0.25	0.31
HC							
Posttest	0.006 (−0.011 to 0.024)	−0.007 (−0.018 to 0.004)	0.23	−0.28	0.001 (−0.022 to 0.024)	0.58	−0.11
3-month FU	0.008 (−0.020 to 0.036)	−0.003 (−0.063 to 0.058)	0.54	−0.20	−0.020 (−0.038 to −0.003)	0.18	−0.59
Executive function							
Posttest	0.39 (0.14 to 0.65)	0.20 (−0.00 to 0.41)	0.34	−0.19	0.30 (−0.09 to 0.69)	0.63	−0.09
3-month FU	0.39 (−0.01 to 0.79)	−0.09 (−0.86 to 0.67)	0.04	−0.46	0.35 (−0.23 to 0.94)	0.65	−0.03
Episodic memory							
Posttest	0.54 (0.28 to 0.81)	0.41 (0.01 to 0.82)	0.62	−0.12	0.12 (−0.27 to 0.52)	0.10	−0.39
3-month FU	1.82 (1.40 to 2.24)	1.62 (0.23 to 3.01)	0.64	−0.17	1.61 (0.86 to 2.37)	0.70	−0.18

[a]*p-value of the Group [Control vs. Cognitive/Physical Training] × Session [pre vs. post and pre vs. 3-month FU] interaction, before adjustment for multiple comparisons.*
[b]*Hedges' g: change in cognitive/physical training minus change in control group divided by the pooled baseline standard deviation corrected for bias in small samples. Positive values indicate beneficial effects of the interventions. gCC, genu of the corpus callosum; FA, fractional anisotropy; FU, follow-up; FX, fornix; HC, hippocampal cingulum; MMSE, Mini Mental State Examination; n, number of participants.*

2014). The estimated effect sizes of the two training programs at the posttest were not of relevance (Hedges' $g < 0.1$), and the two 95% confidence intervals did not include medium effects (Hedges' $g < 0.5$).

The lack of training-induced changes in FA is consistent with several previous findings. For example, for the cognitive training program used in our study, Strenziok et al. (2014) did not find any effect on FA scores compared to two other video games. Moreover, in one of the largest studies in the field, Voss et al. (2012) did not show significant FA increases in a 1-year aerobic fitness training intervention compared to a stretching control intervention.

It is worth to note that physical training has been shown to increase FA in fiber tracts implicated in motor functioning such as the corticospinal tract (Svatkova et al., 2015). These tracts were not of interest in this study and potential effects could not be detected in our ROI analysis.

The lack of a cognitive training effect contrasts with three studies that found significant effects of different working memory training programs on regions of the anterior part of the corpus callosum (Lövdén et al., 2010; Takeuchi et al., 2010; Salminen et al., 2016). These inconsistent results might be explained by the working memory training and by the study population. In contrast to the other studies our working memory training did not include an updating component and our sample comprised older adults at risk of dementia vs. younger adults in Takeuchi et al. (2010) and Salminen et al. (2016), and healthy older adults in Lövdén et al. (2010).

The associations between cognitive training skills and the FA composite, as well as between functional physical fitness with the fornix FA hint at the potential of cognitive and physical activities to improve WMI in these tracts. Correlations between these two training outcomes and FA transfer outcomes allow us to estimate the maximal transfer gains given a specific increase in the training outcomes (Jaeggi et al., 2010; Baniqued et al., 2013; Rode et al., 2014). The higher the association, the higher is the transfer potential. Therefore, long-term rather than short-term training programs and lifestyles that induce larger effects on training outcomes may significantly increase the targeted white matter tracts.

Self-reported lifestyles at baseline were not associated with changes in WMI. In addition, positive associations between cognitive lifestyle and changes in global cognition and episodic memory were not altered after accounting for WMI. To our knowledge, there has been no other study that has assessed the relationship between lifestyles and changes in WMI. Therefore, this is initial evidence that other brain mechanisms than changes

TABLE 3 | Associations with cognitive and physical lifestyles.

Measures	Cognitive lifestyle (n = 39)		Physical lifestyle (n = 39)	
Time point	β[a] (95% CI)	p-value[b]	β[a] (95% CI)	p-value[c]
Composite scores				
FA composite				
Posttest	0.20 (− 0.16 to 0.56)	0.27	−0.04 (− 0.40 to 0.32)	0.80
3-month FU	−0.04 (− 0.54 to 0.45)	0.97	0.15 (− 0.34 to 0.64)	0.69
Global cognition				
Posttest	0.51 (0.23 to 0.80)	0.004	0.12 (− 0.17 to 0.41)	0.49
3-month FU	0.40 (− 0.01 to 0.82)	0.01	0.12 (− 0.29 to 0.54)	0.71
Specific scores				
gCC				
Posttest	0.34 (− 0.00 to 0.69)	0.08	0.02 (− 0.32 to 0.36)	0.92
3-month FU	−0.20 (− 0.68 to 0.29)	0.31	0.12 (− 0.37 to 0.61)	0.71
Fornix				
Posttest	−0.10 (− 0.46 to 0.26)	0.63	0.19 (− 0.17 to 0.55)	0.36
3-month FU	−0.06 (− 0.56 to 0.43)	0.95	0.15 (− 0.34 to 0.64)	0.74
HC				
Posttest	0.18 (− 0.17 to 0.53)	0.30	−0.28 (− 0.64 to 0.07)	0.13
3-month FU	0.16 (− 0.32 to 0.66)	0.33	−0.01 (− 0.50 to 0.48)	0.92
Executive function				
Posttest	0.26 (− 0.08 to 0.60)	0.16	−0.08 (− 0.42 to 0.26)	0.67
3-month FU	0.08 (− 0.39 to 0.54)	0.21	−0.02 (− 0.49 to 0.44)	0.77
Episodic memory				
Posttest	0.45 (0.15 to 0.74)	0.02	0.21 (− 0.09 to 0.50)	0.28
3-month FU	0.41 (0.00 to 0.82)	0.02	0.16 (− 0.25 to 0.57)	0.57

[a]βs represent the standardized regression coefficients of cognitive and physical lifestyles predicting changes in outcomes. [b]p-value of the Cognitive Lifestyle × Session [pre vs. post and pre vs. 3-month FU] interaction. [c]p-value of the Physical Lifestyle × Session [pre vs. post and pre vs. 3-month FU] interaction. gCC, genu of the corpus callosum; FA, fractional anisotropy; FU, follow-up; FX, fornix; HC, hippocampal cingulum; MMSE, Mini Mental State Examination; n, number of participants.

in WMI do underlie lifestyle-related cognitive changes in older adults at risk of dementia.

Limitations

Our use of ROI analyses rather than whole brain-based approaches means that any changes in other brain regions would not be detected. However, in this sample of older adults at risk of dementia, we were particularly interested in the white matter tracts that are affected in cognitive aging and Alzheimer's disease. Importantly, by using ROIs, we limited the problems of alpha-error inflation and a reduction in power through multiple comparisons – an issue that is particularly important in analyses with limited sample sizes. Other limitations include the lack of randomization, which was not feasible due to logistic issues (see above). However, we used a minimization approach instead to prevent group differences in participants' characteristics from inducing bias. The limited sample size likely impeded the detection of very small effects. However, the sample size was sufficient to detect lifestyle-related cognitive changes and to reveal associations between WMI and both cognitive training skills and functional physical fitness. In addition, the confidence intervals of the training effects immediately after the training period were lower than a Hedges' g of 0.5, suggesting that effects of medium size are unlikely. Finally, the lack of a lifestyle intervention prevented a causal inference regarding associations between lifestyles and FA changes. However, before implementing cost-intensive experimental designs, it is a reasonable strategy to initially employ observational designs.

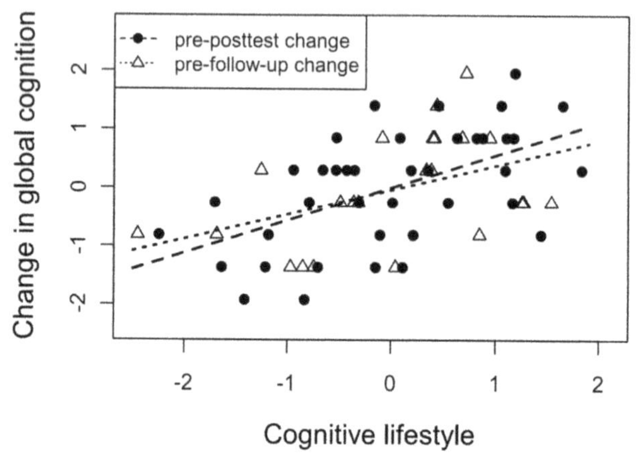

FIGURE 3 | Cognitive lifestyle as a predictor of cognitive change. Association between self-reported cognitive lifestyle at baseline and changes in global cognition from pretest to posttest (β = 0.51, p = 0.004) and from pretest to 3-month follow-up (β = 0.40, p = 0.01).

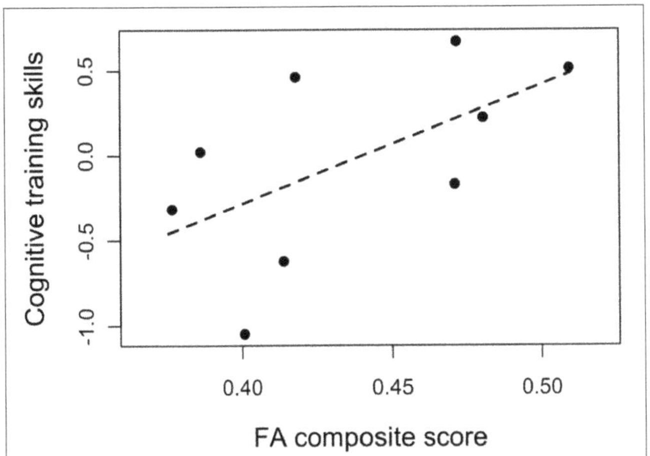

FIGURE 4 | The potential of the cognitive training program to affect white matter integrity. Association between cognitive training skills at the beginning of the training and FA composite score at baseline ($r_S = 0.68$, $p = 0.05$). The cognitive training data from two individuals were not properly stored and could not be included in the analysis.

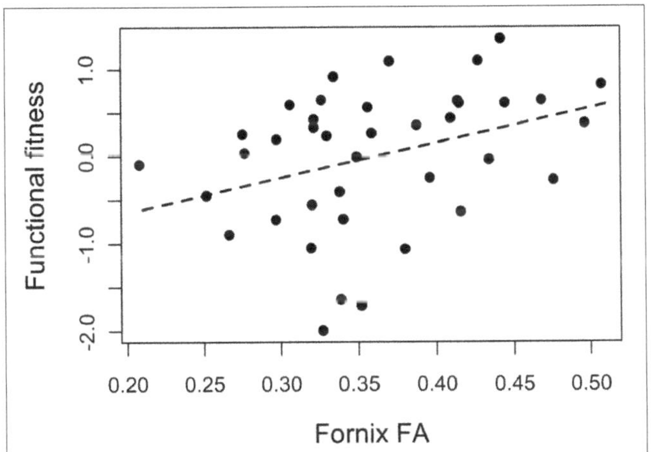

FIGURE 5 | The potential of the physical training program to affect white matter integrity. Association between functional physical fitness and fornix FA at baseline ($r = 0.35$, $p = 0.03$).

Future Perspectives

Future studies should use larger samples to increase the probability of finding small effect sizes; moreover, they should lengthen the training periods to enhance the potential to induce larger effects. In addition, little is known about the time course and maintenance of activity-induced white matter changes, suggesting that future studies should implement multiple assessments during the training regime and after the training period. Activity-related white matter changes may be differential for specific populations; thus, younger participants without cognitive impairments may profit more than older adults at risk of dementia. Future meta-analyses should assess these potential moderators. Interventional studies have only rarely reported the correlation of training outcomes with potential neurobiological mechanisms and have neglected the relation between cognitive and neurobiological changes. Future interventional studies should include these analyses to allow a better understanding of the mediating role of WMI for cognitive benefits. Finally, to our knowledge, cognitive and physical lifestyle-related changes in WMI have not yet been reported. Large-scale studies investigating this association should be conducted as a first step to explore the role of active cognitive and physical lifestyles for WMI.

Conclusion

First, we found no evidence that short-term cognitive and physical training programs do affect the integrity of hippocampus-related and prefrontal white matter tracts in older adults at risk of dementia. Second, we provide first evidence that WMI changes do not underlie the positive association between a cognitive lifestyle and cognitive change. However, as the two training outcomes (cognitive training skills and functional physical fitness) were related to WMI, engagement in long-term cognitive and physical activities might have the potential to affect WMI.

AUTHOR CONTRIBUTIONS

PF contributed to study conception and design, organized study procedures and acquired data, analyzed and interpreted data, and wrote the first draft of the manuscript as well as the paper. H-PM designed the MRI protocol, supervised the DTI analysis, was involved in the interpretation of the imaging results, and critically revised the manuscript for intellectual content. OK and DL contributed to study conception and design, organized study procedures and acquired data, contributed to the data analysis and interpretation of results, and critically revised the manuscript for intellectual content. FT contributed to study conception and design, organized study procedures, acquired data, and critically revised the manuscript for intellectual content. AW designed the physical training program and revised the manuscript. TE contributed to study conception and design and critically revised the manuscript for intellectual content. JK designed the MRI protocol, supervised the DTI analysis, was involved in the interpretation of the imaging results, and critically revised the manuscript for intellectual content. CvA and I-TK conceptualized the study, obtained funding, supervised all phases of the study as principle investigators, and critically revised the manuscript for intellectual content. All authors read and approved the final manuscript.

ACKNOWLEDGMENTS

We thank Anita Stewart for the adaptation of the English CHAMPS questionnaire into German, Claire Bacher for

English proofreading, and Rosine Gröschel, Nelli Hirschauer, Jens Kalchthaler, Anne Korzowski, Claudia Massau, Dörte Polivka, Florentine Jurisch, and Christina Schaldecker for support in subject recruitment, data acquisition, and training implementation.

AVAILABILITY OF DATA AND MATERIALS

Data will be made available upon request. The participants did not approve the unrestricted publication of the data in their informed consents, as this option was not common at the time.

ETHICS STATEMENT

This study was carried out in accordance with the recommendations of the Ethics Committees of the University of Konstanz and Ulm University with written informed consent from all subjects. All subjects gave written informed consent in accordance with the Declaration of Helsinki. The protocol was approved by the Ethics Committees of the University of Konstanz and Ulm University, Germany.

REFERENCES

Allaire, J., and Marsiske, M. (1999). Everyday cognition: age and intellectual ability correlates. *Psychol. Aging* 14, 627–644. doi: 10.1037/0882-7974.14.4.627

Ballesteros, S., Kraft, E., Santana, S., and Tziraki, C. (2015). Maintaining older brain functionality: a targeted review. *Neurosci. Biobehav. Rev.* 55, 453–477. doi: 10.1016/j.neubiorev.2015.06.008

Bamidis, P. D., Fissler, P., Papageorgiou, S. G., Zilidou, V., Konstantinidis, E. I., Billis, A. S., et al. (2015). Gains in cognition through combined cognitive and physical training: the role of training dosage and severity of neurocognitive disorder. *Front. Aging Neurosci.* 7:152. doi: 10.3389/fnagi.2015.00152

Baniqued, P. L., Lee, H., Voss, M. W., Basak, C., Cosman, J. D., DeSouza, S., et al. (2013). Selling points: What cognitive abilities are tapped by casual video games? *Acta psychol.* 142, 74–86. doi: 10.1016/j.actpsy.2012.11.009

Barnes, D. E., and Yaffe, K. (2011). The projected effect of risk factor reduction on Alzheimer's disease prevalence. *Lancet Neurol.* 10, 819–828. doi: 10.1016/S1474-4422(11)70072-2

Bennett, D. A., Arnold, S. E., Valenzuela, M. J., Brayne, C., and Schneider, J. A. (2014). Cognitive and social lifestyle: links with neuropathology and cognition in late life. *Acta Neuropathol.* 127, 137–150. doi: 10.1007/s00401-013-1226-2

Bennett, I. J., Huffman, D. J., and Stark, C. E. (2014). Limbic tract integrity contributes to pattern separation performance across the lifespan. *Cereb. Cortex* 25, 2988–2999. doi: 10.1093/cercor/bhu093

Bennett, I. J., and Stark, C. E. L. (2015). Mnemonic discrimination relates to perforant path integrity: an ultra-high resolution diffusion tensor imaging study. *Neurobiol. Learn. Mem.* 129, 107–112. doi: 10.1016/j.nlm.2015.06.014

Buschkuehl, M., Jaeggi, S. M., and Jonides, J. (2012). Neuronal effects following working memory training. *Dev. Cogn. Neurosci.* 2(Suppl. 1), S167–S179. doi: 10.1016/j.dcn.2011.10.001

Chaddock-Heyman, L., Erickson, K. I., Holtrop, J., Voss, M. W., Pontifex, M. B., Raine, L., et al. (2014). Aerobic fitness is associated with greater white matter integrity in children. *Front. Hum. Neurosci.* 8:584. doi: 10.3389/fnhum.2014.00584

Chapman, S. B., Aslan, S., Spence, J. S., Hart, J. J., Bartz, E. K., Didehbani, N., et al. (2013). Neural mechanisms of brain plasticity with complex cognitive training in healthy seniors. *Cereb. Cortex* 25, 396–405. doi: 10.1093/cercor/bht234

Colcombe, S. J., Erickson, K. I., Scalf, P. E., Kim, J. S., Prakash, R., McAuley, E., et al. (2006). Aerobic exercise training increases brain volume in aging humans. *J. Gerontol. A Biol. Sci. Med. Sci.* 61, 1166–1170. doi: 10.1093/gerona/61.11.1166

Constantinidis, C., and Klingberg, T. (2016). The neuroscience of working memory capacity and training. *Nat. Rev. Neurosci.* 17, 438–449. doi: 10.1038/nrn.2016.43

Cuthbert, B. N., and Insel, T. R. (2013). Toward the future of psychiatric diagnosis: the seven pillars of RDoC. *BMC Med.* 11:126. doi: 10.1186/1741-7015-11-126

Edwards, J. D., Xu, H., Clark, D. O., Ross, L. A., and Unverzagt, F. W. (2016). "The ACTIVE study: what we have learned and what is next? Cognitive training reduces incident dementia across ten years," in *Proceedings of the Alzheimer's Association International Conference 2016*, Toronto, ON. doi: 10.1016/j.jalz.2016.06.373

Engvig, A., Fjell, A. M., Westlye, L. T., Moberget, T., Sundseth, Ø, Larsen, V. A., et al. (2011). Memory training impacts short term changes in aging white matter: a longitudinal diffusion tensor imaging study. *Hum. Brain Mapp.* 33, 2390–2406. doi: 10.1002/hbm.21370

Erickson, K. I., Voss, M. W., Prakash, R. S., Basak, C., Szabo, A., Chaddock, L., et al. (2011). Exercise training increases size of hippocampus and improves memory. *Proc. Natl. Acad. Sci. U.S.A.* 108, 3017–3022. doi: 10.1073/pnas.1015950108

Ezzati, A., Katz, M., Lipton, M., Zimmerman, M., and Lipton, R. (2015). Hippocampal volume and cingulum bundle fractional anisotropy are independently associated with verbal memory in older adults. *Brain Imaging Behav.* 10, 652–659. doi: 10.1007/s11682-015-9452-y

Fields, R. D. (2015). A new mechanism of nervous system plasticity: activity-dependent myelination. *Nat. Rev. Neurosci.* 16, 756–767. doi: 10.1038/nrn4023

Hamer, M., and Chida, Y. (2009). Physical activity and risk of neurodegenerative disease: a systematic review of prospective evidence. *Psychol. Med.* 39, 3–11. doi: 10.1017/S0033291708003681

Head, D., Buckner, R. L., Shimony, J. S., Williams, L. E., Akbudak, E., Conturo, T. E., et al. (2004). Differential vulnerability of anterior white matter in nondemented aging with minimal acceleration in dementia of the Alzheimer type: evidence from diffusion tensor imaging. *Cereb. Cortex* 14, 410–423. doi: 10.1093/cercor/bhh003

Hofer, S., and Frahm, J. (2006). Topography of the human corpus callosum revisited—comprehensive fiber tractography using diffusion tensor magnetic resonance imaging. *Neuroimage* 32, 989–994. doi: 10.1016/j.neuroimage.2006.05.044

Ihl, R., and Weyer, G. (1993). *Die Alzheimer Disease Assessment Scale (ADAS).* Weinheim: Beltz Test.

Ilmberger, J. (1988). *Münchner Verbaler Gedächtnistest.* München: Institut für Medizinische Psychologie.

Jaeggi, S. M., Studer-Luethi, B., Buschkuehl, M., Su, Y. F., Jonides, J., and Perrig, W. J. (2010). The relationship between n-back performance and matrix reasoning – implications for training and transfer. *Intelligence* 38, 625–635. doi: 10.1016/j.intell.2010.09.001

Kantarci, K. (2014). Fractional anisotropy of the fornix and hippocampal atrophy in Alzheimer's disease. *Front. Aging Neurosci.* 6:316. doi: 10.3389/fnagi.2014.00316

Karbach, J., and Verhaeghen, P. (2014). Making working memory work: a meta-analysis of executive-control and working memory training in older adults. *Psychol. Sci.* 25, 2027–2037. doi: 10.1177/0956797614548725

Kattenstroth, J.-C., Kalisch, T., Holt, S., Tegenthoff, M., and Dinse, H. R. (2013). Six months of dance intervention enhances postural, sensorimotor, and cognitive performance in elderly without affecting cardio-respiratory functions. *Front. Aging Neurosci.* 5:5. doi: 10.3389/fnagi.2013.00005

Kunimatsu, A., Aoki, S., Masutani, Y., Abe, O., Hayashi, N., Mori, H., et al. (2004). The optimal trackability threshold of fractional anisotropy for diffusion tensor tractography of the corticospinal tract. *Magn. Reson. Med. Sci.* 3, 11–17. doi: 10.2463/mrms.3.11

Küster, O. C., Fissler, P., Laptinskaya, D., Thurm, F., Scharpf, A., Woll, A., et al. (2016). Cognitive change is more positively associated with an active lifestyle than with training interventions in older adults at risk of dementia: a controlled interventional clinical trial. *BMC Psychiatry* 16:315. doi: 10.1186/s12888-016-1018-z

Lakens, D. (2013). Calculating and reporting effect sizes to facilitate cumulative science: a practical primer for *t*-tests and ANOVAs. *Front. Psychol.* 4:863. doi: 10.3389/fpsyg.2013.00863

Lampit, A., Hallock, H., Suo, C., Naismith, S. L., and Valenzuela, M. (2015). Cognitive training-induced short-term functional and long-term structural plastic change is related to gains in global cognition in healthy older adults: a pilot study. *Front. Aging Neurosci.* 7:14. doi: 10.3389/fnagi.2015.00014

Lampit, A., Hallock, H., and Valenzuela, M. (2014). Computerized cognitive training in cognitively healthy older adults: a systematic review and meta-analysis of effect modifiers. *PLoS Med.* 11:e1001756. doi: 10.1371/journal.pmed.1001756

Lövdén, M., Bodammer, N. C., Kühn, S., Kaufmann, J., Schütze, H., Tempelmann, C., et al. (2010). Experience-dependent plasticity of white-matter microstructure extends into old age. *Neuropsychologia* 48, 3878–3883. doi: 10.1016/j.neuropsychologia.2010.08.026

Madden, D. J., Bennett, I. J., Burzynska, A., Potter, G. G., Chen, N.-K., and Song, A. W. (2012). Diffusion tensor imaging of cerebral white matter integrity in cognitive aging. *Biochim. Biophys. Acta* 1822, 386–400. doi: 10.1016/j.bbadis.2011.08.003

Madden, D. J., Spaniol, J., Costello, M. C., Bucur, B., White, L. E., Cabeza, R., et al. (2009). Cerebral white matter integrity mediates adult age differences in cognitive performance. *J. Cogn. Neurosci.* 21, 289–302. doi: 10.1162/jocn.2009.21047

Madhyastha, T., Mérillat, S., Hirsiger, S., Bezzola, L., Liem, F., Grabowski, T., et al. (2014). Longitudinal reliability of tract-based spatial statistics in diffusion tensor imaging. *Hum. Brain Mapp.* 35, 4544–4555. doi: 10.1002/hbm.22493

Mahncke, H. W., Bronstone, A., and Merzenich, M. M. (2006a). Brain plasticity and functional losses in the aged: scientific bases for a novel intervention. *Prog. Brain Res.* 157, 81–109.

Mahncke, H. W., Connor, B. B., Appelman, J., Ahsanuddin, O. N., Hardy, J. L., Wood, R. A., et al. (2006b). Memory enhancement in healthy older adults using a brain plasticity-based training program: a randomized, controlled study. *Proc. Natl. Acad. Sci. U.S.A.* 103, 12523–12528.

Menke, R. A., Korner, S., Filippini, N., Douaud, G., Knight, S., Talbot, K., et al. (2014). Widespread grey matter pathology dominates the longitudinal cerebral MRI and clinical landscape of amyotrophic lateral sclerosis. *Brain* 137(Pt 9), 2546–2555. doi: 10.1093/brain/awu162

Müller, H. P., and Kassubek, J. (2013). Diffusion tensor magnetic resonance imaging in the analysis of neurodegenerative diseases. *J. Vis. Exp.* 77:50427. doi: 10.3791/50427

Müller, H. P., Unrath, A., Ludolph, A. C., and Kassubek, J. (2007). Preservation of diffusion tensor properties during spatial normalization by use of tensor imaging and fibre tracking on a normal brain database. *Phys. Med. Biol.* 52, N99–N109. doi: 10.1088/0031-9155/52/6/n01

Nagamatsu, L. S., Handy, T. C., Hsu, C. L., Voss, M., and Liu-Ambrose, T. (2012). Resistance training promotes cognitive and functional brain plasticity in seniors with probable mild cognitive impairment. *Arch. Intern. Med.* 172, 666–668. doi: 10.1001/archinternmed.2012.379

Ngandu, T., Lehtisalo, J., Solomon, A., Levälahti, E., Ahtiluoto, S., Antikainen, R., et al. (2015). A 2 year multidomain intervention of diet, exercise, cognitive training, and vascular risk monitoring versus control to prevent cognitive decline in at-risk elderly people (FINGER): a randomised controlled trial. *Lancet* 385, 2255–2263. doi: 10.1016/S0140-6736(15)60461-5

Pinheiro, J., Bates, D., DebRoy, S., Sarkar, D., and R Development Core Team (2000). *nlme: Linear and Nonlinear Mixed Effects Models. R Package Version 3.1-97.* Available at: http://CRAN.R-project.org/package=nlme

R Development Core Team (2015). *R: A Language and Environment for Statistical Computing.* Vienna: R Foundation for Statistical Computing.

Rikli, R. E., and Jones, C. J. (2001). *Senior Fitness Test Manual.* Champaign, IL: Human Kinetics.

Ringman, J. M., O'Neill, J., Geschwind, D., Medina, L., Apostolova, L. G., Rodriguez, Y., et al. (2007). Diffusion tensor imaging in preclinical and presymptomatic carriers of familial Alzheimer's disease mutations. *Brain* 130, 1767–1776. doi: 10.1093/brain/awm102

Rode, C., Robson, R., Purviance, A., Geary, D. C., and Mayr, U. (2014). Is working memory training effective? A study in a school setting. *PLoS ONE* 9:e104796. doi: 10.1371/journal.pone.0104796

Sagi, Y., Tavor, I., Hofstetter, S., Tzur-Moryosef, S., Blumenfeld-Katzir, T., and Assaf, Y. (2012). Learning in the fast lane: new insights into neuroplasticity. *Neuron* 73, 1195–1203. doi: 10.1016/j.neuron.2012.01.025

Salat, D. H. (2014). "Chapter 12 – Diffusion tensor imaging in the study of aging and age-associated neural disease," in *Diffusion MRI*, 2nd Edn, eds H. Johansen-Berg and T. E. J. Behrens (San Diego, CA: Academic Press), 257–281.

Sale, A., Berardi, N., and Maffei, L. (2014). Environment and brain plasticity: towards an endogenous pharmacotherapy. *Physiol. Rev.* 94, 189–234. doi: 10.1152/physrev.00036.2012

Salminen, T., Mårtensson, J., Schubert, T., and Kühn, S. (2016). Increased integrity of white matter pathways after dual n-back training. *Neuroimage* 133, 244–250. doi: 10.1016/j.neuroimage.2016.03.028

Shah, T. M., Weinborn, M., Verdile, G., Sohrabi, H. R., and Martins, R. N. (2017). Enhancing cognitive functioning in healthly older adults: a systematic review of the clinical significance of commercially available computerized cognitive training in preventing cognitive decline. *Neuropsychol. Rev.* doi: 10.1007/s11065-016-9338-9 [Epub ahead of print].

Smith, G. E., Housen, P., Yaffe, K., Ruff, R., Kennison, R. F., Mahncke, H. W., et al. (2009). A cognitive training program based on principles of brain plasticity: results from the improvement in memory with plasticity-based adaptive cognitive training (IMPACT) study. *J. Am. Geriatr. Soc.* 57, 594–603. doi: 10.1111/j.1532-5415.2008.02167.x

Smith, P. J., Blumenthal, J. A., Hoffman, B. M., Cooper, H., Strauman, T. A., Welsh-Bohmer, K., et al. (2010). Aerobic exercise and neurocognitive performance: a meta-analytic review of randomized controlled trials. *Psychosom. Med.* 72, 239–252. doi: 10.1097/PSY.0b013e3181d14633

Sofi, F., Valecchi, D., Bacci, D., Abbate, R., Gensini, G. F., Casini, A., et al. (2011). Physical activity and risk of cognitive decline: a meta-analysis of prospective studies. *J. Intern. Med.* 269, 107–117. doi: 10.1111/j.1365-2796.2010.02281.x

Steele, C. J., Bailey, J. A., Zatorre, R. J., and Penhune, V. B. (2013). Early musical training and white-matter plasticity in the corpus callosum: evidence for a sensitive period. *J. Neurosci.* 33, 1282–1290. doi: 10.1523/JNEUROSCI.3578-12.2013

Stewart, A. L., Mills, K. M., King, A. C., Haskell, W. L., Gillis, D., and Ritter, P. L. (2001). CHAMPS physical activity questionnaire for older adults: outcomes for interventions. *Med. Sci. Sports Exerc.* 33, 1126–1141. doi: 10.1097/00005768-200107000-00010

Strenziok, M., Parasuraman, R., Clarke, E., Cisler, D. S., Thompson, J. C., and Greenwood, P. M. (2014). Neurocognitive enhancement in older adults: comparison of three cognitive training tasks to test a hypothesis of training transfer in brain connectivity. *Neuroimage* 85(Pt 3), 1027–1039. doi: 10.1016/j.neuroimage.2013.07.069

Svatkova, A., Mandl, R. C. W., Scheewe, T. W., Cahn, W., Kahn, R. S., and Hulshoff Pol, H. E. (2015). Physical exercise keeps the brain connected: biking increases white matter integrity in patients with schizophrenia and healthy controls. *Schizophr. Bull.* 41, 869–878. doi: 10.1093/schbul/sbv033

Takeuchi, H., Sekiguchi, A., Taki, Y., Yokoyama, S., Yomogida, Y., Komuro, N., et al. (2010). Training of working memory impacts structural connectivity. *J. Neurosci.* 30, 3297–3303. doi: 10.1523/JNEUROSCI.4611-09.2010

Thurm, F., Scharpf, A., Liebermann, N., Kolassa, S., Elbert, T., and Lüchtenberg, D. (2011). Improvement of cognitive function after physical movement training in institutionalized very frail older adults with dementia. *GeroPsych* 24, 197–208. doi: 10.1024/1662-9647/a000048

Toril, P., Reales, J. M., and Ballesteros, S. (2014). Video game training enhances cognition of older adults: a meta-analytic study. *Psychol. Aging* 29, 706–716. doi: 10.1037/a0037507

Valenzuela, M. J., Matthews, F. E., Brayne, C., Ince, P., Halliday, G., Kril, J. J., et al. (2011). Multiple biological pathways link cognitive lifestyle to protection from dementia. *Biol. Psychiatry* 71, 783–791. doi: 10.1016/j.biopsych.2011.07.036

Valenzuela, M. J., and Sachdev, P. (2006). Brain reserve and cognitive decline: a non-parametric systematic review. *Psychol. Med.* 36, 1065–1073. doi: 10.1017/S0033291706007744

Valenzuela, M. J., Sachdev, P., Wen, W., Chen, X., and Brodaty, H. (2008). Lifespan mental activity predicts diminished rate of hippocampal atrophy. *PLoS ONE* 3:e2598. doi: 10.1371/journal.pone.0002598

Von Aster, M., Neubauer, A., and Horn, R. (2006). *Wechsler Intelligenztest für Erwachsene (WIE). Deutschsprachige Bearbeitung und Adaptation des WAIS-III von David Wechsler [Wechsler Intelligence Scale for adults. German adaptation of the WAIS-III by David Wechsler].* Frankfurt: Harcourt Test Services.

von Bastian, C. C., and Oberauer, K. (2014). Effects and mechanisms of working memory training: a review. *Psychol. Res.* 78, 803–820. doi: 10.1007/s00426-013-0524-6

Voss, M. W., Heo, S., Prakash, R. S., Erickson, K. I., Alves, H., Chaddock, L., et al. (2012). The influence of aerobic fitness on cerebral white matter integrity and cognitive function in older adults: results of a one-year exercise intervention. *Hum. Brain Mapp.* 34, 2972–2985. doi: 10.1002/hbm.22119

Wang, Y., West, J. D., Flashman, L. A., Wishart, H. A., Santulli, R. B., Rabin, L. A., et al. (2012). Selective changes in white matter integrity in MCI and older adults with cognitive complaints. *Biochim. Biophys. Acta* 1822, 423–430. doi: 10.1016/j.bbadis.2011.08.002

Welsh, K. A., Butters, N., Mohs, R. C., Beekly, D., Edland, S., Fillenbaum, G., et al. (1994). The Consortium to Establish a Registry for Alzheimer's disease (CERAD). Part V. A normative study of the neuropsychological battery. *Neurology* 44, 609–614. doi: 10.1212/WNL.44.4.609

Zelinski, E. M., Peters, K. D., Hindin, S., Petway, K. T., and Kennison, R. F. (2014). Evaluating the relationship between change in performance on training tasks and on untrained outcomes. *Front. Hum. Neurosci.* 8:617. doi: 10.3389/fnhum.2014.00617

Zelinski, E. M., Spina, L. M., Yaffe, K., Ruff, R., Kennison, R. F., Mahncke, H. W., et al. (2011). Improvement in memory with plasticity based adaptive cognitive training: results of the 3 month follow up. *J. Am. Geriatr. Soc.* 59, 258–265. doi: 10.1111/j.1532-5415.2010.03277.x

19

The Impact of Aerobic Exercise on Fronto-Parietal Network Connectivity and its Relation to Mobility: An Exploratory Analysis of a 6-Month Randomized Controlled Trial

*Chun L. Hsu[1,2,3,4], John R. Best[1,2,3,4], Shirley Wang[1,2,3,4], Michelle W. Voss[5,6], Robin G. Y. Hsiung[7], Michelle Munkacsy[1,2,3,4], Winnie Cheung[1,2,3,4], Todd C. Handy[8] and Teresa Liu-Ambrose[1,2,3,4]**

[1] *Aging, Mobility, and Cognitive Neuroscience Lab, University of British Columbia, Vancouver, BC, Canada,* [2] *Department of Physical Therapy, University of British Columbia, Vancouver, BC, Canada,* [3] *Djavad Mowafaghian Center for Brain Health, University of British Columbia, Vancouver, BC, Canada,* [4] *Center for Hip Health and Mobility, Vancouver, BC, Canada,* [5] *Health, Brain, and Cognition Lab, University of Iowa, Iowa City, IA, United States,* [6] *Department of Psychology, University of Iowa, Iowa City, IA, United States,* [7] *Department of Medicine, University of British Columbia, Vancouver, BC, Canada,* [8] *Department of Psychology, University of British Columbia, Vancouver, BC, Canada*

Edited by:
Srikantan S. Nagarajan,
University of California,
San Francisco, United States

Reviewed by:
C. J. Boraxbekk,
Umeå University, Sweden
Gary Abrams,
University of California,
San Francisco, United States
Karl Meisel,
University of California,
San Francisco, United States

***Correspondence:**
Teresa Liu-Ambrose
teresa.ambrose@ubc.ca

Impaired mobility is a major concern for older adults and has significant consequences. While the widely accepted belief is that improved physical function underlies the effectiveness of targeted exercise training in improving mobility and reducing falls, recent evidence suggests cognitive and neural benefits gained through exercise may also play an important role in promoting mobility. However, the underlying neural mechanisms of this relationship are currently unclear. Thus, we hypothesize that 6 months of progressive aerobic exercise training would alter frontoparietal network (FPN) connectivity during a motor task among older adults with mild subcortical ischemic vascular cognitive impairment (SIVCI)—and exercise-induced changes in FPN connectivity would correlate with changes in mobility. We focused on the FPN as it is involved in top-down attentional control as well as motor planning and motor execution. Participants were randomized either to usual-care (CON), which included monthly educational materials about VCI and healthy diet; or thrice-weekly aerobic training (AT), which was walking outdoors with progressive intensity. Functional magnetic resonance imaging was acquired at baseline and trial completion, where the participants were instructed to perform bilateral finger tapping task. At trial completion, compared with AT, CON showed significantly increased FPN connectivity strength during right finger tapping ($p < 0.05$). Across the participants, reduced FPN connectivity was associated with greater cardiovascular capacity ($p = 0.05$). In the AT group, reduced FPN connectivity was significantly associated with improved mobility performance, as measured by the Timed-Up-and-Go test ($r = 0.67$, $p = 0.02$). These results suggest progressive AT may improve mobility in older adults with SIVCI via maintaining intra-network connectivity of the FPN.

Keywords: aging, impaired mobility, vascular cognitive impairment, fronto-parietal network, functional connectivity, fMRI

INTRODUCTION

Impaired mobility is a major concern for older adults and is associated with increased risk for disability, institutionalization, and death (Rosano et al., 2008). The prevalence of impaired mobility is 14% at age 75 years and involves half of the population over 84 years (Odenheimer et al., 1994). Falls are a significant consequence of impaired mobility.

Current evidence supports the recommendation of targeted exercise training to improve mobility, prevent major mobility disability, and reduce the risk of future falls (Campbell et al., 1999; Pahor et al., 2014). The widely accepted view is that improved physical function, such as improved balance and increased muscle strength, primarily underlies the effectiveness of the exercise in improving mobility and reducing falls (Layne et al., 2017). However, in a meta-analysis of four randomized trials of exercise, falls were significantly reduced by 35% while postural sway significantly improved by only 9% and there was no significant improvement in knee extension strength (Robertson et al., 2002). Moreover, in a proof-of-concept randomized controlled trial, we demonstrated that a home-based exercise signficantly reduced falls by 47% in older adults - in the absence of significant improvement in physical function (i.e., balance and muscle strength) (Liu-Ambrose et al., 2008). Rather, significant improvement in executive functions were observed in the exercise group as compared with the usual care (i.e., control) group.

These data suggest that exercise may reduce falls in older adults via several mechanisms, not just via improved physical function.

We previously proposed that cognitive and neural plasticity may be an important, yet under-appreciated mechanism by which exercise promotes mobility and reduce falls (Liu-Ambrose et al., 2013). This hypothesis stems from the growing evidence that suggest: (1) cognitive impairment and impaired mobility are associated (Atkinson et al., 2007; Buracchio et al., 2010; Montero-Odasso et al., 2012); (2) reduced executive function, is associated with impaired mobility and increased falls risk (Delbaere et al., 2012; Hsu et al., 2012); (3) aberrant neural network functional connectivity is associated with impaired mobility (Hsu et al., 2014); and (4) targeted exercise training, particulary aerobic-based, promotes cognitive and cortical plasticity, including executive function and its neural correlates, in older adults (Erickson and Kramer, 2009; Voss et al., 2010b).

Despite the growing recognition that targeted exercise training may promote mobility outcomes in older adults via central mechanisms (Liu-Ambrose et al., 2013), few intervention studies of exercise to date have provided direct evidence for this theory (Bolandzadeh et al., 2015). A better understanding of the neural mechanisms underlying exercise-induced improvements in mobility may facilitate the development and refinement of preventative/intervention strategies, as well as identify the populations for whom these effects apply.

Older adults with subcortical ischemic vascular cognitive impairment (SIVCI), the most common form of vascular cognitive impairment (VCI) (Bowler, 2005), are at particular risk for both impaired mobility and dementia secondary to underlying white matter lesions (WMLs) or lacunar infarcts (Roman et al., 2002; Vermeer et al., 2007). VCI is the second most common cause of dementia after Alzheimer's disease (AD) (Desmond et al., 1999; Erkinjuntti et al., 1999; Pantoni et al., 1999; Rockwood et al., 2000). The clinical consequences of covert ischemic strokes are substantial (Roman et al., 2002; Vermeer et al., 2007). These WMLs and lacunar infarcts typically manifest in brain regions such as caudate, pallidum, thalamus, frontal and prefrontal white-matter (Roman et al., 2002). As a result, they may disrupt the integrity of functional neural networks and negatively impact cognitive function, particulary executive functions, and mobility (Kuo and Lipsitz, 2004; O'Brien, 2006).

Among the relevant neural networks, most notably, is the frontoparietal network (FPN). The FPN is involved in top-down attentional control and allocation of available neural resources that contribute to executive processes, such as response anticipation and conflict processing (Fogassi and Luppino, 2005; Seeley et al., 2007; Sridharan et al., 2008), as well as motor planning and motor execution (Wise et al., 1997; Wu et al., 2009; Wymbs et al., 2012). Of particular relevance, previous studies have shown that key regions within the FPN were actively recruited during actual as well as imagined completion of the walking while talking (WWT) test (Holtzer et al., 2011; Blumen et al., 2014). Specifically, neural activity within these FPN regions were positively associated with both task difficulty and cognitive performance of the WWT test (Holtzer et al., 2011; Blumen et al., 2014). Although previous studies have linked aspects of mobility to FPN connectivity, its potential role understanding exercise-induced effects on mobility is unkown.

Thus, we propose FPN connectivity as one of the neural mechanisms by which exercise promotes mobility in older adults with mild SIVCI. Using functional magnetic resonance imaging (fMRI) data from a 6-month single-blind randomized controlled trial (clinicaltrials.gov Identifier: NCT01027858), we conducted a planned secondary analysis to assess the impact of moderate-intensity aerobic exercise training on functional connectivity of FPN among older adults with mild SIVCI. We hypothesized that aerobic exercise-induced increases in FPN connectivity would correlate with improved mobility. The primary results from the parent study have been published (Liu-Ambrose et al., 2016), which provided preliminary evidence that 6 months of thrice-weekly progressive aerobic training (AT) promotes cognitive performance in community-dwelling adults with mild SIVCI, relative to usual care plus education.

MATERIALS AND METHODS

Study Design

This is a secondary analysis of neuroimaging data acquired from a 6-month proof-of-concept RCT (NCT01027858) of aerobic exercise in older adults with mild SIVCI (Liu-Ambrose et al., 2010, 2016). Trained study assessors were blinded to group allocation of participants. Functional MRI (fMRI) data were acquired at baseline prior to randomization and at trial completion (i.e., 6 months) in a subset of eligible participants.

Participants

As the current study was a secondary analysis, we sought to recruit as many eligible and consenting individuals from the parent study as possible. To briefly describe the recruitment process, we recruited from the University of British Columbia Hospital Clinic for Alzheimer's Disease and Related Disorders, the Vancouver General Hospital Stroke Prevention Clinic, and specialized geriatric clinics in Metro Vancouver, BC. Recruitment occurred between December 2009 and April 2014 with randomization occurring on an ongoing basis. Study participants were clinically diagnosed with mild SIVCI as determined by the presence of cognitive syndrome and small vessel ischaemic disease (Erkinjuntti et al., 2000). Small vessel ischemic disease was defined as evidence of relevant cerebrovascular disease by brain computed tomography or MRI defined as the presence of both: (1) Periventricular and deep WMLs; (2) Absence of cortical and/or cortico-subcortical non-lacunar territorial infarcts and watershed infarcts, hemorrhages indicating large vessel disease, signs of normal pressure hydrocephalus, or other specific causes of WMLs (i.e., multiple sclerosis, leukodystrophies, sarcoidosis, brain irradiation). In addition to the neuroimaging evidence, the presence or a history of neurological signs such as Babinski sign, sensory deficit, gait disorder, or extrapyramidal signs consistent with sub-cortical brain lesion(s) was required and confirmed by study physicians (G-YRH and PL). Cognitive syndrome was defined as a baseline Montreal Cognitive Assessment (MoCA) score less than 26/30. However, participants were free of frank dementia (i.e., clinically diagnosis of dementia) as determined by a Mini-Mental State Examination (MMSE) score $\geq$ 20 and the absence of diagnosed dementia. Progressive cognitive decline was confirmed through medical records or caregiver/family member interviews.

The Consolidated Standards of Reporting Trial flowchart shows the number and distribution of participants included in this secondary analysis (**Figure 1**). Of the 38 participants (54% of parent sample) that completed baseline MRI scanning, 7 (18% of the sample) dropped out from the study and 10 (26% of the sample) failed to correctly perform the motor finger tapping task (e.g., finger tapped during resting blocks). Consequently, 21 participants who completed MRI at baseline and trial completion were included in this secondary analysis (30% of parent sample). Ethical approval was provided by the University of British Columbia's Clinical Research Ethics Board (H07-01160). All participants provided written informed consent.

Randomization

The randomization sequence was generated using the web application www.randomization.com with a ratio of 1:1 to AT

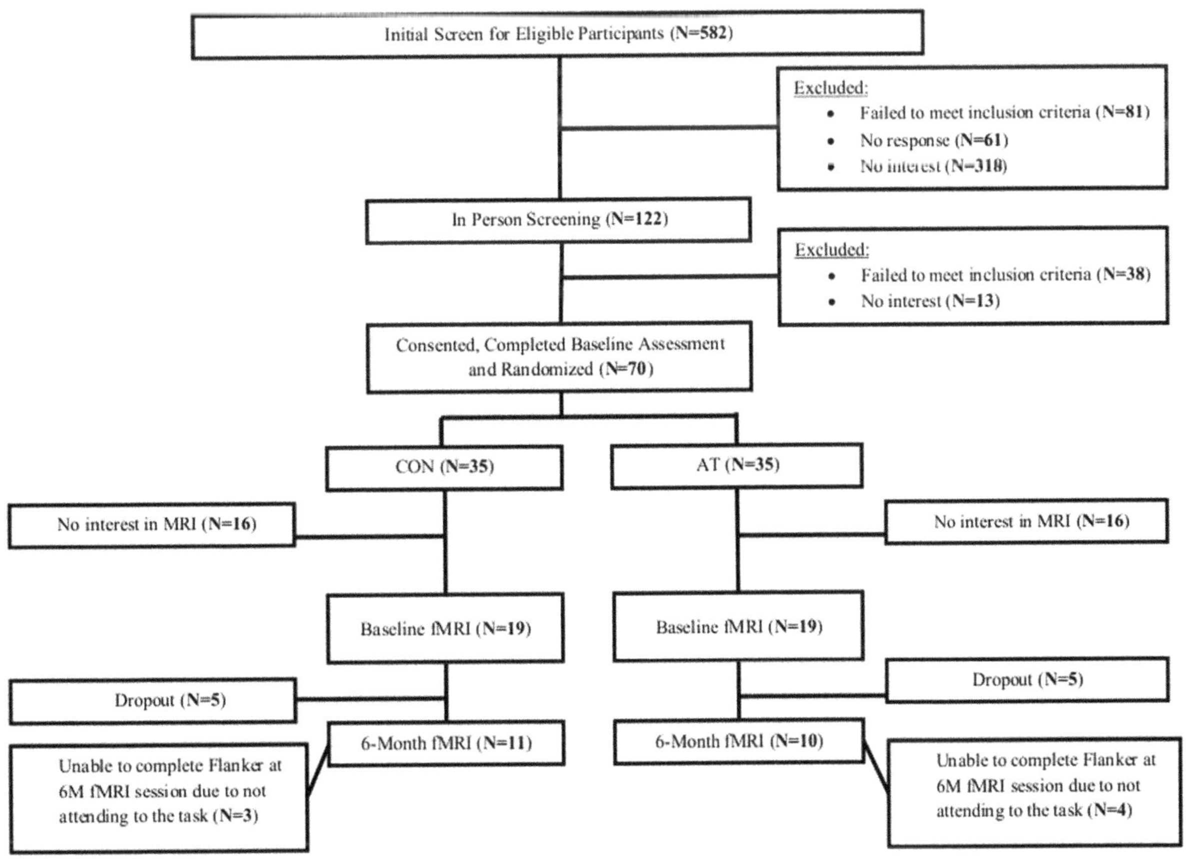

FIGURE 1 | Overview of the flow of study participants through the 6-month study.

or usual care (CON). A research team member not involved with the study held this sequence at a remote location. After the completion of consent and baseline testing, the research coordinator contacted the team member holding the list to determine the next allocation.

Aerobic Training and Compliance

For the AT group, AT consisted of supervised thrice-weekly 60-min classes of walking for the 6-month intervention period. All AT group classes were led by instructors certified to instruct seniors and were delivered in a group setting. Each 60-min class included a 10-min warm-up, 40-min of walking, and a 10-min cool down. Both the warm-up and cool-down included passive and active stretches, as well as range of motion exercise.

Walking occurred outdoors and followed predetermined routes around local areas. The intensity of the AT program was monitored and progressed using three approaches: (1) heart rate monitoring with an initial intensity of 40% of age specific target heart rate (i.e., heart rate reserve; HRR). HRR was calculated by subtracting resting heart rate from maximum heart rate [using the formula: 206.9 − 0.67 × Age (Gellish et al., 2007)] and recalculation each month. Participants progressed over the first 12 weeks to the range of 60–70% of HRR, after which this was sustained for the remainder of the intervention period; (2) subjective monitoring using the Borg's Rating of Perceived Exertion (RPE) (Borg, 1982) with a target RPE of 14 to 15; and (3) the "talk" test (Persinger et al., 2004), starting at a walking pace allowing comfortable conversation and progressing to a walking pace where conversation was difficult. Individual training logs (i.e., target heart rate, heart rate achieved, and rate of perceived exertion) were maintained throughout the intervention period.

The AT group was also given a pedometer to serve as both an incentive and monitoring tool. Participants recorded the number of steps each day taken outside the AT classes on standard logs provided by the research team.

Usual Care

Participants in the CON group received usual care, in which they were provided with monthly educational materials about VCI and healthy diet. However, no specific information regarding physical activity was provided. In addition, research staff phoned the CON participants on a monthly basis to maintain contact and to acquire research data.

Adverse Effects

All participants were instructed to report any adverse effects due to the AT exercises to our research coordinator, such as falls or musculoskeletal pain persisting longer than 48 h. Participants were also questioned about the presence of any adverse effects, such as musculoskeletal pain or discomfort, at each exercise session. All instructors also monitored participants for symptoms of angina and shortness of breath during the exercise classes. External experts from our safety monitoring committee reviewed all adverse events reported on a monthly basis.

Descriptive Variables

At baseline, participants underwent a clinical assessment with study physicians (GYRH and PL) to confirm current health status and study eligibility. Age in years and education level were assessed by self-report. Standing height was measured as stretch stature to the 0.1 cm per standard protocol. Weight was measured twice to the 0.1 kg on a calibrated digital scale. Waist-to-hip ratio was determined by measuring the widest part of the hip circumference and the waist just above the navel in centimeters. The Functional Comorbidity Index (Groll et al., 2005) assessed the number of comorbid conditions related to physical functioning.

Global cognition was assessed using the MMSE (Cockrell and Folstein, 1988) and the MoCA. The MMSE and MoCA are 30-point tests that encompass several cognitive domains. The MoCA has been found to have good internal consistency and test–retest reliability and was able to correctly identify 90% of a large sample of individuals with mild cognitive impairment from two different clinics with a cut-off scores of $\leq$26/30 (Nasreddine et al., 2005).

Functional MRI Acquisition

All MRI was conducted at the University of British Columbia (UBC) MRI Research Center located at the UBC Hospital on a 3.0 Tesla Intera Achieva MRI Scanner (Philips Medical Systems, Markham, ON, Canada) using an 8-channel SENSE neurovascular coil. The fMRI consisted of two successive runs with 165 dynamic images of 36 slices (3 mm thick) with the following parameters: repetition time (TR) of 2000 ms, echo time (TE) of 30 ms, flip angle (FA) of 90 degrees, field of view (FoV) of 240 mm, acquisition matrix 80 × 80, voxel size of 3 mm × 3 mm × 3 mm. High resolution anatomical MRI T1 images were acquired using the following parameters: 170 slices (1 mm thick), TR of 7.7 ms, TE of 3.6 ms, FA of 8 degrees, FoV of 256 mm, acquisition matrix of 256 × 200.

During each scanning session, the study participants were asked to perform a finger tapping motor task that had been previously administered and described (Hsu et al., 2014). Briefly, the task consisted of three conditions: right finger tapping, rest, and left finger tapping. The specific instructions given required the participants to finger tap in a particular sequence regardless of condition: start with the index finger and progress toward the little (pinky) finger continuously until a different condition is presented. For the rest condition, participants were asked to rest with their eyes open. The exact order of motor task blocks was not disclosed to the participants and was counter balanced over two runs as follow:

Run A: Rest, Left Tap, Rest, Right Tap, Rest, Right Tap, Rest, Left Tap, Rest

Run B: Rest, Right Tap, Rest, Left Tap, Rest, Left Tap, Rest, Right Tap, Rest

Total WML volume (in mm^3) at baseline was quantified with structural MRI data acquired on the same MRI scanner (3T Achieva, Philips Medical Systems, Markham, ON, Canada) at the UBC MRI Research Centre. A T2-weighted scan and a proton-density-weighted (PD-weighted) scan were acquired for each subject. For the T2-weighted images, the repetition time (TR) was 5,431 ms and the echo time (TE) was 90 ms, and for the PD-weighted images, the TR was 2,000 ms, and the TE was 8 ms. T2- and PD-weighted scans had dimensions of 256 × 256 × 60 voxels and a voxel size of 0.937 mm × 0.937 mm × 3.000 mm. Briefly, WMLs were identified and digitally marked (i.e., placing seed points) by a radiologist on T2 and PD weighted images. Marked WMLs were automatically segmented by a customized Parzen windows classifier that estimated the intensity distribution of the lesions – which also included heuristics that optimized the accuracy of the estimated distributions (Parzen, 1962; McAusland et al., 2010; Bolandzadeh et al., 2015). WML segmentation was reviewed by a trained technician to ensure accuracy.

Mobility, Cardiovascular Capacity, and Physical Activity

Mobility was assessed with the Timed-Up-and-Go test (TUG) and the Short Physical Performance Battery (SPPB). The TUG required participants to rise from a standard chair, walk a distance of three meters, turn, walk back to the chair and sit down (Shumway-Cook et al., 2000). We recorded the time (s) to complete the TUG, based on the average of two separate trials.

For the SPPB, participants were assessed on performances of standing balance, walking, and sit-to-stand. Each component is rated out of four points, for a maximum of 12 points; a score < 9/12 predicts subsequent disability (Guralnik et al., 1995).

Participant's cardiovascular capacity was assessed using the 6-Minute Walk Test (Enright, 2003). The total distance walked (meters) within the span of 6 min was recorded.

Monthly total physical activity level was determined by the Physical Activities Scale for the Elderly (PASE) self-report questionnaire (Washburn et al., 1999).

Data Analysis

Functional MRI Preprocessing

Image preprocessing was carried out using tools from FSL (FMRIB's Software Library) [78], MATLAB (Matrix Laboratory), and toolboxes from SPM (Statistical Parametric Mapping). Excess unwanted structures (i.e., bones, skull, etc.) in high resolution T1 images were removed via Brain Extraction Tool (BET); rigid body motion correction was completed using MCFLIRT (absolute and relative mean displacement were subsequently extracted and included in the statistical analysis as covariates); spatial smoothing was carried out using Gaussian kernel of Full-Width-Half-Maximum (FWHM) 6.0 mm; temporal filtering was applied with high pass frequency cut-off of 120 s. In addition, a low pass temporal filtering was also included to ensure the fMRI signal fluctuated between $0.008 < f < 0.080$ Hz, the ideal bandwidth to examine functional connectivity. Furthermore, the application of a low pass filter eliminated high frequency signals that could be confounds. Participants' low-resolution functional data were registered to personal high resolution T1 anatomical images, which were subsequently registered to standardized 152 T1 Montreal Neurological Institute (MNI) space.

Noise generated from both physiological and non-physiological sources were removed through regression of the cerebral-spinal fluid (CSF) signal, white matter signal, and global brain signal. Global signal regression had been reported as both valid and useful step in functional connectivity analyses (Fox et al., 2009) that may improve specificity (Murphy and Fox, 2016).

Functional Connectivity Analysis

Previous studies guided our choice of seeds in the whole brain analysis of the FPN (Voss et al., 2010b). The FPN included the inferior parietal sulcus (IPS), ventral visual cortex (VV), supramarginal gyrus (SMG), superior lateral occipital cortex (SLOC), frontal eye field (FEF), as well as overlapping areas in the temporal-parietal junction. The respective MNI space coordinates for each region of interest (ROI) are provided in **Table 1**.

From each ROI, preprocessed time-series data were extracted with 14 mm spherical regions of interest drawn around their respective MNI coordinates in standard space. The different conditions (i.e., left, right, and rest) within each block of the motor task were extracted and compiled together. To concatenate the time-series data, the stimulus onset time for each task condition was acquired from the task program. Each volume of the data was then sorted according to their respective condition. Once the data were properly categorized, the task-specific volumes (e.g., all the "left" volumes) were merged using a script provided in the FSL program. The first three volumes of any condition were discarded to account for delay of the hemodynamic response. Evidence in the literature has demonstrated that functional connectivity derived from temporally spliced/merged resting-state data from blocked fMRI design is not significantly different from connectivity derived from continuous data (Fair et al., 2007). Recent study using motor task fMRI also showed that quantifying functional connectivity via similar seed-based approach using concatenated data is comparable to results from continuous data (Zhu et al., 2017).

Region of interest time-series data were subsequently cross-correlated with every voxel within the brain to establish functional connectivity maps of their associated neural networks,

TABLE 1 | Frontoparietal network regions of interest and relative MNI coordinates.

FPN	ROI	*X*	*Y*	*Z*
	RIPS	25	−62	53
	RVV	36	−62	0
	LVV	−44	−60	−6
	RSMG	32	−38	38
	RSLOC	26	−64	54
	LSLOC	−26	−60	52
	RFEF	28	−4	58
	LFEF	−26	−8	54

RIPS, right inferior parietal sulcus; RVV, right ventral visual; LVV, left ventral visual; RSMG, right supramarginal gyrus; RSLOC, right lateral occipital cortex; LSLOC, left lateral occipital cortex; RFEF, right frontal eye field; LFEF, left frontal eye field.

in which pairwise correlation between time-series extracted from ROI listed above was calculated. Individual-level within-subject results were generated via ordinary least-squares (OLS) regression using FSL's flameo (Beckmann et al., 2003) in FSL by congregating the voxel-wise functional connectivity maps from each condition. Similarly, for group results, a mixed-level OLS analysis was conducted. The statistical map thresholding was set at $Z = 2.33$, with cluster correction of $p < 0.05$.

Statistical Analyses

Statistical analysis was conducted using the IBM SPSS Statistic 23 for Windows (SPSS Inc., Chicago, IL, United States). Statistical significance was set at $p \leq 0.05$ for all analyses. Change in network connectivity strength was computed in SPSS as 6-month FPN connectivity minus baseline FPN connectivity. Linear mixed models with random intercepts and time-varying outcome measures were constructed to statistically test for significant between-group differences in change in network connectivity while adjusting for baseline total WML and age. A group by time interaction indicated group differences in changes in FPN connectivity from baseline to post-intervention. Similar analyses were conducted to determine whether there were group differences in changes in TUG, SPPB, 6MWT, and PASE scores. The primary analyses included the 21 participants with valid baseline and post-intervention fMRI data. Secondary analyses followed the intention-to-treat principle by including nine additional individuals with valid baseline fMRI but were lost to follow-up; maximum likelihood estimation allowed for these individuals to inform the treatment effects, despite having missing follow-up data and to determine whether loss to follow-up might bias the treatment effects estimated with only treatment completers.

Bivariate correlation analyses were performed to determine whether any significant changes in intra-network FPN connectivity (during rest, left tap, and right tap) in the AT group ($n = 12$) correlated with change in mobility, as measured by TUG and SPPB, or change in 6MWT across the 6-month study duration.

RESULTS

Participants and Treatment Fidelity

Among the 70 randomized individuals in the parent study, we observed a significant effect of AT on 6-min walk performance, a well-established tool that accurately evaluates cardiovascular fitness (Cataneo et al., 2010) ($B = 30.34$, $p = 0.02$), indicating that AT had a positive effect on cardiovascular capacity (Liu-Ambrose et al., 2016). Twenty-one participants who completed fMRI scans at both baseline and 6 months were included in the primary analysis (**Figure 1**). Study demographics are reported in **Table 2**, pedometer information over the intervention period is reported in **Table 3**, mobility and cardiovascular capacity measures are reported in **Table 4**; these measures do not differ between groups at baseline nor differ significantly from the 70 eligible participants enrolled in the parent study (Liu-Ambrose et al., 2016). The mean

TABLE 2 | Participant characteristics at baseline ($N = 21$).

Variables	CON group, $n = 9$ Mean (*SD*) or *n*	AT Group, $n = 12$ Mean (*SD*) or *n*
Age (year)	69.9 (9.2)	72.0 (8.6)
Height (cm)	165.4 (11.4)	169.0 (15.9)
Weight (kg)	73.6 (13.1)	73.6 (14.8)
Sex (M/F)	5/4	8/4
MMSE (30 points max)	27.2 (1.9)	26.4 (2.8)
MOCA (30 points max)	24.2 (2.3)	22.5 (2.0)
FCI	3.0 (1.9)	3.1 (1.7)
White matter lesion (mm^3)	1389.5 (2023.4)	3492.8 (3882.1)
Relative head motion (mm)	0.17 (0.09)	0.14 (0.07)

MMSE, Mini-Mental Status Examination; MoCA, Montreal Cognitive Assessment; FCI, Functional Comorbidity Index. All measures were not statistically significant at $p < 0.05$.

TABLE 3 | AT group pedometer information over 6-month intervention period.

	Average pedometer count Mean (*SD*)
Baseline	7002.1 (5496.4)
Month 1	9009.2 (6337.9)
Month 2	9786.3 (6944.2)
Month 3	10713.8 (7209.0)
Month 4	10922.1 (7645.7)
Month 5	11484.8 (8074.6)
Month 6	11552.7 (7411.9)

age of all participants included in this secondary analysis was 71.1 years ($SD = 8.7$ years), which is not significantly different from the mean age of the parent cohort at 74.3 years ($SD = 8.3$ years). Compared to the nine individuals with valid baseline data only, the study sample did not differ on baseline FPN connectivity (all $p > 0.19$) but did have higher average baseline MoCA scores (23.2 versus 20.4; $p = 0.02$). Neither of the mobility measures nor self-reported physical activity differed significantly between groups across the 6 months. However, we observed a trend-level group difference in the change in 6-Minute Walk Test performance ($p = 0.08$; **Table 4**), in which the AT group showed greater improvement (48.6 m) compared with the CON group (−0.3 m).

AT Compliance and Adverse Effects

The average compliance observed in the AT group was 76% for the walking classes and 65% for the nutrition education classes; whereas the average compliance observed in the CON group was 74%. Two study-related adverse events were reported in the AT group and one in the CON group. All three were non-syncopal falls. One of the falls in the AT group resulted in a broken tooth and required assessment in the Emergency Department; the remaining two did not result in injury.

fMRI Results

Results from the seed-based functional connectivity analysis on the FPN (**Figure 2**) showed there were no significant between

TABLE 4 | Mobility and cardiovascular capacity measures ($N = 21$).

	Baseline		Change from baseline to month 6* (end of intervention)		
	Mean (SD)		Adjusted within-group change (SE)		
Variables	**CON**	**AT**	**CON**	**AT**	**Between-group *p*-value**
Timed Up and Go (s)	8.2 (1.3)	7.6 (1.8)	0.16 (0.46)	−0.06 (0.41)	0.73
Short Physical Performance Battery (max 12 points)	10.4 (0.9)	11.2 (1.3)	0.48 (0.34)	−0.23 (0.31)	0.15
Six-Minute Walk Test (meters)	531.2 (56.9)	555.6 (104.3)	−0.30 (19.29)	48.64 (16.57)	0.08
PASE Score	132.2 (61.3)	134.6 (94.0)	−6.05 (39.62)	−4.99 (34.05)	0.99

**Adjusted for baseline WML and age; PASE, Physical Activities Scale for the Elderly.*

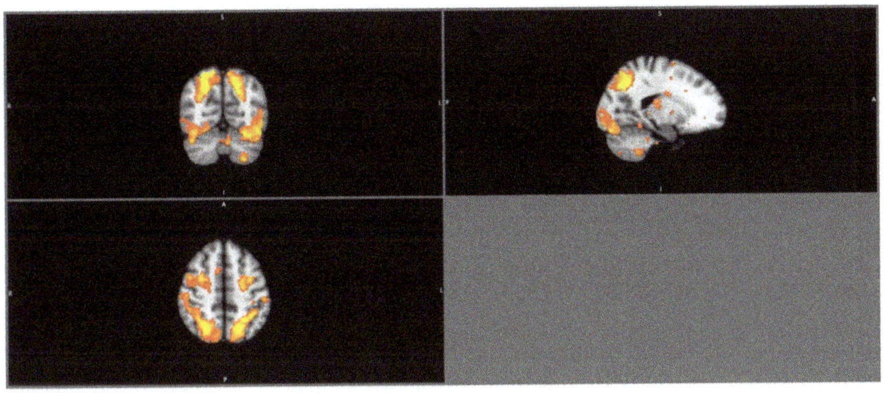

FIGURE 2 | Image of the fronto-parietal network.

TABLE 5 | Frontoparietal network connectivity during task ($N = 21$).

	Baseline		Change from baseline to month 6* (end of intervention)		
	Mean (SD)		Adjusted within-group change (SE)		
Task condition	**CON**	**AT**	**CON**	**AT**	**Between-group *p*-value**
Right Tapping	0.25 (0.28)	0.34 (0.22)	0.25 (0.09)	−0.06 (0.07)	0.02
Rest	0.29 (0.24)	0.26 (0.24)	0.06 (0.09)	−0.02 (0.07)	0.50
Left Tapping	0.35 (0.24)	0.27 (0.20)	−0.05 (0.08)	0.08 (0.07)	0.26

**Adjusted for baseline WML and age.*

group differences in the mean network connectivity strength at baseline, regardless of task conditions (**Table 5**). At trial completion, compared with AT, CON exhibited significantly greater intra-network coupling of the FPN during right finger tapping ($p < 0.02$) after adjusting for baseline WML and age. No AT effects were observed for FPN connectivity during left finger tapping ($p = 0.26$) or during rest ($p = 0.50$). We conducted a secondary, intention-to-treat analysis using all 30 participants with usable baseline data, regardless of loss to follow-up, and observed similar, though weaker, between-group differences in FPN coupling during right finger tapping ($p = 0.08$). As with the primary analyses, CON showed an increase in intra-network coupling of the FPN (mean = 0.18, $SE = 0.09$), whereas AT showed no significant change over time (mean = −0.04, $SE = 0.08$).

Correlation Results

Bivariate correlation across the study sample showed that the change in FPN connectivity during right tapping was significantly associated with change in 6-Minute Walk Test performance ($r = -0.43, p = 0.05$; **Table 6**). Within the AT group ($N = 12$), the change in FPN connectivity during right tapping was significantly associated with change in TUG performance ($r = 0.67, p = 0.02$; **Table 6**). Specifically, reduced FPN connectivity from baseline to post-intervention correlated with improved TUG performance over the same period of time (**Figure 3**).

DISCUSSION

Contrary to our initial hypothesis, we found that a 6-month AT intervention significantly alters FPN connectivity

TABLE 6 | Changes in mobility and changes in FPN connectivity correlation.

	ΔTimed up and go	ΔShort physical performance battery	ΔSix-minute walk test
Group ($N = 21$)			
ΔFPN Connectivity during right tapping	0.14	0.34	−0.43*
AT group ($n = 12$)			
ΔFPN Connectivity during right tapping	0.67*	0.14	−0.37

*Δ = 6-Months – Baseline. *p < 0.05.*

during right finger tapping among older adults with mild SIVCI. The observed effect of aerobic exercise on the FPN during right tapping was significantly associated with improved mobility and cardiovascular capacity. While these results are preliminary, our data suggest aerobic exercise may promote mobility among older adults with mild SIVCI via altering FPN connectivity.

Our findings are in contrast to previous findings that show altered FPN connectivity is associated with aging (Andrews-Hanna et al., 2007) and with cognitive deficits (He et al., 2007; Geerligs et al., 2012; Poppe et al., 2015). Specifically, Poppe et al. (2015) demonstrated that compared with healthy controls, patients with schizophrenia had significantly less connectivity in the FPN during goal-oriented task performance. Compared with controls, task performance was also significantly worse among patients. Similarly, He et al. (2007) found that compared with age-matched healthy controls, individuals who suffered an acute stroke showed significantly less left–right posterior intraparietal sulcus connectivity while performing a spatial-orientation task. Lower connectivity between the left and right posterior intraparietal sulcus were significantly associated with poorer task accuracy and slower task reaction time.

Moreover, current evidence suggests that SIVCI is generally associated with less functional connectivity of neural networks. For example, among those with SIVCI, Yi et al. (2012) found lower functional connectivity in the medial prefrontal cortex and the middle temporal gyrus. Yu et al. (2015) demonstrated that compared with healthy controls, individuals with SIVCI had less network efficiency in the fronto-temporal and parietal regions. Nonetheless, aberrant functional connectivity has been repeatedly observed among those with SIVCI (Yi et al., 2012; Ding et al., 2015; Yu et al., 2015; Zhou et al., 2016), and the pattern (i.e., increased or decreased connectively) is not consistent across studies. For instance, Ding et al. (2015) found increased functional connectivity in the left middle temporal lobe, right inferior temporal lobe, and left superior frontal gyrus among patients with SIVCI as compared with healthy controls.

However, our results do concur with and extend emerging evidence that show less functional connectivity of large-scale networks may be advantageous (Chuang et al., 2014), especially within the context of mobility. In one cross-sectional study, Rosenberg-Katz et al. (2015) demonstrated that compared with

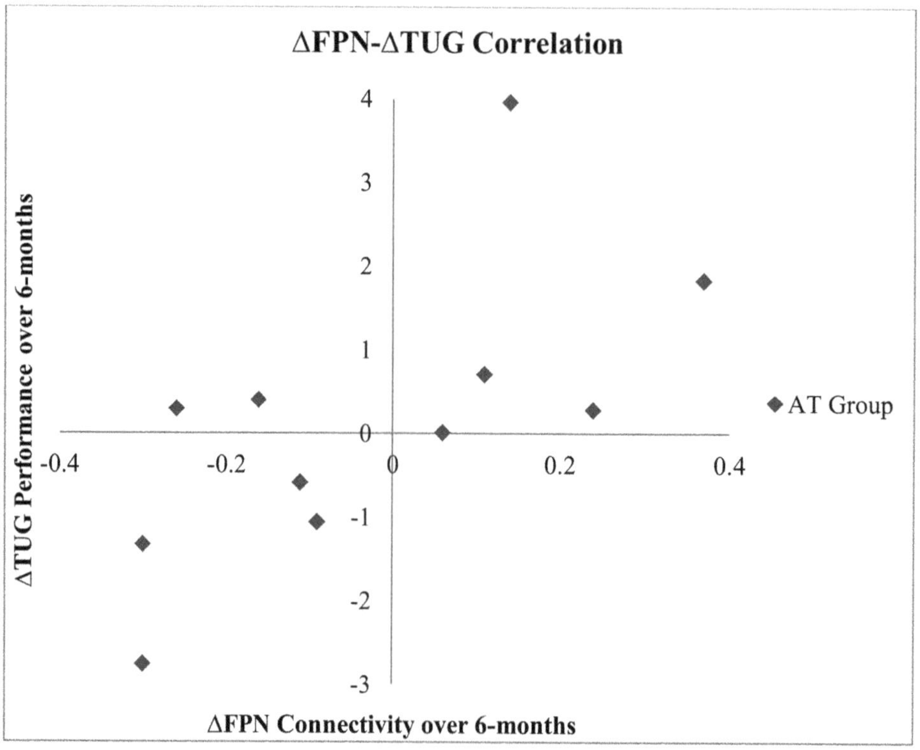

FIGURE 3 | Correlation between change in TUG performance and change in FPN connectivity during right finger tapping within the AT group.

healthy older adults and individuals with Parkinson's disease who were non-fallers, those with Parkinson's disease who were fallers showed significantly greater connectivity between the posterior parietal lobule and the inferior parietal lobule. This data suggest increased connectivity between parietal regions may be associated with more severe motor impairments and more generally, heightened neural activity (e.g., activation or connectivity) may reflect the inability of networks to actively suppress irrelevant neural events, causing regions to compete unnecessarily for available neural resources. In contrast, diminished connectivity may represent greater efficiency as the networks can effectively allocate resources to areas of immediate importance. Certainly, emerging evidence suggests that lifestyle interventions can improve neural efficiency (Smith et al., 2013; Nishiguchi et al., 2015).

Our observation that AT impacted FPN connectivity only during right hand finger tapping concurs with the literature that suggests the FPN connectivity is lateralized (Smith et al., 2009; Pool et al., 2014; Gao et al., 2015). Specifically, using independent component analysis, Smith et al. (2009) revealed that among the neural networks identified, only the FPN exhibit distinct left-right lateralized components. Also, Jancke et al. (2000) found contra-lateralized FPN activation during right index finger tapping task (without visual cue), including the left dorsal lateral premotor cortex and the left inferior parietal lobule. Moreover, Yuan et al. (2015) recently demonstrated that gait velocity among cognitively normal older adults was significantly associated with connectivity of the left-FPN. Therefore, given that our study participants were all right-hand dominant, our results are supported by the literature. We also extend the current state of knowledge by using data generated from a randomized controlled trial to demonstrate the potential impact of aerobic exercise on FPN connectivity during right hand finger tapping and the significant association between FPN connectivity and mobility and cardiovascular capacity. An alternative interpretation of these results may be that aerobic exercise may help maintain mobility and cardiovascular capacity among older adults with SIVCI via reducing cognitive load (i.e., less FPN connectivity) required to perform less attention-demanding motor task (i.e., dominant hand finger tapping). Our own previous work supports this latter concept (Hsu et al., 2017). Critically, in this separate sub-analysis of the same 6-month RCT, we found that after AT, older adults confirmed with SIVCI performed significantly better at the Eriksen flanker task compared with the no-exercise controls. The observed improvement in task performance was associated with overall reduction in activation in the lateral occipital cortex and superior temporal gyrus.

It should be noted that we are aware of only one study in the relevant field in the literature that investigated the association between functional connectivity and cardiorespiratory fitness among older adults (Voss et al., 2010a). While our findings deviate from evidence presented, in which the authors reported greater connectivity is associated with higher fitness among healthy older adults (Voss et al., 2010a), several distinctions from the current study should be considered. Specifically, the differences were: (1) the fMRI task (visual vs. motor); (2) the network examined (default mode network vs. FPN); and (3) study participant (healthy older adults vs. older adults with SIVCI). The combination of these variations could have resulted in disparities in the reported findings.

A few limitations should be taken into consideration. First, our study participants are likely healthier and to have superior physical functioning than average older adults with mild SIVCI. This potential sample bias is somewhat unavoidable given the requirement that participants be able to engage in progressive AT safely. However, it also limits the generalizability of our findings to the population of older adults with mild SIVCI as a whole. Secondly, due to the small sample size of the current study, the current dataset may not possess enough power to detect small differences between the two groups. Provided that the study population is generally frail and older, the occurrence of drop-out from potentially strenuous fMRI session is to be expected. Future studies designed with larger sample sizes are necessary to validate the notion of functional network efficiency/inefficiency by providing sufficient power despite the expectation of drop-out. Thirdly, it is possible that subsets of pairwise connectivity between ROI within the FPN may have driven the effects we observed; however, this was not further investigated due to potential issue with type II error with the current sample size. Moreover, there is much controversy in regards to global signal regression and potential observation of artificial anti-correlations. This may be particularly influential when examining functional connectivity between networks deemed anti-correlated in nature (e.g., default mode network and FPN). In assessing within-network connectivity, it may be that the effects of induced anti-correlation are less significant. However, as stated by Murphy and Fox (Murphy and Fox, 2016) 'there is not a single "right" way to process resting state data that reveals the "true" nature of the brain.' They also summarized the several advantages of global signal regression including removal of motion, cardiac and respiratory signals. In addition, despite evidence supporting its use (Fair et al., 2007; Zhu et al., 2017), we recognize temporally splicing and concatenating data is not recommended and can potentially lead to increase in signal noise. Nevertheless, studies demonstrated that connectivity derived from concatenation does not differ significantly from those acquired from continuous data (Fair et al., 2007; Zhu et al., 2017). In addition, our data is limited by the fact that only the connectivity during right hand tapping was statistically significant while left hand was not. Differences in social interactions experienced by the experimental groups may present addition confounding factors to our data. Specifically, active attention provided by trainers within the AT group may potentially influence our findings. Lastly, the relationship between connectivity and SIVCI status is equivocal with much of the evidence generated from cross-sectional studies. Thus, the inclusion of fMRI data from a healthy-aged matched cohort might have facilitated interpretation of our results. Nevertheless, we highlight the key strengths of our currents study design – a randomized controlled trial – which are: (1) provides evidence of causation; and (2) increased internal validity. Thus, our study provides preliminary evidence to suggest that aerobic exercise may impact functional connectivity in older adults with SIVCI, and this is associated with the maintenance of mobility.

CONCLUSION

Our results demonstrate that neural network functional connectivity may contribute to the effects of aerobic exercise on mobility among older adults with SIVCI. We observed that 6 months of AT maintains motor task-based connectivity within the FPN of older adults with SIVCI, and the degree of decoupling within this region correlates with improvements in mobility. As such, our current findings support emerging results from others that altered functional connectivity within certain neural networks might represent a beneficial change in older adults with mild SIVCI, especially vis-à-vis their mobility. More broadly, these results bring further support to the burgeoning notion that functional neural changes contribute to exercised-induced improvements to mobility among older adults. As extension of these findings, future studies should explore potential interaction between mobility and cognitive outcomes among this population.

DATA ACCESS AND RESPONSIBILITY

TL-A had full access to all the data in the study and takes responsibility for the integrity of the data and the accuracy of the data analysis.

AUTHOR CONTRIBUTIONS

TL-A and RH were involved in the study concept, design, acquisition of data, preparation and critical review of the manuscript. CH, MM, WC, and TL-A were involved in data collection. CH, TL-A, and JB were involved in writing of the manuscript. CH, TL-A, and JB were involved in statistical analyses. CH, TL-A, and JB were involved in interpretation of data. CH and SW were involved in fMRI data analyses. MV and TH were involved in critical review of the manuscript. All authors had full access to all of the data (including statistical reports and tables) in the study and can take responsibility for the integrity of the data and the accuracy of the data analysis.

ACKNOWLEDGMENT

CH is an Alzheimer Society Research Program Doctoral trainee. TL-A is a Canada Research Chair (Tier II) in Physical Activity, Mobility, and Cognitive Neuroscience.

REFERENCES

Andrews-Hanna, J. R., Snyder, A. Z., Vincent, J. L., Lustig, C., Head, D., Raichle, M. E., et al. (2007). Disruption of large-scale brain systems in advanced aging. *Neuron* 56, 924–935. doi: 10.1016/j.neuron.2007.10.038

Atkinson, H. H., Rosano, C., Simonsick, E. M., Williamson, J. D., Davis, C., Ambrosius, W. T., et al. (2007). Cognitive function, gait speed decline, and comorbidities: the health, aging and body composition study. *J. Gerontol. A Biol. Sci. Med. Sci.* 62, 844–850. doi: 10.1093/gerona/62.8.844

Beckmann, C. F., Jenkinson, M., and Smith, S. M. (2003). General multilevel linear modeling for group analysis in FMRI. *Neuroimage* 20, 1052–1063. doi: 10.1016/S1053-8119(03)00435-X

Blumen, H. M., Holtzer, R., Brown, L. L., Gazes, Y., and Verghese, J. (2014). Behavioral and neural correlates of imagined walking and walking-while-talking in the elderly. *Hum. Brain Mapp.* 35, 4090–4104. doi: 10.1002/hbm.22461

Bolandzadeh, N., Tam, R., Handy, T. C., Nagamatsu, L. S., Hsu, C. L., Davis, J. C., et al. (2015). Resistance training and white matter lesion progression in older women: exploratory analysis of a 12-month randomized controlled trial. *J. Am. Geriatr. Soc.* 63, 2052–2060. doi: 10.1111/jgs.13644

Borg, G. (1982). Ratings of perceived exertion and heart rates during short-term cycle exercise and their use in a new cycling strength test. *Int. J. Sports Med.* 3, 153–158. doi: 10.1055/s-2008-1026080

Bowler, J. V. (2005). Vascular cognitive impairment. *J. Neurol. Neurosurg. Psychiatry* 76(Suppl. 5), v35–v44. doi: 10.1136/jnnp.2005.082313

Buracchio, T., Dodge, H. H., Howieson, D., Wasserman, D., and Kaye, J. (2010). THe trajectory of gait speed preceding mild cognitive impairment. *Arch. Neurol.* 67, 980–986. doi: 10.1001/archneurol.2010.159

Campbell, A. J., Robertson, M. C., Gardner, M. M., Norton, R. N., and Buchner, D. M. (1999). Falls prevention over 2 years: a randomized controlled trial in women 80 years and older. *Age Ageing* 28, 513–518. doi: 10.1093/ageing/28.6.513

Cataneo, D. C., Kobayasi, S., Carvalho, L. R., Paccanaro, R. C., and Cataneo, A. J. (2010). Accuracy of six minute walk test, stair test and spirometry using maximal oxygen uptake as gold standard. *Acta Cir. Bras.* 25, 194–200. doi: 10.1590/S0102-86502010000200013

Chuang, Y. F., Eldreth, D., Erickson, K. I., Varma, V., Harris, G., Fried, L. P., et al. (2014). Cardiovascular risks and brain function: a functional magnetic resonance imaging study of executive function in older adults. *Neurobiol. Aging* 35, 1396–1403. doi: 10.1016/j.neurobiolaging.2013.12.008

Cockrell, J. R., and Folstein, M. F. (1988). Mini-mental state examination (MMSE). *Psychophar. Bull.* 24, 689–692.

Delbaere, K., Kochan, N. A., Close, J. C., Menant, J. C., Sturnieks, D. L., Brodaty, H., et al. (2012). Mild cognitive impairment as a predictor of falls in community-dwelling older people. *Am. J. Geriatr. Psychiatry* 20, 845–853. doi: 10.1097/JGP.0b013e31824afbc4

Desmond, D. W., Erkinjuntti, T., Sano, M., Cummings, J. L., Bowler, J. V., Pasquier, F., et al. (1999). The cognitive syndrome of vascular dementia: implications for clinical trials. *Alzheimer Dis. Assoc. Disord.* 13(Suppl. 3), S21–S29. doi: 10.1097/00002093-199912001-00005

Ding, W., Cao, W., Wang, Y., Sun, Y., Chen, X., Zhou, Y., et al. (2015). Altered functional connectivity in patients with subcortical vascular cognitive impairment–a resting-state functional magnetic resonance imaging study. *PLoS ONE* 10:e0138180. doi: 10.1371/journal.pone.0138180

Enright, P. L. (2003). The 6-min walk test: a quick measure of functional status in elderly adults. *Chest* 123, 387–398. doi: 10.1378/chest.123.2.387

Erickson, K. I., and Kramer, A. F. (2009). Aerobic exercise effects on cognitive and neural plasticity in older adults. *Br. J. Sports Med.* 43, 22–24. doi: 10.1136/bjsm.2008.052498

Erkinjuntti, T., Bowler, J. V., Decarli, C. S., Fazekas, F., Inzitari, D., O'brien, J. T., et al. (1999). Imaging of static brain lesions in vascular dementia: implications for clinical trials. *Alzheimer Dis. Assoc. Disord.* 13(Suppl. 3), S81–S90. doi: 10.1097/00002093-199912001-00013

Erkinjuntti, T., Inzitari, D., Pantoni, L., Wallin, A., Scheltens, P., Rockwood, K., et al. (2000). Research criteria for subcortical vascular dementia in clinical trials. *J. Neural Transm. Suppl.* 59, 23–30. doi: 10.1007/978-3-7091-6781-6_4

Fair, D. A., Schlaggar, B. L., Cohen, A. L., Miezin, F. M., Dosenbach, N. U., Wenger, K. K., et al. (2007). A method for using blocked and event-related fMRI data to study "resting state" functional connectivity. *Neuroimage* 35, 396–405. doi: 10.1016/j.neuroimage.2006.11.051

Fogassi, L., and Luppino, G. (2005). Motor functions of the parietal lobe. *Curr. Opin. Neurobiol.* 15, 626–631. doi: 10.1016/j.conb.2005.10.015

Fox, M. D., Zhang, D., Snyder, A. Z., and Raichle, M. E. (2009). The global signal and observed anticorrelated resting state brain networks. *J. Neurophysiol.* 101, 3270–3283. doi: 10.1152/jn.90777.2008

Gao, Q., Wang, J., Yu, C., and Chen, H. (2015). Effect of handedness on brain activity patterns and effective connectivity network during the semantic task of Chinese characters. *Sci. Rep.* 5:18262. doi: 10.1038/srep18262

Geerligs, L., Maurits, N. M., Renken, R. J., and Lorist, M. M. (2012). Reduced specificity of functional connectivity in the aging brain during task performance. *Hum. Brain Mapp.* 35, 319–330. doi: 10.1002/hbm.22175

Gellish, R. L., Goslin, B. R., Olson, R. E., Mcdonald, A., Russi, G. D., and Moudgil, V. K. (2007). Longitudinal modeling of the relationship between age and maximal heart rate. *Med. Sci. Sports Exerc.* 39, 822–829. doi: 10.1097/mss.0b013e31803349c6

Groll, D. L., To, T., Bombardier, C., and Wright, J. G. (2005). The development of a comorbidity index with physical function as the outcome. *J. Clin. Epidemiol.* 58, 595–602. doi: 10.1016/j.jclinepi.2004.10.018

Guralnik, J. M., Ferrucci, L., Simonsick, E. M., Salive, M. E., and Wallace, R. B. (1995). Lower-extremity function in persons over the age of 70 years as a predictor of subsequent disability 10.1056/NEJM199503023320902. *N. Engl. J. Med.* 332, 556–562. doi: 10.1056/NEJM199503023320902

He, B. J., Snyder, A. Z., Vincent, J. L., Epstein, A., Shulman, G. L., and Corbetta, M. (2007). Breakdown of functional connectivity in frontoparietal networks underlies behavioral deficits in spatial neglect. *Neuron* 53, 905–918. doi: 10.1016/j.neuron.2007.02.013

Holtzer, R., Mahoney, J. R., Izzetoglu, M., Izzetoglu, K., Onaral, B., and Verghese, J. (2011). fNIRS study of walking and walking while talking in young and old individuals. *J. Gerontol. A Biol. Sci. Med. Sci.* 66, 879–887. doi: 10.1093/gerona/glr068

Hsu, C. L., Best, J. R., Davis, J. C., Nagamatsu, L. S., Wang, S., Boyd, L. A., et al. (2017). Aerobic exercise promotes executive functions and impacts functional neural activity among older adults with vascular cognitive impairment. *Br J Sports Med* doi: 10.1136/bjsports-2016-096846

Hsu, C. L., Nagamatsu, L. S., Davis, J. C., and Liu-Ambrose, T. (2012). Examining the relationship between specific cognitive processes and falls risk in older adults: a systematic review. *Osteoporos Int.* 23, 2409–2424. doi: 10.1007/s00198-012-1992-z

Hsu, C. L., Voss, M. W., Handy, T. C., Davis, J. C., Nagamatsu, L. S., Chan, A., et al. (2014). Disruptions in brain networks of older fallers are associated with subsequent cognitive decline: a 12-month prospective exploratory study. *PLoS ONE* 9:e93673. doi: 10.1371/journal.pone.0093673

Jancke, L., Loose, R., Lutz, K., Specht, K., and Shah, N. J. (2000). Cortical activations during paced finger-tapping applying visual and auditory pacing stimuli. *Brain Res. Cogn. Brain Res.* 10, 51–66. doi: 10.1016/S0926-6410(00)00022-7

Kuo, H.-K., and Lipsitz, L. A. (2004). Cerebral white matter changes and geriatric syndromes: is there a link? *J. Gerontol. A Biol. Sci. Med. Sci.* 59, M818–M826. doi: 10.1093/gerona/59.8.m818

Layne, A. S., Hsu, F. C., Blair, S. N., Chen, S. H., Dungan, J., Fielding, R. A., et al. (2017). Predictors of change in physical function among older adults in response to long-term, structured physical activity: the LIFE Study. *Arch. Phys. Med. Rehabil.* 98, 11.e3–24.e3. doi: 10.1016/j.apmr.2016.07.019

Liu-Ambrose, T., Nagamatsu, L. S., Hsu, C. L., and Bolandzadeh, N. (2013). Emerging concept: 'central benefit model' of exercise in falls prevention. *Br. J. Sports Med.* 47, 115–117. doi: 10.1136/bjsports-2011-090725

Liu-Ambrose, T., Best, J. R., Davis, J. C., Eng, J. J., Lee, P. E., Jacova, C., et al. (2016). Aerobic exercise and vascular cognitive impairment: a randomized controlled trial. *Neurology* 87, 2082–2090. doi: 10.1212/WNL.0000000000003332

Liu-Ambrose, T., Donaldson, M. G., Ahamed, Y., Graf, P., Cook, W. L., Close, J., et al. (2008). Otago home-based strength and balance retraining improves executive functioning in older fallers: a randomized controlled trial. *J. Am. Geriatr. Soc.* 56, 1821–1830. doi: 10.1111/j.1532-5415.2008.01931.x

Liu-Ambrose, T., Eng, J. J., Boyd, L. A., Jacova, C., Davis, J. C., Bryan, S., et al. (2010). Promotion of the mind through exercise (PROMoTE): a proof-of-concept randomized controlled trial of aerobic exercise training in older adults with vascular cognitive impairment. *BMC Neurol.* 10:14. doi: 10.1186/1471-2377-10-14

McAusland, J., Tam, R., Wong, E., Riddehough, A., and Li, D. (2010). Optimizing the use of radiologist seed points for improved multiple sclerosis lesion segmentation. *IEEE Trans. Biomed. Eng.* 57, 2689–2698. doi: 10.1109/TBME.2010.2055865

Montero-Odasso, M., Verghese, J., Beauchet, O., and Hausdorff, J. M. (2012). Gait and cognition: a complementary approach to understanding brain function and the risk of falling. *J. Am. Geriatr. Soc.* 60, 2127–2136. doi: 10.1111/j.1532-5415.2012.04209.x

Murphy, K., and Fox, M. D. (2016). Towards a consensus regarding global signal regression for resting state functional connectivity MRI. *Neuroimage* doi: 10.1016/j.neuroimage.2016.11.052

Nasreddine, Z. S., Phillips, N. A., Bedirian, V., Charbonneau, S., Whitehead, V., Collin, I., et al. (2005). The montreal cognitive assessment, MoCA: a brief screening tool for mild cognitive impairment. *J. Am. Geriatr. Soc.* 53, 695–699. doi: 10.1111/j.1532-5415.2005.53221.x

Nishiguchi, S., Yamada, M., Tanigawa, T., Sekiyama, K., Kawagoe, T., Suzuki, M., et al. (2015). A 12-Week physical and cognitive exercise program can improve cognitive function and neural efficiency in community-dwelling older adults: a randomized controlled trial. *J. Am. Geriatr. Soc.* 63, 1355–1363. doi: 10.1111/jgs.13481

O'Brien, J. T. (2006). Vascular cognitive impairment. *Am. J. Geriatr. Psychiatry* 14, 724–733. doi: 10.1097/01.JGP.0000231780.44684.7e

Odenheimer, G., Funkenstein, H. H., Beckett, L., Chown, M., Pilgrim, D., Evans, D., et al. (1994). Comparison of neurologic changes in 'successfully aging' persons vs the total aging population. *Arch. Neurol.* 51, 573–580. doi: 10.1001/archneur.1994.00540180051013

Pahor, M., Guralnik, J. M., Ambrosius, W. T., Blair, S., Bonds, D. E., Church, T. S., et al. (2014). Effect of structured physical activity on prevention of major mobility disability in older adults: the LIFE study randomized clinical trial. *JAMA* 311, 2387–2396. doi: 10.1001/jama.2014.5616

Pantoni, L., Leys, D., Fazekas, F., Longstreth, WT Jr, Inzitari, D., Wallin, A., et al. (1999). Role of white matter lesions in cognitive impairment of vascular origin. *Alzheimer Dis. Assoc. Disord.* 13(Suppl. 3), S49–S54.

Parzen, E. (1962). On estimation of a probability density function and mode. *Annal. Math. Stat.* 33, 1065–1076. doi: 10.1214/aoms/1177704472

Persinger, R., Foster, C., Gibson, M., Fater, D. C., and Porcari, J. P. (2004). Consistency of the talk test for exercise prescription. *Med. Sci. Sports Exerc.* 36, 1632–1636. doi: 10.1249/01.MSS.0000074670.03001.98

Pool, E. M., Rehme, A. K., Fink, G. R., Eickhoff, S. B., and Grefkes, C. (2014). Handedness and effective connectivity of the motor system. *Neuroimage* 99, 451–460. doi: 10.1016/j.neuroimage.2014.05.048

Poppe, A. B., Carter, C. S., Minzenberg, M. J., and Macdonald, A. W. III. (2015). Task-based functional connectivity as an indicator of genetic liability to schizophrenia. *Schizophr. Res.* 162, 118–123. doi: 10.1016/j.schres.2014.11.022

Robertson, M. C., Campbell, A. J., Gardner, M. M., and Devlin, N. (2002). preventing injuries in older people by preventing falls: a meta-analysis of individual-level data. *J. Am. Geriatr. Soc.* 50, 905–911. doi: 10.1046/j.1532-5415.2002.50218.x

Rockwood, K., Wentzel, C., Hachinski, V., Hogan, D. B., Macknight, C., and Mcdowell, I. (2000). Prevalence and outcomes of vascular cognitive impairment. Vascular cognitive impairment investigators of the canadian study of health and aging. *Neurology* 54, 447–451. doi: 10.1212/WNL.54.2.447

Roman, G. C., Erkinjuntti, T., Wallin, A., Pantoni, L., and Chui, H. C. (2002). Subcortical ischaemic vascular dementia. *Lancet Neurol.* 1, 426–436. doi: 10.1016/S1474-4422(02)00190-4

Rosano, C., Newman, A. B., Katz, R., Hirsch, C. H., and Kuller, L. H. (2008). Association between lower digit symbol substitution test score and slower gait and greater risk of mortality and of developing incident disability in well-functioning older adults. *J. Am. Geriatr. Soc.* 56, 1618–1625. doi: 10.1111/j.1532-5415.2008.01856.x

Rosenberg-Katz, K., Herman, T., Jacob, Y., Mirelman, A., Giladi, N., Hendler, T., et al. (2015). Fall risk is associated with amplified functional connectivity of the central executive network in patients with Parkinson's disease. *J. Neurol.* 262, 2448–2456. doi: 10.1007/s00415-015-7865-6

Seeley, W. W., Menon, V., Schatzberg, A. F., Keller, J., Glover, G. H., Kenna, H., et al. (2007). Dissociable intrinsic connectivity networks for salience processing and executive control. *J. Neurosci.* 27, 2349–2356. doi: 10.1523/JNEUROSCI.5587-06.2007

Shumway-Cook, A., Brauer, S., and Woollacott, M. (2000). Predicting the probability for falls in community-dwelling older adults using the Timed Up & Go Test. *Phys. Ther.* 80, 896–903.

Smith, J. C., Nielson, K. A., Antuono, P., Lyons, J. A., Hanson, R. J., Butts, A. M., et al. (2013). Semantic memory functional MRI and cognitive function after exercise intervention in mild cognitive impairment. *J. Alzheimers. Dis.* 37, 197–215. doi: 10.3233/JAD-130467

Smith, S. M., Fox, P. T., Miller, K. L., Glahn, D. C., Fox, P. M., Mackay, C. E., et al. (2009). Correspondence of the brain's functional architecture during activation and rest. *Proc. Natl. Acad. Sci. U.S.A.* 106, 13040–13045. doi: 10.1073/pnas.0905267106

Sridharan, D., Levitin, D. J., and Menon, V. (2008). A critical role for the right fronto-insular cortex in switching between central-executive and default-mode networks. *Proc. Natl. Acad. Sci. U.S.A.* 105, 12569–12574. doi: 10.1073/pnas.0800005105

Vermeer, S. E., Longstreth, W. T. Jr., and Koudstaal, P. J. (2007). Silent brain infarcts: a systematic review. *Lancet Neurol.* 6, 611–619. doi: 10.1016/S1474-4422(07)70170-9

Voss, M. W., Erickson, K. I., Prakash, R. S., Chaddock, L., Malkowski, E., Alves, H., et al. (2010a). Functional connectivity: a source of variance in the association between cardiorespiratory fitness and cognition? *Neuropsychologia* 48, 1394–1406. doi: 10.1016/j.neuropsychologia.2010.01.005

Voss, M. W., Prakash, R. S., Erickson, K. I., Basak, C., Chaddock, L., Kim, J. S., et al. (2010b). Plasticity of brain networks in a randomized intervention trial of exercise training in older adults. *Front. Aging Neurosci.* 2:32. doi: 10.3389/fnagi.2010.00032

Washburn, R. A., Mcauley, E., Katula, J., Mihalko, S. L., and Boileau, R. A. (1999). The physical activity scale for the elderly (PASE): evidence for validity. *J. Clin. Epidemiol.* 52, 643–651. doi: 10.1016/S0895-4356(99)00049-9

Wise, S. P., Boussaoud, D., Johnson, P. B., and Caminiti, R. (1997). Premotor and parietal cortex: corticocortical connectivity and combinatorial computations. *Annu. Rev. Neurosci.* 20, 25–42. doi: 10.1146/annurev.neuro.20.1.25

Wu, T., Wang, L., Chen, Y., Zhao, C., Li, K., and Chan, P. (2009). Changes of functional connectivity of the motor network in the resting state in Parkinson's disease. *Neurosci. Lett.* 460, 6–10. doi: 10.1016/j.neulet.2009.05.046

Wymbs, N. F., Bassett, D. S., Mucha, P. J., Porter, M. A., and Grafton, S. T. (2012). Differential recruitment of the sensorimotor putamen and frontoparietal cortex during motor chunking in humans. *Neuron* 74, 936–946. doi: 10.1016/j.neuron.2012.03.038

Yi, L., Wang, J., Jia, L., Zhao, Z., Lu, J., Li, K., et al. (2012). Structural and functional changes in subcortical vascular mild cognitive impairment: a combined voxel-based morphometry and resting-state fMRI study. *PLoS ONE* 7:e44758. doi: 10.1371/journal.pone.0044758

Yu, Y., Zhou, X., Wang, H., Hu, X., Zhu, X., Xu, L., et al. (2015). Small-world brain network and dynamic functional distribution in patients with subcortical vascular cognitive impairment. *PLoS ONE* 10:e0131893. doi: 10.1371/journal.pone.0131893

Yuan, J., Blumen, H. M., Verghese, J., and Holtzer, R. (2015). Functional connectivity associated with gait velocity during walking and walking-while-talking in aging: a resting-state fMRI study. *Hum. Brain Mapp.* 36, 1484–1493. doi: 10.1002/hbm.22717

Zhou, X., Hu, X., Zhang, C., Wang, H., Zhu, X., Xu, L., et al. (2016). Aberrant functional connectivity and structural atrophy in subcortical vascular cognitive impairment: relationship with cognitive impairments. *Front. Aging Neurosci.* 8:14. doi: 10.3389/fnagi.2016.00014

Zhu, Y., Cheng, L., He, N., Yang, Y., Ling, H., Ayaz, H., et al. (2017). Comparison of functional connectivity estimated from concatenated task-state data from block-design paradigm with that of continuous task. *Comput. Math. Methods Med.* 2017:4198430. doi: 10.1155/2017/4198430

Permissions

All chapters in this book were first published in CBPIPECTVGCI, by Frontiers; hereby published with permission under the Creative Commons Attribution License or equivalent. Every chapter published in this book has been scrutinized by our experts. Their significance has been extensively debated. The topics covered herein carry significant findings which will fuel the growth of the discipline. They may even be implemented as practical applications or may be referred to as a beginning point for another development.

The contributors of this book come from diverse backgrounds, making this book a truly international effort. This book will bring forth new frontiers with its revolutionizing research information and detailed analysis of the nascent developments around the world.

We would like to thank all the contributing authors for lending their expertise to make the book truly unique. They have played a crucial role in the development of this book. Without their invaluable contributions this book wouldn't have been possible. They have made vital efforts to compile up to date information on the varied aspects of this subject to make this book a valuable addition to the collection of many professionals and students.

This book was conceptualized with the vision of imparting up-to-date information and advanced data in this field. To ensure the same, a matchless editorial board was set up. Every individual on the board went through rigorous rounds of assessment to prove their worth. After which they invested a large part of their time researching and compiling the most relevant data for our readers.

The editorial board has been involved in producing this book since its inception. They have spent rigorous hours researching and exploring the diverse topics which have resulted in the successful publishing of this book. They have passed on their knowledge of decades through this book. To expedite this challenging task, the publisher supported the team at every step. A small team of assistant editors was also appointed to further simplify the editing procedure and attain best results for the readers.

Apart from the editorial board, the designing team has also invested a significant amount of their time in understanding the subject and creating the most relevant covers. They scrutinized every image to scout for the most suitable representation of the subject and create an appropriate cover for the book.

The publishing team has been an ardent support to the editorial, designing and production team. Their endless efforts to recruit the best for this project, has resulted in the accomplishment of this book. They are a veteran in the field of academics and their pool of knowledge is as vast as their experience in printing. Their expertise and guidance has proved useful at every step. Their uncompromising quality standards have made this book an exceptional effort. Their encouragement from time to time has been an inspiration for everyone.

The publisher and the editorial board hope that this book will prove to be a valuable piece of knowledge for researchers, students, practitioners and scholars across the globe.

List of Contributors

Katarzyna Paluch, Katarzyna Jurewicz, Jacek Rogala, Andrzej Wróbel and Ewa Kublik
Department of Neurophysiology, Nencki Institute of Experimental Biology of Polish Academy of Science, Warsaw, Poland

Rafał Krauz
Centre for Physical Education and Sport, Military University of Technology, Warsaw, Poland

Marta Szczypińska and Mirosław Mikicin
Department of Physical Education, University of Physical Education, Warsaw, Poland

Kathrin Rehfeld, Norman Aye and Milos Dordevic
German Center for Neurodegenerative Diseases, Magdeburg, Germany
Institute for Sport Science, Otto von Guericke University Magdeburg, Magdeburg, Germany

Patrick Müller
German Center for Neurodegenerative Diseases, Magdeburg, Germany
Medical Faculty, Otto von Guericke University Magdeburg, Magdeburg, Germany

Marlen Schmicker
German Center for Neurodegenerative Diseases, Magdeburg, Germany

Jörn Kaufmann
Department of Neurology, Otto von Guericke University Magdeburg, Magdeburg, Germany

Anita Hökelmann
Institute for Sport Science, Otto von Guericke University Magdeburg, Magdeburg, Germany

Notger G. Müller
German Center for Neurodegenerative Diseases, Magdeburg, Germany
Medical Faculty, Otto von Guericke University Magdeburg, Magdeburg, Germany
Center for Behavioral Brain Sciences, Magdeburg, Germany

Yusuf O. Cakmak
Department of Anatomy, School of Biomedical Sciences, University of Otago, Dunedin, New Zealand

Gazanfer Ekinci
Radiology Department, School of Medicine, Marmara University, Istanbul, Turkey

Armin Heinecke
Brain Innovation BV, Biopartner Center, Maastricht, Netherlands

Safiye Çavdar
Department of Anatomy, School of Medicine, Koc University, Istanbul, Turkey

Harry Hallock, Daniel Collins, Michael Valenzuela
Regenerative Neuroscience Group, Brain and Mind Centre, University of Sydney, Sydney, NSW, Australia

Amit Lampit
Regenerative Neuroscience Group, Brain and Mind Centre, University of Sydney, Sydney, NSW, Australia
School of Psychology, University of Sydney, Sydney, NSW, Australia

Kiran Deol
Sydney Medical School, University of Sydney, Sydney, NSW,Australia

Jennifer Fleming
School of Health and Rehabilitation Sciences, University of Queensland, Brisbane, QLD, Australia
Occupational Therapy Department, Princess Alexandra Hospital, Brisbane, QLD, Australia
Centre for Functioning and Health Research, Metro South Hospital and Health Service, Brisbane, QLD, Australia

Aaron Kandola
Brain and Mental Health Lab, School of Psychological Sciences and Monash Institute of Cognitive and Clinical Neurosciences, Monash University, Melbourne, VIC, Australia
Amsterdam Brain and Cognition, University of Amsterdam, Amsterdam, Netherlands

Joshua Hendrikse, and Murat Yücel
Brain and Mental Health Lab, School of Psychological Sciences and Monash Institute of Cognitive and Clinical Neurosciences, Monash University, Melbourne, VIC, Australia,

Paul J. Lucassen
Centre for Neuroscience, Swammerdam Institute of Life Sciences, University of Amsterdam, Amsterdam, Netherlands

Anita Hökelmann
Institute of Sports Science, Otto von Guericke University, Magdeburg, Germany

Jacek Rogala, Katarzyna Jurewicz, Katarzyna Paluch, Ewa Kublik, Ryszard Cetnarski and Andrzej Wróbel
Laboratory of Visual System, Nencki Institute of Experimental Biology, Polish Academy of Sciences, Warsaw, Poland

Maike M. Kleemeyer and Nils C. Bodammer
Center for Lifespan Psychology, Max Planck Institute for Human Development, Berlin, Germany

Thad A. Polk
Computational and Cognitive Neuroscience Laboratory, Department of Psychology, University of Michigan, Ann Arbor, MI, USA

Sabine Schaefer
Institute of Sport Science, Saarland University, Saarbruecken, Germany

Lars Brechtel
Berlin Academy of Sports Medicine, Berlin, Germany

Ulman Lindenberger
Center for Lifespan Psychology, Max Planck Institute for Human Development, Berlin, Germany
European University Institute, San Domenico di Fiesole (FI), Italy

I-Wen Su
Graduate Institute of Linguistics, National Taiwan University, Taipei, Taiwan
Neurobiology and Cognitive Science Center, National Taiwan University, Taipei, Taiwan
Graduate Institute of Brain and Mind Sciences, National Taiwan University, Taipei, Taiwan

Fang-Wei Wu
Department of Psychology, National Taiwan University, Taipei, Taiwan

Keng-Chen Liang
Neurobiology and Cognitive Science Center, National Taiwan University, Taipei, Taiwan
Graduate Institute of Brain and Mind Sciences, National Taiwan University, Taipei, Taiwan
Department of Psychology, National Taiwan University, Taipei, Taiwan

Kai-Yuan Cheng
Institute of Philosophy of Mind and Cognition, National Yang-Ming University, Taipei, Taiwan

Sung-Tsang Hsieh
Neurobiology and Cognitive Science Center, National Taiwan University, Taipei, Taiwan
Graduate Institute of Brain and Mind Sciences, National Taiwan University, Taipei, Taiwan
Department of Neurology, National Taiwan University Hospital, Taipei, Taiwan

Wei-Zen Sun
Neurobiology and Cognitive Science Center, National Taiwan University, Taipei, Taiwan
Graduate Institute of Brain and Mind Sciences, National Taiwan University, Taipei, Taiwan
Department of Anesthesiology, National Taiwan University Hospital, Taipei, Taiwan

Tai-Li Chou
Neurobiology and Cognitive Science Center, National Taiwan University, Taipei, Taiwan
Department of Psychology, National Taiwan University, Taipei, Taiwan

Mark A. Fletcher, Benjamin Zimmerman
Beckman Institute, University of Illinois, Urbana, IL, USA
Neuroscience Program, University of Illinois, Urbana, Illinois,USA

Kathy A. Low
Beckman Institute, University of Illinois, Urbana, IL, USA

Rachel Boyd, Chin H. Tan and Nils Schneider-Garces
Beckman Institute, University of Illinois, Urbana, IL, USA
Department of Psychology, University of Illinois, Urbana, IL, USA

Bradley P. Sutton
Beckman Institute, University of Illinois, Urbana, IL, USA
Neuroscience Program, University of Illinois, Urbana, Illinois, USA
Department of Bioengineering, University of Illinois at Urbana-Champaign, Urbana, IL, USA

Gabriele Gratton and Monica Fabiani
Beckman Institute, University of Illinois, Urbana, IL, USA
Neuroscience Program, University of Illinois, Urbana, Illinois, USA
Department of Psychology, University of Illinois, Urbana, IL, USA
Department of Bioengineering, University of Illinois at Urbana-Champaign, Urbana, IL, USA

Brian A. Gordon
Department of Radiology, Washington University in St. Louis, Saint Louis, MO, USA

Milos Dordevic
Department of Neuroprotection, German Center for Neurodegenerative Diseases, Magdeburg, Germany,
Institute of Sports Science, Otto von Guericke University, Magdeburg, Germany

Patrick Müller
Department of Neuroprotection, German Center for Neurodegenerative Diseases, Magdeburg, Germany

Kathrin Rehfeld
Institute of Sports Science, Otto von Guericke University, Magdeburg, Germany

Notger G. Müller
Department of Neuroprotection, German Center for Neurodegenerative Diseases, Magdeburg, Germany
Center for Behavioral Brain Sciences, Magdeburg, Germany

Justin Hudak, Friederike Blume
LEAD Graduate School & Research Network, University of Tübingen, Tübingen, Germany

Thomas Dresler and Ann-Christine Ehlis
LEAD Graduate School & Research Network, University of Tübingen, Tübingen, Germany
Department of Psychiatry and Psychotherapy, University Hospital Tübingen, Tübingen, Germany

Florian B. Haeussinger
Department of Psychiatry and Psychotherapy, University Hospital Tübingen, Tübingen, Germany

Tobias J. Renner
Department of Child and Adolescence Psychiatry, University Hospital Tübingen, Tübingen, Germany

Andreas J. Fallgatter
LEAD Graduate School & Research Network, University of Tübingen, Tübingen, Germany
Department of Psychiatry and Psychotherapy, University Hospital Tübingen, Tübingen, Germany
Center for Integrative Neuroscience, University of Tübingen, Tübingen, German

Caterina Gawrilow
LEAD Graduate School & Research Network, University of Tübingen, Tübingen, Germany
Department of Psychology, University of Tübingen, Tübingen, Germany
Center for Individual Development andAdaptive Education of Children at Risk, Goethe University Frankfurt, Frankfurt, Germany

Rajanikant Panda and Rose D. Bharath
Cognitive Neuroscience Center, National Institute for Mental Health and Neurosciences, Bangalore, India
Department of Neuroimaging and Interventional Radiology, National Institute for Mental Health and Neurosciences, Bangalore, India

Neeraj Upadhyay
Department of Neurology and Psychiatry, Sapienza University of Rome, Rome, Italy

Sandhya Mangalore
Department of Neuroimaging and Interventional Radiology, National Institute for Mental Health and Neurosciences, Bangalore, India

Srivas Chennu
School of Computing, University of Kent, Chatham Maritime, UK
Department of Clinical Neurosciences, University of Cambridge, Cambridge, UK

Shobini L. Rao
Cognitive Neuroscience Center, National Institute for Mental Health and Neurosciences, Bangalore, India

Alexandra Nadeau and Catherine Duchesne
Research Center of the University Institute of Geriatrics of Montreal, Montreal, QC, Canada
Functional Neuroimaging Unit, Montreal, QC, Canada
Department of Psychology, University of Montreal, Montreal, QC, Canada

Ovidiu Lungu
Research Center of the University Institute of Geriatrics of Montreal, Montreal, QC, Canada
Functional Neuroimaging Unit, Montreal, QC, Canada
Department of Psychiatry, University of Montreal, Montreal, QC, Canada
Centre for Research in Aging, Donald Berman Maimonides Geriatric Centre, Montreal, QC, Canada

Marie-Ève Robillard and Arnaud Bore
Research Center of the University Institute of Geriatrics of Montreal, Montreal, QC, Canada
Functional Neuroimaging Unit, Montreal, QC, Canada

Florian Bobeuf
Research Center of the University Institute of Geriatrics of Montreal, Montreal, QC, Canada
PERFORM Centre, Concordia University, Montreal, QC, Canada

Réjean Plamondon
Department of Electrical Engineering, Polytechnique Montreal, Montreal, QC, Canada

Anne-Louise Lafontaine
Research Center of the University Institute of Geriatrics of Montreal, Montreal, QC, Canada
Functional Neuroimaging Unit, Montreal, QC, Canada
McGill Movement Disorder Clinic, McGill University, Montreal, QC, Canada

Louis Bherer
Research Center of the University Institute of Geriatrics of Montreal, Montreal, QC, Canada
PERFORM Centre, Concordia University, Montreal, QC, Canada
Department of Medicine, University of Montreal, Montreal, QC, Canada
Montreal Heart Institute, Montreal, QC, Canada

Julien Doyon
Research Center of the University Institute of Geriatrics of Montreal, Montreal, QC, Canada
Functional Neuroimaging Unit, Montreal, QC, Canada
Department of Psychology, University of Montreal, Montreal, QC, Canada

Eivind Wengaard, Morten Kristoffersen and Hilde Gundersen
Department of Sport and Physical Education, Western Norway University of Applied Sciences, Bergen, Norway

Anette Harris
Department of Psychosocial Science, Faculty of Psychology, Institute of Psychosocial Science, University of Bergen, Bergen, Norway

Benjamin Cowley
BrainWork Research Centre, Finnish Institute of Occupational Health, Helsinki, Finland
Cognitive Brain Research Unit, Cognitive Science, Institute of Behavioural Sciences, University of Helsinki, Helsinki, Finland

Édua Holmström and Levas Kovarskis
Formally affiliated with Faculty of Behavioural Sciences, University of Helsinki, Helsinki, Finland

Kristiina Juurmaa and Christina M. Krause
Cognitive Brain Research Unit, Cognitive Science, Institute of Behavioural Sciences, University of Helsinki, Helsinki, Finland

Bettina Pollok, Ariane Keitel and Vanessa Krause
Medical Faculty, Institute of Clinical Neuroscience and Medical Psychology, Heinrich-Heine University Duesseldorf, Duesseldorf, Germany

Katharina Stephan and Nora K. Schaal
Department of Experimental Psychology, Heinrich-Heine University Duesseldorf, Duesseldorf, Germany

Freja Gheysen
Department of Movement and Sport Sciences, Ghent University, Ghent, Belgium

Robin G. Y. Hsiung
Department of Medicine, University of British Columbia, Vancouver, BC, Canada

Giancarlo Condello and Laura Capranica
Sport Performance Laboratory, Department of Movement, Human and Health Sciences, Italian University of Sport and Movement "Foro Italico", Rome, Italy

Caterina Pesce, Roberta Forte and Simone Falbo
Exercise and Cognition Laboratory, Department of Movement, Human and Health Sciences, Italian University of Sport and Movement "Foro Italico", Rome, Italy

John B. Shea
Ergonomics Laboratory, School of Public Health, Indiana University Bloomington, Bloomington, IN, USA

Angela Di Baldassarre
Department of Medicine and Aging Sciences, School of Medicine and Health Sciences, "G. d'Annunzio" University of Chieti-Pescara, Chieti, Italy

Patrick Fissler and Olivia C. Küster
Clinical and Biological Psychology, Institute of Psychology and Education, Ulm University, Ulm, Germany
Department of Neurology, University Hospital Ulm, Ulm, Germany

Jan Kassubek, Christine A. F. von Arnim and Hans-Peter Müller
Department of Neurology, University Hospital Ulm, Ulm, Germany

Iris-Tatjana Kolassa and Daria Laptinskaya
Clinical and Biological Psychology, Institute of Psychology and Education, Ulm University, Ulm, Germany
Department of Neurology, University Hospital Ulm, Ulm, Germany

Franka Thurm
Department of Psychology, Technische Universität Dresden, Dresden, Germany

Alexander Woll
Institute of Sports and Sports Science, Karlsruhe Institute of Technology, Karlsruhe, Germany

Thomas Elbert
Department of Psychology, University of Konstanz, Konstanz, Germany

Michelle W. Voss
Health, Brain, and Cognition Lab, University of Iowa, Iowa City, IA, United States
Department of Psychology, University of Iowa, Iowa City, IA, United States

Chun L. Hsu, John R. Best, Shirley Wang, Michelle Munkacsy, Winnie Cheung and Teresa Liu-Ambrose
Aging, Mobility, and Cognitive Neuroscience Lab, University of British Columbia, Vancouver, BC, Canada
Department of Physical Therapy, University of British Columbia, Vancouver, BC, Canada
Djavad Mowafaghian Center for Brain Health, University of British Columbia, Vancouver, BC, Canada
Center for Hip Health and Mobility, Vancouver, BC, Canada

Todd C. Handy
Department of Psychology, University of British Columbia, Vancouver, BC, Canada

Index

CPSIA information can be obtained
at www.ICGtesting.com
Printed in the USA
LVHW062010100122
708212LV00002B/148

9 781639 891160